THE RED BLOOD CELL

A Comprehensive Treatise

CONTRIBUTORS TO THIS VOLUME

David W. Allen

Nathaniel I. Berlin

Charles Bishop

Myron Brin

J. de Gier

Zacharias Dische

John G. Gibson II

Ernst R. Jaffé

Paul A. Marks

Hermann Passow

Robert B. Pennell

Max M. Strumia

Douglas M. Surgenor

James L. Tullis

L. L. M. van Deenen

Winifred M. Watkins

THE RED BLOOD CELL

A Comprehensive Treatise

EDITED BY

CHARLES BISHOP

BUFFALO GENERAL HOSPITAL
BUFFALO, NEW YORK

DOUGLAS M. SURGENOR

SCHOOL OF MEDICINE
STATE UNIVERSITY OF NEW YORK AT BUFFALO
BUFFALO, NEW YORK

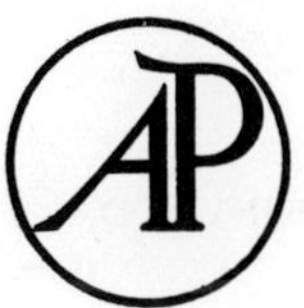

1964

ACADEMIC PRESS New York and London

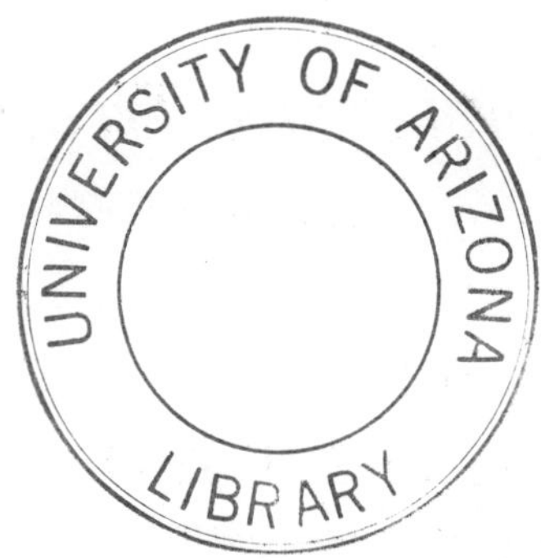

ACADEMIC PRESS INC.
111 Fifth Avenue, New York, New York 10003

United Kingdom Edition published by
ACADEMIC PRESS INC. (LONDON) LTD.
Berkeley Square House, London W.1

LIBRARY OF CONGRESS CATALOG NUMBER: 64-21665

PRINTED IN THE UNITED STATES OF AMERICA

List of Contributors

Numbers in parentheses indicate the page on which the authors' contributions begin.

DAVID W. ALLEN, *The John Collins Warren Laboratories of the Huntington Memorial Hospital of Harvard University at the Massachusetts General Hospital, Boston, Massachusetts* (*309*)

NATHANIEL I. BERLIN, *National Cancer Institute, National Institutes of Health, Bethesda, Maryland* (*423*)

CHARLES BISHOP, *Department of Medicine, State University of New York at Buffalo and Buffalo General Hospital, Buffalo, New York* (*147*)

MYRON BRIN, *Upstate Medical Center, State University of New York, Syracuse, New York* (*451*)

J. DE GIER, *Department of Biochemistry, Laboratory of Organic Chemistry, State University, Utrecht, Holland* (*243*)

ZACHARIAS DISCHE, *Department of Ophthalmology, College of Physicians and Surgeons, Columbia University, New York, New York*, (*189*)

JOHN G. GIBSON II, *Blood Characterization and Preservation Laboratory, Protein Foundation, Jamaica Plain, Massachusetts* (*447*)

ERNST R. JAFFÉ, *Department of Medicine, Albert Einstein College of Medicine and Bronx Municipal Hospital Center, New York, New York* (*397*)

PAUL A. MARKS, *Department of Medicine, Columbia University, College of Physicians and Surgeons, New York, New York* (*211*)

HERMANN PASSOW, *Physiologisches Institut der Universität des Saarlandes, Homberg/Saar, Germany* (*71*)

ROBERT B. PENNELL, *Blood Characterization and Preservation Laboratory, Protein Foundation, Jamaica Plain, Massachusetts* (*29*)

MAX M. STRUMIA, *Laboratory of Clinical Pathology, The Bryn Mawr Hospital, Bryn Mawr and Graduate School, University of Pennsylvania, Philadelphia, Pennsylvania* (*1*)

DOUGLAS M. SURGENOR, *School of Medicine, State University of New York at Buffalo, Buffalo, New York* (*340*)

JAMES L. TULLIS, *Blood Characterization and Preservation Laboratory, Protein Foundation, Jamaica Plain, Massachusetts* (*491*)

L. L. M. VAN DEENEN, *Department of Biochemistry, Laboratory of Organic Chemistry, State University, Utrecht, Holland* (*243*)

WINIFRED M. WATKINS, *The Lister Institute of Preventive Medicine, London, England* (*359*)

Preface

The red blood cell is used nowadays for such diverse studies as osmotic pressure and related phenomena, active transport of ions and non-ionic compounds, special aspects of metabolism, protein synthesis, oxygen and carbon dioxide carriage, acid-base balance, hemoglobin and enzyme isolation, and for a host of other applications. It is not surprising that this is so since the red cell, particularly the mammalian (nonnucleated) red cell, is easily obtained and manipulated, metabolically simpler than other body cells, and has been better characterized than almost any other cell. However, despite an extensive literature in hematology and in special areas of interest in the red cell, there has not been available in English any recent critical compendium dealing with the biology of the mature, mammalian red blood cell. In brief, much has been written about certain aspects of the red blood cell but no one seems to have really looked at the whole cell in all its aspects. Initial optimism on our part that such a volume could be put together by one or two authors soon gave way to the realization that no one person could be critically knowledgeable in more than one small area. The job then became an editorial one, of surveying the field and finding an approachable expert in each area. To find authors who are thoroughly competent in their area, critical of both their own and other's work, able to express themselves without glossing over significant details and yet simply enough that the neophyte can follow, conform to an Editor's demands as to coverage and conventions and submit a manuscript by the deadline set—this is an Editor's dream. We feel fortunate in having succeeded so well in enlisting the collaboration of such competent authors as make up this treatise.

The Editors feel that they have, for the first time, brought together much knowledge concerning many aspects of the red blood cell. The knowledge so collected is not merely compiled but has been critically assembled by persons pursuing active and noteworthy research in each area. These experts were asked to present their own best judgment as to the significant experimental data from the past and a frame of reference for the future developments in their area. They were encouraged to select what they considered to be solid and consistent information and reject what in their opinion was spurious or factitious. Insofar as the experts have guessed well, so shall this volume serve the present and future investigator and knowledge-seeker. Some aspects of the red blood cell have not been as well covered as might have been hoped. In part this results from incomplete comprehension on the part of the Editors of the task we were starting, a task which was better appreciated at the end as the various chapters began to fall into place. Some deficiencies also arose because we could not secure experts in certain areas—oftentimes because an area was poorly defined or poorly covered in the literature or because such an expert was already occupied. In any event, the Editors felt that there was need to sift fact from fancy in order that our knowledge of red cells be established on firm ground and ignorance be revealed wherever it existed. Thus the reader may come away feeling less sure of his "knowledge" than when he started. Such is the tortuous path of science!

CHARLES BISHOP
DOUGLAS M. SURGENOR

April, 1964

Contents

Chapter 1
Historical Introduction

MAX M. STRUMIA

Chapter 2
Composition of Normal Human Red Cells

ROBERT B. PENNELL

Chapter 3

Ion and Water Permeability of the Red Blood Cell

HERMANN PASSOW

Chapter 4

Overall Red Cell Metabolism

CHARLES BISHOP

Chapter 5

The Pentose Phosphate Metabolism in Red Cells

ZACHARIAS DISCHE

Chapter 6

Glucose-6-Phosphate Dehydrogenase: Its Properties and Role in Mature Erythrocytes

PAUL A. MARKS

Chapter 7

Chemical Composition and Metabolism of Lipids in Red Cells of Various Animal Species

L. L. M. VAN DEENEN AND J. DE GIER

Chapter 8

Hemoglobin Metabolism within the Red Cell

DAVID W. ALLEN

Chapter 9

Transport of Oxygen and Carbon Dioxide

DOUGLAS M. SURGENOR

Chapter 10

Blood-Group Substances: Their Nature and Genetics

WINIFRED M. WATKINS

Chapter 11

Metabolic Processes Involved in the Formation and Reduction of Methemoglobin in Human Erythrocytes

ERNST R. JAFFÉ

Chapter 12

Life Span of the Red Cell

NATHANIEL I. BERLIN

Chapter 13

Use of the Erythrocyte in Functional Evaluation of Vitamin Adequacy

MYRON BRIN

Chapter 14

Approaches to Red Cell Preservation in the Liquid State

JOHN G. GIBSON II

Chapter 15

Red Cell Storage in the Frozen State

JAMES L. TULLIS

CHAPTER 1

Historical Introduction

Max M. Strumia

I. Development of Knowledge of the Red Cells, Circulation, and Transfusion before 1900

While blood has been identified with life from remotest antiquity, scientific anatomical and physiological inquiries on circulation and on the red cell awaited the coming of the sixteenth century. Fundamental discoveries of this period were part of a scientific renaissance characterized by a rebellion against the Galenic tradition and leading to the foundation of scientific societies, beginning with the *Accademia dei Lincei* in Rome in 1603.

A. Discovery of Circulation and of the Red Cells

Vesalius in 1543[1] laid the anatomical basis for the study of circulation; Columbus (1516–1559) correctly described the pulmonary circulation; Caesalpinus (1519–1603) anticipated the basic principles of circulation. William Harvey (1578–1657) studied at Padua under Fabricius of Aquapendente and continued the work on returning to England, leading to the publication of "Exercitatio de Motu Cordis" in 1628, which constitutes a milestone in the progress of medical knowledge.

The discovery of the microscope sometime around 1650 made possible the recognition of red cells by Jan Swammerdam (1658). Shortly after Marcello Malpighi discovered the capillary circulation of the lung (1661) and again described red cells, Giovanni Borelli (1680) advanced the knowledge of circulation by demonstrating the mechanism of the steady flow of blood from the arteries through the capillaries and into the veins. In 1674 Anton Van Leeuwenhoek described in detail the red cells of various animal species, and

[1] All literature references prior to 1900 have been omitted from the bibliography since a number of the original articles were not available for consultation by the author. Some of the references after 1900 have been omitted since the full historical meaning of the contribution is implied in the notation.

established their size at about 1/3000 of an inch by comparing them with the known size of a grain of sand.

B. *Respiration*

The first definitive recognition of the relationship of the red cells to respiration was not to come for another century. Lavoisier (1777), two years after the discovery of oxygen, described the nature of oxidation and identified this process with respiration. Additionally he recognized that two factors are involved in respiration: oxidation, with disappearance of "oxigine" or "vital air" (the igneo-aeral salt of Mayow), and appearance of "aeriform acid" carbon dioxide (the "fixed air" of Black, the *gas sylvestre* of Helmont).

Lavoisier's concept of oxidation was that it took place in the tubes of the lungs, at the expense of a substance secreted in the lungs and containing carbon and hydrogen. This theory was rejected on theoretical grounds by Lagrange (1791). It remained for Spallanzani, towards the end of the eighteenth century, to establish another milestone by demonstrating that all body tissues consume oxygen and produce carbonic acid, that is, respire (1803).

C. *Hemopoietic Function of the Bone Marrow; Early Studies of Hemoglobin and Red Cells*

Menghini (1747) showed that iron was present in the ash of red cells; Reichert crystallized hemoglobin in 1849; Justus von Liebig proposed in 1852 that the red cells contain a compound of iron which can combine with oxygen or carbon dioxide in a reversible reaction. Hoppe-Seyler (1802) demonstrated the oxidation-reduction potential of hemoglobin.

Another epochal contribution was made in 1868, when Neumann and Bizzozzero, simultaneously and independently, discovered the hemopoietic function of the bone marrow. Methodology of measure of red cells and hemoglobin made rapid progress in the last part of the nineteenth century. Vierordt (1851) described an exact method for enumerating red blood corpuscles; Welcher (1863) determined the total blood volume and the volume of normal red blood cells; Malassez (1874) designed the first hemocytometer; Hayem (1877) introduced the color index.

D. *Early Recorded Transfusions*

Books on the history of medicine are replete with references to "transfusion" of blood. Actually in most instances it is not clear whether the blood was introduced into the vascular system, or was simply drunk, a procedure known to antiquity for the cure of many ailments. A definite description of transfusion was first given by Giovanni Francesco Colle in 1628. The names and deeds of Francesco Foli (1654), Richard Lower (1655), Jean Baptiste Denis (1667), and others were well recorded and subjected to many comments: success was claimed for the administration of animal blood, more rarely of human blood, under conditions where we consider with wonderment the fact that a life was not lost. That transfusions, during this period, were not more frequently followed by death is probably due to the small volume of blood generally transfused. The choice of patients and conditions for transfusion were entirely empirical, and the patient was almost invariably bled before he was transfused, the purpose being to remove bad blood to let in good blood. The most common indication for blood transfusion, as stated by Andrea Libavius, was weakness due to old age, when the use of blood from a vigorous young man was recommended. Transfusion was also used to change the humor of individuals; thus the blood of a lamb would be suitable for a choleric man. Success of transfusion in a dog performed by Richard Lower in 1666 led Pepys to write, "It gave rise to many pretty wishes as of the blood of a Quaker to be let into an archbishop and such like." It was not until 1783 that Rosa and Scarpa proved that phlebotomy need not precede transfusion. Later (1788) these same investigators gave, for the first time, blood transfusion to treat anemia.

Blundell in 1824 came to the conclusion that transfusion of blood could be performed only between animals of the same species and that humans should receive blood only from another human. A suggestion to explain failure of transfusions is contained in the observation of Landois (1875), who demonstrated that heterologous blood transfusion could lead to dangerous reaction and that if blood from an animal was mixed with that of another species, agglutination or hemolysis of the red cells could occur. It is not surprising that transfusion of blood became a discredited procedure and that civil and religious authorities banned its use. Thus, before 1900 over a period of a little more than three centuries, knowledge of the red cell and its functions and knowledge of the circulation progressed sufficiently to establish most of the knowledge required for the proper use of transfusion. Ignorance of the antigenic constitution of human and animal red cells, and of humoral factors, kept transfusion at near pre-Homeric level.

II. Fundamental Discoveries of Blood Groups and Isoimmunization; Heredity Laws Applied to Blood Groups; Limited Use of Direct Transfusion (1900–1913)

The beginning of the twentieth century marks the dawn of blood transfusion in the sense which we accept today. Between 1900 and 1911 fundamental discoveries and rediscoveries were made which laid the scientific basis for blood transfusion. Landsteiner (1900) repeated in human blood what Landois had done in animal blood and discovered three blood groups on the basis of the determination of two antigens, A and B, in the red cells, and anti-A and anti-B agglutinins in blood sera. DeCastello and Sturli (1902) discovered blood group O, which contained neither antigen A nor B, but both anti-A and anti-B agglutinins. At the same time Ehrlich and Morganroth demonstrated the phenomenon of isoimmunization in goats, and Epstein and Ottenberg (1908) described practical methods for grouping of blood as a prerequisite for blood transfusion. Finally, Mendel's law of heredity, first presented in 1865, was shown to apply to the blood groups by Dungern and Hirszfeld (1911); it remained for Bernstein (1924) to demonstrate that the inheritance of antigens A, B, and O as Mendelian characters was based on the occurrence of three allelomorphic genes, A, B, and O.

In the period immediately following the discovery of blood groups, acceptance and diffusion of the use of transfusion were very slow. George Nuttall (1904) in his treatise on "Blood Immunity and Blood Relationship" makes no mention of Landsteiner's findings published in 1900, although referring to Landsteiner's work published in 1901 on stability of the agglutination of red cells by sera. Ottenberg (1911) and Ottenberg and Kaliski (1913) proved the essential importance of studies preliminary to transfusion, and reported results in 128 cases.

Transfusions were invariably given by the direct method: Carrel, Crile, and many others devised a variety of instruments more or less suited for the purpose. Major problems in the technique of direct transfusion were the inherent danger of thrombosis and embolism and the difficulty in evaluating the volume of blood transfused.

Blood transfusion is seldom mentioned in medical textbooks before 1918; Rous and Turner (1916a) in discussing the necessity to keep red cells alive *in vitro* for longer periods of time, stated as the purpose of their investigation, "Cells could be utilized for serum reactions, or for culture media, or even under certain circumstances for transfusion." As late as 1917 Klinger denied the importance of proper choice of blood for transfusion. Knowledge of the chemical nature of the ABO blood factors was not to come until the work of Kabat (1956). We now know that all are mucopolysaccharides, and that the antigenic specificity is dependent upon variations in the carbohydrate end group.

III. Sodium Citrate Introduced as an Anticoagulant; Sugars as Preservative Agents (1914–1916)

The modern technique of transfusion by the indirect method dates to the introduction by Hustin (1914) of sodium citrate as anticoagulant. Levinshon and Agote confirmed and applied the finding of Hustin; Weil (1915) outlined a simple procedure for the use of citrated blood.

The use of additives to improve red cell preservation was introduced by Rous and Turner (1916a). These authors found that sugars added to rabbit citrated cells suspended in Locke's solution acted as a preservative. Both saccharose and dextrose were found to be effective. When citrate only was added to blood, hemolysis was well marked after little more than a week. However, on storage of 3 parts human blood mixed with 2 parts 3.8% sodium citrate and 5 parts 5.4% dextrose in water, the red cells remained intact for about 4 weeks. The same authors (1916b) found that rabbit erythrocytes preserved in a mixture of sodium citrate, saccharose, and water for 14 days remained in circulation and functioned well.

Considering the mechanism of the effect of sugars, Rous and Turner expressed the view that they possess power to prevent the injurious effect of Locke's solution and, "They (the sugars) possess, in addition, preservative qualities." This preservative action is attributed to retardation of proteolytic action.

The observation of Rous and Turner was applied by Robertson (1918) to the need for preservation of human blood. During the first world conflict Robertson used a mixture of 350 ml. isotonic citrate and 850 ml. isotonic dextrose; these solutions were separately sterilized to avoid caramelization. They were mixed before collection of 500 ml. blood, giving a total volume of 1700 ml. The citrate–dextrose blood thus obtained was preserved at refrigerator temperature for as long as 26 days, the average length of storage being 10 days to 2 weeks. The bulk of the supernatant was removed before transfusion. Twenty-two transfusions were given to 20 patients, and the results were considered comparable to those obtained with fresh blood.

It is interesting to compare these pioneering efforts with the development of transfusion thirty years later, during World War II, when in four and one-half years the American Red Cross collected 13,326,242 units of blood. How much of this amount was actually distributed to troops in the form of freeze-dried plasma, concentrated albumin solution, or whole blood is a military figure.

IV. Nomenclature of Blood Groups

Much confusion was created at this time by the use of conflicting nomenclatures of blood groups proposed by Jansky and by Moss, in addition to the original nomenclature which named the blood groups with the letters identifying the agglutinogens present in each group. This confusion lasted for many years, with most scientific publications adhering to the Landsteiner grouping, later adopted by the League of Nations, and most of the laboratories in the

United States using the Moss classification. As late as 1921 a joint committee representing the American Association of Immunologists, the Society of American Bacteriologists, and the Association of Pathologists recommended the Jansky classification, on the basis of priority! Much later, somewhere between 1930 and 1940, the ABO classification of blood groups became universally adopted.

V. Growth of Blood Transfusion and Establishment of Blood Banks (1921–1937)

In the years following World War I, between 1921 and 1929, the practice of blood transfusion made slow progress. The lesson of Rous and Turner was forgotten; plain citrated blood was used almost exclusively for transfusion. The technique was very simple: blood was collected in an open sterile vessel containing the citrate; it was filtered through gauze in a funnel and transfused immediately. This technique assured fresh red cells and although the technique exposed the blood to bacterial contamination, major reactions due to bacterial growth were not encountered because the blood was not stored. Minor febrile reaction due to contamination of glassware and water with pyrogen occurred at a much higher rate than prevails today. Unfortunately poor technique of grouping and compatibility tests, and ignorance of the Rh factor and other red cell agglutinogens, caused an incidence of hemolytic posttransfusion reactions variously estimated, but generally 0.2% or higher.

In the thirties the practice of blood transfusion received impetus from the contributions of a group of Russian workers experimenting with animal and human blood, from living donors and from cadavers. In this group we need mention Burdenko, Shamoff, Samov and Kostrjakov, and Judine and his co-workers. The use of cadaver blood, outside of Russia, did not attain any degree of popularity.[1] During this period of time trisodium citrate was practically the only anticoagulant used.

Between 1934 and 1937 the limits of useful preservation of red cells for the purpose of transfusion were set arbitrarily. Lindebaum and Stroikova set the maximum limit at 12 days; Doepp at 10 days; Jeanneney and Vieroz at 20 days; others, like Grozdoff, found very little difference in the effect of storage from a few days to over 15 days; Gnoinski used blood 66, 75, and 85 days old; some of these transfusions consisted of only a few milliliters of blood and the criterion of successful transfusion was often the absence of overt reactions. Bagdassarov set for blood stored in plain citrate a limit of 13–21 days, and for blood stored in citrate–dextrose a limit of 20–34 days. In this country at about

[1] At present it is used almost solely in Moscow at the Sklifosovsky Institute for Traumatic Diseases.

the same time, Belk set a limit for blood stored in citrate at 14 days. This confused status continued well after the report of Fantus (1937) on blood banks; Fantus and Shermer recommended a limit of 10 days for plain citrate blood.

The definitions of the useful lifespan of red cells were largely based on studies *in vitro*. Among these, visible hemolysis and changes in osmotic fragility were the most commonly employed.

With the institution of blood banks some of the defects of the previous decade remained, such as the use of plain citrate. Additionally, blood was stored often too long, resulting in little benefit to the patient and carrying a higher rate of severe reactions from bacterial contamination.

VI. World War II: The Use of Plasma, Development of Plasma Fractionation, and Acidification of Citrate–Dextrose Solution

Between 1939 and 1943 two unrelated events created a major turn in the history of blood transfusion. The first was the occurrence of World War II which created, through necessity, impetus for the study and diffusion of blood transfusion. The results were expansion of the use of plasma, practical development of plasma fractionation, and introduction of the acidification of citrate–dextrose solution. The second event was the discovery of the Rh factor.

A. Evaluation of Survival of Stored Red Cells

Strumia (1939) in discussing the rationale of blood transfusion called attention to the evidence of accelerated blood destruction following transfusion of citrated blood preserved for more than 4 or five days. The criteria for estimation of damage to red cells *in vitro* were those previously used, namely, determination of the amount of plasma hemoglobin, obtained after thorough mixing of the blood, and of the osmotic fragility of erythrocytes. Additionally, *in vivo* studies were carried out, which included erythrocyte counts, hemoglobin content, and serum bilirubin level of the recipient's blood before and after transfusion. On the basis of the findings, citrated refrigerated blood was considered unfit for transfusion after 5 days of storage.

Similar conclusions were reached by DeGowin *et al.* (1940). This investigator critically analyzed the composition of blood preservatives, and recommended a modification of the Rous and Turner dextrose–citrate mixture which did not require removal of the supernatant prior to transfusion. Although with the addition of dextrose the limits of preservation of blood could be extended to approximately 10 days, the large volume of blood–dextrose–citrate mixture (1250 ml.) made the application of the method impractical.

In the following years a number of investigators commented on the inadequacies of the *in vitro* studies to determine the degree of survival of the transfused red cells. Mollison and Young (1942) and Maizels among others reduced the significance of the *in vitro* studies to a negative value, that is, the red cells were sure not to survive posttransfusion if the *in vitro* studies showed significant deterioration, but the opposite was not found to be true.

Additionally, Mollison and Young (1942), using the Ashby method, determined that posttransfusion survival of stored red cells was satisfactory for limits of optimal preservation up to 6 days in plain citrate, but that after 14 days the blood was useless, thus confirming Strumia's findings. With the addition of glucose, as with use of the Rous–Turner solution, blood was considered usable for 21 days.

The pressure of World War I was a stimulus for Robertson's first using, for the purpose of blood storage, the preservation properties of dextrose, suggested by Rous and Turner; during World War II the same pressure led to rapidly expanding work on the physiology of red cells *in vitro*.

B. Acid–Citrate–Dextrose Solution

Loutit *et al.* (1943) commented on the phenomenon of caramelization of dextrose solutions at 120°C. in the presence of alkaline solutions of citrate with pH in the neighborhood of 8.5–9. This change did not appear to alter appreciably the effectiveness of the glucose solution, but was noted and avoided by Robertson by separate sterilization of the citrate and the sugar solutions. This required an additional step and, what is more objectionable, risk of contamination in the mixing of the two separately sterilized solutions.

It was noted that caramelization did not occur when acidification to pH below 7.4 was obtained by replacing a portion of the alkaline trisodium citrate with citric acid. It was found that hemolysis of red cells of blood preserved in this solution was retarded. This led the authors to study the survival *in vivo*, using a large transfusion of packed red cells in anemic patients and determining the survival with the Ashby technique. This procedure was carried out in 35 patients and established that the red cells of blood stored with acid–citrate–dextrose (ACD) solution survived better than red cells stored in other solutions. Important observations were also obtained by *in vitro* studies: release of inorganic phosphorus, potassium shift outside of red cells, glycolysis, and alteration in osmotic fragility were different from those obtained with other preservative solutions. These changes did not appear to be correlated with ability of the erythrocytes to survive, except for the delayed spontaneous hemolysis. The ACD solution for preservation of blood proposed by Loutit and Mollison was composed of 100 ml. 2% disodium citrate and 20 ml. 15% glucose for addition to 420–430 ml. of blood. With various modifications this solution became of general use. It constitutes today the almost universally used preservative for whole blood.

Thus by 1943 a much improved method of blood preservation was brought about, while basic knowledge of the relationship between red cell energy requirements, glycolysis, and metabolism of organic phosphate compounds was being accumulated.

C. Use of Blood Plasma for Transfusion

In May 1940, in order to choose and make available a satisfactory "blood substitute" for treatment of shock, the Surgeons General of the Army and Navy of the United States requested advice from the National Research Council. The reports of the Committee on Transfusion,[1] and of the Subcommittee on Blood Procurement and Blood Substitutes, from the first meeting on 31 May, 1940, faithfully reflect the progress in development of practical methods of transfusion for the treatment of shock.

The use of plasma received immediate attention, because its effectiveness in treatment of shock and burns in man had been previously documented by Strumia *et al.* (1940a, b). Vasteenberghe in 1903 and Bordas and d'Arsonval in 1906 laid the basic foundation for the process of drying in the frozen state of labile organic substances for the purpose of preservation. By 1940 numerous other contributors had advanced the technical knowledge of the process; control of production and development of equipment for administration of freeze-dried plasma were immediately considered.

By the end of 1940 the first dry plasma kit for field use was demonstrated; this led rapidly to trials and adoption of standard equipment (Strumia *et al.*, 1942). Simultaneously the question of whole blood preservation and transportation was considered.

D. Plasma Fractionation

In a thorough review of the history of blood proteins, Cohn (1939) credited Mulder in 1838 with the concept that proteins are chemical substances. Fractionation of plasma proteins was first done by Denis in 1841. Mellanby in 1908 and Hardy and Gardiner in 1910 proposed the low temperature, alcohol precipitation procedure for separation of proteins. Ferry and Green in 1929 further pursued this method; there followed a number of contributions from investigators in the Department of Physical Chemistry of Harvard University, whereby knowledge was gained of the isoelectric and neutral salt precipitation methods for proteins. Cohn standardized the method and made it capable

[1] Membership of the original committee included: Doctors Walter B. Cannon, Alfred Blalock, E. D. Plass, Max M. Strumia, and Cyrus C. Sturgis.

of large-scale production. The methodology and identification of protein fractions thus separated were presented in a series of papers (Cohn *et al.*, 1940, *et seq.*).

In the spring of 1941 Cohn presented to the Committee on Transfusion and Subcommittee on Blood Procurement and Blood Substitutes the result of his work with fractionation of human plasma and a program for preparation of purified human albumin in concentrated form for use in the field as a plasma volume expander. Under pressure of rapidly deteriorating international relations, commercial preparation and distribution of dried plasma and concentrated human albumin for treatment of shock due to lost blood volume proceeded rapidly.

VII. Rh Factor and Other Blood Systems

A. Rh Factor

Twenty-seven years after the original description of blood groups, Landsteiner and Levine discovered the factors M, N, and P. The practical importance of these groups was not immediately evident.

The Rh factor of human red cells was discovered by Landsteiner and Wiener (1941) through the finding that the red cells in 85% of a Caucasian population were agglutinated by sera of rabbits and guinea pigs sensitized by injection of Rhesus monkey red cells. Recognition of the importance of this factor in the production of intragroup hemolytic reactions by Wiener and Peters (1940), and in the mechanism of production of erythroblastosis fetalis by Levine *et al.* (1941), brought about considerable reduction in the incidence of posttransfusion hemolytic reaction, and led to the treatment of erythroblastotic infants by exchange transfusion first introduced by Allen *et al.* (1949).

The reduction of mortality due to hemolytic posttransfusion reactions from sensitization to the Rh factor is well exemplified by the record of the transfusion service in our institution. Prior to 1941 the rate of death attributable directly to blood transfusion in the Bryn Mawr Hospital was 0.2%; Tiber reported a rate of 0.13% and DeGowin 0.2%. The last death attributable to transfusion of incompatible blood in the Bryn Mawr Hospital occurred in April 1941. The incompatibility in this patient was apparently the result of Rh sensitization in a woman who had three erythroblastotic newborns, and who was transfused for treatment of severe postpartum hemorrhage with the group-compatible husband's blood. The incomplete Rh antibodies escaped detection because only the saline crossmatch test was performed at that time. From April 1941 through December 1962, 46,479 transfusions of whole blood or packed red cells were performed. No death resulted and only the following untoward results were observed:

A patient who was E-negative and C-negative received emergency transfusion and was later found to be sensitized to both these factors, but no hemolytic reaction occurred.

An emergency transfusion of A_2, Rh-positive blood was given to a patient who was O-positive but because of poorly developed anti-A, no reaction occurred.

A group-B Rh-negative patient received in an emergency a unit of B Rh-positive blood and within 3 days developed anti-D antibodies with a mild hemolytic phenomenon. Complete recovery was observed after 1 week.

Six D-positive patients were given D-negative blood, with only one sensitization of clinical importance.

B. Other Blood Systems

In the years following discovery of the Rh factors, beginning with Mourant's (1946) discovery of the Le antigen, a number of blood group systems, other than ABO, appeared in the literature: Kell, Duffy, Kidd, Lutheran, Diego, and Sutter. Additionally a number of group factors have been described, occurring in only a few families. To these antigens the name of "private" has been applied. In contrast, antigens have been described which are present in the vast majority of individuals. These factors are referred to as "public."

As knowledge of the Rh and other newly discovered factors progressed, it became evident that, in contrast to the ABO system with "natural" or "isoantibodies," the antibodies to these factors or "immune antibodies" did not produce agglutination in saline media. To these antibodies the name of "incomplete" was given.

C. Anti-Human Globulin Test

Moreschi (1908) had demonstrated that erythrocytes exposed to proteins of heterogeneous sera become modified, or sensitized. When exposed subsequently to sera of animals injected with the heterologous protein, agglutination occurs.

This procedure, rediscovered by Coombs *et al.* (1945) is now generally known as the "antiglobulin test" or Coombs test, and has been extensively used for detection of "incomplete" antibodies.

The test, while subject to many pitfalls, has been of great value in the diagnosis and study of acquired hemolytic anemia; it has been invaluable for the detection of incompatibilities due to immune antibodies acquired through transfusion or pregnancy.

The use of albumin in a slide test by Diamond and Abelson (1945), and of enzymatic modification by Morton and Pickles (1947) have added very valuable tools to the methodology of the modern blood bank technique.

History is repeating: in the absence of definitive knowledge of essential immunological data, the perplexing complexity of the Rh system has been considerably aggravated by the existing notation systems. This problem was discussed by a group of investigators interested in the Rh factor problem at a meeting held in Princeton, New Jersey, under the auspices of the Committee on Blood and Related Problems of the National Research Council, with support by a grant from the National Institutes of Health. The meeting succeeded in emphasizing the complexity of the problem, but came to no practical conclusion. Rosenfield *et al.* (1962), in proposing a new Rh numerical notation system, have presented an excellent critical summation of our knowledge of the complex status of the Rh factors in relation to the very practical and essential problem of determining by available serological methods and materials if a person is D-negative (Rh-negative) or D-positive.

VIII. Red Cell Energy Requirement, Glycolysis, and Effect of Purine Nucleosides

A. Glycolysis and Red Cell Metabolism

Lavaczeck in 1924 investigated the influence of acidity on blood glycolysis. Guest (1932) found in defibrinated blood that sugar concentration decreases and, when the glycolytic activity is nearly spent, inorganic phosphate increases from breakdown of organic phosphate of the red cell. It was also pointed out that addition of sugar extends the period of glycolysis, hence retards breakdown of inorganic phosphate. Thus the basic principle of the favorable effect of dextrose on viability of red cells was described sixteen years after the introduction of sugars as preservative for red cells stored *in vitro*.

In 1939, Rapaport and Guest anticipated the role of acidification in the breakdown of diphosphoglycerate, and its important relationship to the glycolytic cycle. Maizels and Whittaker (1940) and Maizels (1941, 1943) made additional contributions on the fundamental role of phosphorus compounds in the metabolism of red cells *in vitro*.

Rapaport published a series of articles (1947, *et seq.*) in which knowledge of the dimensional and chemical changes which characterize the erythrocytes during storage was greatly extended.

Rapaport emphasized that dimensional changes in the red cell imply functional changes, and that the functional status of the cells becomes the limiting factor in red cell survival. Glycolysis is definitely recognized as the energy-yielding process in the red cell, and its great dependence on pH was defined: at pH values above 7.3 inorganic phosphorus increases rapidly at the expense primarily of adenosine triphosphate (ATP), later also of diphosphoglyceric acid. The rationale of the ACD solution becomes more evident.

Ponder (1940), speculating on the mechanism of maintenance of the biconcave shape of red cells, suggested two possible theories: a rigid structure of a dynamic balance of forces, hence an energy requirement. Rapaport's work confirmed the dynamic nature of the factors maintaining red cell shape, and estimated the amount of energy required for maintenance of the dimensional characteristics of the red cell.

The effect of purine nucleosides on the metabolism of red cells was extensively investigated, particularly by groups at the University of Seattle and McGill University. Results appearing in the literature beginning in 1954 extended the knowledge of the pathway of enzymatic activity. This was amplified in successive years by Gabrio *et al.* (1956a) and Rubenstein and Denstedt (1956). These studies led to the concept that the intermediates of the glycolytic process occur as phosphorylated sugars, and that the formation of each of these substances is catalyzed by a specific and a nonspecific coenzyme. Two high-energy compounds are produced during glycolysis, and serve as coenzymes: ATP and reduced diphosphopyridine nucleotide (DPNH, more recently abbreviated NADH). ATP is essential for various phosphorylation processes, those occurring during glycolysis, and those leading to resynthesis of DPN (NAD). The effect of ATP begins with entry of glucose into the red cell and conversion of the glucose to glucose-6-phosphate, which is catalyzed by hexokinase and requires ATP as coenzyme. For an extensive synthetic analysis of this subject the reader is referred to the work of London (1961), and Chapters 4, 5, and 6.

B. *Adenosine, Inosine, Adenine as Red Cell Preservatives*

It was noted that the level of ATP in red cells declines and is parallel to loss of the normal biconcave form and viability of stored red cells. Donohue *et al.* (1956) initially used adenosine as an additive to stored ACD blood to maintain a high concentration of ATP. As a consequence of the improved metabolism, satisfactory posttransfusion survival of erythrocytes was extended to approximately twice that generally obtained with plain ACD solution.

Gabrio *et al.* (1956b), postulated that the effect of adenosine is mediated by an initial conversion to inosine, and inosine was proposed as the additive of choice. Extended use of inosine by other laboratories (Lange *et al.*, 1958) failed to confirm the earlier satisfactory results.

Nakao and co-workers reported (1959) that the addition of both adenine and inosine to blood maintained normal dimensional and osmotic properties of red cells during storage, through regeneration of ATP. An additive containing adenine and inosine was successfully used to improve the posttransfusion survival of stored erythrocytes by Wada and co-workers (1960) (see Chapter 4).

More recently Simon *et al.* (1962) used small amounts of adenine to extend the useful storage period of blood to at least 5 weeks. The very small amount of adenine used (0.75 ± 0.25 μmole/ml. ACD blood), compared with the relatively large amounts of inosine (13 μmoles/ml. ACD blood) used in the extended studies, may explain the variations in results obtained at various times and by various investigators with the addition of inosine. In retrospect it is surmised that the various lots of "inosine" may have contained varying amounts of adenine, small enough to escape detection by the methods used, large enough to exert a protective action on red cell preservation.

The benefits to be derived by extension of the period of useful storage of red cells of blood are considerable. The addition of adenine, and the use of citrate–phosphate–dextrose solution proposed by Gibson and co-workers in 1957 on the basis of some of Parpart's finding ten years previously, need confirmation by other investigators. A major difficulty in such studies is the variety of procedures used and results obtained in determining the life span of transfused red cells. This variable may cause a difference of as much as 20% when the storage of blood is prolonged. The main difficulty is in establishment of the theoretical expected 100%, which in turn depends on an accurate method of blood volume measurement (see Chapter 12).

It is hoped that investigators will agree on some procedure whereupon the *relative* value of the various methods can be determined. This approach may be somewhat less desirable than acceptance of a standard method, but is certainly of far easier achievement.

IX. Blood Volume; Red Cell Tagging; Life Span of Red Cells

Quantitative data on erythrokinesis could not develop until it became possible to measure the mass of the circulating erythron, and the life span of red cells in circulation.

A. Blood Volume Determination

The measure of the blood volume, introduced by Welcker in 1854, was very slow in becoming of general use, because the only "direct" method, that of exsanguination used by Welcker, is hardly applicable to human subjects, and the "indirect" methods carried for a long time numerous sources of error, with poor to fair reproducibility.

The first indirect method, employing carbon monoxide to tag red cells, was introduced by Gréhaut and Quinquad in 1882. The dye dilution method, developed by Keith, Rowntree, and Geraghty in 1915 represents a milestone in the progress of this determination. Replacement of brilliant vital red with the blue diazo dye T-1824 by Gregersen, Gibson, and Stead in 1935 greatly improved the procedure, by virtue of the slower diffusibility of the blue dye and the accuracy with which its concentration could be measured photometrically.

B. Red Cell Tagging

The introduction of isotopic tagging of the globin moiety introduced by Gray and Sterling (1950) constituted a major contribution, and made possible the direct determination of the red cell mass. The use of P^{32}, described by Chaplin (1954), proved to be less accurate than tagging with radioactive sodium chromate because the radioactive phosphorus tag is more labile and errors are introduced by some rapid elution after transfusion of the tagged cells.

The introduction of tagging of plasma albumin with I^{131} did not offer essential improvement over the use of T-1824 dye, as both of these methods have in common the diffusion of the albumin in the extravascular spaces. An additional difficulty with I^{131} is that a portion of the iodine is loosely attached to the albumin, becomes eluted, and is rapidly taken out of circulation by the thyroid.

Determination of the blood volume has been the subject of a great deal of criticism, some of which is inherent in the methodology and much more in the improper consideration of biological variables. Perhaps the major difficulty has been the time of sampling, after transfusion of the tag, particularly when the material tagged is the plasma component albumin. This can be well eliminated by multiple sampling in rapid succession beginning immediately after transfusion of the tagged material, so that a sample may be chosen after complete mixing has taken place but before an appreciable amount of the tag has been lost either through elution, diffusion outside the vascular bed, or, in the case of red cells, by destruction of damaged cells (Strumia *et al.*, 1958a).

C. Red Cell Life Span

Prior to 1919 the life span of red blood cells had been, more or less arbitrarily, estimated as 30 days. Ashby (1919), using the differential agglutination method, established the life span of transfused erythrocytes at 30–100 days, with an average of 83 days. This method, with technical modifications by several investigators, remained the basic method for estimation of life span of transfused red cells until the introduction of isotopic tagging of red cells in 1942.

Sophistication of the differential agglutination technique has resulted in fairly reproducible results, and by this method the life span of red cells has been estimated in our laboratory at 118 days. Notwithstanding inevitable damage related to the extracorporeal phase of the process, these results compare reasonably well with those obtained with N^{15} tagging *in vivo*.

The first accurate measure of red cell life span was obtained in 1938, by an indirect method utilizing the measure of bilirubin output. Hawkins and Whipple (1938) produced a hemolytic crisis by administration of phenylhydrazine to dogs with a bile fistula. Due to severe reduction of the red cell population and entrance into the circulation of numerous young cells, the bile pigment output fell to low values. The subsequent rise in bile output indicated the senescence of the generation of cells newly produced after the hemolytic crisis. The time, measured from the midpoint of the rapid increment of red cell population to the beginning of the increment of bile output, was determined as 112, 120, 126, and 133 days, an average for the life span of dog red cells in circulation of 124 days.

The values obtained by Shemin and Rittenberg (1946) for human red cells nineteen years later, by a direct method, was 127 days. These investigators found that glycine labeled with N^{15} is the nitrogenous precursor of the four pyrrole nuclei of protoporphyrin. Acetic acid or a closely related compound participates in the synthesis. Isotopic N^{15}, incorporated in protoporphyrin, tags limited generations of red cell, for the entire life span. Upon breakdown of the cells and separation of the heme components, the N^{15} tag follows the pathway of pigment to excretion as stercobilinogen, thus permitting quantitative studies of heme anabolic and catabolic phenomena. The method has been applied to study survival of red cells in a number of diseases.

Practically all other methods of evaluation of life span of red cells have graver limitations than those so far mentioned; results under optimal conditions have been similar to those already mentioned. Radioactive iron, introduced by Ross and Chaplin (1943), for tagging of red cells, was applied by Gibson, Evans, Aub, Sack, and Peacock (1947) to study survival of transfused cells, and by Finch, Wolff, Rath, and Fluharty, (1949a) to tag *in vivo* a limited generation of erythrocytes.

Tagging of red cells with radioisotopes of iron for the purpose of measuring lifespan or survival has the limitation of rapid reutilization of the iron.

Commenting on comparative studies of methods of estimating the life span of red cells, Berlin and co-workers in 1957 noted that, because of the large reutilization of iron, the red cell survival curves with the Fe^{59} method did not show the sharp fall associated with the N^{15} or C^{14} studies, and that analysis of the lifespan by this method was not too satisfactory (compare Chapter 12).

The use of C^{14}-tagged glycine, introduced by Berlin, Lawrence, and Lee (1951), has so far been limited to study of patients with incurable diseases. The effect of continual synthesis of labeled hemoglobin from the preceding labeled glycine tends to alter the slope of the curve of C^{14}-hemoglobin and make interpretation somewhat difficult.

The use of sodium chromate containing radioactive Cr^{51} was extended to measure the life span of a mixed generation of red cells by tagging *in vitro* by Ebaugh *et al.* (1953). This method has received wide acceptance because of simplicity, ease of counting, and the fact that radioactivity disappears completely from the body with the loss of the last tagged cell. It has the limitations of inevitable damage to cells during the extracorporeal handling and of elution of the tag from the red cells.

A fundamental requirement for determination of the red cell life span, which applies to all red cell tagging methods, is that the subject must be in a steady state as far as red cell population is concerned, i.e., as many red cells must enter the circulation as are lost or destroyed per unit of time. Any alteration of the steady state may considerably alter the meaning of the regression curves of labeled cells. Thus a patient who has reduced output of red cells and progressive reduction of the red cell mass would have an apparently extended survival of tagged cells, whereas the patient with increased erythropoiesis, following an acute loss, would have an apparently accelerated reduction of tagged cells, suggesting a more rapid loss of red cell population.

X. Erythrokinetics

A. Measures of Red Cell Turnover Rate

The functional integrity of the erythron is based on the maintenance of a steady state through the activity of a complex homeostatic mechanism. This mechanism has been the subject of a very large number of contributions of relatively recent date, although bone marrow was identified as the erythropoietic organ in 1868, and numerous observations of the morphology of bone marrow cells accumulated in ensuing years. The advent of accurate methods for determining the volume of circulating red cells and the life span of red cells in circulation made possible an indirect and reasonably accurate quantitative evaluation of red cell production before direct methods became available. With these data the overall average rate of red cell production is obtained by the formula:

$$\frac{\text{Total number of red cells in circulation}}{\text{Life span of red cells in circulation (days)}} = \text{Number of red cells produced daily}$$

The limitation of this approach is that it is restricted to the measure of cells delivered to the circulation and surviving in the circulation for at least long enough to be counted.

The total stercobilinogen output, when done simultaneously, offers a means for semiquantitative measure of the total heme production. Merits and limitations of this method will be briefly discussed later.

Direct quantitative studies of cell proliferation may be based on the determination of mitosis. The mitotic index, i.e., the ratio of number of cells in mitosis over total number of cells in the population, offers a quantitative measure of cell production. Applied to the red cells this method, even with the sophistication of the colchicine technique as described by Dustin in 1943 and Astaldi and Mauri (1954) does not give information on the rate of delivery of red cells from the bone marrow to the circulation, a datum of basic importance.

The daily turnover of red cells has been measured with the radioiron technique in animal and man by a number of investigators, among them Finch *et al.* (1949b), Huff *et al.* (1952e).

Giblett and co-workers (1956) used the bone marrow differential count (erythroid–myeloid ratio), measure of plasma radioiron turnover and red cell utilization as described by Huff in 1950, and measure of stercobilinogen output to determine the red cell turnover of normal and anemic subjects.

Using a technique introduced by Suit (1957), Donohue *et al.* (1958) determined in animals and man the total amount of cells in a sample of bone marrow, and the distribution of various nucleated cell types in the sample. The relation of this aliquot to total bone marrow was determined by using an Fe^{59} tag for measure of the erythroid cells. Thus a measure of the total cellularity of the bone marrow was obtained, with the exclusion of megakaryocytes.

Finch (1959) in a critical summary of data obtained in his laboratory reported the transit time of Fe^{59} radioactivity in rabbit bone marrow to be 24 hours, and 82 hours in man. Fractional turnover of four types of cell was calculated from data on the cellular composition of the erythron in relation to body weight and the relative ratio between the various categories of cells; time for complete turnover of human reticulocytes in the bone marrow was found to be 44 hours and in the circulating blood 29 hours, based on a mean life span of red cells of 120 days.

B. Humoral Control of Erythropoiesis

The radioiron red cell turnover studies left many questions largely unanswered. Particularly important is the nature of the processes involved in differentiation, maturation, and release of the erythron, in the normal individual and in the presence of abnormal conditions.

A fundamental contribution was the discovery and study of the humoral factor or factors which control erythropoiesis. The existence of such a humoral factor was first intuitively described by Carnot and DéFlandre in 1906. A definite outline of function and properties has been the work of a number of investigators, beginning with Reissman in 1950, and followed by Erslev; Gordon and co-workers; Borsook and co-workers; and Stohlman and co-workers. The results of these and other studies point to the importance of pO_2 in a site, or sites, of the body as stimulus to production of erythropoietin; the mechanism of this action is unknown.

Erythropoietin has been established by Borsook as being a mucoprotein; salic acid is essential for its activity. The renal origin of erythropoietin proposed by Jacobson is not compatible with the observations of Erslev. There is more agreement on the mode of action of erythropoietin on bone marrow cells, which appears to be largely on differentiation, whereas the subsequent maturation of the erythron is more or less automatic (see Scheme 1).

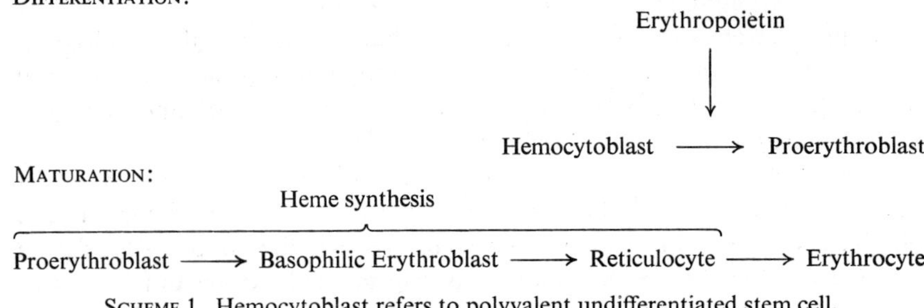

SCHEME 1. Hemocytoblast refers to polyvalent undifferentiated stem cell.

The observations of Fisher and London in 1961, Gordon *et al.* in 1959, and Alpen *et al.* (1959) question the validity of the conclusion that erythropoietin acts solely on differentiation. For the time being it seems better to interpret available data as indicating that erythropoietin is essentially concerned with differentiation of the basophilic proerythroblast from the stem cell, and that the role of erythropoietin in subsequent steps towards maturation is as yet undetermined.

The work of Leblond, Hughes, Cronkite, Bond, and co-workers, using tritiated thymidine in animals and man to tag deoxyribonucleic acid (DNA) at the time of synthesis, before cellular division, has introduced a specific label highly suitable for autoradiography. The β particles emitted by tritium are of low energy, permitting high resolution for radiographic identification of specific cells. By this method, the percentage of labeling reaches a maximum in the entire erythrocytic series in 12–24 hours, and eosinophilic normoblasts are shown to be nondividing cells, requiring only completion of maturation by disposal of nuclei. After 5 days no further labeling occurs.

C. *Significance of Stercobilinogen Output*

The value of the measure of stercobilinogen excretion in the stool as a measure of erythropoiesis has been the subject of considerable controversy.

The importance of the relationship of stercobilinogen output to total amount of circulating hemoglobin was first pointed out by Greppi (1926). He measured blood volume by the CO method and accurately estimated total circulating hemoglobin. The significance of this observation was not appreciated; one of the reasons for lack of interest in the measure of stercobilinogen output as a measure of erythropoiesis was the usage of expressing stercobilinogen values without consideration of circulating hemoglobin. Miller *et al.* (1942), proposed anew this concept and introduced use of the hemolytic index to express the relationship.

Since in a steady state the amount of red cells produced equals the amount destroyed, the basic formula (a) may be changed to (b):

$$\text{(a)}\quad \frac{\text{Total number of red cells in circulation}}{\text{Number of red cells produced daily}} = \text{Life span of red cells in circulation}$$

$$\text{(b)}\quad \frac{\text{Total number of red cells in circulation}}{\text{Number of red cells destroyed daily}} = \text{Life span of red cells in circulation}$$

The work of Shemin and Rittenberg and of Gray has shown that within the first few days following administration of N^{15}-tagged glycine an excess of N^{15}-tagged stercobilinogen is excreted in the stools, at a time when there should be minimal or no destruction of the newly formed cells. Some of the experimental data of Stohlman on rats (1959) also suggest that a significant number of erythrocyte precursors are destroyed in the marrow. However, no definition of the amount of heme involved is available. It may be assumed that no cellular division, and no cell elimination, occur after the stage of polychromatophilic normoblasts. A very marked disproportion between amount of stercobilinogen output and lifespan of red cells in circulation has been noted in some hemopathies, such as thalassemia and pernicious anemia. The hemoglobin lost through destruction of the erythron, other than in circulation, has been referred to as "wasted hemoglobin."

These observations may be the subject of several interpretations: the excess stercobilinogen may be due to (1) breakdown of heme in the bone marrow, (2) myoglobin breakdown, or (3) elimination of excess porphyrins. London (1951) has taken the view that such an excess of stercobilinogen loss can be explained only by the destruction of hemoglobin-containing cells in the bone marrow itself or immediately after entry into the circulation, so that the loss of these cells cannot be measured by the means employed to measure the life-span of red cells in circulation. Actually, no direct definitive evidence is available to support any of the possible explanations of the phenomena noted. Whichever the mechanism of the abnormalities in output, the measure of stercobilinogen output in relation to total circulating hemoglobin, if not a quantitative measure of erythropoiesis, is a convenient semiquantitative estimation of turnover of the porphyrins, if not of heme.

Practically, we need be concerned with the amount of total hemoglobin in circulation and the total amount of stercobilinogen in the stool. On the basis of a lifespan of 128 days, in the normal individual, we have found that for each gram of hemoglobin lost from circulation, 23 mg. stercobilinogen are eliminated in the stools. A working formula is then obtained:

$$\frac{\text{Total hemoglobin in circulation (gm.)}}{\text{Total daily stercobilinogen output (mg.)}} \div 23 = \begin{array}{c}\text{Apparent turnover of porphyrins}\\ \text{(or heme) (days)}\end{array}$$

Unfortunately, several factors related to transformation of bilirubin into stercobilinogen may introduce errors. Amongst these vitiating factors one need note diarrhea and constipation, resulting in an apparent diminished output; drugs capable of reducing the coliform flora of the intestine, likewise resulting in an apparent reduced output and consequently in an underestimation of red cell destruction.

Since only an error in dating of stool specimens can result in overestimation of the stercobilinogen output, all values in excess of normal may be considered significant if the stool collection is carried out over a period of 4 days or more.

XI. Hemoglobinopathies (Molecular Diseases)

A. Biosynthesis of Heme and Globin

The pathway of biosynthesis of heme has been elucidated by the work of Shemin, Rittenberg, London, Granick, Neuberger, Rimington, and others, beginning with publications in 1946. For a complete review of the subject, the reader is referred to the excellent critical presentation of London (1961) and Chapter 8.

Briefly, it has been clearly shown that biosynthesis of heme requires an intact Krebs tricarboxylic acid cycle, mitochondria, and ribonucleic acid (RNA); the complex molecule is synthesized from glycine and succinate, by action of specific enzymes; iron is incorporated when coproporphyrinogen III is oxidized and decarboxylated to yield protoporphyrin IX.

The synthesis of globin was a subject of later studies, beginning with Shemin and co-workers in 1950. Synthesis of globin occurs in ribosomes, and proceeds at a parallel rate with the formation of heme. However, synthesis of heme and of globin follow two different and independent pathways. Synthesis of heme and of globin, while occurring at parallel rates, are not interdependent in the individual. There are many conditions where such a parallel relationship is lost.

B. Identification of Sickle Cell Hemoglobin

Pauling and Itano in 1949 opened a new era in the physiopathology of red cells by the fundamental observation that in sickle cell disease there is present in the red cells a hemoglobin different from the normal. The difference was first revealed by the electrophoretic mobility; difference in isoelectric point of adult hemoglobin (A) and sickle cell hemoglobin (S) suggested that the latter has 2–4 more net positive charges per molecule than normal hemoglobin. Ingram (1956) discovered that sickle cell hemoglobin differs from normal hemoglobin in having a residue of valine instead of glutamic acid in its β-polypeptide chain. From these and other studies has emerged the concept of molecular disease as one in which the change in protein responsible for the hemoglobinopathy is at the molecular level. It has been argued that a mutant gene may act by producing a different amino acid composition, resulting in the production of an abnormal hemoglobin. This subject is developed thoroughly in Chapter 8.

C. Hemoglobin Patterns

In addition to electrophoresis, column chromatography, and alkali denaturation rate, the amino acid composition, the amino acid sequence, and the two-dimensional study by paper electrophoresis and paper chromatography of peptides obtained by trypsin digestion of globin (Ingram, 1956) have led to the present concept of globin pattern. It is now accepted that globin of hemoglobin A is composed of two pairs of polypeptide chains, α and β. Fetal (F) hemoglobin differs with respect to the β chain; this chain is called the γ chain. The polypeptide and amino acid composition has been applied to the characterization of an increasing number of abnormal hemoglobins; further enumeration is beyond the scope of this review.

In 1955 Kunkel, by starch block electrophoresis, identified a slow moving component of normal hemoglobin A, now known as hemoglobin A_2. Column chromatography has shown that hemoglobin A is heterogeneous, containing in addition to A_2 at least seven other components. Hemoglobin A_2 is composed of two normal α chains and of two chains designated as δ in place of the β chains. Hemoglobin A_2 has been found to be increased in the majority of cases of thalassemia minor, fetal hemoglobin being more often increased in thalassemia major. The ever increasing number of hemoglobinopathies have been characterized by absence of one or more of the normal hemoglobin chains and/or by abnormalities in amino acid sequence of one of the peptides separated from the main polypeptide chain.

D. *Genetic Control of Hemoglobinopathies; Structure and Function of Red Cells*

Since 1949, study of the genetic control of hemoglobinopathies has grown into a field of ever increasing importance to human pathology and anthropology. It is now hypothesized that a gene can be represented as a molecule of DNA. The linear sequence of basic pairs in this double-stranded, helicoidal molecule determines the linear sequence of amino acids in the structure of the protein which it controls genetically. By virtue of its easy availability the red cell has been the subject of an astonishing amount of investigative work. The application of electron microscopy has already made major contributions, and many more are to come. The knowledge of the ultrastructure of the red cell surface, the complexity of the genetic determinants, the enzymatic potential are in themselves the results of thousands of investigative efforts by competent workers.

Outstanding has been the identification of the role of the various structures of normoblasts and reticulocytes with the proliferative and functional capacities. Normoblasts can synthesize DNA and RNA and possess proliferative capacity as well as hemoglobin-synthesizing activity. With loss of the nucleus, the resulting reticulocyte retains endoplasmic reticulum and mitochondria essential to total biosynthesis of heme (Krueger *et al.*, 1956, Schwartz *et al.*, 1959, 1961; Granick and Sano, 1961). Ribosomes, present in nucleated erythroblasts as well as reticulocytes, have been identified with the production of globin (Rabinovitz and Olson, 1956).

E. *Use of Water-Repellent Surfaces*

The use of water-repelling surfaces is hardly a recent development. Paraffined glass containers were in use for collection of blood for direct transfusion in the early part of the century.

The introduction of silicone by Jacques and co-workers in 1946 and of plastic containers by Walter (1951) permitted expansion of experimental work which culminated in general acceptance of these containers, in preference to glass, for storage of blood. The improved preservation of red cells stored in plastic containers is due according to Strumia *et al.* (1955) essentially to the fact that conventional glass containers release a substance or substances toxic to red cells, which action is less pronounced with the use of polyvinyl containers.

Great differences between grades of plastic material were noted initially; now most containers available commercially have a fairly uniform composition, resulting in a dependable favorable effect on stored red cells. Under optimal conditions, 80% of transfused red cells of blood stored in plastic containers survive in the circulation 24 hours after transfusion; with glass containers the survival is approximately 70%.

F. Preservation of Red Cells in the Frozen State

Storage of red cells at low temperature is readily suggested by the dependence of their metabolic integrity on enzymatic activity and the depressing effect of lowered temperature on enzymatic activity. In this respect storage of food in the frozen state is considerably ahead of the storage of red cells. It may be safely stated that at about −40°C. all enzymatic activity is virtually stopped; but at this temperature the growth of ice crystals continues, and with it progressive deterioration of the red cells. Early work of Luyet (1937) and Luyet and Gehenio (1940) has shown that ultrarapid freezing, of the order of 100° per second, resulting in microcrystalline ice formation ("vitrification"), and equally rapid warming, result in preservation of a major portion of the cell population. For many reasons this method is not applicable to the quantities of blood involved in ordinary transfusions.

Polge and collaborators in 1950 introduced the use of glycerol to bind water and thereby control the formation of ice crystals. The principle was applied to erythrocytes by Smith (1950). This problem is extensively discussed in Chapter 15.

Strumia *et al.* (1958b) introduced a method which combines relatively rapid freezing, compatible with large volumes of blood, with addition of a modifying agent, such as a sugar. With this method it has been shown that blood can be preserved in the frozen state for periods of at least three years, with a recovery of better than 90% of the red cells and a survival, 24 hours after transfusion, of 77% of the original amount, including all losses *in vivo* and *in vitro*. The work was recently extended to the use of a modifying agent, such as lactose, and a macromolecular substance, such as human albumin or dextran, to obtain a practical method of freezing and storing red cells for the purpose of transfusion (Strumia, 1962).

XII. Possible Future of Blood Preservation

Looking to the future, I can conclude only by quoting from the Ninth J. G. Gibson Lecture, given recently at Columbia-Presbyterian Medical Center:

"It is evident from the complexity of the factors which determine the usefulness of a transfusion and from the vast difference of methodology required to preserve each of these factors optimally that an ideal system will consist of immediate fractionation of blood upon collection, each of the separate components being stored with the technique best suited for the longest period of storage.

"This ideal goal would do away with the enormous waste of material implied with the present system of blood preservation, which should actually be more properly called delayed deterioration. At present, platelet-rich fresh plasma, freeze-dried fresh plasma, plasma preserved in various ways, purified human albumin, γ-globulin, fibrinogen, and packed red cells comprise the components more readily available. Other components, particularly red cells and platelets, must be the subject of extensive investigation to achieve a longer life span *in vitro*.

"Such methods of component therapy are not expected to replace whole blood therapy as we understand it; simply to make it better in specific cases."

References

Allen, F. N., Jr., Diamond, L. K., and Watrous, J. B., Jr. (1949). *New Engl. J. Med.* **241**, 779.

Alpen, E. L., and Cranmore, D. (1959). "The Kinetics of Cellular Proliferation," p. 290. Grune and Stratton, New York.

Ashby, W. (1919). *J. Exptl. Med.* **29**, 267.

Astaldi, G., and Mauri, C. (1954). *Haematol. Latina (Milan)* **38**, 535.

Berlin, N. I., Lawrence, J. H., and Lee, H. C. (1951). *Science* **114**, 385.

Bernstein, F. (1924). *Klin. Wochschr.* **3**, 1495.

Chaplin, H., Jr., (1954). *J. Physiol. (London)* **123**, 22.

Cohn, E. J. (1939). *Harvey Lectures Ser.* **34,** 124.

Cohn, E. J., Luetscher, J. A., Oncley, J. L., Armstrong, S. H., Jr., and Davis, B. D. (1940). *J. Am. Chem. Soc.* **62**, 3396.

Coombs, R. R. A., Mourant, A. E., and Race, R. R. (1945). *Lancet* **2**, 15.

DeCastello, A. V., and Sturli, A. (1902). *Muench. Med. Wochschr.* **49,** 1090.

DeGowin, E. L., Harris, J. E., and Plass, E. D. (1940). *J. Am. Med. Assoc.* **114**, 850.

Diamond, L. K., and Abelson, N. M. (1945). *J. Lab. Clin. Med.* **30**, 204.

Donohue, D. M., Finch, C. A., and Gabrio, B. W. (1956). *J. Clin. Invest.* **35**, 562.

Donohue, D. M., Gabrio, B. W., and Finch, C. A. (1958). *J. Clin. Invest.* **37**, 1564.

Dungern, E. V., and Hirszfeld, L. (1911). *Z. Immunitaetsforsch.* **8**, 526.

Dustin, A. P. (1943). *Arch. Biol. (Liége)* **54**, 111.

Ebaugh, F. G., Jr., Emerson, C. P., and Ross, J. F. (1953). *J. Clin. Invest.* **32**, 1260.

Epstein, A. A., and Ottenberg, R. (1908). *Proc. N. Y. Pathol. Soc.* **8**, 117.

Fantus, B. (1937). *J. Am. Med. Assoc.* **109**, 128.

Finch, C. A. (1959). *Ann. N.Y. Acad. Sci.* **77,** 410.

Finch, C. A., Wolff, J. A., Rath, C. E., and Fluharty, R. G. (1949a). *J. Lab. Clin. Med.* **34,** 1480.

Finch, C. A., Gibson, J. G., II, Peacock, W. C., and Fluharty, R. G. (1949b). *Blood* **4,** 905.

Gabrio, B. W., Finch, C. A., and Huennekens, F. M. (1956a). *Blood* **11**, 103.

Gabrio, B. W., Donohue, D. M., Huennekens, F. M., and Finch, C. A. (1956b). *J. Clin. Invest.* **35**, 657.

Giblett, E. H., Coleman, D. H., Pirzio-Biroli, G., Donohue, D. M., Motulsky, A. G., and Finch, C. A. (1956). *Blood* **11**, 291.

Gibson, J. G., II, Evans, R. D., Aub, J. C., Sack, T., and Peacock, W. C. (1947). *J. Clin. Invest.* **26,** 715.

Granick, S., and Sano, S. (1961). *Federation Proc.* **20**, 64.

Gray, S. J., and Sterling, K. (1950). *Science* **112**, 179.

Greppi, E. (1926). *Arch. patol. e clin. med.* **5**, 459.

Guest, G. M. (1932). *J. Clin. Invest.* **11**, 555.

Hawkins, W. B., and Whipple, G. H. (1938). *Am. J. Physiol.* **122,** 418.

Huff, R. L., Emlinger, P., Mortimer, R., Anger, H., and Tobias, C. A. (1952). *J. Clin. Invest.* **31**, 640.

Hustin, A. (1914). *Bull. Soc. Roy. Sci. Med. Nat. Bruxelles*, April.

Ingram, V. M. (1956). *Nature* **178**, 792.

Kabat, E. A. (1956). "Blood Group Substances." Academic Press, New York.

Krueger, R. C., Melnick, I., and Klein, J. R. (1956). *Arch. Biochem. Biophys.* **64**, 302.

Landsteiner, K. (1900). *Zentr. Bakteriol. Parasitenk.* **27**, 357.

Landsteiner, K. (1901). *Wien. Klin. Wochschr.* **14**, 1132.

Landsteiner, K., and Wiener, A. S. (1941). *J. Exptl. Med.* **74**, 309.

Lange, R. D., Crosby, W. H., Donohue, D. M., Finch, C. A., Gibson, J. G. II, McManus, T. J., and Strumia, M. M. (1958). *J. Clin. Invest.* **37**, 1485.

Levine, P., Katzin, E. M., and Burnham, L. (1941). *J. Am. Med. Assoc.* **116**, 825.

London, I. M. (1951). *Proc. 3rd Congr. Intern. Soc. Hematol.* p. 79. Grune & Stratton, New York.

London, I. M. (1961). *Harvey Lectures, Ser.* **56**.

Loutit, J. F., Mollison, P. L., and Young, I. M. (1943). *Quart. J. Exptl. Physiol.* **32**, 183.

Luyet, B. J. (1937). *Biodynamica.*

Luyet, B. J., and Gehenio, P. M. (1940). *Biodynamica.*

Maizels, M. (1941). *Lancet* **1**, 722.

Maizels, M., and Whittaker, N. (1940). *Lancet* **1**, 113.

Maizels, M. (1943). *Quart. J. Exptl. Physiol.* **32**, 143.

Miller, E. B., Singer, K., and Dameshek, W. (1942). *Arch. Internal Med.* **70**, 722.

Mollison, P. L., and Young, I. M. (1942). *Quart. J. Exptl. Physiol.* **31**, 359.

Moreschi, C. (1908). *Zentr. Bakteriol. Parasitenk.* **46**, 49.

Morton, J. A., and Pickles, M. M. (1947). *Nature* **159**, 779.

Mourant, A. E. (1946). *Nature* **158**, 237.

Nakao, M., Nakao, T., Tatibana, M., Yoshikawa, H., and Abe, T. (1959). *Biochim. Biophys. Acta* **32**, 564.

Nuttall, G. H. (1904). "Blood Immunity and Blood Relationship." Cambridge Univ. Press, London and New York.

Ottenberg, R. (1911). *J. Exptl. Med.* **13**, 425.

Ottenberg, R., and Kaliski, D. J. (1913). *J. Am. Med. Assoc.* **61**, 2138.

Ponder, E. (1940). *Cold Spring Harbor Symp. Quant. Biol.* **8**, 133.

Rabinovitz, M., and Olson, M. E. (1956). *Exptl. Cell Res.* **10**, 747.

Rapaport, S. (1947). *J. Clin. Invest.* **26**, 591.

Robertson, O. H. (1918). *Brit. Med. J.* **1**, 691.

Rosenfield, R. E., Allen, F. H., Swisher, S. N., and Kochwa, S. (1962). *Transfusion* **2**, 287.

Ross, J. F., and Chaplin, M. A. (1943). *J. Am. Med. Assoc.* **123**, 827.

Rous, P., and Turner, J. R. (1916a). *J. Exptl. Med.* **23**, 219.

Rous, P., and Turner, J. R. (1916b). *J. Exptl. Med.* **23**, 239.

Rubenstein, D., and Denstedt, O. F. (1956). *Can. J. Biochem. Physiol.* **34**, 927.

Schwartz, H. C., Cartwright, G. E., Smith, E. L., and Wintrobe, M. M. (1959). *Blood* **14**, 486.

Schwartz, H. C., Goudsmith, R., Hill, R. L., Cartwright, G. E., and Wintrobe, M. M. (1961). *J. Clin. Invest.* **40**, 188.

Shemin, D., and Rittenberg, D. (1946). *J. Biol. Chem.* **166**, 627.

Simon, E. R., Chapman, R. G., and Finch, C. A. (1962). *J. Clin. Invest.* **41**, 351.

Smith, A. U. (1950). *Lancet* **2**, 910.

Stohlman, F., Jr. (1959). "The Kinetics of Cellular Proliferation," p. 318. Grune and Stratton, New York.

Strumia, M. M. (1939). *Surg. Clin. North Am.* **22**, 1693.
Strumia, M. M. (1962). Meeting Intern. Soc. Blood Transfusion, Mexico City.
Strumia, M. M., Colwell, L. S., and Ellenberger, K. (1955). *J. Lab. Clin. Med.* **46**, 225.
Strumia, M. M., Wagner, J. A., and Monaghan, J. F. (1940a). *J. Am. Med. Assoc.* **114**, 1337.
Strumia, M. M., Wagner, J. A., and Monaghan, J. F. (1940b). *Ann. Surg.* **111**, 623.
Strumia, M. M., Newhouser, L. R., Kendrick, D. G., Jr., and McGraw, J. J. (1942). *War Med.* **2**, 102.
Strumia, M. M., Colwell, L. S., and Dugan, A. (1958a). *Blood* **8**, 128.
Strumia, M. M., Colwell, L. C., and Strumia, P. V. (1958b). *Science* **128**, 1002.
Suit, H. D. (1957). *J. Clin. Pathol.* **10**, 267.
Wada, T., Takaku, F., Nakao, K., Nakao, M., Nakao, T., and Yoshikawa, H. (1960). *Proc. Japan Acad.* **36**, 618.
Walter, C. W. (1951). *Surg. Forum, Proc. 36th Congr. Am. Coll. Surgeons, 1950.*
Weil, R. (1915). *J. Am. Med. Assoc.* **64**, 425.
Wiener, A. S., and Peters, H. R. (1940). *Ann. Internal Med.* **13**, 2306.

CHAPTER 2

Composition of Normal Human Red Cells

Robert B. Pennell

I. Introduction

Strictly speaking, the term "normal human erythocyte" is an abstraction of convenience made necessary to permit intelligible consideration of these vital cells. There is ample evidence, however, that any erythrocyte population consists of cells of all stages of aging and that the composition of the cell is often dependent on its relative age (Prankerd, 1961–1962; Mandel *et al.*, 1961–1962; Bertolini *et al.*, 1961b; Lohr and Waller, 1961; Quarto di Palo *et al.*, 1960). There is also ample evidence of variation in composition between the "normal cells" of different donor age groups (Corsini *et al.*, 1959a; Massari *et al.*, 1960a,b; Guardamagna *et al.*, 1960; Chow, 1960; Bertolini *et al.*, 1960a,b,e; DeSantis and Pisconti, 1961). This variation is particularly evident in cells of the very young and of the very old (Massari *et al.*, 1960a; Bertolini *et al.*, 1961e).

In many, perhaps most, instances precise data on the donor population on which given values are based are not reported. This leads to some uncertainty in assessing the validity of the value. However, variation in composition of erythrocytes arising from the age of the donor or the age of the cell itself may be small relative to changes seen in cells from many pathological states, and the values for "normal cells" do thus provide an essential tool for revelation of truly abnormal cells or of abnormal distribution of cells.

Recent compilations of the composition of human erythrocytes are to be found in "Blood and Other Body Fluids" (published by the Federation of American Societies for Experimental Biology in 1961) and in the "Biochemists' Handbook" (edited by Cyril Long in 1961). Appreciable additions to the literature of red cell components have been made, however, since these references were compiled. Rather than to cite only the data more recent than or additional to the above compilations, the tabular material of this chapter attempts to be inclusive, hopefully making it unnecessary to consult several sources for a complete picture of the composition of the "normal" human erythrocyte. Attention should also be called to the comprehensive review of human erythrocyte enzymes by Cartier and Leroux (1962).

The data are presented in several forms, tabular listing of components in somewhat arbitrary groups, brief consideration of the state of knowledge as to the probable location of the component within the cells, and discussion of documented changes influenced by the age of the donor and the relative age of the cell. Consideration of components in groups related to function has been omitted inasmuch as this is covered in the appropriate sections of this book.

In some instances, primarily that of the enzymes, components are listed which have not been isolated but the presence of which has been demonstrated clearly by biological activity. Enzymes have not been listed, however, which might be presumed present because in other tissues they have been found essential to certain processes known to transpire in the erythrocyte, but which have not been specifically identified in the human erythrocyte. It has been assumed that, even when not identified by isolation, all enzymes are protein in nature.

It has been considered impractical to attempt to list all references pertinent to a given component. In most instances the references given are those from which the listed values have been taken. Consultation of such references will lead the investigator to the pertinent earlier literature.

II. Components of the Erythrocyte Membrane

Certain of the components of the erythrocyte can be shown to exist essentially in entirety in the structural portion of the cell. Others would appear to occur in both the membrane and the free fluid of the cell. In some instances the method of separation of the cell membrane determines whether or not a cell component appears as part of the structure or free in the cellular fluid, suggesting that some cell components may be associated with but may not be an integral part of the "ghost."

Though details of the intimate structure of the erythrocyte membrane are unknown, complex mixtures of fibrous protein, lipid, and mucopolysaccharides can be prepared from red cell ghosts. The best characterized of such complexes is the elinin of Moskowitz and his collaborators (1950). Studies of elinin led to the proposal (Moskowitz and Calvin, 1952) that the cell membrane could be considered composed of long, fibrillar elinin molecules, arranged so that the fibrils lie side by side and parallel to the surface of the cell. These fibrils are joined together by the ether-extractable lipids to form the framework of the membrane which was given the name of stromin. The framework so formed may contain its own protoplasm (Bartlett, 1958).

The necessity for the use of alcohol-ether for complete extraction of the lipid of elinin suggested part of the lipid to be bound in the form of lipoprotein. Lipoprotein complexes can seldom be lyophilized without major change, and since lyophilization was employed in the preparation of elinin it is probable that the complex was appreciably altered from its native state.

The Rh, A, and B activities of the erythrocyte are all found in the elinin moiety. The Rh antigen and Lutheran antigen are destroyed by ribonuclease, which does not affect A, B, M, N, P, or I antigens (Hackel and Smolker, 1960). This would suggest the presence of nucleotides in elinin.

All of the blood group antigens must be considered to be components of the cell membrane. Predominantly lipid Forssman hapten and "blood group-active lipid" have been isolated by Yamakawa *et al.* (1960). Cook (1962) has isolated a sialomucopeptide which is linked to a galactosamine residue in an alkali-labile saccharide moiety. It resembles the M and N mucoids extracted by phenol. Papain is reported to liberate the M and N mucoids but does not alter the antigen responsible for influenza virus hemagglutination (Klenk and Uhlenbruck, 1960). On the other hand, neuraminadase destroys M and N as well as the influenza virus antigen (Kathan *et al.*, 1961). The latter has been reported by Kathan to contain 10.1% N, 12.4% protein-bound hexose, 12.1% P, 1.2% fucose, 22–24% sialic acid. The surface charge of the cell is primarily associated with neuraminic acid (Eylar *et al.*, 1962) and probably the carboxyl group of this acid (Cook *et al.*, 1961).

It is probable that essentially the total lipid of the erythrocyte lies within the membrane, though recent work by Cacciari and his colleagues (1959b) reports less than the total value for lipid, phosphatide, and glycerides in the isolated stroma. The question of losses during the preparation of the stroma is, however, always present (Hogeboom *et al.*, 1957). Boyer, by electron microscopy, has reported the lipid of the membrane to have a myelin structure (1961). Platelet-like activity has been shown to be associated with a stroma lipid fraction (Tropeano *et al.*, 1958).

Some of the cholesterol of the stroma is firmly bound to protein. Other cholesterol is loosely associated. It is the latter which exchanges freely with plasma cholesterol (Blagorazumova, 1959).

About half the free amino acids are associated with the cell membrane (Corsini *et al.*, 1959b).

It is generally held that hemoglobin is in part bound to membrane substances. Klipstein and Ranney (1960) found hemoglobins A_1, A_2, and A_3 in stroma. The relative amounts in the membrane differ, however, from the distribution in the soluble portion of the hemolysate, A_2 being relatively higher in the stroma.

ATPase activity is believed to be associated only with the stroma although, if it is prepared by freezing and thawing, some of the ATPase may appear with the soluble proteins (Clarkson and Maizels, 1952; Caffrey *et al.*, 1956; Bartlett, 1958). The phosphatidic acid cycle enzymes, phosphatidic acid phosphatase and diglyceride kinase, occur in the erythrocyte membrane (Hokin and Hokin, 1961). One effect of these enzymes is hydrolysis of ATP, and they must be recognized as accounting for at least part of the ATPase activity. The factors responsible for Na and K transport are also exclusively in the cell membrane, and may be identical with the ATPase factors since both are influenced similarly by the same variables (Post and Albright, 1961).

Other enzyme activities reported to reside exclusively in the cell membrane are acetylcholinesterase (Carta and Vivaldi, 1958; Vincent *et al.*, 1961), catalase, triose phosphate dehydrogenase, and DPNase (Prankerd, 1961–1962; Alivasatos *et al.*, 1956). Cholinesterase distribution in the membrane has been studied by electron microscopy (Shinagawa and Ogura, 1961). An acid phosphomonoesterase optimally active at about pH 5.7 (Tsuboi and Hudson, 1953–1954), a specific phosphatase for 2,3-diphosphoglycerate (Clarkson and Maizels, 1952; Rapoport and Luebering, 1951), and probably TPNase (Prankerd, 1956) exist in stroma as do three proteases (Morrison and Neurath, 1953). Although the enzyme itself is essentially in the soluble portion of hemolysates, an activator of glucose-6-phosphate dehydrogenase has been isolated from stroma (Ramat *et al.*, 1961).

Enzymes which are predominantly in the soluble portion of hemolysates but which have been found as well in carefully prepared and washed stroma include glutamic-pyruvic and glutamic-oxaloacetic transaminases (Massari *et al.*, 1960b), aldolase (Corsini *et al.*, 1959a), glyceraldehyde phosphate dehydrogenase, lactic dehydrogenase, and 3-phosphoglycerate kinase (Bartlett, 1958), lipase (Cacciari *et al.*, 1959a), and nucleoside phosphorylase (Lionetti *et al.*, 1961). The last mentioned, nucleoside phosphorylase, was considered by Prankerd (1961–1962) to be completely stroma-bound.

III. Variation in Composition with Age of Donor

In consideration of the possible effect of the age of the donor and of the age of the cell itself on cell composition, one may be confronted with conflicting data. Recent studies are considered in this section and the succeeding one and conflicts of opinion are noted. One can, however, certainly find differences of reported values in the earlier literature.

Many enzyme activities have been reported to vary with the age of the donor. Lipase and amylase are higher in adults than in juveniles (Cacciari *et al.*, 1959a). Stromal and total glutamic-pyruvic and glutamic-oxaloacetic transaminases decrease progressively with the age of the donor, whereas cholinesterase is appreciably lower in the newborn (Sabine, 1955), rises in middle age, and falls in old age (Massari *et al.*, 1960b; Bertolini *et al.*, 1961b,c). Carbonic anhydrase is lower in infants than in adults (DeSantis and Pisconti, 1961). Stromal aldolase is higher in children than in adults but the total aldolase activity does not change with age of the donor (Corsini *et al.*, 1959a; Bertolini *et al.*, 1961e). Cholesterol esterase differs in the nature of its activity, being hydrolytic in the young and esterifying in the old (Guardamagna *et al.*, 1960).

A decline in erythrocyte Cu can be noted in the fifth decade of life (Massari *et al.*, 1960a; Herring *et al.*, 1960). Nickel is lowest during the second decade (Herring *et al.*, 1960). Total P, inorganic P, and phosphoglyceric acid are found to increase with age of the individual (Quarto di Palo *et al.*, 1960). Guardamagna *et al.* (1960) report a rise in total cholesterol from 0.39 mg./mg. N in young subjects to 0.47 mg./mg. N in adults. In the senile, free erythrocytic porphyrin is moderately increased. The increase is predominantly coproporphyrin (Bertolini *et al.*, 1960).

IV. Variation in Composition with Age of Cell

As the erythrocyte ages *in vivo* its composition changes. Generally, enzyme activities are higher in younger cells and decrease as the cell ages. Thus, Lohr and Waller (1961) have reported phosphoglyceraldehyde dehydrogenase, glucose-6-phosphate dehydrogenase, hemoglobin reductase, and lactic dehydrogenase activities to decrease as the cell ages. A similar finding is reported for glucose-6-phosphate dehydrogenase by Marks *et al.* (1958). Bertolini *et al.* (1961d) and Marks *et al.* (1958), however, found no difference in lactic dehydrogenase activity with the age of the cell. Cholinesterase, catalase, triose phosphate dehydrogenase, and DPNase also decrease as the cell ages (Prankerd, 1961–1962; Bertolini *et al.*, 1961c). Phophohexose isomerase and 6-phosphogluconic dehydrogenase are relatively high in young cells and diminish with age of the cell (Marks *et al.*, 1958). Acid phosphatase activity (Valentine *et al.*, 1961) and glutamic-pyruvic transaminase (Bertolini *et al.*, 1961b) are higher in young than in old cells.

In contrast, aldolase activity has been reported to increase as the cell grows older (Bertolini *et al.*, 1961e). Purine nucleoside phosphorylase shows no change with the age of the cell (Marks *et al.*, 1958).

The ADP/ATP ratio is 1:5 for young cells and remains so for the first 50 days of the cell's life. Thereafter it declines and is 1:1.15 at 90 days. Mg^{++} and DPN also decrease with cell age (Lohr and Waller, 1961; Quarto di Palo *et al.*, 1960).

TABLE 1

HUMAN ERYTHROCYTE PROTEINS: NOT RECOGNIZED AS ENZYMES[a, b]

Constituent	Value	Remarks	Reference
Choleglobin	17.66 μg./gm. Hb	Measured as biliverdin	Nakagawa (1960)
Cu-containing protein	—	Differs from erythrocuprein	Shields *et al.* (1961)
Elinin	—	Contains 2–5% carbohydrate and Rh, A, and B factors	Moskowitz *et al.* (1950)
Erythrocuprein	16±2.9 mg./100 ml. cells	Contains 60% of total erythrocyte Cu	Shields *et al.* (1961)
Eosinophil-stimulating substance	—	Perhaps a glycoprotein	J. Chapman (1961)
Fe-containing fraction (hematin ?)	456 μg. Fe/100 ml. cells	Binds Fe in stroma	Faber and Falbe-Hansen (1959)
Hemoglobin	33.5 gm./100 ml. cells	—	Osgood (1935)*
HbA (HbA_{II}, Clegg; HbA_1, Haut)	—	Approx. 88% of total Hb	Derrien *et al.* (1961); Haut *et al.* (1962); Clegg and Schroeder (1959); Huisman and Meyering (1960)
HbA_2 (HbA_{III}, Clegg)	2.54±0.35% of total Hb	—	Kunkel *et al.* (1957); Huisman and Meyering (1960); Haut *et al.* (1962); Clegg and Schroeder (1959)
HbA_{Ia}	—	HbA_I(a–e)+HbA_{III} represents 12% of total Hb	Clegg and Schroeder (1959)
Hba_{Ib}	—	—	Clegg and Schroeder (1959)
HbA_{Ic}	—	—	Clegg and Schroeder (1959)
HbA_{Id}	—	—	Clegg and Schroeder (1959)
HbA_{Ie}	—	—	Clegg and Schroeder (1959)
Hemoprotein	—	Differs from catalase, Hb, myeloperoxidase, cytochromes, and TPNH oxidase	M. Morrison (1961)
Methemoglobin	<0.4%	—	Van Slyke *et al.* (1946)
S-Protein	—	—	Moskowitz *et al.* (1950, 1952)
Stroma protein?	—	—	Kunzer and Schutz (1959)

[a] *Editor's note*: The values compiled in the tables in this chapter were derived from the literature and from other compilations already in print. Dr. Pennell did not have available to him at the time of writing the other chapters of this book. It is therefore not improbable that some of the data he cites will differ in varying degrees from similar data appearing elsewhere in this book

[b] *Single asterisk* (*) denotes values derived from "Blood and Other Body Fluids," Federation of American Societies for Experimental Biology, Washington, D.C. (1961).

Double asterisks (**) denotes values derived from Long, C. (ed.), "Biochemists' Handbook" Van Nostrand, Princeton, New Jersey (1961).

TABLE 2

Human Erythrocyte Proteins: Enzymes

Enzyme	Value	Enzyme activity units	Remarks	Reference
Acetylcholinesterase	19.06 ± 3.28	μliters CO_2/mg. dry cells/hr.	0.0184 *M* acetylcholine substrate	DeSandre and Chiotto (1960)
	876 (725–1024)	μmoles/acetylcholine hydrolyzed/min./100 ml. cells	0.012 *M* acetylcholine substrate	Sawitsky *et al.* (1948)*
	501 (335–638)	μmoles/acetylcholine hydrolyzed/min./100 ml. cells	0.01 *M* acetylcholine substrate	Calloway *et al.* (1951)*
	1190 (910–1370)	μmoles/acetylcholine hydrolyzed/min./100 ml. cells	0.002 *M* acetylcholine substrate	Sabine (1955)*
	547 (437–660)	μmoles/acetylcholine hydrolyzed/min./100 ml. cells	0.00025 *M* acetylcholine substrate	Sabine (1940)*
	1.08 ± 0.18	moles acetylcholine hydrolyzed/min./red cell $\times 10^{15}$	Acetylthiocholine substrate	Ellman and Calloway (1961)
Acid phosphatase	543 ± 264	Bücher units/10^{11} erythrocytes	Bücher unit is that amount of enzyme producing a turnover of 1 μmole substrate per hr. under the test conditions prescribed (Czok and Bücher, 1960)	Lohr and Waller (1961)
	21.5 (8.9–35.4)	mg. *p*-nitrophenol liberated/10^{10} erythrocytes/hr. (pH 5.7, 37°C.)	—	Valentine *et al* (1961)
Aconitase	—	—	—	Beutler and Yeh (1959)
Adenosine deaminase	90	mmoles/liter/hr.	—	Rapoport (1961) Clark *et al* (1952)

TABLE 2—*cont.*

Enzyme	Value	Enzyme activity units	Remarks	Reference
Adenosine monophosphate deaminase	—	—	—	Conway and Cooke (1939)
Adenosine monophosphate synthetase	—	—	—	Liebermann (1956)
ATPase	0.013	μmoles P_i/mg. dry wt./hr.	—	Post and Albright (1961)
	1620 ± 254	Bücher units/10^{11} cells	—	Lohr and Waller (1961)
Adenylate deaminase	23	μmoles/ml. cells/hr.	—	Hennessey *et al.* (1962)
Adenylate kinase (myokinase)	124	μg. glucose phosphorylated/hr./0.5-ml. cell suspension (37°C., 5 mmoles added ADP)	—	Kashkett and Denstedt (1958)*
	5570	Bücher units/10^{11} cells	—	Lohr and Waller (1961)
	1.23	μmoles ADP converted/ 8 min./ml. hemolysate cont'g 10% Hb (37°C.)	—	Cerletti and DeRitis (1962)
Adenylosuccinate synthetase	—	—	—	Liebermann (1956)
Alanine aminopeptidase	—	—	—	Klaus (1961)
Aldolase	1.4–5.2	μmoles fructose-1,6-diphosphate hydrolyzed/ml. packed cells/hr. (37°C.)	—	Bruns *et al.* (1958b)
	1010	cu. mm. HDP split/hr./ml. cells as hemolysate (37°C.)	—	Corsini *et al.* (1959a)
	31	μmoles substrate converted/ml. cells/hr. (pH 8.1)	—	Hennessey *et al.* (1962)
	1.2 ± 0.4	μmoles substrate converted/gm. Hb/min.	—	Heller *et al.* (1960a)
	561 ± 48	Bücher units/10^{11} cells	—	Lohr and Waller (1961)

Alkaline phosphatase	1.48	mg. P_i liberated/hr (pH 8.6, 37°C.)	—	Cacciari *et al.* (1959a)
Amino acid-activating enzyme	35.4	mμmoles ATP/mg. protein/hr.	—	Izak et al. (1960)
5-Amino-4-imidazole carboxamide ribotide transformylase	—	—	—	Hartman and Buchanan (1959); Bishop (1960); Lowy *et al.* (1962)
δ-Aminolevulinic acid dehydrase	1.01 ± 0.124	μmoles porphyrin/ml./hr. (pH 7, 38°C.)	35 Subjects	Rubino *et al.* (1960); Rimington and Booij (1957); Fallot *et al.* (1956)
Amylase	4.7	Starch units	—	Cacciari *et al.* (1959a)
Arginase	5100 (2500–7700)	units/100 ml. (as described by Kochakian)	—	Edebacher and Rothler (1925)*; Kochakian *et al.* (1944, 1948)*
	11.7 ± 2.5	μmoles arginine hydrolyzed/hr.	—	Nikkila *et al.* (1960)
Aspartic transcarbamylase	100–200	mμmoles/10^9 cells/hr. (37°C.)	—	Smith *et al.* (1961)
Carbonic anhydrase	73,000	number of erythrocytes that will halve the time of uncatalyzed reaction at 3°C. under special conditions	Parallels erythrocyte zinc concentration	Ashby (1943)*
	2.5	mg./ml. red cells	—	Roughton and Rupp (1958)
Carboxylic esterases				
Aliesterase	—	—	Single band chromatographically	Shinagawa and Ogura (1961); Tashian (1961)
Arylesterases	—	—	8 Bands chromatographically	Tashian (1961)
Catalase	0.1	gm./100 gm. dry wt.	—	Herbert and Pinsent (1948)*
	3220×10^3	μmoles/ml. cells/hr.	—	Hennessey *et al.* (1962); Higashi *et al.* (1961)

TABLE 2—*cont.*

Enzyme	Value	Enzyme activity units	Remarks	Reference
Catalase (*cont.*)	3.65 (2.74–4.75)	$K_{cat} = 10^3(1/t \, . \log_{10} X_0/X_t)$ $X_o = \mu$moles H_2O_2 at time 0 $X_t = \mu$moles H_2O_2 at time t	—	Haut *et al.* (1962)
Cholesterol esterase	—	—	Hydrolytic in young subjects, esterifying in old subjects	Guardamagna *et al.* (1960)
Cysteine aminopeptidase	—	—	—	Klaus (1961)
Cytochrome oxidase	6.9	mmoles/liter/hr.	—	Rapoport (1961)
Cytochrome reductase	6	mmoles/liter/hr.	—	Rapoport (1961)
Diglyceride kinase	—	—	Present in membranes	Hokin and Hokin (1961)
Dihydroorotase	95–185	mμmoles/10^9 cells/hr. (37°C.)	—	Smith *et al.* (1961)
Dipeptidase	6±2.9	Proteolytic coefficient × 10^4	(See prolidase)	Adams *et al.* (1952); Panagopoulus *et al.* (1957)
Diphosphoglycerate mutase	0.46	mmoles/liter/hr.	—	Rapoport (1961)
Diphosphoglycerate phosphatase	2.1×10^{-3}	μmoles substrate used/10^{10} red cells/hr.	—	Manyai and Varady (1956)
DPN diaphorase	147	mmoles/liter/hr.	Absent in hereditary methemoglobinemia	Rapoport (1961); Scott (1960); Scott and McGraw (1962)
DPN nucleosidase	1.14	μmoles nucleotide/ml. cells/hr.	—	Hofmann and Noll (1961)
	28 (20–35)	μmoles DPN split/100 ml. blood/hr. (37°C., pH 6.5)	—	Alivasatos *et al.* (1956)
DPN phosphorylase	—	—	—	Preiss and Handler (1958)
DPN synthetase	—	—	—	Preiss and Handler (1958)
Enolase	95	μmoles substrate converted/ml. hemolyzed cells/hr.	—	Chapman *et al.* (1962)
			—	
	1032±121	Bücher units/10^{11} erythrocytes	—	Lohr and Waller (1961)

	About 600	μmoles/ml. packed cells/hr. (37°C.)	—	Bruns *et al.* (1958b); Blostein and Denstedt (1962)
Formate-activating enzyme	48	mμmoles/mg. Hb/hr.	—	Bertino *et al.* (1962)
Fumarase	—	—	—	Rubenstein (1952–1953); Quastel and Wheatley (1931)
Galactose-1-phosphate uridine transferase	—	—	Absent in galactosemia	Kalckar *et al.* (1956); Hugh-Jones *et al.* (1960)
Galactokinase	—	—	—	Kalckar and Maxwell (1958)
Glucose-6-phosphate dehydrogenase	720 ± 70	mmoles/liter/hr.	Deficient in certain anemias	Rapoport (1961)
	5.6 ± 1.4	μmoles/gm. Hb/min.	—	Heller *et al.* (1960a)
	70	Bücher units/10^{11} cells	—	Lohr and Waller (1961)
	74	μmoles/ml. hemolyzed cells/hr.	—	Hennessey *et al.* (1962)
	18.6 ± 4.3	Change in O.D./10^8 cells/min.	—	Pitkanen and Nikkila (1960); Nikkila *et al.* (1960)
	550 ± 39	Bücher units/10^{11} cells	—	Manganelli and Grimaldi (1962)
Glucose-6-phosphate dehydrogenase activator	—	—	Purification	Kirkman (1962)
	—	—	Occurs in cell stroma	Ramat *et al.* (1961)
Glutamic-oxaloacetic transaminase	374 ± 110	Bücher units/10^{11} cells	—	Lohr and Waller (1961)
	40	mmoles/liter/hr.	—	Rapoport (1961)
	10.1 ± 3.5	change in O.D./10^8 cells/min.	—	Pitkanen and Nikkila (1960); Nikkila *et al.* (1960)

TABLE 2—*cont.*

Enzyme	Value	Enzyme activity units	Remarks	Reference
Glutamic-oxaloacetic transaminase (*cont.*)	347	Bruns units/ml. cells	Bruns unit = μmoles substrate/ml. packed cells/hr. (pH 7.4, 37°C.)	Corsini *et al.* (1959a)
	22.3	μmoles glutamate formed/gm. cells/hr. (pH 7.4, 37°C.)	—	Fessler (1959)
Glutamic-pyruvic transaminase	11	mmoles/liter/hr.	—	Rapoport (1961)
	78 ± 24	Bücher units/10^{11} cells	—	Lohr and Waller (1961)
	63	Bruns units/ml. cells	—	Corsini *et al.* (1959a); Mauri and Torelli (1959)
Glutaminase	15	mmoles/liter/hr.	—	Rapoport (1961)
Glutathione peroxidase	—	—	Starch block separation	Haut *et al.* (1962)
Glutathione reductase	295 ± 133	Bücher units/10^{11} cells	—	Lohr and Waller (1961)
	28	μmoles/ml. cells/hr.	—	Hennessey *et al.* (1962)
	0.37 ± 0.08 (0.29–0.05)	μmoles GSH formed/ml. 1:10 hemolysate/6 min.	—	Jocelyn (1960)
	32.4	μmoles substrate/10^{11} cells/hr.	—	Lohr *et al.* (1958)
	4.4 ± 2.1	Change in O.D./10^8 cells/min.	—	Nikkila *et al.* (1960)
Glycine aminopeptidase	—	—	—	Klaus (1961)
Glycogen phosphorylase	—	—	—	Cornblath *et al.* (1960)
Glycyl-L-leucine dipeptidase	1800	μmoles substrate split/10^{11} cells/hr.	—	Haschen (1961a)
Glyoxalase	61.4	mg. methylglyoxal split/10^{10} cells/hr. (37°C.)	—	Valentine and Tanaka (1961)
	1398 (1320–1500)	ml. CO_2/100 ml. cells/20 min. (26°C., pH 7.2 in presence of glutathione)	—	Cohen and Sober (1945)*

Guanase	—	—	—	Herschko *et al.* (1962)
Hexokinase	10	μmoles substrate converted/ml. hemolyzed cells/hr.	—	Chapman *et al.* (1962)
	212	Bücher units/10^{11} cells	—	Lohr and Waller (1961)
	3	mmoles/liter/hr.	—	Rapoport (1961)
	1.5–2.5	μmoles/ml. packed cells/hr. (37°C.)	—	Bruns *et al.* (1958b)
	2	μmoles substrate/10^{10} cells/hr.	—	Bartlett and Marlow (1951)
Hydroxysteroid (17β-estradiol) dehydrogenase	0.8±0.11	μg. estradiol formed at 2.5% Hb	—	Portius and Repke (1960); Brown *et al.* (1961)
Inorganic pyrophosphatase	35±7.5	μg. P_i liberated/30 min. (pH 5.6)	—	Pitkanen and Nikkila (1960)
	39.4±10.2	μg. P_i liberated/30 min. (pH 7.2)	—	
	40.7±13	μg. P_i liberated/30 min. (pH 9.4)	—	
	—	—	—	Carta and Vivoldi (1957)
	300	mmoles P_i/liter/hr.	—	Rapoport (1961)
	212	μmoles P_i/ml. dialyzed hemolysate/hr. (pH 7.5, 37°C.)	—	Malkin and Denstedt (1956)*
Isocitric dehydrogenase	1.5±0.5	μmoles/gm. Hb/min.	—	Heller *et al.* (1960a, b)
	68±11	Bücher units/10^{11} cells	—	Lohr and Waller (1959, 1961)
Lactic acid dehydrogenase	55 (42.5–73.5)	mg. DPNH/ml. packed cells/min. (37°C., pH 7.2)	—	Hill (1956)*
	230	μliters O_2/gm. Hb/100 min. (37.5°C., pH 7.4)	—	Blanchaer *et al.* (1951)*
	87	μliters O_2/ml./100 min. (37.5°C., pH 7.4)	—	Kohn and Klein (1939)*
	30	μliters O_2/ml./30 min. (38°C., pH 7.4)	—	Quastel and Wheatley (1938)*
	396	μliters CO_2/ml./30 min. (38°C., pH 7.4)	—	Quastel and Wheatley (1938)*

TABLE 2—*cont.*

Enzyme	Value	Enzyme activity units	Remarks	Reference
Lactic acid dehydrogenase (*cont.*)	1020	μmoles substrate/10^{10} cells/hr.	—	Lohr *et al.* (1958)
	60 ± 18	μmoles/gm. Hb/min.	—	Heller *et al.* (1960a)
	500–1140	μmoles/ml. packed cells/hr. (37°C.)	—	Bruns *et al.* (1958b)
	1257	μmoles substrate converted/ml. cells/hr.	—	Chapman *et al.* (1962)
	9320 ± 1040	Bücher units/10^{11} cells	—	Lohr and Waller (1961)
	21.2	mmoles/liter/hr.	—	Rapoport (1961)
	87.3 ± 23.8	change in O.D./10^7 cells/min.	—	Pitkanen and Nikkila
	183 ± 25	change in O.D./10^8 cells/min.		(1960)
	—	—	—	Nikkila *et al.* (1960)
	—	—	4 Peaks electrophoretically	Vesell and Bearn (1961)
Leucine aminopeptidase	21.4 ± 6.2	μmoles/ml. cells/hr.	At substrate concn. of 5×10^{-3} M; if 5×10^{-2}, value is higher by factor of 1.57	Haschen (1961b)
	5 ± 3.2	proteolytic coefficient $\times 10^4$	See prolidase	Adams *et al.* (1952)
Lipase	1.86	ml. 0.02 N acid liberated/3 hr. (38°C.)	—	Cacciari *et al.* (1959a)
Malic dehydrogenase	6830 ± 890	Bücher units/10^{11} cells	—	Lohr and Waller (1961)
	208	μmoles/gm. Hb/min.	—	Heller *et al.* (1960a)
	97 ± 3.15	change in O.D./10^7 cells/min.	—	Pitkanen and Nikkila
	180 ± 28	change in O.D./10^8 cells/min.		(1960); Nikkila *et al.* (1960)
Methemoglobin reductase	134 ± 11	Bücher units/10^{11} cells	TPNH dependent	Lohr and Waller (1961)
	0.14	E/mg. protein of hemolysate	E = μl. O_2 min./of purified reductase	Kiese *et al.* (1957)

	7.7	μmoles/ml. cells/hr.	DEAE cellulose isolation, minimum molecular wt. 68,000	Hennessey *et al.* (1962); Huisman and Meyering (1960)
Methemoglobin reductase	—	—	(See DPN diaphorase)	
N^5,N^{10}-Methylenetetra-hydroformate dehydrogenase	8.2	mμmoles/mg. Hb/hr.	—	Bertino *et al.* (1962)
Nicotinamide mono-nucleotide synthetase	—	—	—	Haberman and Habermanova (1962); Preiss and Handler (1958)
Nicotinamide mono-nucleotide nucleotidase	1.86	μmoles nucleotide/ml. cells/hr.	—	Hofmann and Noll (1961)
Nucleotide diphosphatase	—	—	—	Banaschak (1961)
Orotodylic decarboxylase	10–17	mμmoles/10^9 cells/hr. (37°C.)	—	Smith *et al.* (1961)
Orotodylic pyrophosphorylase	7–17	mμmoles/10^9 cells/hr. (37°C.)	—	Smith *et al.* (1961)
Oxaloacetate decarboxylase	—	—	—	Nossal (1948)
Palmitate oxidase	—	—	—	Hrachovec *et al.* (1961)
Phosphatidic acid phosphatase	approx. 5	mμmoles ortho-P formed/mg. dry wt. of ghost	—	Hokin and Hokin (1961)
	approx. 9	mμmoles ortho-P formed/mg. dry wt. of ghost	In presence of added Mg^{++}	
Phosphoenol pyruvate kinase	242	μmoles/substrate/10^{10} cells/hr.	—	Lohr *et al.* (1958)
Phosphofructokinase	974 ± 147	Bücher units/10^{11} cells	—	Lohr and Waller (1961)
	2.13	mmoles/liter/hr.	—	Rapoport (1961)
	82	μmoles substrate/ml. cells/hr.	—	Chapman *et al.* (1962)
	38.4	μmoles substrate/10^{10} cells/hr.	—	Blanchaer *et al.* (1955)
Phosphogluconate dehydrogenase	390 ± 42	Bücher units/10^{11} cells	—	Lohr and Waller (1961)
	3 ± 0.8	μmoles/gm. Hb./min.	—	Heller *et al.* (1960a)

TABLE 2—*cont.*

Enzyme	Value	Enzyme activity units	Remarks	Reference
Phosphogluconate dehydrogenase (*cont.*)	49.4	μmoles substrate/10^{10} cells/hr.	—	Lohr *et al.* (1958)
Phosphoglucomutase	27–35	μmoles/ml. cells/hr. (37°C.)	Not on cell membrane	Bruns *et al.* (1958b)
	28.1	μmoles substrate/10^{10} cells/hr.	—	Noltmann and Bruns (1958)
Phosphoglucose isomerase	151	μmoles substrate/ml. cells/hr.	—	Chapman *et al.* (1962)
	3200 (3100–3300)	units/100 ml. (as described by Bodansky)	—	Bodansky (1954)*
	30 ± 7	μmoles/gm. Hb/min.	—	Heller *et al.* (1960a)
	900–1090	μmoles/ml. cells/hr. (37°C.)	—	Bruns *et al.* (1958b)
	4301 ± 248	Bücher units/10^{11} cells	—	Lohr and Waller (1961)
	28.2 ± 4.9	μg. fructose-6-phosphate formed/10^{8} cells/30 min.	—	Nikkila *et al.* (1960)
	—	—	Starch block electrophoretic separation	Haut *et al.* (1962)
Phosphoglyceraldehyde dehydrogenase (triose phosphate dehydrogenase	$10,830 \pm 1600$	Bücher units/10^{11}/cells	—	Lohr and Waller (1961)
	800	μmoles substrate converted/ml. cells/hr.	—	Chapman *et al.* (1962)
	13.9	mmoles/liter/hr.	—	Rapoport (1961)
	261	μmoles substrate/10^{10} cells/hr.	—	Lohr *et al.* (1958)
Phosphoglycerate kinase	287	mmoles/liter/hr.	—	Rapoport (1961)
	163	μmoles substrate/10^{10} cells/hr.	—	Lohr *et al.* (1958)
	1910	μmoles substrate/ml. cells/hr.	—	Chapman *et al.* (1962)
	$15,800 \pm 2470$	Bücher units/10^{11} cells	—	Lohr and Waller (1961)
	24.6	μmoles 1,3-diphosphoglycerate used/mg. Hb/hr. (pH 8.3, 37°C.)	—	Blostein and Denstedt (1960)*

Phosphoglycerate mutase	3510 ± 580	Bücher units/10^{11} cells	—	Lohr and Waller (1961)
	228	μmoles substrate/ml. cells/hr.	—	Chapman *et al.* (1962)
	140	mmoles/liter/hr.	—	Rapoport (1961)
	0.33	μmoles 1,3-diphosphoglycerate used/mg. Hb/hr. (pH 8.3, 37°C.)	—	Blostein and Denstedt (1960)*
Phosphomonoesterase	—	—	—	Buruiana *et al.* (1961)
		2 μmoles cysteamine formed from cysteamine-5-phosphate/0.25 ml. packed cells/30 min. (37°C.)		Akerfeldt (1960)
Phosphoribose isomerase	3000–5500	μmoles/ml. cells/hr. (37°C.)	—	Bruns *et al.* (1958a, b)
	3.6	μmoles ketopentose formed/gm. Hb/hr. (37°C., pH 7.4)	—	Brownstone *et al.* (1958*, 1961a)
	—	—	From stroma	Micheli and Grabar (1961)
Prolidase	19 ± 3.7	Proteolytic coefficient × 10^4	Proteolytic coefficient = K_1/E; K_1 is first order constant, E is mg. protein N/ml. test solution	Adams *et al.* (1952)
Proteases				
Cathepsin	0.5	mmoles/liter/hr.	Decreases in activity with maturation of the cell	Rapoport (1961); Kuenzel (1961)
I	—	—	Stromal enzyme activated by Zn^{++}, Fe^{++}, reducing agents; opt. pH 7.4	Morrison and Neurath (1953)
II	—	—	Stromal enzyme activated by Zn^{++}, Fe^{++}, not activated by reducing agents; opt. pH 7.4	Morrison and Neurath (1953)

TABLE 2—*cont.*

Enzyme	Value	Enzyme activity units	Remarks	Reference
Proteases (*cont.*)				
III	—	—	Stromal enzyme, not activated by reducing agents; opt. pH 3.2	Morrison and Neurath (1953)
Purine nucleoside phosphorylase	1610	μmoles/ml. cells (hemolysate)	Recovery from DEAE cellulose	Hennessey *et al.* (1962)
	—	—	Purification and kinetics	Tsuboi and Hudson (1957)
Pyrophosphorylase	—	—	Catalyzes reaction of nicotinic acid with 5-phosphoribose-1-pyrophosphate	Preiss and Handler (1958)
Pyruvic kinase	5.3	mmoles/liter/hr.	—	Rapoport (1961)
	158	μmoles substrate/ml. cells/hr.	—	Hennessey *et al* (1962)
	1790 ± 320	Bücher units/10^{11} cells	—	Lohr and Waller (1961)
Serine hydroxylmethylase	—	—	—	Bertino *et al.* (1962)
Succinic dehydrogenase	5	mmoles/liter/hr.	—	Rapoport (1961)
Tetrahydrofolate formylase	approx. 8.5	μmoles substrate/ml. cells/hr.	—	Hennessey *et al.* (1962)
	—	—	Purification	Lowy *et al.* (1962); Bertino *et al.* (1962); Donohue (1962)
Transaldolase	40	moles/gm. Hb/hr. (37°C.)	—	Brownstone *et al.* (1958,* 1961b)
Transketolase	33	μmoles sedoheptulose-7-P formed/gm. Hb/hr. (pH 7.4, 37°C.)	—	Brownstone (1958)*
	4.7 (2.7–6.9)	μmoles/ml. cells/hr. (37°C.)	—	Bruns *et al.* (1958b); Brin (1962); Mircevova (1958)

Triose phosphate isomerase	5100	μmoles substrate/ml. cells/hr.	—	Chapman *et al.* (1962)
	52,300 ± 7650	Bücher units/10^{11} cells	—	Lohr and Waller (1961)
	4600	μmoles/10^{10} cells/hr.	—	Lohr *et al.* (1958)
Tripeptidase	900	μmoles/10^{10} cells/hr.	—	Haschen (1962); Panagopoulos *et al.* (1957)
	10 ± 3.7	proteolytic coefficient × 10^4	(See prolidase)	Adams *et al.* (1952)
TPN nucleosidase	0.36	μmoles nucleotide/ml. cells/hr.	—	Hofmann and Noll (1961)
Uridyl diphosphoglucose pyrophosphatase	1.1	μmoles substrate/10^{10} cells/hr.	—	Kalckar and Maxwell (1958)

TABLE 3

HUMAN ERYTHROCYTE LIPIDS

Lipid	Value	Reference
Total lipid	427.9[a]	Gerstl *et al.* (1961)
	846.7[a]	Cacciari *et al.* (1959b)
	392 ± 65[a] (adults)	Maggioni *et al.* (1960)
	464 ± 86[a] (children)	Maggioni *et al.* (1960)
	596[a] (411–781)	Boyd (1934)*
	510 ± 51[a]	Farquhar (1962)
Phosphorus	11.9 ± 0.8[a]	Farquhar (1962)
	13.3[a] (12–14.5)	Munn and Crosby (1961)
Phospholipid	298 ± 20[a]	Farquhar (1962)
Plasmalogen	56[a]	Farquhar (1962)
Total cholesterol	120 ± 8.7[a]	Farquhar (1962)
	132[a] (117–158)	Munn and Crosby (1961)
Fatty acids	200[a]	Farquhar (1962)
	170[a] (120–220)	Munn and Crosby (1961)
Other	92 ± 18[a]	Farquhar (1962)
Fatty acids as % total fatty acid		
Lauric (n-C_{12})	0.3	Kates *et al.* (1961)
	0.23[b]	Manfredi *et al.* (1962)
Myristic (n-C_{14})	0.8	Kates *et al.* (1961)
	0.48[b]	Manfredi *et al.* (1962)
Pentoenoic (15:1)	3.7[c] (2.7–4.4)	Munn and Crosby (1961)
(n-C_{15})	0.3	Kates *et al.* (1961)
	0.16[b]	Manfredi *et al.* (1962)
Palmitoleic (16:1)	1:1	Kates *et al.* (1961)
	1.5	Kogl *et al.* (1960)
	1.68[b]	Manfredi *et al.* (1962)
	3.9[c] (2.1–6.1)	Munn and Crosby (1961)
Palmitic (n-C_{16})	41	Kates *et al.* (1961)
	37.5	Kogl *et al.* (1960)
	23.6[b]	Manfredi *et al.* (1962)
(C_{17}) branched	0.3	Kates *et al.* (1961)
(17:1)	3.6[b]	Manfredi *et al.* (1962)
(n-C_{17})	0.3	Kates *et al.* (1961)
	0.22[b]	Manfredi *et al.* (1962)
Linoleic ($18{:}2^{9,12}$)	15.3	Kates *et al.* (1961)
	17	Kogl *et al.* (1960)
	12[b]	Manfredi *et al.* (1962)
	5.8[c] (4.5–7.3)	Munn and Crosby (1961)
Linolenic ($18{:}3^{9,12,15}$)	2	Kogl *et al.* (1960)
	0.57[b]	Manfredi *et al.* (1962)
Oleic (18:1)	18.9	Kates *et al.* (1961)
	26.5	Kogl *et al.* (1960)
	19.8[b]	Manfredi *et al.* (1962)
	48.2[c] (41.8–57.5)	Munn and Crosby (1961)

TABLE 3—*cont.*

Lipid	Value		Reference
Oleic isomer	trace		Kates *et al.* (1961)
cis-Octadecanoic	—		Baufeld and Luther (1961)
Stearic (n-C_{18})	7.9		Kates *et al.* (1961)
	15.5		Kogl *et al.* (1960)
	16.5 [b]		Manfredi *et al.* (1962)
(20:3)	1.5		Kates *et al.* (1961)
	7.11 [b]		Manfredi *et al.* (1962)
Arachidonic (20:4)	7.9		Kates *et al.* (1961)
			deGier *et al.* (1961)
(n-C_{20})	2.14 [b]		Manfredi *et al.* (1962)
(C_{22} unsat. a)	2.5		Kates *et al.* (1961)
(C_{22} unsat. b)	2.0		Kates *et al.* (1961)
(22:6)	5.11 [b]		Manfredi *et al.* (1962)
Long chain aldehydes as % total aldehyde			Kates *et al.* (1961)
n-C_{14}	trace		
Branched C_{15}	0.8		
n-C_{15}	0.6		
Highly branched C_{16}	trace		
C_{16} monoene	0.4		
n-C_{16}	24.2		
Highly branched C_{17}	1.7		
Branched C_{17}	7.5		
n-C_{17}	1.3		
C_{18} monoene	6.0		
Isomeric C_{18} monoene	2.8		
n-C_{18}	42.5		
Unknown C_{19}	2.9		
Unknown C_{20}	3.1		
Unknown C_{21}	5.6		
Neutral Lipid			
Unesterified cholesterol	80% of total		Hanahan *et al.* (1960)
Long-chain fatty acid cholesterol esters	4% of total		Hanahan *et al.* (1960)
Triglycerides	10% of total		Hanahan *et al.* (1960)
Free fatty acid	0.5% of total		Hanahan *et al.* (1960)
Total cholesterol	173 (118–228)	mg./100 ml.	Foldes and Murphy (1946)*
Unesterified cholesterol	140 (119–161)	mg./100 ml.	Brun (1939)*
Cholesta-3,5-diene-7-one	—	—	Irie *et al.* (1961)
7-Oxycholesterol	—	—	Irie *et al.* (1961)
7-Hydroxycholesterol	—	—	Irie *et al.* (1961)
Fatty acids as % total fatty acids of neutral lipid			James *et al.* (1959)
n-C_{10}	0–0.6		
n-C_{12}	1.1–2.2		

TABLE 3—*cont.*

Lipid	Value	Reference
Fatty acids as % total fatty acids of neutral lipid—cont.		
n-C_{14}	5.9–17.3	
16:1	3.2–6.0	
n-C_{16}	15.2–22.6	
18:2 and 3	11.4–21.1	
18:1	28.8–29.1	
n-C_{18}	5.7–10.7	
Unsat. $C_{19}A$	trace	
Arachidonic (20:1)	7.4–8.3	
Polyunsat. (C_{20})	trace	
Phospholipids		
Total	196 (26–297) mg./100 ml.	Kirk (1938)*
	337.5 mg./100 ml.	Cacciari *et al.* (1959b)
	298 ± 20 mg./100 ml.	Farquhar and Oette (1961)
Cephalin	117 (38–191) mg./100 ml.	Kirk (1938)*
	42.4 ± 1% total phospholipid	Phillips and Roome (1962)
Ethanolamine phosphoglyceride	30% total phospholipid	Hanahan *et al.* (1960)
	11.9% total phospholipid P	Blomstrand *et al.* (1962)
	29% total phospholipid	Farquhar and Oette (1961)
Mean plasmologen content	67% (of ethanolamine phosphoglyceride)	Farquhar and Oette (1961)
Serine phosphoglyceride	2% total phospholipid	Hanahan *et al.* (1962)
	12.4% total phospholipid P	Blomstrand *et al.* (1962)
	10% total phospholipid	Farquhar and Oette (1961)
Mean plasmalogen content	8% (of serine phosphoglyceride)	Farquhar and Oette (1961)
Lecithin	32 (3–95) mg./100 ml.	Kirk (1938)*
	36.5% total phospholipid P (includes lysolecithin)	Blomstrand *et al.* (1962)
	32.7 ± 2% total phospholipid	Phillips *et al.* (1962)
	38.5% total phospholipid	de Gier *et al.* (1961)
Sphingomyelin	12–113 mg./100 ml.	Kirk (1938)
	23.1 ± 1.9% total phospholipid	Phillips and Roome (1962)
Lysolecithin	1.8 ± 0.2% total phospholipid	Phillips and Roome (1962)

Fatty Acid Composition of Phospholipids[d]

Fatty acid	Mixed (mole %)	Individual (mole %)		
		Ethanol amine	Serine	Choline
12:0	0.1, 0–0.2[e]	—	—	0.1
14:0	0.5, 1.2–2.5[e]	0.2	trace	0.5
15:0	0.3	0.2	trace	0.3

TABLE 3—*cont.*

	Fatty acid	Mixed (mole %)		Individual (mole %)		
				Ethanol amine	Serine	Choline
	16:0	28.8, 23–25.2[e]		18.9	7.1	33.0
cis	16:1[9]	0.7, trace–1.6[e]		0.6	0.4	1.0
	17:0 iso or ante-iso	—		—	—	—
	17:0	0.4		trace	0.3	0.5
	18:0	15.1, 16.6–17.7[e]		8.0	41.6	11.7
cis	18:1[9]	18.3	17–25.5[e]	21.6	7.9	17.9
trans	18:1[9]	2.9		3.6	5.1	2.7
cis,cis	18:2[9,12]	10.6	8.6–12.3[e]	7.0	2.8	18.2
cis,cis,cis	18:3[9,12,15]	—		trace	—	—
	18:4	—		—	—	—
	19:0 iso or ante-iso	trace		0.2	—	—
	20:0	0.1		—	trace	0.2
	20:1[11]	0.2		0.2	trace	0.2
	20:2[8,11]	—		trace	—	—
	20:2[11,14]	0.1	2.4–4.1[e]	0.1	—	0.2
	20:3[5,8,11]	1.6		1.0	2.1	1.6
	20:4[5,8,11,14]	10.8		21.9	19.7	5.0
	20:5[5,8,11,14,17]	0.8		1.4	0.3	0.5
	Unknown (22:unsat?)	1.7		4.7	2.2	0.3
	22:5	0.7		0.8	0.9	1.7
	22:5	2.3		2.3	2.0	2.7
	22:5[7,10,13,16,19]	1.0		—	—	1.0
	22:6[4,7,10,13,16,19]	2.1		3.9	4.2	1.1

Fatty Aldehyde Compositions of Phospholipids[d]

	Fatty aldehyde	Mixed (mole %)	Individual (mole %)		
			Ethanol amine	Serine	Choline
	14:0	trace	—	—	0.8
branched	15:0	2.8	2.6	5.5	—
	15:0 iso *or* ante-iso	0.1	—	0.4	—
	15:0	0.2	0.3	—	—
	Unknown	0.1	—	1.6	1.0
	Unknown	trace	—	1.0	—
cis	16:1[9]	trace	—	—	0.2
	16:0	18.2	15.9	17.1	49.8
branched	17:unsat?	0.9	1.5	—	—
branched	17:unsat?	2.4	3.0	—	—
branched	17:0	5.8	5.5	11.3	6.9
	17:0 iso or ante-iso	1.1	0.8	0.7	2.9
cis,cis	18.2[9,12]	trace	—	1.4	1.9
cis	18:1[9]	6.8	7.0	5.4	5.3
	18:1 isomer	13.2	18.8	10.5	7.7

TABLE 3—*cont.*

Fatty aldehyde		Mixed (mole %)	Individual (mole %)		
			Ethanol amine	Serine	Choline
	18.0	37.1	40.4	32.3	19.2
	Unknown	1.3	2.1	—	—
branched	19:0	—	—	—	—
	19:0	—	—	—	—

[a] In mg./100 ml.
[b] Children 2–3 years.
[c] In % of total unsaturated fatty acid.
[d] Farquhar (1962) except as noted.
[e] Phillips and Roome (1962).

TABLE 4

Human Erythrocyte Polysaccharides

Polysaccharide	Value	Remarks	Reference
Sialomucopeptide	—	Structure similar to M and N specific mucoids extracted by phenol. The sialomucopeptide is liberated by trypsin. Contains 10.1% N, 12.4% protein-bound hexose, 12.1% hexosamine, 0.25% P, 1.12% fucose, and 22–24% sialic acid. Contains galactose, galactosamine, lysine, arginine, aspartic acid, glutamic acid, glycine, serine, alanine, proline, valine, histidine, leucine, isoleucine, methionine, threonine. Inhibits influenza virus and M and N hemagglutination. Inhibition of influenza virus hemagglutination destroyed by trypsin, receptor-destroying enzyme of *Vibrio comma*, and active influenza virus. Removal of neuraminic acid destroys M and N specificity and influenza virus hemagglutination. Papain destroys M and N but not influenza specificity	Cook *et al.* (1960); Cook (1962); Klenk (1959); Kathan *et al.* (1961)
Sialic acid	19.2 mg./100 ml. cells	15 normal children	Manfredi (1960)
	135 ± 22 (86–182) μg./ml. cells	—	Yachnin and Gardner (1961)
	—	Treatment with neuraminadase liberated *N*-glycolyl- and *N*-acetylneuraminic acids and altered electrophoretic mobility of cells	Cook *et al.* (1961); Eylar *et al.* (1962)
A and B substance	—	Contains galactosamine, glucosamine, galactose, sphingosine, and higher fatty acids; has no H or O specificity	Koscielak and Zakrzewski (1960)
Platelet-agglutinating polysaccharide	—	—	Ollgaard (1961)

TABLE 5

HUMAN ERYTHROCYTE NUCLEOTIDES

Nucleotide	Value	Units	Remarks	Reference
Adenosine monophosphate	2.6 ± 1.13	μmoles/100 ml. cells	Donor age 30–45 yr.	Mandel *et al.* (1961–1962)
	2.0 ± 0.3	10^{-6} moles/10^{11} cells	—	Waller and Lohr (1961–1962)
	6.2 (50) [a]	μmoles/liter whole blood	Males, hematocrit 47	Bishop *et al.* (1959)
	5.1 (25.5) [a]	μmoles/liter whole blood	Female, hematocrit 42	Bishop *et al.* (1959)
	0.01–0.02	μmoles P/ml. red cells	—	Bartlett (1959)
	< 0.10	μmoles/gm. cell mass	—	Gerlach *et al.* (1958)
	0.3–2.3	μmoles/100 ml. blood	—	Yoshikawa *et al.* (1960)
Adenosine diphosphate	17.2 ± 4.5	μmoles/100 ml. cells	Donor age 30–45 yr.	Mandel *et al.* (1961–1962)
	0.3	μmoles/gm. cell mass	—	Gerlach *et al.* (1958)
	3.9 ± 0.4	10^{-6} moles/10^{11} cells	—	Waller and Lohr (1961–1962)
	47.8 (27.2) [a]	μmoles/liter whole blood	Males, hematocrit 47	Bishop *et al.* (1959)
	46.6 (15.0)	μmoles/liter whole blood	Females, hematocrit 42	Bishop *et al.* (1959)
	0.38–0.49	μmoles P/ml. red cells	—	Bartlett (1959)
	2.9–8.1	μmoles/100 ml. blood	—	Yoshikawa *et al.* (1960)
Adenosine triphosphate	85.6 ± 7.3	μmoles/100 ml. cells	Donor age 30–45 yr.	Mandel *et al.* (1961–1962)
	0.68	μmoles/gm. cell mass	—	Gerlach *et al.* (1958)
	69.2 ± 14.3	μmoles/100 ml. cells	Adult	DeLuca *et al.* (1962)
	86.4	μmoles/100 ml. cells	Newborn	DeLuca *et al.* (1962)
	0.15	mμmoles/10^{10} cells	—	Jorgensen (1957)
	14.6 ± 1.7	10^{-6} moles/10^{11} cells	—	Waller and Lohr (1961–1962)
	0.12	mμmoles/10^{10} cells	—	Mandel and Chambon (1959)
	2.7–3.7	μmoles P/ml. red cells	—	Bartlett (1959)
	433.2 (16.9) [a]	μmoles/liter whole blood	Males, hematocrit 47	Bishop *et al.* (1959)
	424.8 (13.4) [a]	μmoles/liter whole blood	Females, hematocrit 42	Bishop *et al.* (1959)
	43	μmoles/100 ml. blood	—	Yoshikawa *et al.* (1960)

Diphosphopyridine nucleotide	1.4–2.1	μmoles/100 ml. blood	—	Yoshikawa *et al.* (1960)
	0.66 ± 0.15	10^{-6} moles/10^{11} cells	—	Waller and Lohr (1961–1962)
	29.8 (17.1)[a]	μmoles/liter whole blood	Males, hematocrit 47	Bishop *et al.* (1959)
	32.4 (16.4)[a]	μmoles/liter whole blood	Females, hematocrit 42	Bishop *et al.* (1959)
Guanosine diphosphate	1.6 ± 0.52	μmoles/100 ml. cells	Donor age 30–45 yr.	Mandel *et al.* (1961–1962)
Guanosine triphosphate	5.7 ± 0.96	μmoles/100 ml. cells	Donor age 30–45 yr.	Mandel *et al.* (1961–1962)
	26.4 (8.0)[a]	μmoles/liter whole blood	Females, hematocrit 42	Bishop *et al.* (1959)
	24.5 (26)[a]	μmoles/liter whole blood	Males, hematocrit 47	Bishop *et al.* (1959)
5-Inosine monophosphate	3.1 ± 1.48	μmoles/100 ml. cells	Donor age 30–45 yr.	Mandel *et al.* (1961–1962)
	0.1–1.1	μmoles/100 ml. blood	—	Yoshikawa *et al.* (1960)
Rh antigen Lutheran antigen	—	—	Separated by anion-exchange chromatography; both antigens lowered by ribonuclease	Hackel and Smolker (1960)
Total nucleotide	1534 ± 33	μmoles/liter cells	—	Overgaard-Hansen and Jorgensen (1960)
Total pyridine nucleotide	7700 (6100–9300)	μg./100 ml.	—	Levitas *et al.* (1947)
Triphosphopyridine nucleotide	0.3–2.3	μmoles/100 ml. blood	—	Yoshikawa *et al.* (1960)
	0.32 ± 0.14	10^{-6} moles/10^{11} cells	—	Waller and Lohr (1961–1962)
	1.1 ± 0.4 (0.5–1.7)	μmoles/100 ml. cells	—	Jocelyn (1960)
	11.2 (10.7)[a]	μmoles/liter whole blood	Males, hematocrit 47	Bishop *et al.* (1959)
	11.6 (14.7)[a]	μmoles/liter whole blood	Females, hematocrit 42	Bishop *et al.* (1959)
	2.3	μmoles/100 ml. cells	Donor age 30–45 yr.	Mandel *et al.* (1961–1962)
5-Uridine diphosphoglucose	3.1 ± 1.48	μmoles/100 ml. cells	Donor age 30–45 yr.	Mandel *et al.* (1961–1962)
	—	—	Separated by anion-exchange chromatography	Mills (1960)
Uridine diphospho-*N*-acetyl glucosamine	—	—	Separated by anion-exchange chromatography	Mills (1960)

[a] (Standard deviation/median) × 100.

TABLE 6

NONPROTEIN NITROGENOUS COMPONENTS OF THE RED CELL

Component	Value	Units	Remarks	Reference
Amino acids				
Total	12.15	mg./100 ml.	Whole cells	Corsini *et al.* (1959b)
	6.38	mg./100 ml.	Stroma	
α-Alanine	2.56–5.6	mg./100 ml.	—	Gutman and Alexander (1947)*; Wiss and Kruger (1948)*
	427 ± 25	μmoles/kg. water	—	McMenamy *et al.* (1960)
γ-Amino-*n*-butyric acid	25 ± 2	μmoles/kg. water	—	McMenamy *et al.* (1960)
Arginine	0.3 (0.1–0.6)	mg./100 ml.	—	Hier and Bergeim (1946)*
	0.27 ± 0.14	mg./100 ml.	—	Johnson and Bergeim (1951)**
	12	μmoles/kg. water	—	McMenamy *et al.* (1960)
Cystine	0.4 (0.3–0.5)	mg./100 ml.	—	Johnson and Bergeim (1951)*
Glutamic acid	374 ± 33	μmoles/kg. water	—	McMenamy *et al.* (1960)
Glutamine	601 ± 46	μmoles/kg. water	—	McMenamy *et al.* (1960)
	8 ± 0.9	mg./100 ml.	—	Iyer (1956)**
Glycine	1.6–3.5	mg./100 ml.	—	Alexander *et al.* (1954)*; Christensen *et al.* (1946*, 1947)*; Gutman and Alexander (1947)*
Histidine	2.2–2.8	mg./100 ml.	—	von Euler and Heller (1947)*
	1.09 ± 0.25	mg./100 ml.	—	Johnson and Bergeim (1951)**
	131 ± 8	μmoles/kg. water	—	McMenamy *et al.* (1960)
Isoleucine	0.9 (0.5–1.4)	mg./100 ml.	—	Johnson and Bergeim (1951)*
Leucine	1.5 (1.0–1.8)	mg./100 ml.	—	Hier (1947)*
	1.54 ± 0.18	mg./100 ml.	—	Johnson and Bergeim (1951)**
Leucine + isoleucine	211 ± 21	μmoles/kg. water	—	McMenamy *et al.* (1960)
Lysine	1.4 (0.9–1.8)	mg./100 ml.	—	Johnson and Bergeim (1951)*
	223 ± 24	μmoles/kg. water	—	McMenamy *et al.* (1960)
Methionine	0.5 (0.3–0.8)	mg./100 ml.	—	Johnson and Bergeim (1951)*
	30 ± 4	μmoles/kg. water	—	McMenamy *et al.* (1960)

Phenylalanine	1.0 (0.7–1.3)	mg./100 ml.	—	Johnson and Bergeim (1951)*
	59 ± 4	μmoles/kg. water	—	McMenamy *et al.* (1960)
Proline	191 ± 11	μmoles/kg. water	—	McMenamy *et al.* (1960)
Serine + glycine	948 ± 48	μmoles/kg. water	—	McMenamy *et al.* (1960)
Threonine	1.6 (1.3–2.1)	mg./100 ml.	—	Johnson and Bergeim (1951)*
	157 ± 9	mg./100 ml.	—	McMenamy *et al.* (1960)
Tryptophan	0.3	mg./100 ml.	—	Dunn *et al.* (1945)*; Hier and Bergeim (1946)*; Steele *et al.* (1950)
	0.29 ± 0.07	mg./100 ml.	—	Johnson and Bergeim (1951)**
	21 ± 4	μmoles/kg. water	—	McMenamy *et al.* (1960)
Tyrosine	1.1 (0.7–1.5)	mg./100 ml.	—	Johnson and Bergeim (1951)*
	72 ± 5	μmoles/kg. water	—	McMenamy *et al.* (1960)
Valine	2.0 (1.6–2.5)	mg./100 ml.	—	Henderson *et al.* (1949)*; Johnson and Bergeim (1951)**
	223 ± 12	μmoles/kg. water	—	McMenamy *et al.* (1960)
Coproporphyrin	0.5 (0–2.0)	μg/100 ml.	—	Watson (1950)*
	0.5 ± 0.54	μg/100 ml.	Adults	Bertolini *et al.* (1960)
	0–0.004	μmoles/100 ml.	Whole blood	Rubino *et al.* (1960)
Creatine	8.1 (6.0–10.2)	mg./100 ml.	—	Jellinek and Looney (1939)*; Looney (1924)*
	5.62	mg./100 ml.	—	Sandberg *et al.* (1953)**
Creatinine	1.8 (1.7–1.9)	mg./100 ml.	—	Jellinek and Looney (1939)*; Looney (1924)*
Ergothioneine	458 ± 51	μmoles/kg. water	—	McMenamy *et al.* (1960)
Ethanolamine	10	μmoles/kg. water	—	McMenamy *et al.* (1960)
Glutathione	87	mg./100 ml.	Total	Jellinek and Looney (1939)*
	8.5	mg./100 ml.	Oxidized	Looney and Childs (1934)*
	79	mg./100 ml.	Reduced	Looney and Childs (1934)*
	5 ± 1.3 (0–15)	μmoles/100 ml. packed cells	Oxidized	Jocelyn (1960)
	220 ± 41 (160–300)	μmoles/100 ml. packed cells	Reduced	Jocelyn (1960)
	280	μmoles/100 ml.	—	Chow (1960)

TABLE 6—*cont.*

Component	Value	Units	Remarks	Reference
Glutathione (*cont.*)				
	1.5	μmoles/gm. packed cells	—	Koz (1962)
	74.5 ± 4.8	mg./100 ml. cells	—	Tada (1961)
	44–71	mg./100 ml. cells	—	Swarup *et al.* (1961)
Protoporphyrin	35 (13–140)	μg./100 ml.	—	Cartwright *et al.* (1948)*
	35.1 ± 7.7	μg./100 ml.	—	Bertolini *et al.* (1960)
	0.018–0.110	μmoles/100 ml. blood	—	Rubino *et al.* (1960)
	38.8	μg./100 ml.	—	Darocha (1958)
Taurine	< 70	μmoles/kg. water	—	McMenamy *et al.* (1960)
Tripeptide	3.9	mg./100 ml. cells	Hydroxyamino acid-cysteine-glycine	Bittner *et al.* (1961)
Urea	6000 ± 370	μmoles/kg. water	—	McMenamy *et al.* (1960)
Uric acid	1.9 (0.8–3.0)	mg./100 ml.	—	Folin and Svedberg (1930a, b)*; Jellinek and Looney (1939)*; Looney (1924)*
	2.5	mg./100 ml.	—	Jorgensen and Nielsen (1956)**
	140.9 (16.1)[a]	μmoles/liter whole blood	Males	Bishop *et al.* (1959)
	135.1 (19.8)[a]	μmoles/liter whole blood	Females	Bishop *et al.* (1959)

[a] (Standard deviation/median) × 100.

TABLE 7

Human Erythrocyte Coenzymes and Vitamins

Substance	Value	Units	Remarks	Reference
Ascorbic acid	0.69 ± 0.12	mg./100 ml.	—	Barkham and Howard (1958)**
	1000 (500–2800)	IU/100 ml.	—	Sargent (1947)*
	1100 (500–1700)	IU/100 ml.	—	Butler and Cushman (1940)*
Choline (free)	4.7–7.5	IU/100 ml.	—	Luecke and Pearson (1944)*
				Schlegel (1949)*
Cocarboxylase	10.2 (7–14)	μg./100 ml.	Males	Beerstecher and Spangler (1961)*
	6.5 (5–8)	μg./100 ml.	Females	
	2.1	μg./10^{11} cells	—	Smits and Florijn (1949)**
Coenzyme A	210–280	μg./100 ml.	As bound pantothenic acid	Kaplan and Lipmann (1948)*
	7.05	Lipmann units/gm.	—	Causi (1958); Axelrod and Elvehjem (1939)**
	4.32 ± 0.64	Lipmann units/ml.	—	Chiarini and Melani (1960)
Nicotinic acid (niacin)	135	IU/100 ml.	—	Klein *et al.* (1945)*
Pantothenic acid	25 (15–30)	μg./100 ml.	Microbiological assay	Pearson (1941)*
Pyridine nucleotide (total)	7700 (6100–9300)	μg./100 ml.	—	Levitas *et al.* (1947)*
DPN	5.5	μmoles/ml. cells	—	Hofmann and Noll (1961)
	0.66 ± 0.15	10^{-6} moles/10^{11} cells	—	Waller and Lohr (1961–1962)
	29.8 (17.1)[a]	μmoles/liter whole blood	Males, hematocrit 47	Bishop *et al.* (1959)
	32.4 (16.4)[a]	μmoles/liter whole blood	Females, hematocrit 42	Bishop *et al.* (1959)
TPN	4.5	μmole/ml. cell	—	Hofmann and Noll (1961)
	0.32 ± 0.14	10^{-6} moles/10^{11} cells	—	Waller and Lohr (1961–1962)
	1.1 ± 0.4 (0.5–1.7)	μmoles/100 ml. cells	—	Jocelyn (1960)
	11.2 (10.7)[a]	μmoles/liter whole blood	Males, hematocrit 47	Bishop *et al.* (1959)
	11.6 (14.7)[a]	μmoles/liter whole blood	Females, hematocrit 42	Bishop *et al.* (1959)
	2.3	μmoles/100 ml. cells	Donor age 30–45 yr.	Mandel *et al.* (1961–1962)
Pyridoxine (pyridoxal, pyridoxamine)	3.8–21.1	—	—	Greenberg and Rinehard (1949)**
Riboflavin	22.4 (18–26)	IU/100 ml.	—	Burch *et al.* (1948)*
	17.77 ± 0.56 (10.5–25)	μg./100 ml.	—	Payva *et al.* (1961)
Thiamine	8.0 (6.6–9.4)	IU/100 ml.	—	Burch (1952)*
	4.45	IU/100 ml.	—	Yamadori (1949)*

[a] (Standard deviation/Mean) × 100.

TABLE 8

Human Erythrocyte Carbohydrates, Organic Acids, and Metabolites

Substance	Value	Units	Remarks	Reference
Deoxyribonucleic acid	trace	—	—	Metais and Mandel (1950)
2,3-Diphosphoglycerate	360–500	μmoles/100 ml.	—	Vanderheiden (1961)
	3520	mμmoles/10^{10} cells	—	Gerlach *et al.* (1958)
Fructose-6-phosphate	—	—	Formed by ghosts	Lionetti *et al.* (1961)
	9–17	mμmoles/10^{10} cells	—	Bartlett (1959)
Fructose diphosphate	—	—	Formed by ghosts	Lionetti *et al.* (1961)
	50–100	mμmoles/10^{10} cells	—	Bartlett (1959)
	410	mμmoles/10^{10} cells	—	Gerlach *et al.* (1958)
Galactose-1-phosphate	—	—	—	Inouye *et al.* (1962)
Galactose-6-phosphate	—	—	—	Inouye *et al.* (1962)
Galactose diphosphate	—	—	—	Inouye *et al.* (1962)
Glucuronic acid	0.6 (0.2–2.0)		—	Deichman and Dierker (1946)
Glucose	74 (46–102)	mg./100 ml.	—	Somogyi (1928)
	3700	mμmoles/10^{10} cells	—	Cartier and Leroux (1962)
Glucose-6-phosphate	—	—	Formed by ghosts	Lionetti *et al.* (1961)
	69–86	mμmoles/10^{10} cells	—	Bartlett (1959)
Glucose 1,6-diphosphate	18–30	μmoles/100 ml.	—	Vanderheiden (1961)
	180	mμmoles/10^{10} cells	—	Bartlett (1959)
Lactic acid	12	mg./100 ml.	—	Johnson *et al.* (1945)
	7800	mμmoles/10^{10} cells	—	Behrendt (1957)
Octulose-1,8-diphosphate	—	—	—	Bartlett and Bucolo (1960)
Phosphoglycerate	—	—	Formed by ghosts	Lionetti *et al.* (1961)
Phosphoglyceraldehyde	360	mμmoles/10^{10} cells	—	Gerlach *et al.* (1958)
Ribonucleic acid	135.5 (101.5–169.5)	mg./100 ml.	—	Mandel *et al.* (1948)
Ribose-1,5-diphosphate	<1	μmoles/100 ml.	—	Vanderheiden (1961)
Ribulose-5-phosphate	—	—	—	Bruns *et al.* (1958a)
Sedoheptulose-7-phosphate	—	—	—	Bruns *et al.* (1958a)
Sedoheptulose diphosphate	—	—	—	Bucolo and Bartlett (1960)
Uridine diphospho-*N*-acetylglucosamine	—	—	—	Mills (1960)
Uridine diphosphoglucose	52	mμmoles/10^{10} cells	—	Mills (1960); Mandel and Chambon (1959)

TABLE 9

HUMAN ERYTHROCYTE ELECTROLYTES

Constituent	Value	Units	Reference
Aluminum	7	μg./100 ml.	Kehoe *et al.* (1940)*
Bromine	0.98 (0.92–1.40)	mg./100 ml.	Hunter (1955)*
Calcium	0.6–1.4	meq./liter	Sobel *et al.* (1941)*
Chloride	78	meq./liter	Berstein (1954)*
Chromium	0.02 (0.005–0.054)	parts per million	Herring *et al.* (1960)
Cobalt	1.2	μg./100 ml.	Heyrovsky (1952)*
Copper	115 (84–159)	μg./100 ml.	Lahey *et al.* (1953)*
	105	μg./100 ml. (males)	Gisinger (1960)
	107	μg./100 ml. (females)	Gisinger (1960)
	0.82 (0.22–2.8)	parts per million	Herring *et al.* (1960)
Fluorine	25 (9–40)	μg./100 ml.	Largent and Cholak (1961)*
Iodine-protein bound	4.9–5.2	μg./100 ml.	McClendon and Foster (1944)*
Iron (nonhemoglobin)	2.48 (1.58–5.30)	μg./100 ml.	Alcuin-Arens (1940, 1941)*
	104	mg./100 gm.	McCance and Widdowson (1956)**
Lead	57 (29–86)	μg./100 ml.	Kehoe *et al.* (1940)*
	40	μg./100 ml. (infants)	Jensovsky and Roth (1961)
	25	μg./100 ml. (age 60 yr.)	Jensovsky and Roth (1961)
Magnesium	3.4–5.6	mg./100 ml.	Streef (1939)*
	74.3 (26–131)	parts per million	Herring *et al.* (1960)
Manganese	19	μg./100 ml.	Kehoe *et al.* (1940)*
	0.2 (0–0.48)	parts per million	Miller and Yoe (1962)
Nickel	0.053 (0.00–0.31)	parts per million	Herring *et al.* (1960)
Phosphorus			
Total	597	μmoles/100 ml.	Bartlett (1953)**
Inorganic	2.41 (0.9–3.3)	mg./100 ml.	Helve (1946)*
	4.0	mg./100 ml.	Gabrio *et al.* (1956)**
	21	μmoles/100 ml.	Bartlett (1953)**
Organic acid-soluble	49.7 (38.5–58.7)	mg./100 ml.	Helve (1946)*
Adenosine monophosphate P	1.1	μmoles/100 ml.	Bartlett (1953)**
Adenosine diphosphate P	11.6	μmoles/100 ml.	Bartlett (1953)**
Adenosine triphosphate P	45.2	μmoles/100 ml.	Bartlett (1953)**
Diphosphoglycerate P	29.2 (19.0–40.4)	mg./100 ml.	Helve (1946)*
	157	μmoles/100 ml.	Bartlett (1953)**

TABLE 9—*cont.*

Constituent	Value	Units	Reference
Phosphorus (*cont.*)			
Fructose monophosphate P	1	μmoles/100 ml.	Bartlett (1953)**
Fructose diphosphate P	10.5	μmoles/100 ml.	Bartlett (1953)**
Glucose monophosphate P	2	μmoles/100 ml.	Bartlett (1953)**
Hexose phosphate P	7.5 (3.5–10.7)	mg./100 ml.	Helve (1946)*
Nucleotide P	6.2 (5.1–7.1)	mg./100 ml.	Kerr and Daoud (1935)*
Lipid P	11.9	mg./100 ml.	Ferranti and Gianetti (1933)*
Unidentified phosphate P	43	mg./100 ml.	Bartlett (1953)**
Potassium	437 (425–444)	mg./100 ml.	Overman and Davis (1947)*
	371 ± 11.2	mg./100 ml.	Hald (1946)**
	605		Widdowson and McCance (1956)**
Silicon	< 1	mg./ml.	Baumann (1960)
	3% (in red cell ash)		Kehoe *et al.* (1940)*
Silver	trace		Kehoe *et al.* (1940)*
Sodium	14 (trace–31)	mg./100 ml.	Overman and Davis (1947)*
	48		McCance and Widdowson (1956)**
Sulfur (ethereal)	0.015	mg./100 ml.	Reed and Denis (1927)*
Tin	26	μg./100 ml.	Kehoe *et al.* (1940)*
Zinc	1440 (900–1980)	μg./100 ml.	Vallee and Gibson (1948)
	10 (3.6–25.4)	parts per million	Herring *et al.* (1960)
	206.9 (118–288)	μg./100 ml.	Zak *et al.* (1962)

References

Adams, E., McFadden, M., and Smith, E. L. (1952). *J. Biol. Chem.* **198**, 663.

Akerfeldt, S. (1960). *Acta Chem. Scand.* **14**, 1019.

Alcuin-Arens, M. (1940–1941). *Am. J. Med. Technol.* **6–7**, 203.

Alexander, B., Landvehr, G., and Seligman, A. (1945). *J. Biol. Chem.* **160**, 51.

Alivisatos, S. G. A., Kashket, S., and Denstedt, O. F. (1956). *Can. J. Biochem. Physiol.* **34**, 46.

Ashby, W. (1943). *J. Biol. Chem.* **151**, 521.

Axelrod, A. E., and Elvehjem, C. A. (1939). *J. Biol. Chem.* **131**, 77.

Banaschak H. (1961). *Acta Biol. Med. Ger.* **7**, 216.

Barkhan, P., and Howard, A. N. (1958). *Biochem. J.* **70**, 163.
Bartlett, G. R. (1953). *J. Appl. Physiol.* **6**, 51.
Bartlett, G. R. (1958). *Ann. N. Y. Acad. Sci.* **75**, 110.
Bartlett, G. R. (1959). *J. Biol. Chem.* **234**, 449.
Bartlett, G. R., and Bucolo, G. (1960). *Biochem. Biophys. Res. Commun.* **3**, 474.
Bartlett, G. R., and Marlow, A. A. (1951). *Bull. Scripps Metabolic Clinic* 2, No. 5.
Baufeld, H., and Luther, P. (1961). *Klin. Wochschr.* **39**, 444.
Baumann, H. (1960). *Z. Physiol. Chem.* **320**, 11.
Beerstecher, E., Jr., and Spangler, S. (1961). *In* "Blood and Other Body Fluids" (D. S. Dittmer, ed.), p. 108. Fed. Am. Soc. Exptl. Biol., Washington, D.C.
Behrendt, H. (1957). "Chemistry of Erythrocytes." Thomas, Springfield, Illinois.
Berstein, R. E. (1954). *Science* **120**, 459.
Bertino, J. R., Simmons, B., and Donohue, D. M. (1962). *J. Biol. Chem.* **237**, 1314.
Bertolini, A. M., Massari, N., and Guardamagna, C. (1960). *Acta Gerontol.* **10**, 3.
Bertolini, A. M., Quarto di Palo, F. M., and Agugini, G. (1961a). *Giorn. Gerontol.* **9**, 529.
Bertolini, A. M., Massari, N., and Civardi, F. (1961b). *Giorn. Gerontol.* **9**, 537.
Bertolini, A. M., Massari, N., and Guardamagna (1961c). *Giorn. Gerontol.* **9**, 543.
Bertolini, A. M., Massari, N., and Civardi, F. (1961d). *Giorn. Gerontol.* **9**, 547.
Bertolini, A. M., Massari, N., Civardi, F., and Tenconi, L. (1961e). *Giorn. Gerontol.* **9**, 551.
Beutler, E.. and Yeh, M. K. Y. (1959). *J. Lab. Clin. Med.* **54**, 456.
Bishop, C. (1960). *J. Biol. Chem.* **235**, 3228.
Bishop, C., Rankin, D. M., and Talbott, J. H. (1959). *J. Biol. Chem.* **234**, 1233.
Bittner, J., Rapoport, S., and Suchrow, D. (1961). *Acta Biol. Med. Ger.* **6**, 31.
Blagorazumova, M. A. (1959). *Sb. Nauchn. Rabot. Stalingrad Med. Inst.* **12**, 27.
Blanchaer, M. C., Weiss, P., and Bergsogel, D. E. (1951). *Can. J. Med. Sci.* **29**, 108.
Blanchaer, M. C., Brownstone, S., and Williams, H. (1955). *Am. J. Physiol.* **183**, 95.
Blomstrand, R., Nakayama, F., and Nilsson, I. M. (1962). *J. Lab. Clin. Med.* **59**, 771.
"Blood and Other Body Fluids", D. S. Dittmer, Editor (1961) *Fed. Am. Soc. Exptl. Biol.* Washington, D.C.
Blostein, R., and Denstedt, O. F. (1962). *Can. J. Biochem. Physiol.* **40**, 1005.
Bodansky, O. (1954). *Cancer* **7**, 1191.
Boyd, E. M. (1934). *J. Clin. Invest.* **13**, 347.
Boyer, M. (1961). *Proc. European Reg. Conf. Electron Microscopy, Delft 1960*, p. 726.
Brin, M. (1962). *Ann. N. Y. Acad. Sci.* **97**, 528.
Brown, B. T., Golder, W. S., and Wright, S. E. (1961). *Australian J. Exptl. Biol. Med. Sci.* **39**, 345.
Brownstone, Y. S. (1958). Ph.D. Thesis, McGill Univ., Montreal, Canada.
Brownstone, Y. S., and Denstedt, O. F. (1961a). *Can. J. Biochem. Physiol.* **39**, 527.
Brownstone, Y. S., and Denstedt, O. F. (1961b). *Can. J. Biochem. Physiol.* **39**, 533.
Brun, G. C. (1939). *Acta Med. Scand. Suppl.* **99**.
Bruns, F. H., Noltmann, E., and Vahlhaus, E. (1958a). *Biochem. Z.* **330**, 483.
Bruns, F. H., Dunwald, E., and Noltmann, E. (1958b). *Biochem. Z.* **330**, 497.
Bucolo, G., and Bartlett, G. R. (1960). *Biochem. Biophys. Res. Commun.* **3**, 620.
Burch, H. B. (1952). *J. Biol. Chem.* **198**, 486.
Burch, H. B., Bessey, O. A., and Lowry, O. H., (1948). *J. Biol. Chem.* **175**, 457.
Buruiana, I. M., Hadarag, E., Dema, A., and Dema, I. (1961). *Acad. Rep. Populare Romine, Studii Cercetari Biochim.* **4**, 463.
Butler, A. M., and Cushman, M. (1940). *J. Clin. Invest.* **19**, 459.
Cacciari, E., Corsini, F., Manfredi, G., and Pintozzi, P. (1959a). *Boll. Soc. Ital. Biol. Sper.* **35**, 395.

Cacciari, E., Corsini, F., Manfredi, G., and Pintozzi, P. (1959b). *Boll. Soc. Ital. Biol. Sper.* **35**, 404.
Caffrey, R., Trembley, R., Gabrio, B., and Huennekens, F. (1956). *J. Biol. Chem.* **223**, 1.
Calloway, S., Davies, D. R., and Rutland, J. P. (1951). *Brit. Med. J.* **2**, 812.
Carta, S., and Vivaldi, G. (1957). *Boll. Soc. Ital. Biol. Sper.* **33**, 1454.
Cartier, P., and Leroux, J. P. (1962). *Ann. Biol. Clin. Paris* **20**, 273.
Cartwright, G. E., Huguley, C. M., Jr., Ashenbrucker, H., Fay, J., and Wintrobe, M. M. (1948). *Blood* **3**, 501.
Causi, N. (1958). *Policlinico (Rome), Sez. Med.* **65**, 179.
Cerletti, P., and Marchesini, B. M. (1960). *Boll. Soc. Ital. Biol. Sper.* **36**, 1965.
Cerletti, P., and DeRitis, G. (1962). *Clin. Chim. Acta* **7**, 402.
Chapman, J. (1961). *Proc. Soc. Exptl. Biol. Med.* **108**, 566.
Chapman, R. G., Hennessey, M. A., Waltersdorph, A. M., Huennekens, F. M., and Gabrio, B. W. (1962). *J. Clin. Invest.* **41**, 1257.
Chiarini, P., and Melani, F. (1960). *Sperimentale* **5**, 364.
Chow, B. F. (1960). *Am. Inst. Biol. Sci. Publ.* **6**, 153.
Christensen, H. N., and Lynch, E. L. (1946). *J. Biol. Chem.* **163**, 741.
Christensen, H. N., Cooper, P. F., Jr., Johnson, R. D., and Lynch, E. L. (1947). *J. Biol. Chem.* **168**, 191.
Clarke, D., Davoll, J., Phillips, F., and Brown, G. (1952). *J. Pharmacol. Exptl. Therap.* **106**, 291.
Clarkson, M., and Maizels, M. (1952). *J. Physiol. (London)* **116**, 112.
Clegg, M. D., and Schroeder, W. A. (1959). *J. Am. Chem. Soc.* **81**, 6065.
Cohen, P. P., and Sober, E. K. (1945). *Cancer Res.* **5**, 631.
Conway, E., and Cooke, R. (1939). *Biochem. J.* **33**, 457.
Cook, G. M. W. (1962). *Nature* **195**, 159.
Cook, G. M. W., Heard, D. H., and Seaman, G. V. F. (1960). *Nature* **188**, 104.
Cook, G. M. W., Heard, D. H., and Seaman, G. V. F. (1961). *Nature* **191**, 44.
Cornblath, M., Levin, E. Y., Marquetti, E., and Hause, E. Y. (1960). *Federation Proc.* **19**, 68.
Corsini, F., Cacciari, E., Manfredi, G., and Pintozzi, P. (1959a). *Boll. Soc. Ital. Biol. Sperm.* **35**, 393.
Corsini, F., Pintozzi, P., Cacciari, E., and Manfredi, G. (1959b). *Boll. Soc. Ital. Biol. Sper.* **35**, 398.
Czok, R., and Bücher, T. H. (1960). *Advan. Protein. Chem.* **15**, 315.
Darocha, T. (1958). *Polski Tygod. Lekar. Wiadomosci Lekar.* **13**, 1141.
DeGier, J., Mulder, I., and Van Deenen, L. L. M. (1961). *Naturwissenschaften* **48**, 54.
Deichmann, W. B., and Dierker, M. (1946). *J. Biol. Chem.* **163**, 753.
DeLuca, C., Stevenson, J. H., and Kaplan, E. (1962). *Anal. Biochem.* **4**, 39.
Derrien, Y., Laurent, G., Depieds, R., and Borgomano, M. (1961). *Bull. Soc. Chim. Biol.* **43**, 43.
DeSandre, G., and Chiotto, G. (1960). *Brit. J. Haematol.* **6**, 39.
DeSantis, U., and Pisconti, G. (1961). *Minerva Pediat.* **13**, 504.
Dunn, M. S., Schott, H. F., Frankl, W., and Rockland, L. B. (1945). *J. Biol. Chem.* **157**, 387.
Edebacher, S., and Rothler, H. (1925). *Z. Physiol. Chem.* **148**, 264.
Ellman, G. L., and Calloway, E. (1961). *Nature* **192**, 1216.
Eylar, E. H., Madoff, M. A., Brody, O. V., and Oncley, J. L. (1962). *J. Biol. Chem.* **237**, 1992.
Faber, M., and Falbe-Hansen, I. (1959). *Nature* **184**, 1034.
Fallot, P., Canivet, J., Moudet, M., and Poidaz, J. (1956). *Compt. Rend.* **242**, 2668.
Farquhar, J. W. (1962). *Biochim. Biophys. Acta* **55**, 80.

Farquhar, J. W., and Oette, K. (1961). *Federation Proc.* **20**, 279.
Ferranti, F., and Giannetti, O. (1933). *Diagnos. tec. lab. Napoli, Riv. mens.* **4**, 664.
Fessler, A. (1959). M.Sc. Thesis, McGill Univ., Montreal, Canada.
Foldes, F. F., and Murphy, A. J. (1946), *Proc. Soc. Exptl. Biol. Med.* **62**, 215.
Folin, O., and Svedberg, H. (1930a). *J. Biol. Chem.* **88**, 85.
Folin, O., and Svedberg, H. (1930b). *J. Biol. Chem.* **88**, 715.
Gabrio, B. W., Donohue, D. M., and Finch, C. A. (1956). *J. Clin. Invest.* **35**, 657.
Gerlach, E. Fleckenstein, A., and Gross, E. (1958). *Arch. Ges. Physiol.* **266**, 528.
Gerstl, B., Athineos, E., Kahnke, M. J., Davis, W. E., Jr., and Smith, J. K. (1961). *Lab. Invest.* **10**, 76.
Gisinger, E. (1960). *Wien. Z. Inn. Med. Grenzg.* **41**, 1.
Greenberg, L. D., and Rinehard, J. F. (1949). *Proc. Soc. Exptl. Biol. Med.* **70**, 20.
Guardamagna, C., Massari, N., and Santambrogio, C. (1960). *Giorn. Gerontol.* **8**, 161.
Gutman, G. E., and Alexander, B. (1947). *J. Biol. Chem.* **168**, 527.
Haberman, V., and Habermanova, S. (1962). *Folia Haematol.* **78**, 690.
Hackel, E., and Smolker, R. E. (1960). *Nature* **187**, 1036.
Hald, P. M. (1946). *J. Biol. Chem.* **163**, 429.
Hanahan, D. J., Watts, R. M., and Pappajohn, D. (1960). *J. Lipid Res.* **1**, 421.
Hartman, S. C., and Buchanan, J. M. (1959). *J. Biol. Chem.* **234**, 1812.
Haschen, R. J. (1961a). *Biochem. Z.* **334**, 560.
Haschen, R. J. (1961b). *Biochem. Z.* **334**, 569.
Haschen, R. J. (1962). *Acta Biol. Med. Ger.* **8**, 209.
Haut, A., Tudhope, G. R., Cartwright, E. E., and Wintrobe, M. M. (1962). *J. Clin. Invest.* **41**, 579.
Heller, P., Weinstein, H. G., West, M., and Zimmerman, H. J. (1960a). *Ann. Internal. Med.* **53**, 898.
Heller, P., Weinstein, H. G., West, M., and Zimmerman, H. J. (1960b). *J. Lab. Clin. Med.* **55**, 425.
Helve, O. (1946). *Acta Med. Scand.* **125**, 505.
Henderson, L. M., Schurr, P. E., and Elvehjem, C. A. (1949). *J. Biol. Chem.* **177**, 815.
Hennessey, M. A., Waltersdorph, A. M., Huennekens, F. M., and Gabrio, B. W. (1962). *J. Clin. Invest.* **41**, 1249.
Herbert, D., and Pinsent, J. (1948). *Biochem. J.* **43**, 203.
Herring, W. B., Leavell, B. S., Paixao, L. M., and Yoe, J. H. (1960). *Am. J. Clin. Nutr.* **8**, 846.
Herschko, A., Wind, E., and Mager, J. (1962). *Bull. Res. Council Israel, Sect. A* **11**, No. 1.
Heyrovsky, A. (1952). *Casopis Lekaru Ceskych* **91**, 680.
Hier, S. W. (1947). *J. Biol. Chem.* **171**, 813.
Hier, S. W., and Bergeim, O. (1946). *J. Biol. Chem.* **163**, 129.
Higashi, T., Yogi, M., and Hirai, H. (1961). *J. Biochem. (Tokyo)* **49**, 707.
Hill, B. R. (1956). *Cancer Res.* **16**, 460.
Hofmann, E. C. G., and Noll, F. (1961). *Acta Biol. Med. Ger.* **6**, 1.
Hogeboom, G. H., Kuff, E. L., and Schneider, W. C. (1957). *Intern. Rev. Cytol.* **6**, 425.
Hokin, L. E., and Hokin, M. R. (1961). *Nature* **189**, 836.
Hrachovec, J. P., LeBlanc, M., and Rockstein, M. (1961). *Proc. Soc. Exptl. Biol. Med.* **107**, 205.
Hugh-Jones, K., Newcomb, A. L., and Hsia, D. Y. (1960). *Arch. Disease Childhood* **35**, 521.
Huisman, T. H. J., and Meyering, C. A. (1960). *Clin. Chim. Acta* **5**, 103.
Hunter, G. (1955). *Biochem. J.* **60**, 261.
Inouye, T., Tannenbaum, M., and Hsia, D. Y. (1962). *Nature* **193**, 67.
Irie, R., Iwanaga, M., and Yamakawa, T. (1961). *J. Biochem. (Tokyo)* **50**, 122.

Iyer, G. Y. N., (1956). *Ind. J. Med. Res.* **44,** 201.
Izak, G., Wilner, T., Mager, J., and Karshai, A. (1960). *J. Clin. Invest.* **39**, 1763.
James, A. T., Lovelock, J. E., and Webb, J. P. W. (1959). *Biochem. J.* **73**, 106.
Jellinek, E. M., and Looney, J. M. (1939). *J. Biol. Chem.* **128**, 621.
Jensovsky, L., and Roth, Z. (1961). *Naturwissenschaften* **48**, 382.
Jocelyn, P. C. (1960). *Biochem. J.* **77**, 363.
Johnson, C. A., and Bergeim, O. (1951). *J. Biol. Chem.* **188**, 833.
Johnson, R. E., Edwards, H. T., Dill, D. B., and Wilson, J. W. (1945). *J. Biol. Chem.* **157**, 461.
Jorgensen, S. (1957). *Acta Pharmacol. Toxicol.* **13**, 102.
Jorgensen, S., and Nielsen, A. A. T. (1956). *Scand. J. Clin. Lab. Invest.* **8**, 108.
Kalckar, H. M., and Maxwell, E. S. (1958). *Physiol. Rev.* **38**, 77.
Kalckar, H. M., Anderson, E. P., and Isselbacher, K. J. (1956). *Proc. Natl. Acad. Sci. U.S.* **42**, 49.
Kaplan, N. O., and Lipmann, F. (1948). *J. Biol. Chem.* **174**, 37.
Kashket, S., and Denstedt, O. F. (1958). *Can. J. Biochem. Physiol.* **36**, 1057.
Kates, M., Allison, A. C., and James, A. T. (1961). *Biochim. Biophys. Acta* **48**, 571.
Kathan, R. H., Winzler, R. J., and Johnson, C. A. (1961). *J. Exptl. Med.* **113**, 37.
Kehoe, R. A., Cholak, J., and Story, R. V. (1940). *J. Nutr.* **19**, 579.
Kerr, S. E., and Daoud, L. (1935). *J. Biol. Chem.* **109**, 301.
Kirk, E. (1938). *J. Biol. Chem.* **123**, 637.
Kirkman, H. N. (1962). *J. Biol. Chem.* **237**, 2364.
Kiese, M., Schneider, C., and Waller, H. D. (1957). *Arch. Exptl. Pathol. Pharmakol.* **231,** 158.
Klaus, D. (1961). *Aerztl. Forsch.* **15**, 548.
Klein, J. R., Perlzweig, W. A., and Handler, P. (1945). *J. Biol. Chem.* **158**, 561.
Klenk, E. (1959). *Intern. Symp. Biol. Active Mucoids, Warsaw, Poland 1959* p. 35.
Klenk, E., and Uhlenbruck, G. (1960). *Z. Physiol. Chem.* **319**, 151.
Klipstein, F. A., and Ranney, H. M. (1960). *J. Clin. Invest.* **39**, 1894.
Kochakian, C. D. (1944). *J. Biol. Chem.* **155**, 579.
Kochakian, C. D., Keutman, E. H., and Garber, E. E. (1948). *Conf. Metab. Aspects Convalescence Trans. 17th* p. 187.
Kogl, F., deGier, J., Mulder, I., and van Deenen, L. L. M. (1960). *Biochim. Biophys. Acta* **43**, 95.
Kohn, H. I., and Klein, J. P. (1939). *J. Biol. Chem.* **130**, 1.
Koscielak, J., and Zakrzewski, K. (1960). *Intern. Symp. Biol. Active Mucoids, Warsaw, Poland, 1959* p. 2108.
Koz, A. (1962). *Acta Biochim. Polon.* **9**, 11.
Kuenzel, W. (1961). *Folia Haematol.* **78**, 362.
Kunkel, H. C., Ceppellini, R., Müller-Eberhard, V., and Wolf, J. (1957). *J. Clin. Invest.* **36**, 1615.
Kunzer, W., and Schutz, E. (1959). *Folia Haematol.* **76**, 303.
Lahey, M. E., Gubler, C. J., Cartwright, G. E., and Wintrobe, M. M. (1953). *J. Clin. Invest.* **32**, 322.
Largent, E. J., and Cholak, J. (1961). *In* "Blood and Other Body Fluids" (D. S. Dittmer, ed.), p. 21. Fed. Am. Soc. Exptl. Biol., Washington, D.C.
Levitas, N., Robinson, J., Rosen, F., Huff, J. W., and Perlzweig, W. A. (1947). *J. Biol. Chem.* **167**, 169.
Liebermann, I. (1956). *J. Biol. Chem.* **223**, 327.
Lionetti, F. J., McLellan, W. L., Fortier, N. L., and Foster, J. M. (1961). *Arch. Biochem. Biophys.* **94**, 7.

Lohr, G. W., and Waller, H. D. (1959). *Klin. Wochschr.* **37**, 833.

Lohr, G. W., and Waller, H. D. (1961). *Folia Haematol.* **78**, 384.

Lohr, G. W., Waller, H. D., Karges, O., Schlegel, B., and Muller, A. A. (1958). *Klin. Wochschr.* **36**, 1008.

Long, C. (ed.) (1961). "Biochemists' Handbook." Van Nostrand, Princeton, New Jersey.

Looney, J. M. (1924). *Am. J. Psychiat.* **4**, 34.

Looney, J. M., and Childs, H. M. (1934). *J. Clin. Invest.* **13**, 963.

Lowy, B. A., Williams, M. K., and London, I. M. (1962). *J. Biol. Chem.* **237**, 1622.

Luecke, R. H., and Pearson, P. B. (1944). *J. Biol. Chem.* **153**, 259.

McCance, R. A., and Widdowson, E. M. (1956). *Clin. Sci.* **15**, 409.

McClendon, J. F., and Foster, W. C. (1944). *Am. J. Med. Sci.* **207**, 549.

McMenamy, R. H., Lund, C. C., Neville, G. J., and Wallach, D. F. H. (1960). *J. Clin. Invest.* **39**, 1657.

Maggioni, G., Bottini, E., Joppolo, C., and Antognoni, G. (1960). *Boll. Soc. Ital. Biol. Sper.* **36**, 904.

Malkin, A., and Denstedt, O. F. (1956). *Can. J. Biochem. Physiol.* **34**, 121.

Mandel, P., and Chambon, P. (1959). *Bull. Soc. Chim. Biol.* **41**, 989.

Mandel, P., Metais, P., and Beith, R. (1948). *Compt. Rend. Soc. Biol.* **142**, 241.

Mandel, P., Chambon, P., Karon, H., Kulic, I., and Seter, M. (1961–1962). *Folia Haematol.* **78**, 525.

Manfredi, G. (1960). *Boll. Soc. Ital. Biol. Sper.* **36**, 447.

Manfredi, G., Corsini, F., Paolucci, G., Salvioli, G. P., and Babini, B. (1962). *Boll. Soc. Ital. Biol. Sper.* **38**, 726.

Manganelli, G., and Grimaldi, N. V. (1962). *Biochim. Appl.* **9**, 53.

Manyai, S., and Varady, Z. (1956). *Biochim. Biophys. Acta* **20**, 594.

Marks, P. A., Johnson, A. B., Hirschberg, E., and Banks, J. (1958). *Ann. N. Y. Acad. Sci.* **75**, 95.

Massari, N., Guardamagna, C., and Bertolini, A. M. (1960a). *Giorn. Gerontol.* **8**, 21.

Massari, N., Guardamagna, C., and Tenconi, L. (1960b). *Giorn. Gerontol.* **8**, 155.

Mauri, C., and Torelli, V. (1959). *Klin Wochschr.* **37**, 769.

Metais, P., and Mandel, P. (1950). *Compt. Rend. Soc. Biol.* **144**, 277.

Micheli, A., and Grabar, P. (1961). *Ann. Inst. Pasteur* **100**, 569.

Miller, D. O., and Yoe, J. H. (1962). *Anal. Chim. Acta* **26**, 224.

Mills, G. C. (1960). *Texas Rept. Biol. Med.* **18**, 446.

Mircevova, L. (1958). *Acta Univ. Carolinae Med. 1958*, p. 793.

Morrison, M. (1961). *Nature* **189**, 765.

Morrison, W. L., and Neurath, H. (1953). *J. Biol. Chem.* **200**, 39.

Moskowitz, M., and Calvin, M. (1952). *Exptl. Cell. Res.* **3**, 33.

Moskowtiz, M., Dandliker, W. B., Calvin, M., and Evans, R. S. (1950). *J. Immunol.* **65**, 383.

Munn, J. I., and Crosby, W. H. (1961). *Brit. J. Haematol.* **7**, 523.

Nakagawa, S. (1960). *Okayama Igakkai Zasshi* **72**, 1695.

Nikkila, E. A., Pitkanen, E., Viropio, P., and Forsell, O. (1960). *Ann. Med. Intern. Fenniae* **49**, 187.

Noltmann, E., and Bruns, F. H. (1958). *Z. Physiol. Chem.* **313**, 194.

Nossal, P. M. (1948). *Australian J. Exptl. Biol. Med. Sci.* **26**, 123, 531, 533.

Ollgaard, E. (1961). *Thromb. Diath. Haemorrhag.* **6**, 68.

Osgood, E. E. (1935). *Arch. Internal. Med.* **56**, 849.

Overgaard-Hansen, K., and Jorgensen, S. (1960). *Scand. J. Clin. Lab. Invest.* **12**, 10.

Overman, R. R., and Davis, A. K. (1947). *J. Biol. Chem.* **168**, 641.

Panagopoulos, K., Kovatsis, A., and Karavouas, G. (1957). *Chronica, Spec. ed.* **63.**

Payva, C. A., Sendon, E., and Ortiz, R. (1961). *Bol. Soc. Quim. Peru* **27**, 179.
Pearson, P. B. (1941). *J. Biol. Chem.* **140**, 423.
Phillips, G. B., and Roome, N. S. (1962). *Proc. Soc. Exptl. Biol. Med.* **109**, 360.
Pitkanen, E., and Nikkila, E. A. (1960). *Ann. Med. Internae Fenniae* **49**, 197.
Portius, H. J., and Repke, K. (1960). *Arch. Exptl. Pathol. Pharmakol.* **239**, 184, 299.
Post, R. L., and Albright, C. D. (1961). *Membrane Transport Metab. Proc. Symp. Prague 1960*, p. 219.
Prankerd, T. A. J. (1956). *Intern. Rev. Cytol.* **5**, 279.
Prankerd, T. A. J. (1961–1962). *Folia Haematol.* **78**, 382.
Preiss, J., and Handler, P. (1958). *J. Biol. Chem.* **233**, 493.
Quarto di Palo, F. M., Gastoldi, L., and Bertolini, A. M. (1960). *Atti Accad. Med. Lombarda* **15**, 97.
Quastel, J. H., and Wheatley, A. H. M. (1931). *Biochem. J.* **25**, 117.
Quastel, J. H., and Wheatley, A. H. M. (1938). *Biochem. J.* **32**, 936.
Ramat, B., Ashkenazi, I., Reinon, A., Adam, A., and Sheba, C. (1961). *J. Clin. Invest.* **40**, 611.
Rapoport, S. (1961). *Folia Haematol.* **78**, 364.
Rapoport, S., and Luebering, J. (1951). *J. Biol. Chem.* **189**, 683.
Reed, L., and Denis, W. (1927). *J. Biol. Chem.* **73**, 623.
Rimington, C., and Booij, H. L. (1957). *J. Biol. Chem.* **3**, 65.
Roughton, F. J. W., and Rupp, J. C. (1958). *Ann. N. Y. Acad. Sci.* **75**, 156.
Rubenstein, D. (1952–1953). Ph.D. Thesis, McGill Univ., Montreal, Canada.
Rubino, G. F., Teso, G., and Rosetti, L. (1960). *Acta Haematol.* **24**, 300.
Sabine, J. C. (1940). *J. Clin. Invest.* **19**, 833.
Sabine, J. C. (1955). *Blood* **10**, 1132.
Sandberg, A. A., Hecht, H. H., and Tyler, F. H. (1953). *Metabolism* **2**, 22.
Sargent, F. (1947). *J. Biol. Chem.* **171**, 471.
Sawitsky, A., Fitch, H., and Meyer, L. M. (1948). *J. Lab. Clin. Med.* **33**, 203.
Schlegel, J. V. (1949). *Proc. Soc. Exptl. Biol. Med.* **70**, 695.
Scott, E. M. (1960). *J. Clin. Invest.* **39**, 1176.
Scott, E. M., and McGraw, J. C. (1962). *J. Biol. Chem.* **237**, 249.
Shields, G. S., Markowitz, H., Klassen, W. H., Cartwright, G. E., and Wintrobe, M. M. (1961). *J. Clin. Invest.* **40**, 2007.
Shinagawa, Y., and Ogura, M. (1961). *Kagaku (Tokyo)* **31**, 554.
Smith, L., Jr., Sullivan, M., and Huguley, C. M., Jr. (1961). *J. Clin. Invest.* **40**, 656.
Smits, G., and Florijn, E. (1949). *Biochim. Biophys. Acta* **3**, 44.
Sobel, A. E., Kraus, G., and Kramer, B. (1941). *J. Biol. Chem.* **140**, 501.
Somogyi, M. (1928). *J. Biol. Chem.* **78**, 117.
Steele, B. F., Reynolds, M. S., and Baumann, C. A. (1950). *J. Nutr.* **40**, 145.
Streef, G. M. (1939). *J. Biol. Chem.* **129**, 667.
Swarup, S., Ghosh, S. K., and Chatterjea, J. B. (1961). *Bull. Calcutta School Trop. Med.* **9**, 152.
Tada, K. (1961). *Tohoku J. Exptl. Med.* **75**, 263.
Tashian, R. C. (1961). *Proc. Soc. Exptl. Biol. Med.* **108**, 364.
Tropeano, L., Cacciola, E., and Ferranto, A. (1958). *Boll. Soc. Ital. Biol. Sper.* **34**, 1179.
Tsuboi, K. K., and Hudson, P. B. (1953). *Arch. Biochem. Biophys.* **43**, 399.
Tsuboi, K. K., and Hudson, P. B. (1954). *Arch. Biochem. Biophys.* **53**, 341.
Tsuboi, K. K., and Hudson, P. B. (1957). *J. Biol. Chem.* **224**, 879, 889.
Valentine, W. N., and Tanaka, K. R. (1961). *Acta Haematol.* **26**, 303.
Valentine, W. N., Tanaka, K. R., and Fredericks, R. E. (1961). *Am. J. Clin. Pathol.* **36**, 328.
Vallee, B. L., and Gibson, J. G. II (1948). *J. Biol. Chem.* **176**, 445.

Vanderheiden, B. S. (1961). *Biochem. Biophys. Res. Commun.* **6**, 117.

Van Slyke, D. D., Hiller, A., Weissiger, J. R., and Cruz, W. O. (1946). *J. Biol. Chem.* **166**, 121.

Vesell, E. S., and Bearn, A. G. (1961). *J. Clin. Invest.* **40**, 586.

Vincent, D., Segonzac, G., and Sesque, G. (1961). *Compt. Rend. Soc. Biol.* **155**, 662.

von Euler, H., and Heller, L. (1947). *Ark. Kemi.* **25A**, 10.

Waller, H. D., and Lohr, G. W. (1961–1962). *Folia Haematol.* **78**, 588.

Watson, C. J. (1950). *Arch. Internal Med.* **86**, 797.

Widdowson, E. M., and McCance, R. A. (1956). *Clin. Sci.* **15**, 361.

Wiss, O., and Kruger, R. (1948). *Helv. Chim. Acta* **31**, 1774.

Yachnin, S., and Gardner, F. H. (1961). *Brit. J. Haematol.* **7**, 464.

Yamadori, M. (1949). *Kitasato Arch. Exptl. Med.* **22**, 281.

Yamakawa, T., Irie, R., and Iwanaga, M. (1960). *J. Biochem.* (*Tokyo*) **48**, 490.

Yoshikawa, H., Nakao, M., Miyamoto, K., and Tachibana, M. (1960). *J. Biochem.* (*Tokyo*) **47**, 635.

Zak, B., Nalbandian, R. M., Williams, L. A., and Cohen, J. (1962). *Clin. Chim. Acta* **7**, 634.

CHAPTER 3

Ion and Water Permeability of the Red Blood Cell

Hermann Passow

I. Development of Present Concepts of Ion and Water Permeability in Red Cells

The basic information on the permeability of the red cell membrane to solutes and water was obtained by studies of its osmotic properties. The rates and magnitudes of the water movements, induced by transfer of the cells from plasma to solutions containing a test substance, were measured. In isotonic solutions of a large variety of solutes such as urea, ethylene glycol, glycerol, etc., the water content of the cells increased more or less rapidly and eventually hemolysis occurred (Gryns, 1896; Hedin, 1897, 1898). From such observations it was inferred that the membrane allows the passage of water and the examined substances. If, however, sucrose, mannitol, or electrolytes like NaCl were used as test substances, the cell volume increased in hypertonic and decreased in hypotonic solutions (Hamburger, 1902; Ege, 1922). A new steady state was quickly attained, and the volume changes in response to the variations in concentration (tonicity) of these substances could be calculated under the assumption that the cells behaved like nearly perfect osmometers. It was concluded that the erythrocyte membrane is impervious to sucrose and electrolytes, and that the water movements across the membrane lead to the establishment of osmotic equilibria between cells and media containing nonpenetrating solutes.

On closer examination it became apparent that the membrane was also permeable to at least the anions of an electrolyte. Shortly after Arrhenius (1887) discovered electrolytic dissociation, the famous "chloride shift," the one-to-one exchange of chloride with bicarbonate across the cell membrane, was described (Hamburger, 1891, von Limbeck, 1895); soon afterwards it was shown that during the process of "anion exchange" virtually no net cation movements take place (Gürber, 1895; Doisy and Eaton, 1921; Mukai, 1921). One could therefore attribute to the red cell membrane the property of selective anion permeability (Koeppe, 1897).

In ordinary electrolyte solutions, the negative and positive charges of anions and cations balance each other. There are no net charges present in the solutions and they appear electrically neutral. It is generally assumed that electroneutrality obtains also in biological fluids, and studies were undertaken to establish the chemical nature of the anions and cations balancing each other in red cells and plasma. Besides the nonpenetrating phosphoric acid esters, the highly negatively charged hemoglobin was also found to contribute appreciably to this balance in spite of its low concentration on a molar basis. It was realized (Warburg, 1922; Barcroft *et al.*, 1922) that in the presence of nondiffusible anions the equilibrium distribution of the diffusible anions can be predicted on the basis of the thermodynamic theory of membrane equilibria developed by Donnan in 1911. Van Slyke *et al.* (1923) derived an equation describing the relationship between the composition of the medium and the ion distribution across a membrane permeable to water and small anions like Cl^-, HCO_3^-, and OH^-, and impermeable to cations and a limited number of anions, such as negatively charged proteins. The calculations were based on three assumptions:

(1) Electroneutrality on both sides of the membrane.
(2) Donnan equilibrium of diffusible anions.
(3) Osmotic equilibrium.

The validity and applicability of their calculations have, in the main, been confirmed by the work of many subsequent investigators (Van Slyke *et al.*, 1925; Hastings *et al.*, 1928; Harkins and Hastings, 1931; Dill *et al.*, 1937; Rapoport and Guest, 1939; Fitzsimons and Sendroy, 1961).

The establishment of Donnan equilibria for diffusible ion species depends solely on the presence of nondiffusible ions, regardless of whether the latter are confined to the inside of the cell either by a membrane or by attachment to an immobile protoplasmic jelly. An explanation of the selective anion permeability depends therefore on the question of whether or not the red cell is surrounded by an effective permeability barrier. Among the many arguments in favor of the existence of such a barrier, an especially interesting one was contributed by Höber (1910, 1913). Using alternating currents of high frequency, he measured the internal conductivity of intact red cells and found its value similar to that of 0.1–0.5 isotonic NaCl solution. Since electrostatic interactions with the highly charged hemoglobin molecules are likely to reduce the conductivity coefficient of the small ions present in the cell interior (c.f. Schwan, 1957), these and similar results of other authors (Fricke and Morse, 1926; Fricke and Curtis, 1935; Cook, 1952; Schwan, 1957, Pauly and Schwan, 1958) were considered to be satisfactory evidence for the absence of appreciable binding of KCl to cell proteins. Consequently the large concentration gradients for K^+ and Na^+ between the inside and outside of the cell could be explained only by postulating the existence of a cation-impermeable membrane.

In view of the latter observations and other relevant evidence, it was asked how the red cell membrane discriminates between small cations and anions of similar size. At the time when this problem began to attract general attention, Michaelis and Fugita (1925) and Michaelis and Perlzweig (1927) had just published their now famous studies on the selective cation permeability of collodion membranes. They assumed that cations penetrate through water-filled channels across the membrane, whereas anions are prevented from passing by the presence of cations adsorbed inside the pores. Impressed by their results, Mond tried to find out whether Michaelis' concepts of the nature of selectivity could be applied to the red cell membrane as well. By incorporating basic dyes into collodion, he first showed (1928) that selective anion permeability could also be demonstrated in artificial membranes. Mond concluded that fixed charges instead of adsorbed ions would also be capable of rendering a membrane selectively permeable, and suggested that the amino groups of proteins may play a role in the erythrocyte membrane similar to that of basic dyes in collodion. Since amino groups are dissociable, their concentration ought to decrease at increasing pH values, and the normally positively charged membrane proteins should be left with a negative net charge. Consequently, raising the pH of the medium must lead to reduction in the rate of anion permeability, until the isoelectric point has been exceeded whereupon the membrane should become impermeable to anions and permeable to cations. Mond (1927) actually discovered drastic diminution in the rate of anion exchange at high pH values, and above pH 8.1 even observed rapid potassium loss.

The use of Michaelis' theory for the explanation of selective anion permeability tacitly assumes that anions penetrate through water-filled channels. The fact that many hydrophilic molecules readily pass the cell membrane was taken as evidence by Mond and Hoffmann (1928) for the existence of "pores." They tried to obtain information on the dimensions of the pores by studying the permeability to hydrophilic probing molecules of varying size. Erythritol and substances of similar or lower molar volume were found to penetrate easily through the membrane, whereas bigger molecules including glucose and sucrose were observed to penetrate much more slowly or not at all. It was inferred that the red cell membrane possesses pores of molecular dimensions and thus fulfills another essential requirement of Michaelis' theory. This conclusion was supported by the observation of Jacobs *et al.* (1936) that the temperature coefficient (Q_{10}) for water transfer through the red cell membrane is close to 1.3, a value to be expected if water moves by viscous flow through pores.

Mond's suggestions concerning the nature of the anion permeability were initially accepted enthusiastically, but later met with increasing criticism. His observation of a reversal of the selectivity of the membrane above pH 8.1 could not be confirmed by Danielli and Davson (1936), who measured net potassium movements at various pH values in cells suspended in buffered saline solutions. On account of their results, Mond's theory was largely abandoned. Wilbrandt (1940a) later pointed out that Mond had performed his experiments with red cells suspended in nonelectrolyte solutions and that—as was discovered by Davson (1939) and Maizels (1935) and confirmed by Wilbrandt—under these conditions, red cells may become permeable to K^+ regardless of the pH employed. In isotonic solutions of low electrolyte content, the Donnan distribution of anions markedly deviates from normal and the red cell interior, which is normally negative with respect to the medium, becomes positive. Davson and Wilbrandt therefore assumed that the reversal of potential increases the driving force by the concentration difference of K^+ between the inside and outside of the cell, and thus forces K^+ to leak out.

Since it is difficult to explain the normally observed selective anion permeability of a porous membrane without assuming the existence of fixed positive charges, Wilbrandt (1942a, b) still maintained that such charges played a major part in governing the ion permeability of the red cell membrane. Stimulated by the well-known theoretical considerations of Teorell (1935) and Meyer and Sievers (1936), he made extensive calculations on the interrelationship between diffusion potentials, fixed charges, and rates of anion exchange across the red cell membrane. He emphasized that complete impermeability to cations does not exist, unless the concentration of fixed charges approaches infinity. Since any exchange of sodium with potassium across the membrane is necessarily associated with water uptake, which will eventually lead to colloid osmotic hemolysis, Wilbrandt suggested that the life span of the red cell is limited by the rate of cation passage through a membrane of imperfect selectivity.

Wilbrandt realized, however, that other factors besides fixed charges must play an important role in maintaining the unequal cation distribution between cells and medium. Ørskov (1935) demonstrated a drastic increase in K^+ permeability by minute amounts of lead and other heavy metals; Davson (1940) published observations on the effects of anesthetics on sodium permeability of cat red cells, which hardly fitted into the concept of a fixed charge model of the red cell membrane. Wilbrandt (1937,1940b) discovered that human red cells poisoned with fluoride lost their impermeability to cations, and he drew the important conclusion that the resistance the membrane offers to the diffusion of cations may diminish under abnormal metabolic conditions. Although this work received much attention, it was only recently resumed (Eckel, 1958; Lindemann and Passow, 1960c) and extended by other workers (Kregenow and Hoffman, 1962; Passow, 1961), who tried to accumulate evidence for a metabolic control of passive cation permeability.

With the discovery of active transport, the question of pores, fixed charges, and metabolic control of diffusion processes received much less attention. Shortly after radioisotopes became available, it was found that the red cell membrane is permeable to cations in spite of the persistence of large concentration gradients (Dean *et al.*, 1941; Mullins *et al.*, 1941). In human red cells, 50% each of cellular K and Na was found to exchange within about 43 hours (Raker *et al.*, 1950; Sheppard and Martin, 1950) and 20 hours (Solomon, 1952), respectively, and similar data were obtained with red cells of many other animal species (Sheppard *et al.*, 1951). These results could not be reconciled with the assumption that Na^+ and K^+ of cells and plasma are at thermodynamic equilibrium, since with a membrane freely permeable to both anions and cations, the establishment of a Donnan equilibrium would inevitably result in colloid osmotic hemolysis. Therefore, in order to explain an ion exchange without concomitant net movements across the membrane, one had to assume that the unequal distribution of at least one ion species between cells and medium is the result of a balance between two processes: active transport against and passive diffusion down an electrochemical potential gradient.

It had been suggested that only sodium ions were actively extruded, and that it is the unequal distribution of these ions only which determines the equilibrium position for the passively penetrating K ions (Maizels, 1949). However, in contrast to the requirements of the Donnan theory, the distribution ratio of neither K nor Na is inversely related to those of the anions. One had to conclude, therefore, that both alkali metal ion species are actively transported.

Under steady state conditions, the time course of the diminution in concentration of labeled cations in plasma could be approximately fitted to a single exponential curve (Raker *et al.*, 1950; Sheppard and Martin, 1950, Solomon, 1952). This could be readily explained by assuming the existence of only two compartments in the system: two solutions separated by an infinitely thin rate-limiting membrane.

With the increasing accuracy of the experimental methods employed, more or less pronounced deviations from this simple behavior were detected (Gold and Solomon, 1955; Solomon and Gold, 1955). In order to evalute these data, additional assumptions regarding the nature of the factors governing cation permeability in red cells were introduced into the mathematical treatment of isotope exchange reactions. The influence of the heterogeneity of the cell population with respect to size or cation content of individual cells was considered (Sheppard and Householder, 1951), as well as the effects of the existence of more than two compartments in each cell (e.g. a membrane with finite capacity to bind cations would be an additional compartment) on the kinetics of K^{42} and Na^{24} movements (for summary see Solomon, 1960a). The solution of Fick's second law for diffusion in convection-free media yields mathematical expressions (series of exponentials) similar to those reported to be adequate for describing actual observations on red cells. It was therefore suggested that certain deviations from the kinetics expected for a two compartment system may be explained simply by the slow rate of diffusion through the convection-free interior of the cell (Harris and Prankerd, 1958).[1]

The rate of cation transfer across the membrane, the concentration ratios of Na^+ and K^+, and the anion distribution ratios (allowing estimation of the membrane potential) being known, it was possible to calculate the minimum energy the cell must provide for maintenance of the nonequilibrium distribution of the cations. Applying a formula first used by Ussing (1949b),[2] the energy necessary to transfer ions across concentration and potential gradients was calculated by Solomon (1952), who found that human erythrocytes must expend about 9 cal./liter cells/hr. for maintenance of a Na^+ flux of 3.1 meq./liter cells/hr. and a K^+ flux of 1.7 meq./liter cells/hr. They metabolize some 2.3 mmoles glucose/liter cells/hr., thereby liberating about 110 cal./liter cells/hr. Hence only about 8% of the total metabolic energy is required for active transport.

At the same time that the foregoing studies on the kinetics of cation transport were undertaken, the question was raised as to what part of red cell metabolism supplies the energy for active cation transport. Such investigations

[1] It appears unlikely that the diffusion in the red cell interior is rate-limiting. As has been pointed out by Harris and Prankerd themselves, small anions like Cl^- or HCO_3^-, having diffusion coefficients similar to those of K^+ and Na^+ may reach diffusion equilibrium at the red cell membrane within about $1/10^6$ the time necessary for the cation exchange. Moreover, the isotopically measured exchange with sulfate ions follows a single exponential as closely as the conventional methods employed enable one to determine (Passow, 1961).

[2] The equation used by Solomon (1952) applies strictly only to systems far from equilibrium. For more general cases the following equation should be used:

$$\dot{w} = \dot{n}[1 - \exp(-zF\Delta\psi/RT)]RT \ln C_i/C_o + zF\Delta\psi)$$

where $\dot{w}$ = osmotic work in cal./min./kg. cells, $\dot{n}$ = isotopically measured unidirectional flux, and z = valency. The other symbols have the usual meaning. This equation allows for the fact that only the passive *net* movements of an ion have to be compensated for by active transport, and not the *total* unidirectional passive flux which is usually measured with isotopes.

began with Harris' (1941) discovery that the interruption of metabolism by cooling cells to 4°C. induces K loss and Na uptake. These ion movements are readily reversed after rewarming and addition of suitable substrates, whence sodium and potassium ions migrate against the electrochemical potential gradient. The most important energy-supplying substrates for this accumulation process are glucose (Maizels, 1951) and nucleosides such as adenosine or inosine (Harris and Prankerd, 1955; Gabrio *et al.*, 1955). In mature erythrocytes these substances are metabolized almost entirely by anaerobic processes with lactic acid as an end product. While glucose is metabolized via the well-known glycolytic pathway, the nucleosides are phosphorolytically cleaved (Huennekens *et al.*, 1956; Tsuboi and Hudson, 1957). The resulting pentose phosphate is converted to fructose phosphate and triose phosphate and thus enters the glycolytic reaction sequence (Dische, 1951; Dische *et al.*, 1960; Dische and Iglas, 1961; Bruns *et al.*, 1958). Inhibitors of glycolysis, like NaF or iodoacetate, suppress active transport while substances which poison the respiration of cells, like CN, azide, or dinitrophenol, are ineffective (Flynn and Maizels, 1949).

In summary, the following basic concepts of the water and ion permeability of erythrocytes have emerged in the course of the last 70 years:

The water and anion distribution between cells and media tends to approach a thermodynamic equilibrium at a rapid rate. The equilibrium conditions are determined by a porous membrane carrying fixed positive charges. Its imperfect selectivity to cations is balanced by active transport. Changes in the cell metabolism may affect the cation distribution in two ways: (1) by varying the energy supply for active transport against the electrochemical gradient, and (2) by altering the membrane resistance to passive diffusion.

On the whole, these concepts provide a useful framework for arranging the diversity of newer facts and theories of red cell permeability presented below.

II. Factors Controlling Distribution of Water and Electrolytes between Cells and Media of Varying Composition

A surprisingly large number of distribution phenomena observed in short-term experiments can be explained by the simplifying assumption that the membrane is readily permeable to water and certain but not all solutes, and that the penetrating substances attain a thermodynamic equilibrium distribution before measurable net movements of other substances present occur. This depends on the particular experimental conditions which define the solutes that are prevented from passing. For example in the intact red cell, anions penetrate or even 10^6—10^7 times faster than cations, and it may therefore be reasonable, as a first approximation, to consider the membrane permeable to anions and impermeable to cations. In the presence of certain agents like fluoride or lead, the membrane becomes highly permeable to K^+ but remains nearly as impermeable to Na^+ as in the normal state. With sublytic doses of suitable hemolytic agents, the membrane is rendered permeable to both K^+ and Na^+. A fairly general treatment of the ionic and osmotic equilibria at selectively permeable membranes can be given, and is readily adapted to special assumptions regarding the permeability to various solutes present in the system if the following propositions are made:

(a) the chemical potential of water is the same on both sides of the membrane, i.e.:

$$\mu_{H_2O_i} = \mu_{H_2O_o} \qquad \text{(osmotic equilibrium)}$$

(b) the chemical (μ) or electrochemical ($\bar{\mu}$) potential of each penetrating solute is the same on both sides of the membrane, e.g.:

$$\bar{\mu}_{Cl_i} = \bar{\mu}_{Cl_o}; \qquad \bar{\mu}_{HCO_{3i}} = \bar{\mu}_{HCO_{3o}}; \qquad \text{etc.}$$

or more generally

$$\bar{\mu}_{aji} = \bar{\mu}_{ajo}; \qquad \bar{\mu}_{bki} = \bar{\mu}_{bko} \qquad \text{(Donnan equilibrium)}$$

where the aj's and bk's refer to the jth anion and the kth cation species respectively.

These assumptions are supplemented by the obvious restriction that:

(c) the electrical balance between anions and cations is always maintained

$$\sum^{j} z_j a_j + \sum^{k} z_k b_k = 0 \qquad \text{(electroneutrality)}$$

Although the erythrocyte membrane is permeable to cations, their distribution obeys the Donnan law only under certain abnormal conditions. Nevertheless, any variation in composition of the medium leading to changes in cell volume or anion distribution ratios alters the driving forces for the cations, and thereby affects the balance between active transport and passive diffusion. Slow redistribution of the cations is thus induced which eventually leads to establishment of a new stationary state. This process, in turn, produces a shift in the water and anion equilibrium which originally brought about the redistribution of cations. Hence, if the period of experimental observation is sufficiently long, these events cannot be neglected and allowance must be made for them by introducing suitable assumptions about the conditions governing the stationary cation distribution. Tosteson and Hoffman (1960), who dealt with this situation, presume that:

(d) water and penetrating anions are at thermodynamic equilibrium in the system, i.e. propositions (a) and (b) remain valid, and

(e) in the stationary state, the flux ratios of passive K^+ and Na^+ movements conform to the Ussing equation (Ussing, 1949a, b):

$$\frac{m_{\text{in}}}{m_{\text{out}}} = \bar{\mu}_i - \bar{\mu}_o$$

It should be noted that the use of these equations does not refine the treatment based on assumptions (a)–(c). Instead, it allows one to deal with the special case in which the measurements are made after the cation permeability has attained a new steady state.

For the actual calculations, the differences of the standard chemical potentials for water and each diffusible solute on both sides of the membrane are usually assumed to be zero. This assumption is justified if the system is isothermal and the pressure difference between cells and medium can be neglected. Although the existence of pressure differences cannot wholly be excluded, the mechanical strength of the membrane would seem to be insufficient to allow the development of pressure differences large enough to affect measurably the distribution equilibrium.

Now assumptions (a)–(e) may be rewritten using the more conventional quantities, concentration and activity, instead of chemical potential. In addition, the activity of water is expressed in terms of osmolarity of the solute.

Osmotic equilibrium:

$$\frac{1}{V}\sum^{g} g_{xg} X_g + \sum^{k} g_{ik} b_{ik} + \sum^{j} g_{ij} a_{ij} = \sum^{k} g_{ok} b_{ok} + \sum^{j} g_{oj} a_{oj} + \sum^{l} g_{ol} M_{ol} \qquad (1)$$

Electroneutrality:

$$\frac{1}{V}\sum^{n} z_n Y_n + \sum^{k} b_{ik} - \sum^{j} a_{ij} = 0 \qquad (2)$$

Donnan equilibrium:

$$f_{a1}\frac{a_{i1}}{a_{o1}} = f_{a2}\frac{a_{i2}}{a_{o2}} = \ldots = f_{aj}\frac{a_{ij}}{a_{oj}} = r$$
$$f_{b1}\frac{b_{i1}}{b_{o1}} = f_{b2}\frac{b_{i2}}{b_{o2}} = \ldots = f_{bk}\frac{b_{ik}}{b_{ok}} = \frac{1}{r} \qquad (3)$$

Ussing equation:

$$\frac{m_{\text{in}1}\cdot f_{o1}\cdot b_{o1}}{m_{\text{out}1}\cdot f_{i1}\cdot b_{i1}} = \frac{m_{\text{in}2}\cdot f_{o2}\cdot b_{o2}}{m_{\text{out}2}\cdot f_{i2}\cdot b_{i2}} = \ldots = \frac{m_{\text{in}\,k}\cdot f_{ok}\cdot b_{ok}}{m_{\text{out}k}\cdot f_{ik}\cdot b_{ik}} = r \qquad (4)$$

EXPLANATION OF SYMBOLS

X_g = amount of indiffusible ions or molecules of g'th species

g_{Xg} = osmotic coefficient of X_g

b_{ik}, b_{ok} = concentration of diffusible cations of kth species within or outside the cells, respectively

g_{ik}, g_{ok} = osmotic coefficient of b_{ik} and k_{ok}, respectively
a_{ij}, a_{oj} = concentration of diffusible anions of jth species within or outside the cells, respectively
g_{ij}, g_o = osmotic coefficient of a_{ij} and a_{oj}, respectively
M_{ol} = concentration of indiffusible nonelectrolyte of lth species outside the cells.
Y_n = amount of nonpenetrating ions of nth species inside the cells
z_n = valency of Y_n (positive for cations, negative for anions)
f_{bk}, f_{aj} = ratio of activity coefficients f_{ik}/f_{ok} of diffusible cations (anions) of kth (jth) species inside and outside the cells
$m_{\text{in}\,k}, m_{\text{out}\,k}$ = passive influx and outflux of kth cation species
V = volume of cell water

Combining these equations allows the elimination of the concentrations of all diffusible intracellular ion species, and the calculation of cell volume and distribution ratios from extracellular concentrations and the constant amounts of nonpenetrating substances (provided their state of ionization is known) inside the cells. The general solution for short-term experiments where the membrane must be considered impermeable to cations or where, besides the anions, a limited number or all of the cations present also attain a true (i.e. Donnan) equilibrium, has been derived by Jacobs and Stewart (1947). Tosteson and Hoffman (1960), on the other hand, dealt with the other special case where the cations reached a new stationary nonequilibrium state after the composition of the medium had been changed. Both groups of authors were content to predict the nature and the order of magnitude of the observed effects, and made no attempt to elaborate their mathematical treatment by taking into account the deviations of isotonic electrolyte solutions from ideal behavior.

Since a more general description of water and electrolyte distribution between cells and media necessarily rests on the above assumptions, emphasis in the following pages is on discussion of quantitative studies undertaken in order to test their validity. Subsequently, the simplified theories of Jacobs and Stewart, and of Tosteson and Hoffman, will be outlined and some special cases frequently encountered in experimental work with red cells will be presented.

A. Osmotic Equilibrium

The osmotic properties of the red cells have been studied mainly under conditions in which the distribution of anions and water, but not that of the cations, attained a new steady state. Measurements of freezing point depression or vapor pressure lowering have been employed, and volume changes in response to variations in osmotic pressure of the medium have been measured.

Although it has occasionally been claimed that the water distribution between tissue cells and medium depends on metabolic factors (Aebi, 1952; Bartley *et al.*, 1954; Opie, 1954; Robinson, 1953) and that large osmotic gradients across the membrane of animal cells can be maintained, there is a wealth of evidence showing that if such differences exist, they can be only very small. The freezing point depression (or thawing point) of red cells and whole blood were found to be equal by Tammann (1896) and Hedin (1897, 1898), and these early observations were later confirmed by a large number of investigators (e.g. Hamburger, 1897; Collins and Scott, 1932; Hill and Kupalov, 1930; the latter authors measured vapor pressure lowering). Applying very sensitive techniques, many authors observed the freezing point depression of whole blood or whole blood plus saline to be slightly less after hemolyzing the cells in their own surrounding fluid than previously. This difference increased upon addition of nonpenetrating substances to the medium but was unaffected by addition of penetrating solutes (urea), regardless of the final osmolarity reached (Williams *et al.*, 1959). These findings were not regarded as incompatible with the hypothesis that red cells remain in osmotic equilibrium with their surroundings. It was suggested that the results merely reflect the decrease in the osmotic coefficient of hemoglobin which takes place if the cell content is diluted upon hemolysis (Roepke and Baldes, 1942; Williams *et al.*, 1959).

These contentions were supported by measurements of red cell volume in media of varying tonicity. Combining (1) and (2) and neglecting deviations of the osmotic coefficients from unity, the following equation relating cell volume to external concentrations may be derived:

$$V = W\left(\frac{1}{T}-1\right)+1 \tag{5}$$

where V = cell volume in percent of its value in isotonic solution, W = water content of the cells at $T = 1$, and T = tonicity (osmolarity of medium in percent of the osmolarity of an isotonic solution).

The straight line relationship, which according to Eq. (5) should obtain if the volume is plotted against the reciprocal of tonicity, was actually observed but the slope was found to be slightly smaller than expected. To account for this deviation, Ponder introduced the empirical constant R:

$$V = RW\left(\frac{1}{T}-1\right)+1 \tag{6}$$

R values were estimated by many authors with a variety of different methods: hematocrit (Ørskov, 1946; Guest, 1948; Ponder, 1950), dilution of nonpenetrating substances like Evan's blue (Ponder, 1944) or plasma proteins (Hendry, 1954), diffractometry (Ponder, 1951a), and immersion refractometry (Dick and Lowenstein, 1958), to mention some of the more accurate ones (for a more complete compilation of older data see Ponder, 1948). The most reliable values for corpuscles from heparinized blood suspended in saline solution or diluted plasma lie in the range 0.9–1.0. In the small range of tonicities used, any tonicity-dependent variation of R would have been obscured by inaccuracies of the techniques employed for measuring red cell volume. It seems possible, however, that R decreases at decreasing tonicities (Ørskov, 1946).

Several possible explanations for the physical meaning of the factor R have been discussed by Ponder (1948, 1955), Dick and Lowenstein (1958), and others:

(1) Leakage of ions from red cells into the medium.
(2) Binding of water of solvation to red cell proteins.
(3) The concentration dependence of the osmotic coefficient of hemoglobin.
(4) A rigidity of cell membrane which may resist changes in volume.

These will now be discussed briefly:

(1) Any leakage of ions from the cell into the hypotonic media would reduce the amount of osmotically active substances inside the cell and thus diminish the value of R. Although potassium leaves the cell in the absence of substrates, the amount lost during the 1–2 hours of experimental observation is far too small to account for the observed deviation from the simplified formula. Moreover, any K loss is largely balanced by the uptake of an almost equivalent amount of sodium ions from the medium.

(2) V in Eq. (5) is the volume of the solvent and not that of the solution. If part of the cell water should be bound to the cell protein as water of solvation, W of Eq. (5) (i.e., the cell water available to act as solvent either to the macromolecules themselves, or to the other small molecular solutes) is reduced. Correspondingly, R would assume values less than 1.0. Drabkin (1950), who measured the water-binding capacity of hemoglobin, assumes that about 16% of the red cell water is not available for dissolving solutes. Hutchinson (1952), on the other hand, found that C^{14}-labeled alcohols or H_2O^{18} rapidly equilibrate with the red cell interior and that all the cell water acts as "free" water with respect to these substances. In view of these divergent results, it should be emphasized that the bound water concept depends on the sense in which this term is used. Following Dick and Lowenstein (1958), it seems most reasonable to assume that the question of bound water is in fact only one aspect of explanation (3), since the water of solvation may drastically affect the osmotic coefficients of the solutes.

(3) Williams *et al.* and Dick and Lowenstein suggest in the papers cited that the osmotic "anomalies" of red cells are mainly due to an exceptionally large concentration dependence of the osmotic coefficient of hemoglobin.

The osmotic coefficient of many proteins, including hemoglobin (Adair, 1928), rises sharply with concentration. Although the hemoglobin concentration in erythrocytes is only 5 mM, its partial osmotic pressure lies at 17.5 mOsm., corresponding to an osmotic coefficient of about 3.55, thus contributing measurably to the total intracellular osmolarity of about 300 mOsm.

After transfer of the cells from an isotonic to a hypotonic medium, when the intracellular hemoglobin concentration falls due to swelling of the cells, a decrease in its osmotic coefficient occurs. At low tonicities, where the "critical" hemolytic volume is nearly reached, the osmotic coefficient may assume a value of about 2.0 instead of the previous 3.5. This decrease in the contribution of hemoglobin to the total osmolarity of the cell makes the apparent cell water content, as determined by measurements of osmotic equilibria, appear smaller than the water content estimated by direct methods. Dick and Lowenstein (1958) could show that this effect explains most of the deviations of the osmotic behavior of red cells from the simplified formula, and calculated from Adair's data that, in the range of tonicities used in their experiments, R should vary slightly with tonicity and assume values between 0.93 and 0.97. These figures are to be compared with the experimentally observed R values which lie in the range 0.9–1.0.

Obviously, the described changes in the osmotic coefficient of hemoglobin are even more pronounced if the cell content is diluted by hemolysis. This may easily explain the differences in freezing points of blood containing intact or hemolyzed cells, referred to above.

Although the results described leave little doubt of the preeminence of the hemoglobin in producing the osmotic "abnormalities" of the red cells, one should not forget that in the above treatment the osmotic coefficients of other intracellular solutes have been neglected, and that especially in concentrated protein solutions they also might exhibit unexpected features and measurably affect the osmotic behavior of the cell.

(4) However, certain observations on the osmotic properties of red cell "ghosts" are difficult to interpret in terms of the above hypothesis. In this context the view that the membrane exerts some elastic forces which may counteract the tendency to swell has received some attention.

Red cells that have lost most of their hemoglobin during osmotic hemolysis ("ghosts") regain a high degree of impermeability to cations and continue to exhibit osmotic phenomena. Ponder (1955) and especially Teorell (1952), who thoroughly studied the volume changes of "ghosts" in media of varying tonicity, observed that their behavior may conform even less well to the simplified osmotic law (Eq. 5) than that of whole cells. Teorell was able to fit his data to an empirical equation which contains in addition to b, the nonsolvent volume (which is equal to $1-W$ in Ponder's notation as used above), an additional constant:

$$(T+a)(V-b) = \text{const.} \tag{7}$$

Due to the positive term a, V assumes smaller values than expected from the simplified Eq. (5) even if allowance is made for the nonsolvent volume of the cell. This equation has a somewhat similar mathematical structure to the van der Waals equation. Teorell points out, therefore, that his constant "*a*" shows a certain formal correspondence to the van der Waals *Binnendruck* term, and this led him to discuss the possibility that it represents a measure of elastic forces or a certain rigidity of form which opposes osmotic swelling. Dick and Lowenstein severely criticized Teorell's interpretation of the constant "*a*." They lost sight, however, of the fact that Teorell was as well aware of the limitation of the applicability of the van der Waals equation to his system as they themselves. Teorell only wanted to show that the assumption of an elastic membrane offers a simple but not necessarily convincing explanation for the "abnormal" behavior of hemoglobin-poor ghosts, where concentration-dependent changes in osmotic activity of the remaining intracellular hemoglobin seem to be of little consequence.

B. Donnan Equilibrium

A critical examination of the validity of the Donnan theory requires the measurement of ion activity ratios between cells and media. Unfortunately, however, it is not yet possible, contrary to the situation with nerve or muscle, to insert electrodes sensitive to H^+, K^+, Na^+, or Cl^- into red cells for determination of the activities of these ion species. All that can be achieved is to measure the concentration ratios by analyzing cell contents, or to measure the pH in concentrated hemolysates. Obviously, an accurate estimate of the applicability of the Donnan theory cannot be achieved in this way. Nevertheless, the qualitative agreement of the concentration ratios of penetrating intracellular and extracellular anions, and especially their variation with varying composition of the media, leave little doubt about the usefulness of the Donnan concept. Thus, conforming to the theory, equilibration of blood with added chloride or bicarbonate does not change the similarity of the distribution ratios Cl_i/Cl_o and HCO_{3i}/HCO_{3o}. Moreover, variation in the blood pH, either by oxygenation of the hemoglobin or by adding acid or base, shifts the distribution ratios of all penetrating anion species to the same extent and in a direction that can be easily predicted by applying the Donnan theory to a system where the degree of ionization of indiffusible intracellular anions varies (e.g. Fitzsimons and Sendroy, 1961). Even metabolic changes leading to reduction in the intracellular content of nonpenetrating phosphoric acid esters are reflected by those shifts of the anion distribution which were to be expected from the Donnan theory (Rapoport and Guest, 1939).

A quantitative treatment of the various situations described still presents formidable difficulties, since only little is known about the activity coefficients of electrolytes in the red cell interior. Moreover, in work with weak acids such as H_2CO_3 or H_3PO_4, the calculation of the distribution ratios for the ion species HCO_3^-, $H_2PO_4^-$, and HPO_4^{--} depends decisively on the use of correct values for the apparent dissociation constants in the cell interior. In many cases, as with H_2CO_3 which forms carbamates with hemoglobin, this estimate is affected by the information available about chemical reactions with cell constituents. It is not surprising therefore that the original data of Van Slyke and coworkers (1923, 1925) on the OH^-, Cl^-, and HCO_3^- distribution were repeatedly recalculated and supplemented by studies employing more refined techniques (Rapoport and Guest, 1939; Fitzsimons and Sendroy, 1961). The latter authors observed the following Donnan ratios under a large variety of different experimental conditions:

$$\frac{\alpha H_o}{\alpha H_i} = 0.92\frac{Cl_i}{Cl_o} = 0.93\frac{HCO_{3i}}{HCO_{3o}}$$

Further examples of similar ratios for systems containing sulfate and phosphate ions have been discussed in the literature and will be presented later. (Figs. 1 and 4).

The factors 1.0, 0.92, and 0.93 are generally attributed to differences between activity and concentration ratios. It is rather surprising how small the differences between the distribution ratios for the three ion species are and, instead of looking for an explanation for their existence, it seems more interesting to ask why they are not larger than actually observed.

It is known that the activity coefficients of monovalent ions in isotonic saline are some 20–30% lower than unity, and that under these conditions individual properties of the different ion species become apparent. Thus the similarity of their distribution ratios is most reasonably explained by assuming that for each ion species the activity coefficients for the cell interior and the outside essentially cancel each other. This explanation is not quite self-evident since the ionic strength of the cell interior, which contains polyvalent ions in fairly high concentrations, should be higher by an unknown amount than the ionic strength of the usual immersion media. Moreover, although it has been observed that hemoglobin in dilute solution exerts only little influence on the activity coefficients of monovalent anions and cations like K^+ (Carr, 1953a; Morris and Wright, 1954; Battley and Klotz, 1951) and Cl^- (Carr, 1953b), no factual information on ionic interactions in highly concentrated hemoglobin solution is available. In addition, the effects of intracellular phosphoric acid esters, amino acids, and peptides are difficult to appraise.

Overbeck (1956) has pointed out that the formation of ion clouds is greatly diminished at high concentrations of a polyelectrolyte. The electrical fields of neighboring polyelectrolyte ions overlap, the tendency of the diffusible ions to cluster around widely separated charged particles is thus diminished, and consequently, in spite of a high concentration of charged macromolecules, the activity coefficients of small ions will resume nearly normal values. Even these considerations provide at best some qualitative evidence for a similarity of the activity coefficients inside and outside the cells. It is known, however, that the values for the activity coefficients of monovalent ions pass through a minimum at ionic strengths similar to those of isotonic saline solutions. Consequently, in this concentration range, small changes in ionic strength should be of only little influence on the activity coefficients. This may largely account for the close similarity of the concentration and activity ratios.

In this connection, reference must be made to the view of Donnan and Guggenheim (1932), who maintained that the use of individual ion activity coefficients is not permissible. They pointed out that the measurement of the individual coefficients—which always involves the use of KCl bridges—is influenced to an unknown extent by diffusion potentials. The uncertainties should be particularly great in polyelectrolyte solutions where, as has been emphasized by Overbeck, large diffusion potentials may arise at the liquid junction, if the concentration of the polyelectrolyte and the ionic strength at the low concentration side are small. However, so long as OH distribution ratios are determined by conventional glass electrode systems, the elimination of these uncertainties would be of little help in interpreting biological data.

At first glance, one of the most severe limitations of all examinations of the Donnan theory is the failure so far of all attempts to measure the membrane potential of red cells with KCl-filled microelectrodes. The Donnan concept rests on the assumption that the diffusion of cations down their electrochemical gradients does not appreciably contribute to the transmembrane potential. However, since anions such as Cl^- pass about 1,000,000 times faster through the membrane than do the cations, there seems to be no factual evidence at present for assuming large deviations of the anion distribution from a true Donnan equilibrium.

C. The Ussing Equation

The validity of Ussing's flux equation for describing the stationary cation distribution depends entirely on the applicability of the independence principle to the cation movements across the red cell membrane. Only if the opposing cation fluxes do not interact may Ussing's equation be applied.The evidence for and against the usefulness of this principle in the case of red cells is still meager, and its discussion will be postponed to a later section on the kinetics of cation movements. So far this equation may be considered as a means of illustrating what effects the establishment of new steady states may have on osmotic properties and ion distribution ratios of red cells.

D. Ion and Water Distribution in Complex Media

The main conclusion that can be drawn from the previous sections is that, due to a balance between various counteracting influences, deviations of the ionic and osmotic equilibria from ideal behavior are noted, but are not large enough to invalidate the usefulness of formulas where the osmotic and activity coefficients are set equal to 1.0. Until more information is available on ionic interactions in the cell interior, such simplified formulas may help to predict, in a semiquantitative way, the ion distribution ratios and cell volumes that will be attained in a variety of media by intact and experimentally modified cells.

By assuming the g's and f's to be equal to 1.0, one can derive from Eqs. (1)–(4) the set of formulas presented in Table I. Equations (8) and (9) describe the water and anion distribution in short-term experiments, Eqs. (8) and (8a) for a membrane exclusively permeable to anions, and Eqs. (9) and (9a) for membranes which allow, in addition to anions, the passage of K^+. Eq. (11) applies to experiments of long duration where the membrane can no longer be considered to be impervious to cations, and where the cation distribution, instead of reaching the Donnan equilibrium, attains a new stationary state. If the deviations of the system from the true equilibrium are very small, the flux ratios for K and Na approach 1.0 and Eqs. (10a) and (10b) become identical with Eq. (IIIa, b) of Jacobs and Stewart (1947). Eqs. (8, 8a) are the same as Jacob and Stewart's Eq. (Vd, e). Equations (9) and (9a) describe a situation essentially similar to that dealt with by Boyle and Conway (1941) in their treatment of ionic equilibria in muscle.

A few applications of these expressions to actual experimental situations will be demonstrated in later sections of this paper in connection with the kinetics of ion and water movements leading to the establishment of the steady states described by the formulas. One special case, however, deserves comment. In cells incapable of maintaining, by active transport, a stationary nonequilibrium distribution of the cations, cations and anions tend to assume an equal distribution between the cell interior and outside, and r approaches 1. Due to the impermeability of the membrane to intracellular colloids, the cells take up water and V increases to an infinite extent. Actually, when V reaches the so-called "critical hemolytic volume," the cell perishes. This frequently encountered type of hemolysis, observed for example after exposure of the red cells to ultraviolet light or x-rays or in the presence of high concentrations of alcohol, acetone or chloroform, etc. (for a short review see Wilbrandt, 1953), has been rather thoroughly investigated by Wilbrandt (1941), who applied to it the term "colloid osmotic hemolysis."

The colloid osmotic hypothesis states that a protein-loaded cell rendered freely permeable to both anions and cations is unstable and cannot survive indefinitely. As has been emphasized by Ponder (1948, 1955), the hypothesis does not allow predictions of the time course of hemolysis. To illustrate this point, Ponder refers to his experiments with resorcinol- or *n*-butanol-treated red cells which may exchange about 80–90% of their intracellular K with extracellular Na without undergoing much swelling. He infers that, conversely,

TABLE I

DISTRIBUTION OF WATER AND IONS BETWEEN CELLS AND MEDIA OF VARYING COMPOSITION[a]

Ion distribution ratio r and cell water V:

$$r = \frac{Y_{\mathrm{Na,K}}}{X_{\mathrm{Na,K}} + Y_{\mathrm{Na,K}}} \cdot \frac{c_o}{b_o} \quad (8)$$

$$V = \frac{X_{\mathrm{Na,K}} + Y_{\mathrm{Na,K}}}{c_o} \quad (8a)$$

Membrane permeable to small anions; impermeable to cations, large anions, and nonelectrolytes

$$r = \frac{Y_{\mathrm{Na}}}{X_{\mathrm{Na}} + Y_{\mathrm{Na}}} \cdot \frac{c_o}{2b_o} \pm \sqrt{\frac{4X_{\mathrm{Na}}{}^2 \mathrm{K}_o 4b_o + Y_{\mathrm{Na}}{}^2(c_o{}^2 - 4\mathrm{K}_o b_o)}{4b_o^2(Y_{\mathrm{Na}} + X_{\mathrm{Na}})^2}} \quad (9)$$

$$V = \frac{X_{\mathrm{Na}}\, C_o}{c_o{}^2 - 4b_o \mathrm{K}_o} \pm \sqrt{\frac{Y_{\mathrm{Na}}{}^2 - X_{\mathrm{Na}}{}^2}{c_o{}^2 - 4b_o \mathrm{K}_o} + \left(\frac{X_{\mathrm{Na}}\, c_o}{c_o{}^2 - 4b_o \mathrm{K}_o}\right)^2} \quad (9a)$$

Membrane permeable to K and small anions; impermeable to Na, large anions, and nonelectrolytes

$$r = \frac{Y}{X + Y} \cdot \frac{c_o}{2b_o} \pm \sqrt{\frac{X^2 4b_o b_i + Y^2(c_o{}^2 - 4b_o b_i)}{(X + Y)^2 4b_o{}^2}} \quad (10)$$

$$V = \frac{X\, C_o}{c_o{}^2 - 4b_o b_i} \pm \sqrt{\frac{Y^2(c_o{}^2 - 4b_o b_i) + 4b_o b_i X^2}{(c_o{}^2 - 4b_o b_i)^2}} \quad (10a)$$

$$b_i = \frac{m_{\mathrm{in\,K}}}{m_{\mathrm{out\,K}}} \cdot \mathrm{K}_o + \frac{m_{\mathrm{in\,Na}}}{m_{\mathrm{out\,Na}}}\, \mathrm{Na}_o \quad (10b)$$

Membrane permeable to K, Na, and small anions; impermeable to large anions and nonelectrolytes, K and Na attain a new stationary nonequilibrium distribution

If $b_i = b_o$ (cations at Donnan equilibrium), and $c_o = 2b_o$ (no nonelectrolytes present), then $r = 1$, and $V \to \infty$ (colloid osmotic hemolysis)

---

[a] Explanation of Symbols:

$X_{\mathrm{Na,K}}$ = amount of nonpenetrating osmotically active substances inside the cell, including Na^+ and K^+ (moles)

X_{Na} = amount of nonpenetrating osmotically active substances inside the cell, including Na, but excluding K which is considered to be diffusible (moles)

X = amount of nonpenetrating osmotically active substances inside the cell, excluding Na and K which are assumed to penetrate until a new steady state is attained (moles)

c_o = total concentration in the medium, i.e., anions + cations + nonclectrolytes (moles/liter)

b_o = concentrations of cations in medium (moles/liter)

$Y_{\mathrm{Na,K}}$ = amount of nonpenetrating charges inside the cell, including Na and K (equivalents)

Y_{Na} = amount of nonpenetrating charges inside the cell, including Na, but excluding K (equivalents)

Y = amount of nonpenetrating charges inside the cell, excluding Na and K which are assumed to penetrate until a new steady state is attained (equivalents)

V = cell water

r = Donnan distribution ratio of inside/outside concentration (cf. Eq. 3)

m = passive in- and outfluxes of K^+ and Na^+ (cf. Eq. 4) it may be possible that cation-permeable cells may hemolyze under the influence of an agent before colloid osmotic swelling affects the integrity of the cell membrane. Wilbrandt, who anticipated this criticism, developed methods (1941, 1953) that in many cases permit discrimination between a direct action of the lysin on the membrane and an indirect colloid osmostic effect.

III. Permeability to Water and Hydrophilic Solutes and the Concept of "Pores"

The movement of water and hydrophilic molecules between the cell interior and the surrounding medium conceivably proceeds in two different ways:

(1) The molecules dissolve in the membrane phase and diffuse under their activity gradient from one side of the membrane to the other.

(2) The molecules penetrate by diffusion or by convection through channels, the "pores," which connect extra- and intracellular fluid.

The fact that strongly hydrophilic molecules and ions, particularly inorganic anions, are capable of rapidly crossing the membrane has been taken for many years as evidence for the existence of pores. In the more recent work on water permeability of the red blood cell, the existence of pores is therefore usually taken for granted and the results obtained have been evaluated in terms of pore radii.

A number of different methods were employed for determining pore dimensions (for a short review see Passow, 1963a):

(1) Attempts have been made to refine the classical approach of inferring pore dimensions from the penetration rates of probing molecules of varying size. Giebel and Passow (1960) measured the rate of exchange of a series of dicarboxylic acid anions with intracellular chloride ions across the beef red blood cell membrane. The data were interpreted on the basis of the following hypothesis:

Particles of equal length have similar rotational volumes. Regardless of their shape, so long as they can rotate freely inside a pore, the "hindrance" of their movements through the pores and hence the differences between their penetration rates should be similar to the differences of the diffusion rates in a large volume of water. When, however, the length of a particle is larger than the diameter of the pores, the penetration proceeds preferably in the direction of the longitudinal axis of the diffusing molecule. Under these conditions the "hindrance" of the diffusion for molecules of the same length but of otherwise different shape will differ considerably. The differences between the penetration rates will be much larger than those between the diffusion rates in the bulk phase.

Table II shows molecular lengths, molar volumes, and penetration rates of the dicarboxylic acids investigated. It may be seen that malonic, tartronic, and maleic acid, which are of approximately equal length, have the following molar volumes: 50.8, 54.4, and 59.4 cc. Although the differences between these values indicate that the shapes of these ions must be very different indeed, the half-value times for penetration of these substances are of the same order of magnitude, amounting to 6, 9, and 7 minutes, respectively.

TABLE II

PERMEABILITY OF BEEF ERYTHROCYTES TO DICARBOXYLIC ACIDS[a, b]

Dicarboxylic acid	$t_{1/2}$ (min.)	Molar volume (ml.)	Length (Å)
Oxalate	1	35.8	—
Malonate	6	50.8	7.6
Tartronate	9	54.4	7.6
Maleate	7	59.4	6.9
Fumarate	74	59.8	8.7
Succinate	220	63.8	9.0
Malate	323	72.4	9.0
Tartrate	2200	73.9	9.0
Glutarate	1180	81.0	10.3

[a] Temperature 25°C.
[b] $t_{1/2}$ = half-value time of the anion exchange.

With the C_4 dicarboxylic acids the picture is quite different. Fumaric, succinic, malic, and tartaric acids have about the same length. Their respective molar volumes are 59.8, 63.8, 72.4, and 73.9 cc., the maximum difference (on a percentage basis) being of the same order of magnitude as that between malonic and maleic acids. The half-value times for penetration are 74, 220, 323, and 2200 minutes, respectively. Especially remarkable is the difference between tartaric and malic acids: although the molar volumes differ only slightly, the former penetrates about 67 times faster than the latter.

From these data it appears that molecules up to the length of malonic or tartronic acid can freely rotate in the pores whereas longer molecules cannot. It may be inferred therefore that the diameter of the pores is somewhat larger than the length of malonic acid and somewhat smaller than that of succinic acid, and thus lies in the range 7.6–9 Å.

(2) Another refinement of the classical approach of estimating pore dimensions by means of probing molecules is based on determinations of the osmotic pressure exerted by penetrating solutes (Solomon, 1960b).

The osmotic pressure measured at a membrane should depend on the relative rates of solvent and solute passage. Only if the penetration rate of the solute is zero while the solvent passes freely through the membrane, will the maximum thermodynamic value of the osmotic pressure develop. If, however, the membrane also allows transfer of solute molecules, the osmotic pressure will depend on the restriction offered by the membrane to solvent and solute. Obviously this restriction depends on the relative sizes of pores, solute, and solvent molecules. The ratio between the osmotic pressure calculated by the thermodynamic laws for an ideally semipermeable membrane and that measured at a real membrane is usually designated by the letter σ and called "reflection coefficient" (Staverman, 1952). When the membrane allows only penetration of the solvent, σ is equal to 1 and the osmotic pressure assumes its maximal value; when both solvent and solute move at the same relative rates as in the bulk phase, σ is equal to 0 and there is no osmotic pressure. Intermediate values of σ are a measure of the selectivity of the membrane. Applying the methods of irreversible thermodynamics, Katchalsky (1960) and Kedem and Katchalsky (1961) obtained the following relationship between σ and the parameters describing the properties of the membrane, of solute, and of solvent:

$$\sigma = 1 - \frac{PV_s}{L_p} - \frac{A_s}{A_w} \tag{11}$$

where P = permeability constant of solute at zero volume flow; V_s = partial molar volume of solute; L_p = filtration coefficient; A_w = area available for the diffusion of water; and A_s = area available for the diffusion of solute.

Employing a null method depending upon the determination of that external concentration of penetrating molecules which, at zero time, causes zero water flow, Goldstein and Solomon (1960) measured σ values for a variety of lipid-insoluble molecules at the beef red cell membrane. In order to estimate pore dimensions from their σ values, they introduced into an equation essentially similar to Eq. (11) (Durbin *et al.*, 1956) an expression (Pappenheimer *et al.*, 1951; Renkin, 1954) which relates A_s/A_w to the so-called "equivalent pore diameter" and the dimensions of solute and solvent molecules. In the derivation of this latter expression, hydrodynamic laws governing the movements of macroscopic particles through exactly circular pipes ("equivalent pores") were applied. Inserting their values, Goldstein and Solomon calculated an "equivalent pore diameter" of about 8.4 Å.

(3) Koefoed-Johnson and Ussing (1953) and Pappenheimer *et al.* (1951) have independently pointed out that the equivalent pore radii may be determined from measurements of the relative rates of water movements across the membrane under concentration and osmotic pressure gradients. If D_2O or THO is used as the probing molecule, owing to their similarity to the solvent molecule, σ assumes the value zero. Labeled water molecules thus exert virtually no osmotic pressure at a membrane and hence cannot induce water

flow through pores. They can therefore be used for measuring self-diffusion coefficients in the absence of convection.

The rate of diffusion is proportional to the pore area which is πr^2. If a non-penetrating solute is added to the medium ($\sigma = 1$), water flow under the osmotic pressure gradient is induced. Inside the pores, laminar flow proportional to the fourth power of the pore radius should develop. The proportionality factors depend in both cases, i.e. in diffusion and flow, on parameters related in an unknown way to the membrane structure, e.g. length of pores, tortuosity factors, etc. However, taking the ratio between water transfer by diffusion and by convection these factors largely cancel each other. Besides the square of the pore radius, the resulting expression contains only parameters that characterize the known physical properties of water. Using this method, Paganelli and Solomon (1957) estimated an equivalent pore diameter of about 7 Å in human red blood cells, and Villegas *et al.* (1958) found similar values in beef and dog erythrocytes (8.2 Å and 14.8 Å, respectively).

In order to appraise the studies outlined, it is necessary to distinguish clearly between two questions: (1) are the results compatible with the existence of pores and, if so, (2) are the data on their dimensions reliable?

(1) Each of the three phenomena described, i.e. the "sieve effect" for hydrophilic molecules, the interactions between solute and water flow (i.e. $0 < \sigma < 1$), and the differences between rates of water transport by diffusion and by flow, represents a necessary criterion but not sufficient proof for the existence of pores. Chemical or electrostatic interactions between probing molecules and membrane constituents may completely invalidate the quantitative evaluation of the sieve effect, and hence the above interpretation of the data on dicarboxylate ion permeability. Water and solute movements may influence each other in homogeneous membranes as well as in pores (Kedem and Katchalsky, 1961). Strong interactions like those observed in the red cell, however, point to the existence of pores, since diffusing water molecules should impede the movements of the probing molecules much less than a bulk flow of water. The observed difference between rates of water transfer as measured in the presence and absence of an osmotic pressure gradient is, perhaps, the most convincing piece of evidence for the presence of pores in the red cell membrane.[3]

In common language one usually associates with the term "pore" the idea of a circular pipe. It should be borne in mind, however, that the above considerations are independent of any assumptions concerning the shape and

[3] Measurements by Jacobs *et al.* (1936) of the temperature dependence of water permeability give little information about the mechanism of water transfer, since they are based on the determination of hemolysis. The rate-limiting step in hemolysis is not necessarily the water entry into the cells but probably the release of hemoglobin into the medium. The latter is certainly a diffusion process and would therefore easily explain the observed activation energy of 4 kcal./mole.

dimensions of the channels traversing the membrane. Thus for our present discussion, a broader definition of the term "pore" would seem more useful. It is generally assumed that a diffusing particle migrates by shifting into a gap formed at its surface when a solvent particle moves away (cf. Glasstone *et al.*, 1941). It seems appropriate therefore to speak of a diffusion through "water-filled pores" or "channels" when the rate of penetration of solute within the membrane is limited by the diffusion of water molecules. Obviously in very narrow pores, this process may be greatly modified by electrostatic and chemical interactions between the constituents of the pore wall and the pore contents. It may thus present special physicochemical problems different from those encountered in macroscopic pores.

(2) Although all available data indicate that the sizes of the "pores" are comparable to those of the penetrating small molecules and ions, the numerical values presented above should not be accepted unreservedly.

The usefulness of probing molecules is limited, since their dimensions are accurately known in only a few cases and since it is difficult to decide to what extent allowance must be made for their hydration. Furthermore, the frequency distribution of their various possible configurations should also affect the penetration rate, but has so far never been taken into account. Moreover, the pores themselves may vary in size, either spontaneously under the influence of the Brownian movement of their constituents or induced by chemical or electrostatic interaction with the penetrating particles. Even if the pores were permanent and rigid structures, nothing can be said about the statistical variations in diameter, length, and tortuosity.

Additional problems arise when the evaluation of measurements of pore sizes is based on the macroscopic laws of hydrodynamics, since it is not known down to what dimensions these laws can safely be employed. In artificial membranes they still apply to estimation of pore diameters of about 10–20 Å (Robbins and Mauro, 1960; Durbin, 1960; Pappenheimer *et al.*, 1951). It seems unlikely, however, that Poiseulle's law remains valid at pore radii of about 5 Å, since it is hardly conceivable that a parabolic velocity profile develops in channels containing only 15–20 water molecules over the entire cross section. The application of Stoke's law[4] is equally dangerous even if the correction of Gierer and Wirtz (1953) is applied and wall effects are taken into account. In view of these difficulties, Solomon and his colleagues refer to their data on pore dimensions as "equivalent radii." It seems misleading to calculate, however, from interesting experimental data on solute-water interactions or on water diffusion and flow, figures for "equivalent pore radii" which for the reasons outlined are of limited physical significance.

[4] In Stokes law, the diffusion coefficient D of the solute, and the viscosity η of the solvent, occur as a product. Since, according to Einstein, D is inversely related to η, deviations of the viscosity from the macroscopic behavior are greatly reduced.

IV. Anion Permeability and the Concept of Fixed Charges

If the existence of "pores" is taken for granted, the question arises why the anions but not the cations can readily pass through them. In the absence of any alternative explanation, following Mond (1927) it is usually assumed that the selectivity of the red cell membrane is due to the presence of fixed positive charges. Since the red cell surface is negatively charged, the positive charges are thought to be located at the inside of the "pores."

Investigations of the ultrastructure and biochemistry of the erythrocyte membrane has so far yielded no useful information on the concentration, arrangement, and chemical nature of fixed charges. For the time being therefore one has to rely on inferences drawn from studies on the kinetics of ion permeability. Unfortunately, the experimental data available are still quite unsatisfactory. Systematic studies on the possible role of fixed charges in cation permeability have not yet been published *in extenso*, and investigations of the permeability to the physiologically important anions, Cl^- and HCO_3^-, still encounter formidable technical difficulties. The use of silver chloride electrodes (Luckner and Lo Sing, 1938) for following the net Cl^-/HCO_3^- exchange, and the application of Hartridge and Roughton's (1923) rapid flow technique to the measurement of the unidirectional fluxes of halide anions (Tosteson, 1959) by means of their respective radioisotopes, revealed little more than the fact that HCO_3^- and Cl^- enter the cell in less than a second.

In view of these problems, the more slowly migrating anions, notably SO_4^{--}, have largely been used as a tool for studying the mechanism of anion permeability. Although it remains to be decided whether sulfate ions use the same pathway as do the rapidly moving Cl^- and HCO_3^-, the present considerations on anion permeability are of necessity confined to a discussion of SO_4^{--} permeability.

Sulfate ions enter the red cell in exchange for chloride ions. The half-value time for penetration varies from one species to another (Mond and Gertz, 1929), and even the empirical formulas describing the time course of the concentration change may exhibit characteristic species differences (Dunker and Passow, 1953). For example, in pig erythrocytes the half-value time at 20°C. is about 10 minutes and the chloride and sulfate ion movements follow first order kinetics. In beef erythrocytes, the half-value time at 20°C. is about 40 minutes and the SO_4/Cl exchange obeys second order kinetics.

Immediately after mixing neutral sulfate solutions with slightly alkaline erythrocyte brei, pH values as low as 6.4 may be observed. Then, the pH slowly rises until, at the end of the anion exchange, the medium becomes slightly alkaline. The described pH changes have been explained on the assumption that, at each instant, the fast moving OH and Cl ions attain a "partial ionic equilibrium" (Wilbrandt, 1942a; Schwietzer and Passow, 1953), whereby the position of the equilibrium $OH_i/OH_o = Cl_i/Cl_o$ is determined by the distribution of the slowly migrating sulfate ions. At the beginning of the experiment the extracellular chloride of the erythrocyte brei is diluted by the sulfate solution. Hydroxyl ions therefore rapidly enter the cell in exchange for intracellular Cl ions, whereby the pH of the medium drops until the Cl and OH distribution ratios assume equal values. However, as the SO_4 ions penetrate, the position of the "partial ionic equilibrium" for OH and Cl continuously shifts and the pH slowly rises again. Eventually the SO_4 ions reach the Donnan equilibrium:

$$\frac{Cl_i}{Cl_o} = \frac{OH_i}{OH_o} = \sqrt{\frac{SO_{4i}}{SO_{4o}}}$$

whereby the anion distribution ratio assumes a value of less than 1.0 and the medium a pH of about 7.5 (Fig. 1).

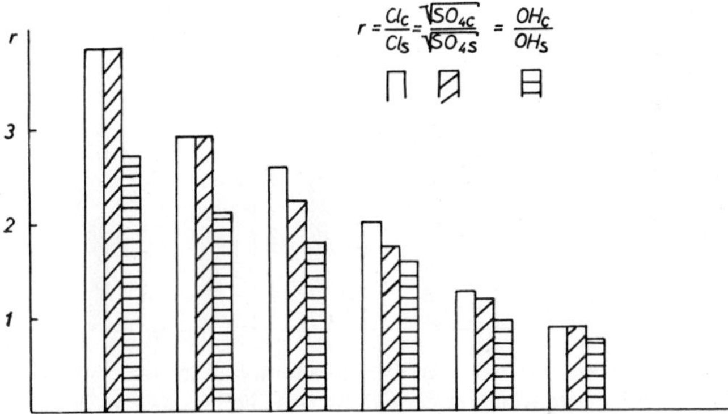

FIG. 1. Anion distribution ratios (r) in horse red blood cells equilibrated with isotonic solutions containing Na_2SO_4, NaCl, and sucrose in varying proportions. The subscripts c and s refer to cell water and suspension medium, respectively. Temperature 32.5°C. (redrawn from Passow, 1961).

The penetration rate of a diffusing anion depends on its concentration within the membrane. This concentration is usually different from that of the medium and at a positively charged membrane is a function of the concentration of nondiffusible cations. Within a highly selective membrane, the concentration of diffusible cations is negligible and the penetrating anions, Cl^- and SO_4^{--}, compete for fixed positive charges. Moreover, if the fixed charges should in fact be dissociable, their number and hence the rate of anion passage should vary with pH, as was suggested by Mond (1927). Any test of the applicability of the fixed charge theory ought to include therefore a study of the effect of pH and Cl^- concentration on sulfate ion permeability.

Due to the establishment of partial ionic equilibria for OH^- and Cl^-, net SO_4 movements are always associated with concomitant changes in pH and

Cl^- concentration. If fixed charges were actually present, the concentration changes in the medium should affect their dissociation as well as any Cl/SO_4 competition. Hence the resistance the membrane offers to the penetration of SO_4 ions should continuously vary in the course of an experiment. Furthermore, since for each two Cl ions moving into the medium only one SO_4 ion enters the cell, the osmolarity of the cell content decreases. A flow of water is thereby induced, which may enhance or retard the penetration of anions through "pores." In addition, the magnitude of the diffusion potential associated with the net anion exchange depends on each of the mutually interdependent effects described and hence varies with time. Obviously, such variations may easily account for the deviations of net SO_4 ion transfer from first order kinetics as

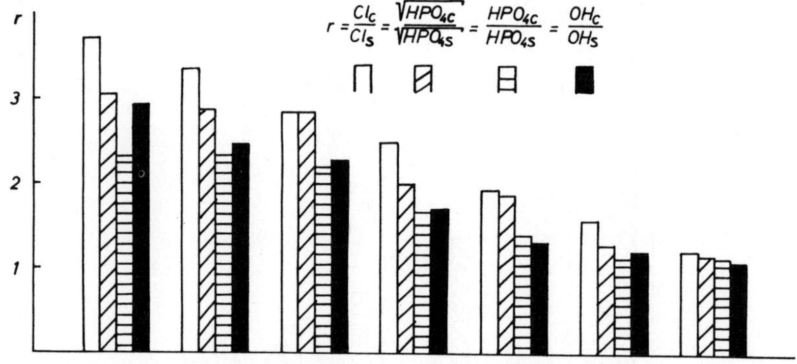

FIG. 2. $S^{35}O_4$ entry into beef red cells. Prior to addition of the radioactivity (= zero time of the graph) the cells were equilibrated with an isotonic $Na_2SO_4/NaCl$ mixture until the Donnan equilibrium was established; pH 7.4; SO_4 concentration of the medium 32 mmoles/liter; temperature 32.5°C. (all values at Donnan equilibrium). The curve was calculated by the method of least squares. $Y_0 = 12{,}229$; $Y_\infty = 8967$; $K = 0.061$. Ordinate: counts/min. in the medium. Abscissa: time in minutes.

observed in beef and horse erythrocytes. Differences in the concentration and arrangement of fixed charges could, perhaps, even explain the species differences. For example, the SO_4/Cl exchange across a membrane of low charge density should give rise to the development of a diffusion potential whereas, at high charge density, diffusion potentials are largely suppressed (cf. Teorell, 1953).

Attempts to elucidate the mechanism of SO_4 transfer are greatly facilitated if SO_4 fluxes are measured in the absence of the described events (net water movements and changes in pH, in chloride and sulfate concentrations, and in membrane potential). Red cells were therefore first equilibrated with isotonic $Na_2SO_4/NaCl$ mixtures until the net movements ceased and the Donnan equilibrium was established. Subsequently, tracer $S^{35}O_4$ was added and the disappearance of radioactivity from the medium was followed (Passow, 1961).

Regardless of the cell origin (beef, horse, pig), the decrease in extracellular $S^{35}O_4$ concentration could be fitted to a single exponential (Fig. 2). This finding showed the unusual kinetic pattern of net SO_4 movements in horse and beef red cells to be in fact largely due to time-dependent variations in the composition of cells and medium. This conclusion was further supported by the observation that the SO_4 influx at Donnan equilibrium (as calculated from the decline in radioactivity in the medium) is a function not only of the SO_4 concentration but is also dependent on the concentrations of Cl^- and H^+.

The effect of pH and Cl^- concentration on SO_4 influx was studied in experiments in which the position of the Donnan equilibrium was varied for the anions. Erythrocytes were suspended in isotonic solutions containing Na_2SO_4, NaCl, and sucrose in varying proportions. Composition and pH of these solutions were such that, at the end of the net anion exchange, the cells were at Donnan equilibrium with media of:

(a) Constant pH and varying SO_4/Cl concentration ratios.
(b) Varying pH and approximately constant SO_4 and Cl concentrations.
(c) Varying pH and varying SO_4/Cl concentration ratio.

(a) The relationship between SO_4 influx and concentration was quite different from either saturation or simple diffusion kinetics. If the SO_4 concentration was raised by replacing NaCl with Na_2SO_4, an approximately linear relation existed up to only 10 mmoles/liter. At higher SO_4 concentrations the flux increased more than the concentration. The data could be fitted to the following equation:

$$m_{SO_4} = a SO_{4o}(1 + b SO_{4o})$$

where $m_{SO_4} = SO_4$ influx at Donnan equilibrium; $SO_{4o} = SO_4$ concentration of the medium at Donnan equilibrium; and a, b = constants.

On the basis of the fixed charge concept, this finding could be explained by assuming a competition of SO_4 with Cl for fixed positive charges within the membrane: under the experimental conditions described an increase in SO_{4o} is associated with a reduction in the Cl/SO_4 ratio. A higher proportion of the given number of fixed positive charges is electrically neutralized by SO_4 anions and hence the SO_4 influx increases more than proportionally to the SO_4 concentration.

(b) If measured at the same sulfate and chloride concentrations, the SO_4 influx, as estimated with $S^{35}O_4$ at Donnan equilibrium, was about 3 times higher at pH 6.8 than at pH 7.6. The relationship between SO_4 influx and pH resembled an S-shaped titration curve with an inflection point at approximately pH 7.2 (Fig. 3). It therefore appeared likely that dissociable ions attached to the cell membrane play a decisive role in the control of anion permeability. Since the pK values of the histidine groups known to be present in the red cell membrane (Sanui *et al.*, 1962) lie in the range 6.8–7.2 one might be tempted to attribute the pH dependence of anion permeability to the dissociation of histidine. However, the pH within the membrane is not necessarily identical with that of the medium, and thus the pK value of dissociable fixed charges might be quite different from the pH at the inflection point of the titration curve.

(c) Generally the described SO_4/Cl competition should be superimposed on pH-dependent variations in the concentration of fixed charges. In order to test this consequence of the fixed charge concept, the cells were equilibrated with solutions of decreasing pH and increasing Cl/SO_4 ratio. In accord with

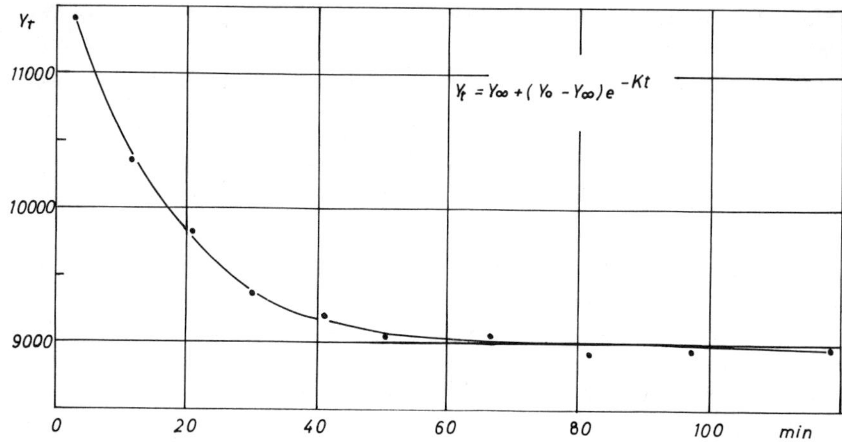

FIG. 3. The pH dependence of SO_4 influx. Cells equilibrated with isotonic Na_2SO_4/NaCl mixtures of varying pH. Addition of $S^{35}O_4$ after the Donnan equilibrium was established. Each point was calculated from a curve similar to that presented in Fig. 2. Temperature 32.5°C. Ordinate: SO_4 influx. Abscissa: pH of medium at Donnan equilibrium (redrawn from Passow, 1961).

the view that increase in the number of fixed charges brought about by acidifying the medium is counteracted by increasing the Cl^- concentration, the pH dependence was suppressed or even reversed (Passow *et al.*, 1960; cf. Passow, 1961).

The results outlined could be used to estimate the concentration and dissociation constant of the fixed charges. This estimate rests on the simplifying assumption that the SO_4 influx is linearly related to the SO_4 concentration within the membrane (SO_{4m}). SO_{4m}, which cannot be measured directly, was calculated on the basis of the following hypothesis:

(1) The distribution of the diffusible anions OH, Cl, and SO_4 between the membrane and the adjacent media follows Donnan's law.

(2) The concentration of diffusible negative charges within the membrane (i.e., $2SO_{4m}^{--}+Cl_{m}^{-}$) is equal to that of the fixed charges (AH^{+}).

(3) The fixed charges are at equilibrium with the hydrogen ions within the membrane: $AH^{+}=A+H_{m}^{+}$.

Applying this hypothesis, it was possible to show that regardless of the experimental conditions the measured SO_4 influx was always nearly proportional to the calculated SO_{4m}, the sulfate concentration within the membrane. The best fit of the data on the pH dependence at different Cl/SO_4 ratios was obtained when the dissociation constant of the fixed ions was chosen to be similar to that of amino groups (viz. 10^{-9}) and when their concentration was put equal to about 3 moles/liter.

The sulfate ion permeability was studied with the limited aim of exploring to what extent the concept of dissociable fixed charges can be applied to the red cell membrane. It should be emphasized, therefore, that the described results could probably as well be explained on the basis of entirely different assumptions about the penetration mechanism. Moreover, the number of variables tested so far is quite insufficient to prove the case in point.[5] Actually, there exist a number of observations which—for the time being—seem to be irreconcilable with the outlined assumptions.

The finding that, unlike Cl ions, neither mono- nor di-valent phosphate ions seem to compete with SO_4 ions for fixed charges must be considered a serious objection. Moreover, the penetration rate of phosphate ions measured under the same conditions as that of SO_4^{--}, shows again an S-shaped curve with an inflection near pH 7.2 (Lohmann and Passow, unpublished). The phosphate ions are dissociable and, in the pH range studied, the ratio between mono- and di-valent anions varies greatly. The pH dependence of PO_4 ion permeability should therefore be different from that of the nondissociable SO_4 ions.

It would be tempting to assume that SO_4 and PO_4 ions move along different pathways through the membrane. There exists, however, an observation that points to a common transfer mechanism for both ion species: the activation energies calculated from the temperature dependence of the ion fluxes at Donnan equilibrium both have the same unusually high value of about 28–30 kcal./mole/degree. This value exceeds by far the highest activation energy reported for the diffusion of ions in ion-exchange resins (about 16 kcal./mole/degree; Soldano and Boyd, 1954).

High activation energies have occasionally been considered to indicate the occurrence of active transport. Sulfate ions always move down their electrochemical potential gradient until the Donnan equilibrium is established. No saturation kinetics could be demonstrated and the common metabolic poisons

[5] Some corroborative evidence for the participation of amino groups in the control of anion permeability may perhaps be seen in Edelberg's (1952, 1953) observation that the net SO_4/Cl exchange across the red cell membrane can be inhibited by tannic acid.

(F, iodoacetate) do not interfere with the penetration process (Lohmann and Passow, unpublished). It seems necessary therefore to reject the idea of active sulfate ion transport in beef or horse red cells, and to attribute the high activation energy of sulfate and phosphate permeability to other causes such as changes in membrane structure with temperature. In this context it will be noted that the pore dimensions are presumably of molecular dimensions. In narrow channels where SO_4 ions moving in opposite directions cannot pass each other, the ions cross the membrane in "single file" (Hodgkin and Keynes, 1955). This particular penetration mechanism is perhaps associated with unusually high activation energies.

In concluding this section, a few remarks may be added concerning the mechanism of phosphate ion permeability. A number of authors (Halpern, 1936; Gourley, 1952; Mueller and Hastings, 1951a, b) believed that—at least in human erythrocytes—phosphate ions are actively transported. They argued that:

(1) The phosphate ion distribution between cells and medium does not obey the Donnan law (Halpern, 1936; Mueller and Hastings, 1951).

(2) Metabolic poisons like F or iodoacetate (IAA) inhibit $P^{32}O_4$ uptake (Gourley, 1952).

(3) The incorporation of inorganic $P^{32}O_4$ from the medium into the inorganic PO_4 pool of the cells is preceded by the labeling of ATP (adenosine triphosphate) (Gourley, 1952; Gerlach *et al.*, 1958).

The view of these authors was not shared by others (Hahn and Hevesy, 1941). Dunker and Passow (1953) demonstrated that the kinetics of the net PO_4/Cl exchange between the red cells of three species (horse, beef, pig) follow the same characteristic pattern as does the purely passive SO_4/Cl exchange. The evidence outlined seems at present insufficient to prove that the phosphate ions do not pass through the same regions of the membrane as do the other anions, notably SO_4^{--}. In particular the above arguments can be challenged for the following reasons:

(1) The observed deviations of the phosphate ion distribution from the Donnan equilibrium are small; they could not be found when exceptional care was taken to prevent PO_4 liberation from acid-labile PO_4 esters. Furthermore, the phosphate ions penetrate relatively slowly. Any rapid change in rate of PO_4 esterification should therefore cause a temporary departure of the phosphate ion distribution from Donnan's law (Vestergaard-Bogind and Hesselbo, 1960) (Fig. 4).

(2) The presence of metabolic poisons (IAA, F) has not yet been shown to inhibit phosphate transfer across the membrane. It blocks to a large extent, however, the incorporation of $P^{32}O_4$ into the intracellular phosphoric acid esters, thereby reducing the total PO_4 uptake by the cells and creating the impression of a diminished rate of transport. This impression is further streng-

thened by the loss into the medium of large quantities of PO_4 liberated from ester bonds. The changes in intracellular esterified PO_4 can be minimized, if the cells are first equilibrated in solutions of high PO_4 content until the Donnan equilibrium is established. The rate of the subsequently measured disappearance of $P^{32}O_4$ from the medium is, under these conditions, not affected by either IAA or F (Lohmann and Passow, unpublished).

(3) If the esterification of inorganic phosphate takes place in the immediate vicinity of the inner membrane surface, PO_4 ions entering the cells should

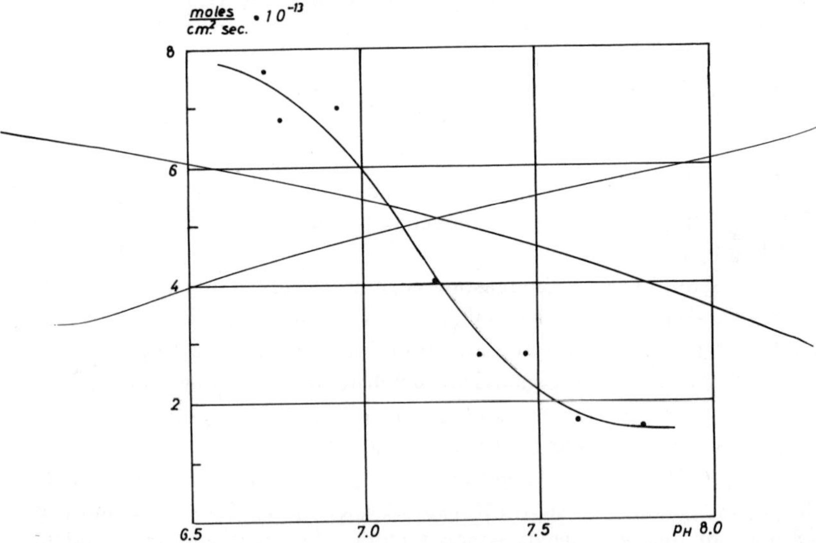

FIG. 4. Anion distribution ratios (r) in horse red blood cells equilibrated with isotonic solutions containing Na_2HPO_4, NaCl, and sucrose in varying proportions. Temperature 32.5°C. The subscripts c and s refer to cell water and suspension medium, respectively (Lohmann and Passow, unpublished).

become incorporated into ATP prior to any appreciable mixing with the intracellular inorganic PO_4 pool. It therefore seems conceivable that the specific activity of ATP may increase faster than that of the intracellular PO_4 although no precursor relationship exists between the two.

V. Cation Permeability

A. *The Pump-Leak Concept*

The red cell membrane is permeable to both K and Na ions. Under physiological conditions, nevertheless, large concentration gradients persist whereby active and passive movements balance each other for each ion species. The kinetics of the cation exchange in the steady state can be followed by measuring unidirectional fluxes with radioactive potassium or sodium. From such measurements more or less plausible estimates of the active and passive components of unidirectional and net fluxes (cf. Fig. 5) can be obtained, provided additional information is available regarding the influence on the total unidirectional fluxes of external cation concentrations, substrates, metabolic inhibitors, etc. Shaw (1955) and Glynn (1956) studied the relationship between total K influx m_K and K concentration K_o of the medium. Their results could be expressed by the following empirical equation:

$$m_K = \frac{\alpha K_o}{1+\beta K_o} + \gamma K_o$$

where α, β, and γ represent constants. They assumed that the first term describes the active component and the second term the passive component of the total K influx.

The latter assumption seemed reasonable, first, because a linear relationship between flux and concentration should exist for a simple diffusion process and, second, because γ, in contrast to α, was found to be independent of the metabolic state of the cell. It was concluded, therefore, that the potassium transfer across the red cell membrane proceeds by way of two different and independent mechanisms, which were referred to as "pump" and "leak."

Although the "pump-leak" concept was very helpful in recent attempts to elucidate the mechanism of active transport, one ought to be aware that it is not self-evident and still needs support from additional and independent experimental evidence.

Thus a linear relationship between flux and concentration can be expected only if ion movements in opposite directions do not influence each other; if, in other words, Ussing's (1949a, b) independence principle applies. Although this principle has occasionally been used (Tosteson and Hoffman, 1960, in sheep; Shaw, 1955, in horse; and Glynn, 1956, and Tosteson *et al.*, 1955, in human erythrocytes), a quantitative appraisal of its validity for the passive cation permeability of red blood cells would be desirable. The available evidence previously discussed suggests the existence in the red cell membrane of pores with radii of the same order of magnitude as those of the alkali metal ions. Since ion movements can proceed only in single file in such narrow pores, large deviations from the independence principle may be expected, whereby—as has recently been shown by Heckmann (1962)—flux and concentration are no longer proportional to each other. Furthermore, the kinetics of passive (downhill) ion penetration may conceivably be affected by electrostatic and chemical interactions with fixed charges or carrier molecules in the membrane.

In human (Hoffman, 1962c) and sheep (Tosteson and Hoffman, 1960) erythrocytes a flux component has in fact been observed which can most conveniently be attributed to exchange diffusion, a carrier transport that requires no metabolic energy. Even if no evidence for the occurrence of a separate exchange diffusion mechanism can be found, it might well be that the same chemical reactions which accomplish active transport may mediate a certain "backwash through the pump." The latter possibility limits the usefulness of metabolic inhibitors as tools for discriminating between the "pump" and "leak" components of cation fluxes. As has been emphasized by Wilbrandt (1963), a backwash through the pump may greatly exceed its normal value in the presence of inhibitors and thus create the impression of an increase in the "leak" flux.

No simple method seems to be presently available permitting an unequivocal decision as to whether an experimentally induced increase in downhill movements is caused by an alteration of either the "pump" or the "leak." Nevertheless, a comparison of the magnitudes of the effects produced by known inhibitors of the pump with those of other agents gives some indication of the nature of the observed changes. All known specific inhibitors of the pump suppress the uphill transport of K and Na, but exert little or no effect on their downhill movements. Thus, the reduction in concentrations of activating cations (K, Na, Mg) on either the inside or outside of the membrane, the depletion of the energy-supplying ATP, or the application to the outside of inhibitory cardiac glycosides never induces downhill movements of either K or Na much in excess of those observed under steady state conditions. It seems reasonable therefore to attribute to an increase in the "leak" flux all those permeability changes in which ion movements down the electrochemical gradient occur at least 10–20 times faster than in the intact cell. Moreover, the physical nature of the agents (e.g. detergents) employed in producing the permeability changes frequently suggests a direct action on the membrane rather than a specific effect on the pump.

Thus in spite of the uncertainties mentioned, the pump-leak concept seems to be the most useful frame of reference available at present for a discussion of the cation permeability of the red cell. On the basis of this concept, the material below may conveniently be arranged in three categories. First, it will be shown how the interrelationship between activity of the "pump" and "size" of the "leak" determines the steady state concentrations of intracellular K and Na, and hence the water content of the cells. Second, a description will be given of a variety of experimentally induced permeability changes allegedly due to modifications of the leak rather than to inhibition of the pump only. Finally, studies will be dealt with that were specifically designed to elucidate the biochemical reaction sequence which accomplishes cation "pumping."

1. Control of Cellular Cation and Water Contents by "Pump" and "Leak"

Tosteson and Hoffman (1960) derived a set of equations which allows the calculation of the steady state concentrations of K and Na and of the water content of the cells, when the composition of the external fluid, the amount of nonpenetrating ions and molecules inside the cell, and the pump and leak fluxes of both K and Na ions are known.

a. Theory. According to Tosteson and Hoffman, the total unidirectional flux of each ion species, as measured with K^{42} or Na^{24}, is made up of a passive

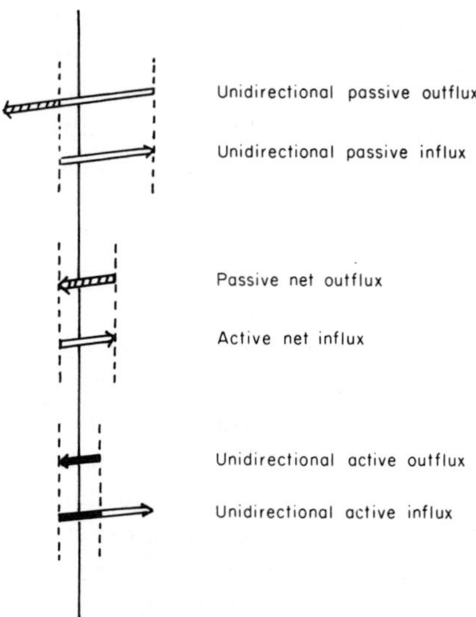

FIG. 5. Fluxes at a membrane.

("leak") and an active ("pump") component, m and M, respectively. In the steady state, influx and outflux balance each other:

$$M_{\text{in K}}+m_{\text{in K}} = M_{\text{out K}}+m_{\text{out K}} \tag{12}$$

$$M_{\text{in Na}}+m_{\text{in Na}} = M_{\text{out Na}}+m_{\text{out Na}} \tag{13}$$

Assuming there to be no active influx of Na or outflux of K, Eqs. (12) and (13) reduce to

$$M_{\text{in K}}+m_{\text{in K}} = m_{\text{out K}} \tag{12a}$$

$$M_{\text{out Na}}+m_{\text{out Na}} = m_{\text{in Na}} \tag{13a}$$

Provided Ussing's independence principle (1949a, b) applies to the passive K and Na fluxes, the following relationships between concentration ratios and passive fluxes exist:

$$\frac{m_{\text{in K}}}{m_{\text{out K}}} = \frac{K_o}{K_i}\exp(-F\Delta\psi/RT) \tag{14}$$

$$\frac{m_{\text{in Na}}}{m_{\text{out Na}}} = \frac{\text{Na}_o}{\text{Na}_i}\exp(-F\Delta\psi/RT) \tag{15}$$

Combining Eqs. (14) and (15) yields:

$$\frac{m_{\text{in K}}\,m_{\text{out Na}}}{m_{\text{out K}}\,m_{\text{in Na}}} = \frac{\text{K}_o\,\text{Na}_i}{\text{K}_i\,\text{Na}_o} \tag{16}$$

By definition:

$$\epsilon = \frac{M_{\text{in K}}}{m_{\text{in K}}}; \qquad \gamma = \frac{M_{\text{out Na}}}{m_{\text{out Na}}} \tag{17}$$

Combining Eqs. (12), (16), and (17) leads to the following relationship:

$$\frac{(1+\gamma)\,\text{Na}_o}{(1+\epsilon)\,\text{K}_o} = \frac{\text{Na}_i}{\text{K}_i} \tag{18}$$

Thus the intracellular K/Na ratio solely depends on the extracellular concentration ratio and the ratios of pump/leak fluxes for both ion species. In the limiting case where the leak fluxes assume very large values compared with the pump fluxes ($\epsilon \approx \gamma \rightarrow 0$), the cations tend to reach a Donnan equilibrium:

$$\frac{\text{K}_i}{\text{K}_o} = \frac{\text{Na}_i}{\text{Na}_o}$$

The rates of alkali metal ion accumulation and back diffusion determine not only the intracellular K and Na concentrations but also the anion distribution ratio and the cell volume. The factors governing the interrelationship between membrane properties and these distribution phenomena have already been outlined and the results of a quantitative description of the situation has been presented. The equations show that, in the steady state, cell volume V and anion distribution ratio r both depend on a factor b_i, which is a function of the passive influxes and outfluxes of K and Na (cf. Eq. 10b):

$$b_i = \frac{m_{\text{in K}}}{m_{\text{out K}}}\,\text{K}_o + \frac{m_{\text{in Na}}}{m_{\text{out Na}}}\,\text{Na}_o$$

Applying Eqs. (12a), (13a), and the definitions of the factors ϵ and γ (Eq. 17), this expression can be transformed to

$$b_i = \frac{\text{K}_o}{1+\epsilon} + \frac{\text{Na}_o}{1+\gamma} \tag{19}$$

If the potassium and sodium leak fluxes are much larger than the pump fluxes, ϵ and γ become small compared with 1, and b_i tends to approach ($\text{K}_o + \text{Na}_o$). Under these conditions $r \rightarrow 1.0$, and $V \rightarrow \infty$ or, in other words, colloid osmotic hemolysis occurs. (cf. p. 87ff.).

b. Experimental Observations. Using sheep red cells, Tosteson and Hoffman tested the validity of the theory outlined. In sheep, two strains of animals occur, one having red blood cells with high (85 mmoles/liter) and the other with low (12 mmoles/liter) potassium content, whereas the sodium concentrations show an inverse variation. In accordance with the theoretical prediction, the values of the pump and leak fluxes observed under a variety of experimental conditions agreed quite well with those calculated by means of the equations derived from the ionic composition of high- and low-K erythrocytes. This suggests that both types of erythrocytes actually control their cation composition and cell volume through the operation of a pump working in parallel with a leak, as postulated by the theory. Interestingly enough, however, in high-K cells not only the pump but also the leak fluxes were larger than in low-K cells. Since the hereditary difference between high- and low-K cells seems to be determined by a single gene (Evans *et al.*, 1956), Tosteson and Hoffman suspected that in spite of their functional independence, pump and leak may be located at the same or adjacent membrane sites.

B. Passive Cation Permeability

In the present section, a number of experimental conditions will be described where K and Na movements down the electrochemical potential gradients greatly exceed the normal rate of cation accumulation, and thus seem to represent a change in membrane resistance to passive penetration rather than a "backwash" through the pump. The effects observed under these conditions may serve as a convenient basis for discussion of a selected number of the more obvious factors that presumably control passive cation permeability: (a) fixed positive charges in the membrane, (b) spatial arrangement of the membrane constituents, (c) presence of specific chemical groups such as SH or S—S or of specific ions such as Ca^{++} and Mg^{++} which stabilize the membrane structure, and (d) metabolic control of membrane resistance to passive penetration.

1. Effect of Variations in Ionic Strength and pH on Potassium and Sodium Permeability of Human Red Cells

Human erythrocytes suspended in isotonic saline solution at room temperature lose K and take up Na. This process, however, is slow (Ponder, 1951b) and, regardless of the pH employed, net changes in intracellular K and Na can hardly be detected within the first 1–2 hours of the experiment. If part of the saline solution is replaced by an isotonic solution of a nonpenetrating nonelectrolyte, such as mannitol or sucrose, both K (Maizels, 1935; Davson, 1939; Wilbrandt, 1940a) and Na (Wilbrandt and Schatzmann, 1960), rapidly leave the cells. The downhill movements may occur at 20–30 times the normal rate, the actual magnitude of the effect greatly depending on the pH of the medium. The permeability change is not related to reduction in external K or Na concentration, since replacing the saline with choline instead of sucrose leaves the cation permeability nearly unaltered. The potassium and sodium movements induced by lowering the ionic strength of the medium are reversible, and can readily be brought to a standstill by the addition of small amounts of an electrolyte.

The rate of K loss increases with decreasing electrolyte concentration of the medium, and plotting the log of the initial rate of K loss against the square root of the ionic strength yields a straight line relationship. Unfortunately, however, it has not yet been possible to compare accurately the effects observed in media containing binary and ternary electrolytes at equal ionic strength.

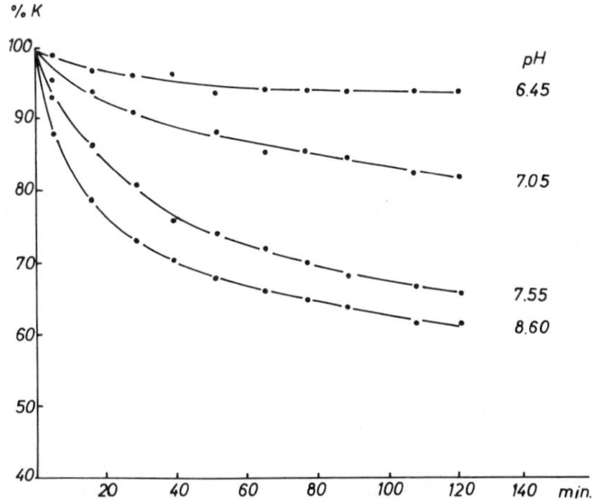

FIG. 6. Effects of pH on K loss at low ionic strength. Human red cells in 0.3 *M* sucrose solution containing 0.016 mole NaCl; temperature 22°C. Ordinate: K content of the cells in percent of initial value. Abscissa: time in minutes (Buchbinder and Passow, unpublished results).

In $MgCl_2$ and $CaCl_2$ solutions, K loss proceeds at approximately the same velocity, but slightly faster than in NaCl solutions. This discrepancy is probably related to the fact that with the divalent cations, twice as much chloride is introduced into the medium as with the monovalent ones. Thus the position of the Donnan equilibrium for the anions, including OH^-, is different in solutions of binary and ternary electrolytes of equal ionic strength. Consequently, differences in pH of the medium obtain, which can obviously not be compensated for by buffering. These differences may greatly affect the permeability change, since increasing the pH at any given ionic strength augments the rate of net K loss. Thus it is possible to induce rapid K loss by raising the pH of a sucrose/NaCl mixture of ionic strength such that at low pH values (say, pH 6.5) net K movements are barely detectable (Fig. 6, Passow, 1960).

The pH of the medium is governed by the Donnan distribution ratio

OH_i/OH_o, which in turn depends on variations in the chloride concentration of the medium. If, for example, packed erythrocytes whose pH lies around 7.4 are mixed with a neutral sucrose solution, the chloride concentration of the medium is reduced, and pH values as low as 5.8 can be observed in the resulting suspension. This shift in the Donnan equilibrium leads to a change in membrane potential whereby the normally negative cell interior may attain potentials up to +100 mV with respect to the outside solution. The relationship between the anion distribution ratio and pH, on the one hand, and the salt concentration of the medium, on the other can be fairly accurately predicted by means of equations based on the Donnon theory.

Subsequent to the described initial decrease in pH, it slowly rises again concomitantly with the cation movements. According to Wilbrandt (1940b), these changes reflect the transition of the ion distribution from that obtained at a cation-impermeable membrane to the distribution existing at a cation-permeable one. During the whole course of the K loss, the rapidly penetrating anions distribute in accordance with the Donnan law, whereby the rate-limiting cations determine the Donnan ratios $Cl_i/Cl_o = OH_i/OH_o$ at each instant (partial ionic equilibrium, Wilbrandt, 1940b).

After a few hours the cations also reach a Donnan equilibrium. Since the red blood cells contain large amounts of indiffusible anions, their internal K content may then still exceed that of the extracellular fluid. Similarly, the H^+ concentration inside the cell will be higher than outside and consequently, at the end of the experiment, the membrane potential regains its original negative sign, the pH of the medium attaining values as high as 8–9.

Several authors have tried to relate the acceleration of cation movements in nonelectrolyte solutions to the discussed changes in membrane potential. Davson (1939) pointed out that the establishment of the positive membrane potential, which occurs immediately after suspending the cells in the medium, increases the electrochemical potential difference for K ions and hence the driving force for their diffusion out of the cell. He rejected, however, the idea of a causal relationship between the increase in driving force and the permeability change, since K loss continues at a rapid rate even after the membrane potential has resumed its original negative sign.

Wilbrandt (1941) later showed that the "driving potential" for the cation transfer is not necessarily identical with the potential differences calculated from the chloride distribution ratios. The potential existing between the bulk phases of the cell interior and the surrounding fluid is composed of at least two interface potentials and the diffusion potential inside the membrane. Only the latter affects the migration rates. Wilbrandt estimated the interface potentials by assuming Donnan equilibria to exist at the two negatively charged membrane surfaces, and subtracted them from the overall potential. He was then able to demonstrate, for a number of those experimental conditions in which the sign of the overall potential did not seem to favor K loss, a parallelism between the K movements and the calculated "driving potentials."

With the discovery of the close relationship between the resistance to cation movements and the membrane potential in excitable tissues, Wilbrandt and Schatzmann (1960) recently extended the original hypothesis. They introduced the assumption that the red cell membrane changes its resistance to diffusion of alkali metal ions under the influence of variations in the membrane potential. Applying Goldman's (1943) equation to their data, they could show that the relationship between membrane potential and membrane resistance to K ions conforms to an S-shaped curve, where the resistance reaches a minimum at high positive potentials with respect to the external solution. Increasing the pH at a given ionic strength enhances the rate of K loss. It also leads to an increase in the dissociation of hemoglobin. As a consequence, the cell interior becomes more negative, and even in nonelectrolyte solutions where the potential is usually positive with respect to the outside, the membrane potential may assume large negative values. Thus the pH dependence of the permeability changes is in contrast to the assumed relationship between potential and membrane resistance. The question may therefore be asked whether other factors, instead of the membrane potential, play a predominant role in the control of passive cation permeability. Actually, the available observations seem to be more consistent with the view that not one but two independent variables, namely, ionic strength and pH, control the situation (Passow, 1960).

Variations in ionic strength and pH could conceivably influence the membrane permeability in many different ways. For example, the degree of polymerization of membrane proteins (as in the transformation of G-actin to F-actin) or the dissociation of fixed charges of the membrane matrix might be affected by the two parameters.

The latter possibility deserves comment since it fits easily into current concepts of the factors controlling the passive ion movements across membranes. If the diffusion of ions through the water-filled channels of the membrane should in fact be governed by the presence of dissociable amino groups, the selectivity of the membrane, and hence its efficiency in preventing the cations from passing, should depend on both pH and ionic strength of the medium.

The pK values of amino groups lie around 9, and thus drastic changes in the selectivity of the membrane can be expected only if the pH inside the membrane exceeds this value. The pH in a positively charged membrane should be higher than that of the adjacent solution. Assuming the establishment of Donnan equilibria between medium and positively charged interior of the membrane, it can be shown that the anion distribution ratio Cl_m/Cl_o, and hence the OH concentration of the membrane, increase with decreasing NaCl content of the medium. Consequently, a lowering of the salt concentration acts in the same direction as an alkalinization of the medium and thus shifts the equilibrium

$$NH_3^+ \rightleftharpoons NH_2 + H^+$$

to the right side. Due to the lowering of the concentration of fixed positive charges, the selectivity of the membrane decreases and net cation movements occur. In addition, variations in ionic strength of the medium affect the activity coefficients of the penetrating ions and thus exert secondary effects on the diffusion of ions through the charged membrane.

In conclusion, the assumption that dissociable fixed charges in the membrane control the passive cation permeability seems to offer the simplest explanation for the observation that variations in pH at high ionic strength have little influence on cation permeability, while increasing the pH at low ionic strength produces drastic effects.

2. Actions of SH Agents

The effect on cation permeability of most of the customary SH agents has been tested. Each substance used showed its own characteristic effects. It is therefore difficult to appraise the role of SH groups or S—S linkages in the control of cation permeability or of stability of the cell membrane.

Substances known to oxidize S—S or SH groups, such as ferricyanide or methylene blue, if applied in concentrations up to a few millimoles/liter seem to affect neither active nor passive cation permeability. Ferricyanide increases the ATP content of the cells presumably by oxidizing DPNH (NADH) to DPN (NAD), the rate-limiting participant of the glyceraldehyde-3-PO_4 dehydrogenase reaction which governs the ATP synthesis of the cell (Passow, 1963b). Active cation transport continues and may even be enhanced. Methylene blue elicits some K loss, but only if present at high concentration (unpublished observations).

Iodoacetate completely blocks active transport by inhibiting generation of the energy-supplying ATP or, after prolonged exposure, by blocking the transport enzyme. The ensuing net K loss does not exceed the normal rate of passive diffusion of about 1–2 mmoles/liter cells/hr. (cf. Fig. 7c).

Although neither ferricyanide nor iodoacetate produces any gross effects on passive cation permeability, both agents are capable of interacting with certain ligands in the cell membrane which play an essential role in maintaining the integrity of the permeability barrier. The latent effects of these interactions become apparent only if IAA and ferricyanide are applied together. The combined actions of both substances evoke rapid K^+ loss with little concomitant Na^+ entry. Ferricyanide cannot enter the red cell. It may be concluded, therefore, that it "conditions" or "sensitizes" membrane constituents located at the outer cell surface.

Inhibition of the glyceraldehyde phosphate dehydrogenase by IAA does not seem to be a necessary prerequisite for the permeability change to occur. At low concentrations of IAA (0.125 mmoles/liter), the formation of lactate from adenosine is not completely interrupted and ATP breakdown proceeds only slowly. No greater K loss than that due to inhibition of the pump can be observed. Under these conditions the generation of ATP can be appreciably enhanced by the addition of ferricyanide, since ferricyanide oxidizes DPNH to DPN and thus stimulates the partially inhibited glyceraldehyde phosphate dehydrogenase. The cellular ATP level may then—at least temporarily—exceed the normal value. Nevertheless rapid K loss occurs, the time course and extent of the permeability change being essentially similar to those observed in the absence of the substrate, adenosine, or in the presence of the high IAA concentrations that completely inhibit glyceraldehyde phosphate dehydrogenase. (Passow, 1963b).

At concentrations exceeding 1 mmole/liter, *N*-ethylmaleimide may produce rapid K loss. With increasing concentration the rates of K loss also increase and may attain 20–30 times the normal values. The K loss there is accompanied by Na uptake, although the latter occurs somewhat more slowly than the former. Since the cation movements tend to establish a Donnan equilibrium, the initially shrunken cells swell and finally disintegrate by colloid osmotic hemolysis. In human blood, about 10% of the cell population seems to maintain the original cation content even in the presence of high concentrations of *N*-ethylmaleimide (Giebel and Passow, 1961).

Most heavy metals have a strong affinity toward SH groups. One would expect, therefore, that when such metals are added to the cells in sufficiently high concentration, nearly all should be capable of inducing permeability changes similar to those seen with *N*-ethylmaleimide. It has in fact been observed that Hg, Au, and Pb evoke a large increase in K turnover (up to several hundred times, Joyce *et al.*, 1954; Grigarzik and Passow, 1958) associated with rapid net K loss. However, other metals like Ni, Co, and Cd exert almost negligible effects. Cu takes an intermediate position. It has been suggested, therefore, that the mode of action of heavy metals is mainly a matter of accessibility of the reactive sites in the cell membrane rather than of reactivity.

The responses to Hg, Au, and Pb show certain characteristic differences. Except in the initial phase, the responses elicited by mercury resemble those produced by *N*-ethylmaleimide in so far as the K loss is accompanied by the uptake of a nearly equivalent amount of Na. In contrast, lead barely enhances the rate of Na entry. Although potassium leaves the cells about 20–25 times faster than normally, the amount of intracellular Na remains nearly constant

(Fig. 7); the Na concentration increases, of course, since the loss of KCl is associated with shrinkage of the cells.

The actions of mercury can be completely prevented if the metal is applied in the presence of equimolar amounts of SH agents (Weed *et al.*, 1962). Lead, on the other hand, evokes rapid K loss, even in the presence of 200-fold excess of cysteine (Passow and Schütt, 1956).

These and other observations suggest that K loss without concomitant Na uptake is caused by interactions with hitherto unidentified ligands other than S—S or SH in the cell membrane. (For a review of the effects of lead, see Passow *et al.*, 1961.) The nonspecific effects of mercury, however, seem to be due to interactions with sulfur-containing compounds (Weed *et al.*, 1962).

In summary, some SH agents are capable of interacting with ligands in the membrane surface and thereby decrease the membrane resistance to diffusion of K and Na, while others produce a latent change in the permeability barrier which manifests itself only if an additional stress is applied.

The chemical nature of the changes induced by the various agents (e.g. oxidation, mercaptide formation, disruption or establishment of S—S linkages, etc.) is still obscure. There remains little doubt, however, that SH or S—S groups are structural elements of functional significance although their exact role remains to be established.

3. Actions of Lytic Agents in Sublytic Doses

Any inhibitor of active transport should, in due course, induce colloid osmotic hemolysis. There exist, however, a large number of substances, e.g., Na-taurocholate, distearyl lecithin (Ponder, 1947a), methanol, ethanol, guaiacol, resorcinol (Ponder, 1947b), *n*-butyl alcohol, etc. (Ponder, 1949), vitamin A (Dingle and Lucy, 1962), and alkyl sulfates (Hutchinson and Bean, 1955), which seem to act by disorienting or removing components of the cell membrane. They either destroy the membrane or induce an alteration in the permeability barrier which eventually leads to colloid osmotic hemolysis. The "prelytic" cation movements occurring in the interval between the addition of a lysin and the ensuing hemolysis consist of a nearly one-to-one exchange of K with Na. According to Ponder (1948), the rate of prelytic cation movements depends on the hemolytic power of the lysins. The more powerful agents usually produce a smaller permeability change than do the weaker ones. For example, with digitonin which acts by removing cholesterol from the membrane, very little K loss precedes the disintegration of the cell, whereas suitable concentrations of resorcinol or butanol cause a nearly complete K/Na exchange without appreciable hemolysis.

The effects of the latter two alcohols are of particular interest since they can be largely reversed by washing the cells free of these agents (Parpart and Green, 1951; Netter, 1959). Within a few hours of incubation following butanol removal, the K outflux returns to nearly normal values while the Na influx falls to about twice the control level (Green and Bond, 1961). The cells regain their capacity for active cation transport. The butanol treatment interferes with neither glucose uptake nor lactate production (Rinehart and Green, 1962). Therefore the action of the alcohol is largely confined to the cell membrane itself.

4. Metabolic Control of Passive Cation Permeability

The cellular cation content is adjusted to physiological requirements by pump and leak. The activity of the pump is governed by the metabolic state of the cell; it varies in response to variations in intra- and extracellular cation concentrations, and is perhaps subject to hormonal control. Control of the rate of active transport is therefore the cell's most obvious means for adapting the cation distribution to functional changes. Nevertheless, the resistance of the membrane to the passive penetration of cations is not fixed at a constant value throughout the life span of the cell, but may vary and thus conceivably support the regulatory function of the pump. The arrangement, spacing, and charge of membrane constituents may be affected by the ionic composition of the medium. Specific poisons, drugs, and hormones, such as vasopressin which increases the passive Na entry into epithelial cells or acetylcholine which reduces the membrane resistance to K and Na of the motor end-plate, may interact with loci at the cell surface which are of special significance for the passage of ions. Moreover, cell membranes are living structures. Many of their constituents are in dynamic equilibrium with their surroundings (e.g. cholesterol (London and Schwarz, 1953; Muir *et al.*, 1951; Zilversmit *et al.*, 1943) and phospholipids[6] (Jones and Gardner, 1962) readily exchange between erythrocytes and plasma) and may undergo metabolic turnover. The cell membrane can thus be regarded as representing a dynamic system rather than a static structure, whose properties should be related to the metabolic events in the cell. One may suspect, therefore, that the cell metabolism also governs the membrane resistance to the passive penetration of ions. There exist, in fact, a number of observations (Passow, 1961, 1963b; Kregenow and Hoffman, 1962; Hoffman, 1962c) concerning the actions of certain substrates and metabolic inhibitors on the cation permeability of the erythrocyte, which indicate a close interrelationship between intermediary metabolism and passive

[6] Altman *et al.* (1951) and Lovelock *et al.* (1960) have suggested that blood cells synthesize many lipids and that there is an exchange of lipids between the blood cells and the plasma. These authors, however, used red cell suspensions which contained platelets, leucocytes, and reticulocytes. Buchanan (1960) has shown that almost all the lipid synthesis in these preparations is brought about by the white cells and not the red cells. In the experiments of Jones and Gardener particular care was taken to remove these cells before measuring the lipid exchange.

permeability, although it remains to be decided whether this interrelationship is of physiological significance.

a. Action of Fluoride on Potassium Permeability. In low concentration (about 1 mmole/liter) fluoride suppresses glycolysis and hence lowers the

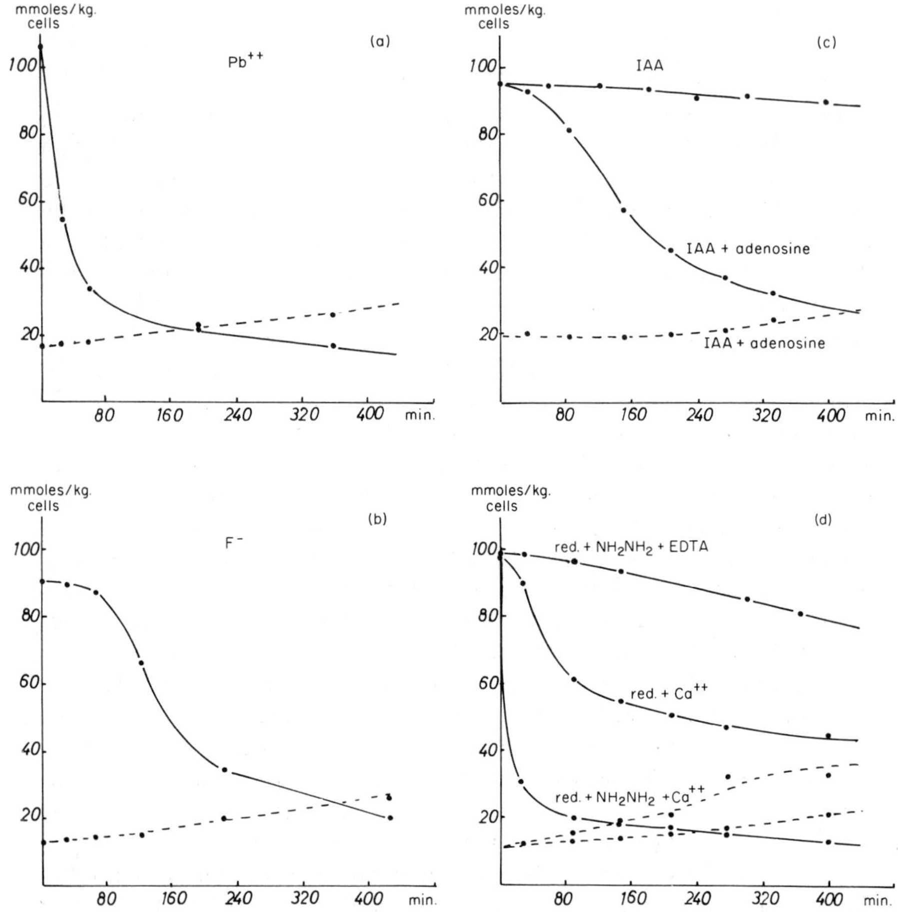

FIG. 7. (*a*) Pb (0.06 mmole/liter, 21°C.); (*b*) fluoride (40 mmoles/liter, 37°C.); (*c*) iodoacetate (2.5 mmoles/liter) and iodoacetate (2.5 mmoles/liter) + adenosine (10 mmoles/liter) + 0.5 mmole/liter $CaCl_2$, 37°C.; (*d*) triose reductone with and without hydrazine (2.5 mmoles/liter triose reductone, 10 mmoles/liter NH_2NH_2, 0.5 mmoles/liter $CaCl_2$, 10 mmoles/liter EDTA, 37°C.).

The lower of the two dashed lines indicates sodium uptake in the presence of reductone, the upper in the presence of both, reductone and hydrazine.

The continuous lines refer to K, the dashed lines to Na concentrations (redrawn from Passow, 1961).

intracellular ATP content. Consequently, active transport of K and Na ceases and net cation movements occur. Under these conditions the rates of K loss (Eckel, 1958) and Na entry (Lepke and Passow, 1960b) do not exceed a few mmoles/liter cells/hr. If the fluoride concentration is raised, however, after a lag period a large increase in the rate of K loss occurs. Both the magnitude of this additional effect and the duration of the lag period depend on the concentration of alkaline earth metal ions in the external solution. In the absence of alkaline earth metal ions, if the medium contains a complexing agent such as ethylenediaminetetraacetic acid, the increase in passive potassium permeability at high F concentrations is completely prevented (Gárdos, 1958; Passow and Lepke, 1959). With up to 0.05 or 0.5 mmoles/liter $CaCl_2$ or $MgCl_2$, respectively, the duration of the lag period preceding the onset of K loss shortens with increasing concentration. The K loss after the latency period is about 20 times faster than normal, while very little sodium is taken up. The cells shrink and attain a high osmotic resistance. Further increasing the concentrations of alkaline earth metal ions reduces the lag period to virtually zero. In addition, the nature of the effect changes. The membrane becomes permeable also to Na ions which enter the cells at about the same rate as K ions leave. The cells swell and eventually disintegrate by colloid osmotic hemolysis (Lepke and Passow, 1960a, b).

The specific effect on potassium permeability alone can be modified by agents which affect the metabolism of the poisoned cells. Addition of substrates such as adenosine or pyruvate, or of oxidizing agents such as methylene blue or ferricyanide, prevents the specific change in membrane resistance to K ions, but exerts little or no influence on the nonspecific damage observed at high Ca or Mg concentrations. It seems reasonable, therefore, to distinguish between two types of fluoride action. One of them apparently represents a direct action on the cell membrane where the changes in cation permeability are comparable to those seen in the presence of lysins at sublytic concentrations. The other seems to be related to the capacity of fluoride to inhibit glycolysis (Lindemann and Passow, 1960a).

As has been stated, certain substrates or intermediates of cell metabolism (e.g., oxidizing agents which act to produce DPN as a substrate for the rate-limiting glyceraldehyde phosphate dehydrogenase) may suppress the specific action of fluoride. Others, like inosine or glucose, however, are without influence or may even slightly enhance the rate of K loss. For a time it was believed therefore that fluoride, by blocking the enolase, diverted the glycolytic reactions into normally less prominent metabolic pathways and thus induced by means of the cell's own enzymes an increase in concentration of an intermediate which controlled the passive potassium permeability (Wilbrandt, 1940b; Gárdos, 1958). It has been observed, however, that cell substrate depletion, obtained by incubating the cells for many hours in saline solutions prior to the addition of fluoride, augments the cell sensitivity to the poison. The lag period shortens and the rate of K loss increases. Obviously, in cells largely devoid of glycolytic intermediates, the occurrence of abnormal side reactions is unlikely. Since the permeability change develops only in the presence of traces of alkaline earth metal ions, which at low concentration penetrate only extremely slowly, it was suggested that the formation of an alkaline earth metal–fluoride complex with ligands in the cell surface is the primary and most important event in fluoride action.

Since the inhibition of glycolysis either by fluoride itself or by substrate deprivation is a prerequisite for the permeability change to occur, it is assumed that only inhibition of glycolysis renders the normally inaccessible surface ligands susceptible to direct interaction with alkaline earth metals and fluoride (Lindemann and Passow, 1960b).

b. Action of Iodoacetate on Potassium Permeability. It has already been mentioned that iodoacetate (IAA), in spite of its strong inhibitory action on glycolysis, evokes no K or Na net movements beyond those to be expected as the result of an interruption of the energy supply to the pump. If, however, suitable substrates and calcium ions are added together with the poison, the net potassium loss after an induction period is greatly enhanced and may exceed 15–25 times the rate observed with IAA-poisoned red cells in the absence of substrates (Gàrdos, 1959, 1961). This effect is again specific for K and not associated with appreciable changes in passive Na permeability (Passow, 1961).

The most effective substrate, adenosine, is readily consumed by IAA-poisoned cells. After deamination and phosphorolytic cleavage, the resulting ribose phosphate is converted via the pentose phosphate pathway to trioses and fructose phosphate. IAA is a very potent inhibitor of the glycolytic enzyme, glyceraldehyde phosphate dehydrogenase. Accordingly, at the fairly high concentration of about 2.5 mmoles/liter where a maximal effect on permeability is elicited, IAA abolishes lactate production while trioses accumulate. Although the esterification of inorganic phosphate under this condition continues for at least 1–2 hours, the ATP content of the cells rapidly decrease to virtually zero.

In contrast to previously expressed views (Passow, 1963b; Gruner and Passow, 1963) the inhibition of glyceraldehyde phosphate dehydrogenase or the ensuing reduction of intracellular ATP content seems to be a necessary prerequisite for the permeability change to occur. This may be inferred from the (unpublished) observation that at low IAA concentrations at which the enzyme is only partially inhibited, any increase of the intracellular DPN content reduces the effect on cation permeability. Thus, addition of pyruvate largely restores the capacity of the poisoned cells to synthesize ATP and simultaneously diminishes the rate of K loss.

The fact that a substrate must be consumed in order to elicit the permeability change seems to indicate that the cellular enzymes are capable of deriving from adenosine a product which specifically controls passive permeability without having any effect on Na transfer. The formation of this product or its capacity to act on the cell membrane depends on the presence of nitrogen-containing compounds. If inosine is added as a substrate, the K loss of the IAA-poisoned cells proceeds much slower than with adenosine. Supplying NH_4Cl together with inosine increases the efficiency of this substrate in enhancing passive K movements. At high NH_4Cl concentrations, inosine may attain an efficiency similar to that of adenosine. A number of other N-containing compounds can be used equally well for supplementing inosine. Hydrazine proved to be the most effective among them, but histidine and histamine (the latter at very low concentrations of about 0.5 mmole/liter) act similarly. Most N-containing substances tested so far (e.g., various amines, amino acids, urea, creatinine, etc.) cannot substitute for NH_4Cl.

The presence of Ca ions in the medium is an essential requirement for the permeability change. Complete removal by EDTA abolishes the specific effect on K permeability. Raising the Ca concentration increases the effect until at about 0.5 mmole/liter a maximal response is reached. Mg cannot replace Ca; instead it has a slightly inhibitory action (Passow, 1963b).

c. Action of Triose Reductone. In order to identify those products of adenosine metabolism responsible for the K loss occurring in the presence of IAA, the change in K permeability was measured after addition to red cells of various possible normal and abnormal intermediates of pentose phosphate metabolism in the presence or absence of IAA, calcium, and a suitable nitrogen-containing substance (usually NH_4Cl or NH_2NH_2). Of a large variety of substances tested (e.g., glyceraldehyde, dihydroxyacetone, etc.) only triose reductone, hitherto not shown to occur in red cells, produced responses to be expected from such a product (Passow, 1961).

Triose reductone is a highly reactive and very unstable compound[7] which may exist as an enediol (HCOH=HCOH—HCHO) (v. Euler and Eistert, 1957). It is thus chemically related to ascorbic acid and certain intermediates formed in the course of enzymatic epimerization and isomerization of sugar esters (Cohen, 1953). In aqueous solution reductone strongly interacts with hydrazine. The reaction rate is greatly enhanced in the presence of red cells, which readily metabolize reductone as well as its hydrazide. Triose reductone induces K loss with little concomitant Na uptake. The magnitude of the effect depends not only on the reductone concentration but also on (1) the

[7] Triose reductone and its hydrazide are fairly stable in acid solution but rapidly decompose in the neutral or alkaline range. The biological effects therefore depend on the time elapsing between preparation of the solutions, the adjustment of the pH, and the addition to the red blood cells. In oxygen-free solutions no decomposition of reductone occurs.

presence of Ca, (2) the concentration of NH_2NH_2 or NH_4Cl, and (3) the metabolic state of the cells. Its actions are thus dependent on factors similar to those in the case of adenosine (Passow, 1963b, and unpublished observations).

Removal of Ca by ethylenediaminetetraacetic acid (EDTA) reduces the net K loss. NH_2NH_2 augments and NH_4Cl diminishes the effects of reductone. The presence of iodoacetate is not essential for the permeability change to develop, although inhibition of the cell metabolism by the poison or by prolonged substrate depletion greatly increases the rate of K loss. Upon addition of 2.5 mmoles/liter reductone and 5.0 mmoles/liter hydrazine, cells preincubated in the absence of substrates for 12–16 hours lose K at about 20–25 times the normal rate. It remains to be decided whether triose reductone or a compound similar to its hydrazine derivative is formed if adenosine-consuming cells are poisoned with IAA. Nevertheless, reductone represents another example of a substrate, readily metabolized by the cells, that acts on K rather than on Na permeability.

5. Role of Alkaline Earth Metal Ions in the Control of Passive Permeability to Alkali Metal Ions

The previously described actions of abnormal substrates and metabolic inhibitors can develop only if traces of alkaline earth metal ions are present. One may now ask what is known of the function of Ca and Mg in the maintenance of the normal membrane resistance to alkali metal ions.

Hoffman and Tosteson (1959; cf. Hoffman, 1962c) recently incorporated Mg or Ca into substrate-free red cell ghosts and followed the effects on K permeability. If Mg was introduced into the "ghosts" the cell membrane regained a high degree of impermeability to K^+, irregardless of the intracellular Mg concentration. Loading the "ghosts" with Ca led also to a reconstitution of the permeability barrier, but only if the Ca concentration was below 0.2 mmoles/liter. At higher concentrations the membrane became leaky and the "ghosts" were incapable of maintaining K^+ concentration gradients (Fig. 8).

Although the ghosts prepared in the absence of alkaline earth metal ions regain a high degree of impermeability to K, the presence in the cell interior of traces of either Mg or Ca is still essential for the control of passive K permeability. This can be inferred from the observation that incorporation of complexing agents such as ATP (or EDTA) prevents the cells from regaining a high diffusional resistance to K after hemolysis. The action of the complexing agent can be overcome, however, if it is incorporated into the ghosts together with an at least equivalent amount of Mg. Calcium, which is less firmly bound to ATP than Mg (cf. Bock, 1960), can replace the latter in restoring a high membrane resistance, provided its concentration does not exceed 25–50% that of ATP. At higher concentration, Ca decreases the membrane resistance to K, just as in the absence of the complexing agent.

Since metabolic inhibitors cause an increase in passive Ca influx into red blood cells (Passow and Wilde, 1961), and at the same time usually reduce the concentration of complexing ATP, their actions on K permeability could

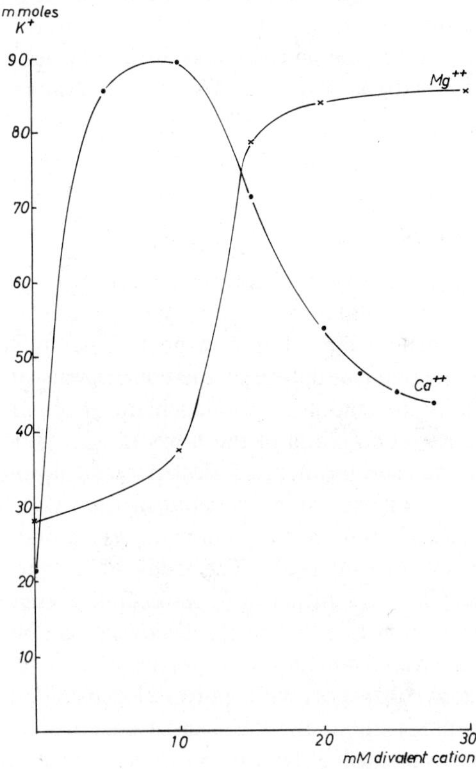

FIG. 8. Effects of Ca^{++} and Mg^{++} on potassium retention by "ghosts." The ghosts were prepared by hemolysis in distilled water containing Ca^{++} or Mg^{++} at the concentration indicated on the abscissa. Ordinate: K concentration of K-loaded ghosts after 3 washes in isotonic NaCl (redrawn from Hoffman, 1962c).

conceivably be interpreted in terms of variations in the concentration of ionized Ca^{++} inside the cells. It may be argued, however, that most metabolic inhibitors induce K loss at extracellular Ca concentrations far below the intracellular concentration required for making the ghosts leaky. Furthermore, under certain experimental conditions the poisons induce K loss while a net synthesis of ATP occurs. Moreover, like ATP or EDTA, penetrating complexing agents such as fluoride ought to increase passive K permeability by precipitating intracellular Mg. This effect should be independent of the external concentrations of alkaline earth metal ions. Yet the presence of traces of extracellular Ca or Mg is essential for the fluoride action to develop, and nonpenetrating complexing agents in the external solution completely prevent the typical fluoride effect on passive K permeability.

At this time it is still unknown why certain metabolic poisons can induce K loss only in the presence of Ca^{++} or Mg^{++}. One may suspect that alkaline earth metal ions modify the actions of surface enzymes which participate in the sequence of metabolic reactions leading to alteration of K permeability, or render structural elements of the membrane susceptible to direct attack by the poison.

C. Active Transport

Until recently it was possible to discuss only in rather general terms the mechanism by which metabolic energy may be transformed into osmotic and electrical work during active ion transport. Due to lack of information concerning the biochemical nature of the constituents of the ion pump, one could only appraise the minimum physicochemical requirements which must be met to bring about coupling of the flows of energy, ions, and "carriers" associated with the establishment of electrochemical potential gradients. In 1960, however, an enzyme was discovered in the red cell membrane which apparently fulfills an important function in active cation transport (Post *et al.*, 1960; Dunham and Glynn, 1961). The study of the mode of action of this enzyme has since played a central role in permeability research. In the following pages, the main steps which led to its discovery will be outlined, and subsequently a detailed account of its properties and of several hypotheses on its function in active transport will be given. Focusing on the vast amount of information available about the "transport enzyme" necessarily limits the space available for describing the transport phenomena observed in the intact red cell. Fortunately, however, a balanced review on this subject has been published by Glynn (1957a) and the reader is referred to this article.

1. Kinetics of Active Transport

If measured under steady state conditions with K^{42} as a tracer, the rate of K uptake by red cells suspended in isotonic solutions containing KCl and NaCl in varying proportions increases with the potassium concentration (Streeten and Solomon, 1954). The slope of the curve relating K concentration to K flux decreases with increasing K concentration of the medium and, at K concentrations above approximately 25 mmoles/liter, assumes a small constant value. The shape of this curve can most conveniently be interpreted by assuming that K enters the cells partly by active transport and partly by passive diffusion. The initial bent part of the curve can be described by an equation similar to that of Michaelis and Menten, thus suggesting that it represents the kinetics of a carrier system. The linear part can be attributed to the proportionality between flux and concentration which is to be expected in simple diffusion processes (Shaw, 1955). This interpretation was supported by the observation that the slope of the linear component is independent of the presence or absence of substrates. Similarly, the parameter corresponding in enzyme kinetics to the Michaelis constant is independent of the metabolic state of the cell, whereas the saturation level, supposed to represent maximum activity of a transport enzyme or the maximum number of carrier molecules available, decreases if the cell metabolism is interrupted by lack of substrates (Glynn, 1956) (Fig. 9).

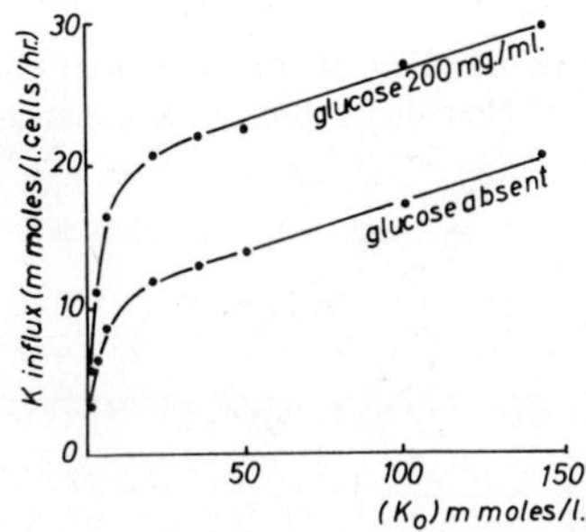

FIG. 9. K influx as measured with K^{42} at increasing K concentrations of the medium Human red cells. 37°C. (redrawn from Glynn, 1956).

Although the explanation of these observations is far from conclusive, it tentatively allows differentiation between the active and passive components of potassium fluxes and is thus a fruitful tool in studies on the relationships between active K and Na transport.

2. Coupling of K and Na Transport

According to Glynn (1956, 1957b), it is also possible to differentiate between two components of the Na flux. One is independent of the K concentration of the medium whereas the other is augmented by increasing the external K concentration. Since the residual sodium flux as measured in the absence of potassium equals that observed in the absence of any substrate, it is concluded that the Na flux is made up of one active and one passive component, the magnitude of the former being dependent on the K concentration of the medium. The activation by K of the sodium transport system can be described by the Michaelis-Menten equation, where the Michaelis constant has the same numerical value as that observed for activation of the K transport system by K ions. This observation was considered to support the hypothesis, first advanced by Harris (1954), that K and Na are pumped by a common mechanism and that a fixed ratio between K and Na transport exists (Figs. 10, 11).

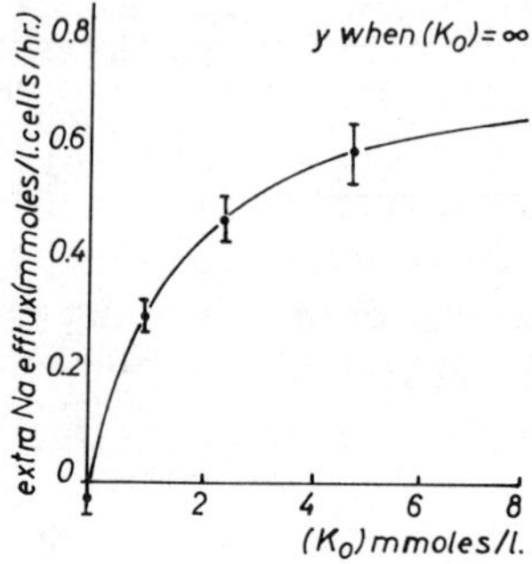

FIG. 10. Sodium outflux as function of the potassium concentration of the medium. Ordinate: active component of Na efflux. Abscissa: K concentration in mmoles/liter.

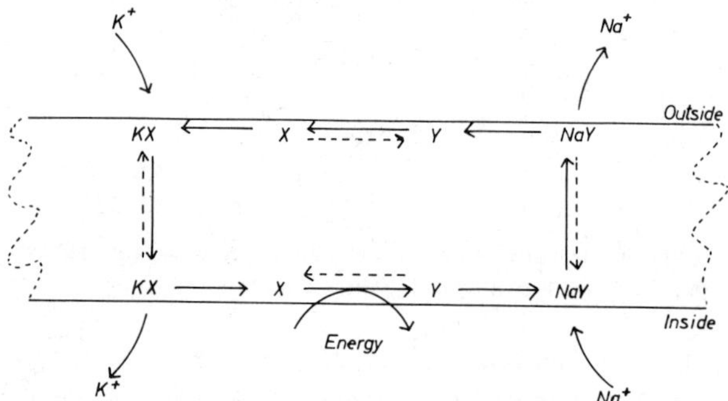

FIG. 11. Coupled carrier transport of K and Na (according to Solomon, 1952, and Glynn, 1955; redrawn from Glynn, 1956).

3. Inhibition of Active Transport by Cardiac Glycoside

Cardiac glycosides have played a key role in the development of present concepts of active transport. They exert little if any effect on the passive components of K and Na transport. Thus the passive cation movements which occur during cold storage of the cells are virtually unaffected by cardiac glycosides, and in studies of their action on K^{42} movements in sheep (Tosteson and Hoffman, 1960) and human (Glynn, 1957b) red cells, only in the latter was a small reduction in the passive fluxes observed.

Cardiac glycosides, however, completely inhibit the active components of cation fluxes and may thus prevent the reaccumulation of cations which takes place if cold-stored cells are rewarmed in the presence of suitable substrates.

These findings were of particular importance since neither glycolysis nor ATP synthesis is decreased by the glycosides. It could therefore be concluded that cardiac glycosides are specific inhibitors of the K-Na pump and that detailed study of their mode of action promised information on the molecular mechanism of active transport (Schatzmann, 1953). This contention was soon supported by the observation that their inhibitory action could be diminished or abolished by increasing the K concentration of the medium. Comparative studies using different glycosides show that their efficiency depends largely on the configuration of the glycoside at C-17 and on the degree of saturation of the lactone ring. The aglycone is less effective (Glynn, 1957b).

4. Role of ATP as Energy Source for Active Cation Transport

It was long suspected that active transport is accomplished at the expense of high-energy phosphate bonds. This view could be confirmed when Straub and co-workers (1953) invented their ingenious methods for introducing non-penetrating substrates of their choice into emptied cells, so-called ghosts. They hemolyzed red cells in hypotonic solutions with a given substrate. During osmotic hemolysis, the contents leave the cell whereas the substrate added to the medium enters the cell. During this process, the membrane seems to suffer no irreversible damage since after hemolysis the substrate is trapped on its inside. The high resistance to the movements of cations (Székely *et al.*, 1953; Teorell, 1952) is regained and, provided adequate substrates are present, active transport occurs. By applying this technique, Straub and co-workers were able to show that ghosts, which—due to the removal of intracellular substrates and enzymes—were incapable of glycolyzing, were still able to accumulate cations provided ATP was introduced into the cells (Gàrdos and Straub, 1956).

Straub's pioneer work has been criticized because, under his experimental conditions, there would have been present in his samples a certain fraction of unhemolyzed cells along with the ghosts. The uncertainty concerning the interpretation of his results was soon removed when Hoffman and Tosteson (1956) repeated and extended Straub's work with more homogeneous ghost preparations. Finally, Hoffman (1960) was able to show with his refined technique that only ATP is a suitable substrate for active transport whereas other nucleotides, like uridine, inosine, guanosine, and cytidine triphosphates, are ineffective.

5. Actions of Alkaline Earth Metal Ions

Studies on the cation accumulation in ATP-loaded ghosts soon revealed that alkaline earth metal ions profoundly influence the transport system. If no magnesium is present in the ghosts or if the complexing agent ethylenediaminetetraacetic acid is incorporated into them, active cation movements cease (Pragay, 1956), whereas maximal activity of the pump is observed if equivalent amounts of ATP and Mg are incorporated into the ghosts. Ca cannot replace Mg, and if Ca enters the cell the pump is inhibited (Rummel *et al.*, 1963; Hoffman, 1962c). Both cation species, Ca and Mg, exert virtually no effect on cation transport if applied to the medium surrounding either intact red cells (Whittam, 1958) or ghosts (Hoffman, 1962c), and the latter have been shown to accumulate alkali metal ions in media containing ethylenediaminetetraacetic acid (Pragay, 1956).

6. K–Na-Sensitive ATPase in the Red Cell Membrane

With the knowledge just described, it appeared reasonable to assume the participation in active cation transport of an enzyme which reacts specifically with ATP. This enzyme should be located in the membrane, be activated by K, Na, and Mg, and be inhibited by cardiac glycosides. ATPase activity has been repeatedly demonstrated in the red cell membrane (Herbert, 1956; Caffrey *et al.*, 1956; Clarkson and Maizels, 1952), and Straub and his group attempted as early as 1953 to correlate ATP breakdown with cation transport in ghosts. ATP breakdown was observed to proceed much faster, however, than ion accumulation and no simple interrelationship between the two processes could be established at that time. It was concluded therefore that nonspecific reactions obscured the true relationship between cation movements and ATP hydrolysis.

The study of this question was resumed along somewhat different lines when Skou (1957) discovered, in submicroscopic particles (supposedly membrane fragments) of leg nerves from the shore crab (*Carcinus maenas*), an enzyme exhibiting many of the properties that one would expect to be typical of a "transport ATPase." Stimulated by Skou's work, Post *et al.* (1960) and Dunham and Glynn (1961) made a successful attempt to prepare a similar ATPase by fragmenting erythrocyte membranes.

They compared substrate specificity, activation requirements, and sensitivity to specific inhibitors of both pump and ATPase, and observed in virtually every detail a quantitative correspondence of the respective properties.

Since the publication of these results, a large number of investigations have revealed the presence of a similar enzyme in membranes (including the endoplasmic reticulum) of many types of cell in many species (e.g., Taylor, 1962; Bonting *et al.*, 1961; Auditore and Murray, 1962; Skou, 1962; Wheeler and Whittam, 1962). It has been shown that in all tissues in which ouabain was reported to block active potassium and sodium movements (including frog skin, brain, cornea, etc.), the ATPase is present and a correlation seems to exist between its activity and the capacity of the respective tissue to transport ions (Bonting *et al.*, 1962).

The study of this enzyme plays a key role in present attempts to elucidate the mechanism of active transport. Its properties as well as the evidence for its participation in the transport processes will therefore be described below in considerable detail. In particular, it will be shown that the effect of the activating alkali metal ions on the ATPase depends on whether they act on the inner, on the outer, or on both surfaces of the membrane, and that active transport may therefore be considered the consequence of an assymetric activation of the enzyme by the two ion species to be transported.

a. Basic Properties of the Enzyme Preparation. The term ATPase as used in this context does not refer to a soluble enzyme preparation, but rather to a suspension of microscopically visible membrane fragments. A convenient way of obtaining an active preparation consists of hemolyzing the cells with digitonin (Tosteson, 1963). Under these conditions, only cholesterol is removed from the membrane (Schmidt Thomé, 1942), which still forms a coherent structure and shows little if any visible alterations under the phase contrast microscope. In spite of many attempts, it has not yet been possible to obtain a solubilized active preparation (Dunham and Glynn, 1961).[8] The main distinction between ghosts obtained by hypotonic hemolysis and the enzyme is therefore that in the former the membrane continues to function as an efficient permeability barrier, whereas in the latter all added substrates and activators have easy access to both sides of the membrane.

b. The Substrate. The membrane preparation converts ATP to AMP (adenosine monophosphate). It is assumed that the liberation of two phosphate ions proceeds in two consecutive steps with ADP (adenosine diphosphate) as an intermediate. ADP is hydrolyzed at about half the rate observed with ATP (Post *et al.*, 1960), and it is tacitly assumed that only the conversion of ATP to ADP is related to active transport. Tosteson (1963) recently indicated that it is possible to study the ATPase under conditions in which the amount of orthophosphate released is equal to the amount of ADP produced. This confirms the idea that the enzyme is a true ATPase and not an apyrase.

The concentration of ATP for half-maximal saturation of the enzyme, in the presence of all activating cations at optimal concentrations, has been estimated by Post *et al.* (1960) and by Tosteson (1963). The former group of authors obtained a figure of about 5×10^{-4} mole/liter (human red cells) whereas Tosteson, who extended the range of measurements to extremely low ATP concentrations, observed a value of about 10^{-6} to 10^{-5} mmoles/liter (sheep red cells). The latter result would imply that the membrane ATPase is saturated with ATP even at intracellular ATP concentrations far below the physiological range.

ITP (inosine triphosphate) is also utilized by the enzyme, but the rate of

[8] Many detergents such as dodecylsulfate or alcohols inhibit the ATPase (Järnefelt, 1961).

hydrolysis is only about 10% that of ATP. Guanosine triphosphate and uridine triphosphate do not seem to be utilized at all. The membrane ATPase thus exhibits the same substrate specificity as does the transport system (Hoffman, 1962c).

Tosteson *et al.* (1961) made the interesting suggestion that the widely distributed alkaline phosphomonoesterase might be identical with the membrane ATPase. They observed a parallelism between ATPase and monoesterase activity in the red cells of various species with widely differing ATPase activities. Furthermore they found that a monoesterase substrate, *p*-nitrophenylphosphate, and its dephosphorylation product inhibited the ATPase, while the esterase was inhibited by ATP and ADP. It would be most remarkable if two substrates of so widely differing structure as ATP and *p*-nitrophenylphosphate were both hydrolyzed by an enzyme exhibiting such unusual discriminating powers with respect to substances as closely related as ATP and ITP or other nucleotides.

c. Activation and Inhibition by Inorganic Cations. ATP hydrolysis is highly dependent on the relative concentration of the four cations K, Na, Mg, and Ca. In the complete absence of alkaline earth metal ions, there is virtually no ATP splitting. Mg activates the enzyme regardless of whether K or Na is present. Addition of either K or Na only slightly augments its activity above that observed in the presence of Mg alone. If, however, both alkali metal ions are added together to the Mg-activated enzyme, its activity increases greatly. At a constant Na concentration of about 160 mmoles/liter the concentration for half-maximal activation (K_m) by potassium was about 3 mmoles/liter compared with 2.1 mmoles/liter for active transport in ghosts or intact cells. Similarly, with sodium in the presence of an excess of potassium, K_m is 24 mmoles/liter compared with 20 mmoles/liter for the transport system.

The activation of the enzyme by the combined action of the two alkali metal ion species depends on the concentration ratio K/Na rather than on absolute values for the concentration of either ion. If the assay is performed in the presence of a large excess of either K or Na, inhibition occurs.

The inhibitory effect of Na on the activation by potassium ions can be counteracted by increasing the potassium concentration. The sodium ions are assumed therefore to compete for the potassium site on the enzyme. In the crab nerve enzyme, potassium ions were shown to displace competitively sodium ions from their site of action. Although the kinetics of the inhibition by potassium of the erythrocyte enzyme have not yet been quantitatively studied, the data presented by Post *et al.* and Dunham and Glynn suggest that a similar effect occurs also in that preparation.

NH_4 ions are a substitute for K but not for Na in both accumulating erythrocytes and enzyme. The corresponding K_m values are 7–16 and 8 mmoles/liter, respectively, in the presence of 160 mmoles/liter Na.

It is not possible to give a generally applicable figure for the Mg concentration which produces maximal activation of the ATPase. Its activity seems to depend on the ratio ATP/Mg rather than on the Mg concentration only.The published data suggest maximal activation at a 1 : 1 ratio of the two substances.

Calcium is incapable of replacing Mg as an activator of the enzyme. In the presence of a given magnesium concentration, Ca stimulates at low, and inhibits at high, concentration. Maximal activation at medium Ca concentration as well as extent of inhibition at high Ca concentration both depend on the Mg concentration. The data suggest, as has been pointed out by Dunham and Glynn, that the inhibitory effect of Ca is due to a Ca-Mg competition. At low Ca concentration the stimulation by K and Na and the inhibition by cardiac glycosides are reduced and, at inhibitory Ca concentrations, virtually absent. In other words, the K–Na-sensitive component of the Mg-activated ATPase is inhibited at all Ca concentrations, whereas the K–Na-insensitive component is stimulated at low and inhibited at high Ca concentration (Hoffman, 1962c).

d. K–Na-Sensitive and -Insensitive ATPase Activity. The difficulties encountered by Straub and co-workers in trying to correlate ATPase activity with transport were obviously due largely to the fact that the ATPase consists of two components of approximately equal size, one of which seems not to be related to active transport. It is not yet clear whether the two components of the ATPase are two separate enzymes.

Hoffman (1962c) postulates the existence of two enzymes. He assumes that the K–Na-sensitive ATPase is located on the inside of the membrane whereas the K–Na-insensitive enzyme is situated on its outside. Tosteson (1963), however, found only small differences between the ATP concentrations required for half-maximal activation of the two components. This observation speaks very much in favor of the existence of only one type of ATP-binding site and therefore for only one single enzyme. This is further supported, as has been pointed out by Dunham and Glynn, by the fact that the ratio between the activities of the two components depends on the Ca concentration. Moreover, slightly different ratios obtain in different preparations, as was also observed with ATPase preparations from crab nerve (Skou, 1960); in a given sample, the ratio of K–Na-insensitive and sensitive activities tends to change if the enzyme is stored in the cold. Furthermore, the activity depends on the mode in which the cell membrane is disrupted. Fragmentation by repeated washings in alkaline buffer solution (Post *et al.*, 1960) and hypotonically (Dunham and Glynn, 1961; Yoshida and Fugisawa, 1962) both increase the activity, and the possibility cannot be excluded that the ATPase preparations studied so far represent fragments in which the enzyme is uncoupled from a more complicated transport system.

e. Action of Inhibitors. The identification of the transport enzyme rested largely on a comparison of the actions of inhibitors, notably cardiac glycosides, on transport and ATPase activity. The same spectacular differences in efficiency of the various glycosides in inhibiting transport in the intact cell were also found with the ATPase preparation. Moreover, the concentration for half-maximal inhibition by ouabain was observed to be virtually the same for both enzyme and transport. Furthermore, at low concentrations of ouabain the inhibition of the ATPase is reduced by increasing the K concentration, just as in the intact cell where the action of glycosides on the ion pump may be overcome by the addition of potassium.

Since the cardiac glycosides inhibit only the K–Na-sensitive component of the enzyme, this component is frequently referred to as "strophanthin-sensitive."

Besides cardiac glycosides, a number of metabolic inhibitors such as iodoacetate, azide, arsenate, dinitrophenol, cyanide, and iodine were tested. They inhibit neither transport nor ATPase (Hoffman, 1962c).

The actions of the sulfhydryl-blocking agents, *N*-ethylmaleimide, chlormerodrin, and $HgCl_2$, were studied by Weed and Berg (1963). Like iodoacetate, *N*-ethylmaleimide, which reacts only with the most readily reactive SH groups (about 7–10% of the total), does not affect the ATPase. The other two agents are, however, capable of abolishing the K–Na-sensitive component of the enzyme if applied at concentrations sufficient to inactivate approximately 10–20% of the total SH content of the membrane.

For practical purposes it is noteworthy that the addition of antibiotics (penicillin and streptomycin) and the presence of leucocytes during preparation of the enzyme inhibit the K–Na-dependent ATPase activity (Weed *et al.*, 1963).

f. Species Differences. The ATPases of erythrocytes from different animal species exhibit more or less pronounced characteristic differences. The differences are accompanied by corresponding variations in their cation transport systems. In rat erythrocytes, cation transport is activated by potassium as is the case with human red cells but, contrary to the behavior of the latter, no active transport occurs until the potassium concentration of the medium exceeds 0.4 mmole/liter. Furthermore, as with human red cells, the K-Na pump can be inhibited by cardiac glycosides but unusually high concentrations must be applied (Pfleger *et al.*, 1961). The ATPase prepared from rat erythrocyte membranes shows similar characteristics: no activation by K at concentrations less than 0.4 mmole/liter and a high degree of insensitivity to heart glycosides (Hoffman, 1962b; Berg *et al.*, 1963).

Even in erythrocytes of different races of the same species, differences in the transport system may be present which are reflected in differences in the ATPase activity. In sheep, two hereditary varieties exist, one having a high proportion of K and the other a high proportion of Na in the erythrocytes.

The ATPase activity in "high-K" erythrocytes was found to be about 4 times that in "low-K" erythrocytes, and these differences almost exactly correspond to those in the transport rates (Tosteson, 1963).

The evidence for participation of the K–Na-sensitive ATPase in active transport thus seems to be fairly conclusive. It remains to be discovered how the enzyme accomplishes the movement of ions across the membrane.

g. Asymmetric Activation of the Enzyme by Inorganic Cations. One of the most important questions in this context is whether the alkali metal ions which activate the ATP-ase represent the ions transported. The similarity of the K_m values for activation by K and Na of transport and enzyme, and the following experiments, support the view that the activating ions are indeed the ones transported.

The ion pump moves K into and Na out of the cell. If the moved ions were the activating ones, one should expect ATP breakdown to be induced if sodium ions are confined exclusively to the inside and K ions to the outside of the membrane. Actually, in ghosts loaded with Na and suspended in K-containing medium, the strophanthin-sensitive ATPase activity was found to be one order of magnitude higher than with K-loaded cells in a K-poor sodium-rich solution. In the unfavorable situation (K inside, Na outside) a small amount of ATPase activity persists. This can probably be explained, however, by the unavoidable leakage of K outwards and Na inwards. Thus, the membrane ATPase is stimulated asymmetrically by Na and K (Glynn, 1962; Whittam, 1962). These observations are in accord with the contention that cation transport and activation of the ATPase by K and Na are identical processes. This conclusion was further supported by the finding that the antagonistic action of Na on the activation produced by K also depends on the location. External Na competitively inhibits activation by external K and thus counteracts the activation of the ATPase by internal Na. In contrast to what one would expect on the basis of Post's observations on the enzyme preparation, variations in internal K from 14–75 mmoles/liter did not affect internal Na activation (Whittam, 1962).

Attempts to measure the stoichiometric ratio of transport to dephosphorylation have been made by Sen and Post (1961) and Glynn (1962). The former authors observed that 3 equivalents of Na plus 2 equivalents of K were transported per mole of ATP split. The latter author reports that 3 Na ions are moved for each ATP molecule. He was unable to provide accurate figures for the K/P ratio but emphasized that it is less than 3. It thus appears that the pump does not operate at a K:Na exchange ratio of 1:1. It should be realized, however, that hydrogen ions are usually capable of competing with metal ions for binding sites. It may well be therefore that changes in pH affect the coupling ratio (Fig. 12).

h. Activation and Inhibition of the ATPase with Physiological Variations in the Alkali Metal Ion Concentrations. One may now ask under what conditions the "pump enzyme" operates in the intact cells. The sites activated by Na and K are located at the inside and outside of the membrane, respectively. The saturation of the enzyme with Na on the inside depends on both the Na and K concentration (Post *et al.*, 1960), although the latter does not seem to play a significant role in the physiological range (Whittam, 1962). At an intracellular Na concentration of about 17 mmoles/liter the enzyme is saturated to about 40%, where a nearly linear relationship exists between the rate of ATP hydrolysis and Na concentration. One may suppose therefore that the rate of net Na transport tends to follow first order kinetics, rising with increasing, and diminishing with decreasing, Na concentration. The effect of internal sodium is modified by external K. At a plasma concentration of about 5 mmoles/liter, the K ions exert about 80% of their maximal effect on the ATPase. Any increase in external K will enhance therefore the rate of ATP splitting and transport, although to a lesser extent than a first order reaction would do.

Variations in intra- and extracellular K concentrations are usually associated with reciprocal changes in Na concentrations. For example, during cold storage the K concentration of the plasma increases while its Na concentration decreases. This has a dual effect on the pumping rate. The augmentation of the plasma K raises the activity of the pump ATPase above its normal level, and the simultaneous lowering of the Na concentration reduces the sodium inhibition of the K-activated sites on the enzyme. Similarly, on the inside, where the Na concentration is above and the K concentration below normal, the K inhibition of Na-activated sites decreases and Na activation increases. Thus, during the reversal of the K/Na exchange between cells and plasma which takes place after cold storage, the rate of pumping is higher than under the usual steady state conditions, as has actually been observed by Ponder (1950b).

Normalization of the ion concentrations brought about by the action of the pump will automatically lead to a reduction in the activity of the pump, until at physiological concentration levels a new steady state is attained where the pumping rate resumes its original low value (Fig. 12).

i. Metabolic Factors Controlling the Activity of the Pump. In the intact cell a variety of reactions compete for ATP as the common substrate. The rate of any ATP-requiring reaction is influenced therefore by that of all others. Dunham (1957) and Hoffman (1962*c*) devised experiments to demonstrate the competition for ATP of the pump with the hexokinase reaction. Hoffman incorporated yeast hexokinase into ATP-loaded ghosts and measured active sodium transport in the presence and absence of glucose. Without glucose the pump operates at normal velocity, but upon addition of the substrate its activity is virtually abolished. Hoffman believes that this is due to the decrease in the

ATP concentration caused by the phosphorylation of glucose brought about by the hexokinase. It should be noted that if such a competition should actually play a role in the intact cell, the affinities for ATP of the transport enzyme and the hexokinase must be similar. Since the present data on ATP binding to the transport enzyme are widely divergent, it is not yet possible to decide whether this is true.

Just as the changes in ATP concentration ought to induce corresponding changes in pump activity, any variation in the latter should alter the intracellular ATP and orthophosphate contents. If the pumping rate is enhanced, ATP utilization should be accelerated and consequently the concentration of inorganic phosphate must increase. Stimulation of the ion pump by augmenting the external potassium concentration actually increased the rate of orthophosphate liberation in intact cells. If the pump was blocked by ouabain, the ATP breakdown occurring in substrate free media was delayed (Whittam, 1958) and the augmentation of the rate of phosphate liberation upon increasing the concentration of pump activating K^+ ions was prevented (Laris and Letchworth, 1962).

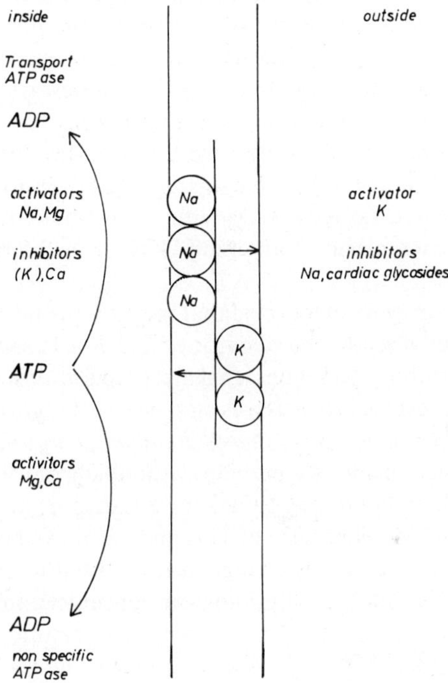

FIG. 12. Factors controlling the K-Na pump.

j. Hormonal Control of Active Transport. The effects of hormones on active cation transport have been studied repeatedly, but no definite results with respect to the K-Na pump of the red cell have yet been obtained. Streeten and Solomon (1954) examined the effects of adrenocorticotropin (ACTH) and adrenal steroids on K^{42} exchange of human red cells. If the hormones were applied *in vivo* prior to withdrawal of the cells for flux measurements in the test tube, a slight reduction in both influx and outflux was observed. There was no net change in cellular cation content. No effect whatsoever could be produced if the free hormones were added to cell suspensions *in vitro*. In view of recent demonstrations of the presence in plasma of phosphatides and sulfatides of the steroid hormones (Oertel, 1962), one is tempted to suspect that the formation of these conjugates from the free steroids is necessary for conversion of the hormones to their physiologically effective forms.

In contrast to human erythrocytes, rat erythrocytes *in vitro* are sensitive to deoxycorticosterone (DOC). Schatzmann (1954) reports that K and Na transport in cold-stored rat red cells is reduced by about 40% if the cells are suspended in their own plasma containing DOC at the high concentration of 1 mg./ml.

In this context, it may be mentioned that recently the hormone thyrotropin was found to affect directly the activity of the K–Na-sensitive "transport ATPase." The hormone stimulates enzyme preparations from the thyroid but not those from several other tissues studied (Turkington, 1962).

k. Efficiency of the Conversion of Phosphate Bond Energy into Osmotic Work. It may be asked whether the free enthalpy available from the splitting of one high-energy phosphate bond may suffice for a transport mechanism working at the proposed stoichiometric ratio of 3 Na and 2 K moved per ATP molecule. In order to check this point, the change in free enthalpy associated with the hydrolysis of 1 mole ATP at physiological concentrations of ATP, ADP, and orthophosphate has to be compared with the osmotic and electric work which must be expended by the cells for transport of 3 moles Na and 2 moles K against their respective electrochemical potential gradients.

According to Gerlach *et al.* (1958), 1 kg. human erythrocytes contains 0.68 mmole ATP, 0.30 mmole ADP, and 0.25 mmole orthophosphate. Since the water content of the cells amounts to approximately 65%, these figures correspond to 1.05, 0.46, and 0.38 mmole/liter of cell water, respectively. Assuming a standard free enthalpy (ΔG_0) of -8.54 kcal./mole for ATP hydrolysis at pH 7.2 [interpolated from Burton's (1957) data], the free enthalpy (ΔG) available under the conditions existing in the red cell interior can be calculated:

$$\Delta G = -8.54 + RT \ln \frac{0.38 \times 0.46 \times 10^{-6}}{1.05 \times 10^{-3}} = -13.9 \text{ kcal./mole}$$

The osmotic and electric work (W) performed at the expense of the free enthalpy change associated with ATP hydrolysis can be estimated by the following equation:

$$W = 3\left(RT\ln\frac{Na_i}{Na_o} + F\Delta\psi\right) + 2\left(RT\ln\frac{K_i}{K_o} - F\Delta\psi\right)$$

Inserting sodium and potassium concentrations of cell water (25 and 140 mmoles/liter respectively) and plasma (140 and 5 mmoles/liter, respectively), and using a value of membrane potential calculated from the chloride distribution ratio (0.65), one obtains $W = 7.55$ kcal.

From the data on ΔG and W, it can be easily calculated that, under the conditions of ATP hydrolysis specified above, 54% of the phosphate bond energy is used for maintenance of the physiological cation distribution ratios. Although this value is subject to considerable uncertainties, mainly because activity coefficients have been neglected and the figure for the standard free enthalpy of ATP is still controversial, it shows that from a thermodynamical point of view a stoichiometric ratio of (2K+3Na):ATP would be possible.

It should be borne in mind that physiological variations in the concentrations of H^+, K^+, Na^+, orthophosphate, ADP, and ATP as well as changes in membrane potential and Na-K coupling ratio will affect the efficiency of the pump.

l. Hypotheses of the Mechanism of Active Alkali Metal Ion Transport. The molecular mechanism by which ATP breakdown brings about the uphill transport of K and Na is still obscure. Nevertheless, several stimulating hypotheses have been published. Although they will almost certainly be replaced by actual knowledge in the near future, it may be worthwhile to outline them below in order to review from a common aspect a few pertinent observations concerning the interactions of the various components of the ion transport system.

In the course of the last few years, two concepts have emerged: (*a.*) ATP breakdown may be accomplished by a single enzyme which is specifically adapted to translocate K and Na by rotation due to thermal agitation (Davies and Keynes, 1960) or by changes in the configuration of the enzyme in the course of the formation and decomposition of the enzyme-substrate complex (Goldacre, 1952). (*b.*) Alternatively, ATP breakdown may be the net result of consecutive actions of several transphosphorylating enzymes and a phosphatase, whereby the ion transport is the consequence of either cyclic translocations of K and Na-sensitive surfaces of the enzymes associated with the catalytic activity or of synthesis and breakdown of a nonenzymatic K-Na carrier which traverses the membrane by diffusion.[9]

[9] It should be emphasized that besides K-Na transport a variety of other seemingly unrelated transport processes, such as iodine accumulation by thyroid tissue (Wolff, 1960), uptake of acidic and basic dyes in the kidney (Braun, 1961), active transfer of sugars, amino

(*i*) It has been suggested by Skou (1960) and Wheeler and Whittam (1962) that at $K_{outside}/Na_{inside}$ ratios of less than 1.0 something like the following reactions may take place.

$$\text{Enzyme} + \text{ATP} + \text{Mg} + \text{K} + \text{Na} \longrightarrow \begin{matrix}\text{K}\\ \text{Enzyme–Mg–ATP}\\ \text{Na}\end{matrix}$$

After rotation by Brownian movement[10] the enzyme-substrate complex breaks down into the free enzyme, ADP, orthophosphate, K, and Na, whereby the latter two ions are trapped on the inside and the outside of the membrane, respectively.

At high potassium concentration inside the cell or at high sodium concentration at the outside, competition between K and Na may lead to the formation of enzyme-substrate complexes which contain either K or Na ions only. Under these conditions the rate of ATP breakdown is reduced, just as in the absence of either of the two activating alkali metal ions (Wheeler and Whittam, 1962).

Obviously an enzyme-substrate complex supposedly containing at least 5 different components cannot be assumed to be formed by the simultaneous collision of all its constituents. Instead a number of consecutive reactions should be involved. Several attempts have been made to elucidate the nature of these hypothetical reactions. In the crab nerve preparation, which closely resembles in most respects the red cell ATPase, Skou (1960) in studying the ADP^{32}/ATP exchange mediated by the enzyme obtained evidence for the following sequence of events:

$$\begin{array}{lcl}
\text{Enzyme} + \text{ATP} & \longrightarrow & \text{Enzyme–ATP} \\
\text{Enzyme–ATP} & \longrightarrow & \text{Enzyme–P} + \text{ADP} \\
\text{Enzyme–P} + H_2O & \longrightarrow & \text{Enzyme} + \text{orthophosphate} \\
\hline
\text{ATP} + H_2O & \longrightarrow & \text{ADP} + \text{orthophosphate}
\end{array}$$

In this concept of the mechanism of ATP breakdown, the phosphorylation of the enzyme plays an essential role. At present, experiments are under way

acids and pyridines across the intestine (Czáky, 1961; Czáky, 1962; Czáky *et al.*, 1961), and incorporation of vanadium into tunicates (Biehlig *et al.*, 1963) can be inhibited by ouabain. It therefore seems feasible that the ouabain sensitive ATPase catalyses a reaction common to many different transport processes. If so, the enzyme could not possibly be involved in the actual translocation of substances across the membrane since the translocation processes are highly specific for the various substrates.

[10] Hypotheses advanced by Goldacre (1952), Koshland *et al.* (1962), and others, on the shape changes in enzyme molecules during formation of the enzyme-substrate complex have served as the basis for other interesting models for explaining the mode in which the cations might be translocated (Hoffman, 1962a; Hokin and Hokin, 1963). Since there is no experimental evidence available to test their validity, discussion seems to be premature and the reader is referred to the original papers.

in many laboratories to demonstrate the existence and, if possible, to determine the chemical nature of the phosphate-accepting groups of the enzyme. Many authors have obtained convincing evidence for the formation of measurable quantities of the postulated intermediate. Nevertheless, disagreement exists concerning the conditions under which phosphorylation and dephosphorylation take place. Charnock *et al.* (1963) report on an enzyme preparation from kidney in which phosphorylation was stimulated by Na, dephosphorylation by K, and action of the latter ions inhibited by ouabain. Working with red cell ghosts, Heinz and Hoffman (1963) on the other hand were unable to observe any consistent effects of K, Na, (Na + K), or strophanthidin on the incorporation of P^{32} from ATP^{32} into the ATPase preparation. Finally, Fahn *et al.* (1963), who used a purified ATPase from the electric organ of *Electrophorus electricus*, found the rate of phosphorylation of the enzyme strongly enhanced by ouabain and variable effects of K and Na.

Skou suggests that magnesium plays a twofold role in the formation of the enzyme-P compound: one Mg ion forms a chelate with ATP and thus establishes an ATP-Mg complex which is the true substrate of the enzyme. A second Mg ion fixes Mg-ATP to the enzyme. Dunham and Glynn concluded, however, that such dual action of Mg does not take place with the red cell ATPase. Nevertheless, the formation of an ATP-Mg-enzyme complex or of an enzyme-P complex may still be a prerequisite for the creation of specific binding sites for the ions to be transported. In rat red cells where enough K is bound to the cell surface or to ghosts to be measurable, Hoffman (1962b) found binding to be dependent on the presence of ATP. Similarly Järnefelt (1962), working with a microsomal preparation from rat brain, observed sodium binding to be dependent on the presence of ATP.

(*ii*) So far the term "adenosine triphosphatase" (ATPase) has been used as a convenient means of designating an enzyme-mediated reaction leading to the liberation of orthophosphate from ATP. A combination of two or more enzymes could clearly produce the same effects. Two hypotheses based on the assumption of the participation in ATP hydrolysis of two enzymes have actually been proposed:

(I) (1) ATP + membrane protein ⟶ phosphoprotein + ADP
(2) Phosphoprotein ⟶ protein + orthophosphate
(Ahmed and Judah, 1962)

(II) (1) ATP + diglycerate ⟶ phosphatidic acid + ADP
(2) Phosphatidic acid ⟶ diglycerate + orthophosphate
(Hokin and Hokin, 1960)

The first hypothesis is based on the observation that the phosphorylation by ATP of the serine of an as yet unidentified protein is activated by K and Na and inhibited by ouabain (Ahmed and Judah, 1962). The experiments presented so far are of a preliminary character and need not be considered here in detail. The second view, although highly controversial, is brought up at present in many discussions on the mechanism of active transport, and will therefore be dealt with at some length below.

It originated from the studies of Hokin and Hokin (1960) on the relation between the metabolism of phosphatides and the secretion of organic substances such as proteins and polypeptides. They found an increase in secretory activity to be always associated with increased turnover of inositol phosphatides and phosphatidic acid. This result led them to ask whether phosphatides may play a role in active transport. In their experiments they used the salt gland of the albatross, an organ which upon stimulation with acetylcholine is capable of producing a practically protein-free 1*M* NaCl solution. The secretion of NaCl after stimulation with acetylcholine was always accompanied by increased turnover of phosphatidic acid and to a lesser degree of inositol phosphatide. These observations suggested that phosphatidic acid may play a role in active sodium transport. Although at first appearing somewhat implausible, this was supported by further studies of the same authors (1961) on a diglyceride kinase in the red cell membrane. This kinase is specific for ATP and is activated by Mg^{++} and K^{+}. The phosphatidic acid which results from phosphorylation of diglyceride is split by a phosphatidic acid phosphatase, which also occurs in the erythrocyte membrane. The latter phosphatase contains two components, one of which is inhibited by Na^{+} while the other is activated by Mg^{++} and Na^{+}. Hokin and Hokin believe the K- and Na-sensitive ATPase, described by Dunham and Glynn and by Post *et al.*, to be not a single enzyme but really diglyceride kinase and phosphatidic acid phosphatase.

Hokin and Hokin first suggested that phosphatidic acid may be a sodium carrier, forming a sodium salt when synthesized at the inner surface of the membrane, and releasing the sodium ions when hydrolyzed at the outer surface. In view of the recent discovery that in tissues which derive their energy from respiration, up to 28 Na ions per molecule of oxygen (Lassen *et al.*, 1960) may be transported as compared with 12, the upper limit compatible with the assumption that phosphatidic acid is the carrier, Hokin and Hokin (1963) modified their original view on the role of phosphatidic acid in Na transport. They suggest that phosphatidic acid is part of a lipoprotein undergoing structural changes in the course of phosphatidic acid synthesis and breakdown. These are thought to be associated with cyclic variations in the affinity of the molecule for K and Na, respectively, and with translocation of the K- and Na-binding sites from one side of the membrane to the other.

The data presented so far by Hokin and Hokin are very stimulating, but do not as yet seem to provide conclusive evidence of the participation of phosphatidic acid in the active transport of K and Na. Further appraisal of this hypothesis would be greatly facilitated by a thorough comparison of the activation by K and Na and the inhibition by cardiac glycosides of both the so-called membrane ATPase and the diglyceride kinase–phosphatidic acid phosphatase system in the red cell membrane.

In this context, it should be pointed out that phosphatidic acid, even though it were not a participant in active transport, might play a significant role in controlling the membrane resistance to the passive permeability of the alkali metal ions. It was shown by Vogt (1958) that an extract from intestinal tissue containing mainly phosphatidic acid (the so-called *Darmstoff*, Vogt, 1957)

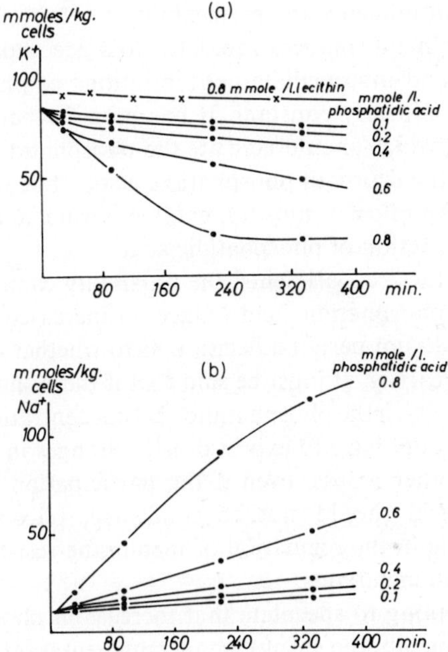

FIG. 13. Effects of phosphatidic acid on (*a*) potassium and (*b*) sodium permeability. The phosphatidic acid was enzymatically prepared from chromatographically purified egg lecithin (x). Human erythrocytes in isotonic NaCl. Temperature 37°C.

produces pharmacological actions which can most conveniently be explained by assuming a direct action of phosphatidic acid on the passive permeability of the cell membrane. In order to obtain preliminary information on the question as to whether phosphatidic acid is actually capable of interfering with permeability processes, it was thought of interest to study the effect of added phosphatidic acid on cell membranes (Passow, 1961) (Fig. 13).

If phosphatidic acid should act exclusively as a specific carrier for Na^+, one would expect that an experimentally produced increase in its concentration in the membrane would augment the rate of exchange diffusion of Na^+ without inducing concomitant net movements. But if phosphatidic acid should decrease the membrane resistance to passive movements of Na^+ and K^+, one ought to observe an acceleration of the net downhill movements of Na^+ and K^+ upon addition of this agent.

In order to decide between these possibilities, the action of phosphatidic acid on the cation permeability of human red cells was studied. The phosphatidic acid used was prepared by incubating chromatographically purified egg lecithin with a phospholipase isolated from Brussels sprouts. Figure 13 shows that the egg lecithin used for preparation of the phosphatidic acid practically does not influence the permeability to Na^+ and K^+. Phosphatidic acid, on the other hand, induces rapid K^+ loss accompanied by uptake of Na^+, and at low and intermediate concentrations of phosphatidic acid the sum Na^+ and K^+ is nearly constant. It has been further demonstrated that addition of Mg^{++}, which should activate the phosphatidic acid phosphatase, hardly diminishes the action of phosphatidic acid, while Ca^{++} exerts a strong inhibitory effect. Addition of inositol, choline, serine, and ethanolamine has no influence on the action of phosphatidic acid.

On the basis of these experiments, the possibility cannot be excluded that small amounts of phosphatidic acid induce an increased exchange diffusion of Na^+; they thus do not permit a decision as to whether or not phosphatidic acid acts as a Na^+ carrier. It must be said that if there should exist abnormal metabolic states in which the phosphatidic acid concentration in the membrane is increased, one would have to expect drastic changes in the permeability to K^+ and Na^+. In other words, even if the participation in active transport of phosphatidic acid should not be confirmed, phosphatidic acid could certainly play a role in the regulation of membrane resistance to the passive movements of alkali metal ions.

It would be tempting to speculate that increase in phosphatidic acid concentration in the membrane brings about augmentation of the passive Na influx and rise of the intracellular Na concentration. This would automatically enhance the rate of pumping, which in turn would stimulate ATP breakdown in the tissue, i.e., active transport and ATP turnover should be accelerated by similar changes in passive Na permeability, as observed in certain epithelia in the presence of vasopressin (Frazier *et al.*, 1962). One should be aware, however, that no net changes in phosphatidic acid concentration have been found so far under conditions where active sodium transport and phosphatidic acid turnover are stimulated (Hokin and Hokin, 1963).

Acknowledgments

My thanks are due to Drs. J. F. Hoffman (Bethesda) and Ch. Weiss (Homburg) for reading the manuscript and offering many helpful suggestions on its content and style. I am indebted to Mrs. H. Zimmermann and Miss E. Lohmeyer for secretarial help.

REFERENCES

Adair, G. S. (1928). *Proc. Roy. Soc.* (*London*) *Ser. A* **120**, 573.

Aebi, H. (1952). *Helv. Physiol. Pharmacol Acta* **10**, 184.

Ahmed, K., and Judah, J. D. (1962). *Biochim. Biophys. Acta* **57**, 245.

Altman, K. J., Whatman, R. N., and Salomo, K. (1951). *Arch. Biochem.* **33**, 168.

Arrhenius, S. (1887). *Z. Physik. Chem.* **1**, 631.

Auditore, J. V., and Murray, L. (1962). *Arch. Biochem. Biophys.* **99**, 372.

Barcroft, J., Bock, A. V., Hill, A. V., Parsons, T. R., Parsons, W., and Skoji, A. (1922). *J. Physiol.* (*London*) **56**, 157.

Bartley, W., Davies, R. E., and Krebs, H. A. (1954). *Proc. Roy. Soc.* (*London*) *Ser. B* **142**, 187.

Battley, E. H., and Klotz, I. M. (1951). *Biol. Bull.* **101**, 215.

Berg, G., Rothstein, A., and Chapman. (1963). In press.

Biehlig, H. J., Rüdiger, W., Forth, W., and Rummel, W. (1963). personal communication.

Bock, R. M. (1960). *In* "The Enzymes" (P. D. Boyer *et al.*, eds.), Vol. II. Academic Press, New York. p. 3.

Bonting, S. L., Simon, K. A., and Hawkins, N. M. (1961). *Arch. Biochem. Biophys.* **95**, 416.

Bonting, S. L., Caravaggio, L. L., and Hawkins, N. M. (1962). *Arch. Biochem. Biophys.* **98**, 413.

Boyle, P. J., and Conway, E. J. (1941). *J. Physiol.* (*London*) **100**, 1.

Braun, W. (1961). unpublished observations.

Bruns, F. H., Noltman, E., and Valhaus, E. (1958). *Biochem. Z.* **330**, 483.

Buchanan, A. A. (1960). *Biochem. J.* **75**, 315.

Burton, K. (1957). *Ergeb. Physiol. Biol. Chem. Exptl. Pharmakol.*, **49**, 275.

Caffrey, R. W., Trembelay, R., Gabrio, B. W., and Huennekens, F. M. (1956). *J. Biol. Chem.* **223**, 1.

Carr, C. W. (1953a). *Arch. Biochem. Biophys.* **46**, 417.

Carr, C. W. (1953b). *Arch. Biochem. Biophys.* **46**, 424.

Carr, C. W. (1956). *Arch. Biochem. Biophys.* **62**, 476.

Charnock, J. S., Rosenthal, A. S., and Post, R. L. (1963). *Federation Proc.* **22**, 212.

Clarkson, E. M., and Maizels, M. (1952). *J. Physiol.* (*London*) **116**, 112.

Cohen, S. S. (1953). *J. Biol. Chem.* **201**, 71.

Collins, D. A., and Scott, F. H. (1932). *J. Biol. Chem.* **97**, 189.

Cook, H. F. (1952). *Brit. J. Appl. Phys.* **3**, 249.

Czáky, T. Z. (1961). *Biochem. Pharmakol.* **8**, 38.

Czáky, T. Z. (1962). *Proc. 1st Intern. Pharmacol. Meeting* **3**, 225

Czáky, T. Z., Hartzog, H. G., and Fernald, G. W. (1961). *Am. J. Physiol.* **200**, 459.

Danielli, J. F., and Davson, H. (1936). *J. Cellular Comp. Physiol.* **7**, 393.

Davies, R. E., and Keynes, R. D. (1960). *In* "Membrane Transport and Metabolism" (A. Kleinzeller and A. Kotyk, eds.), p. 336. Academic Press, New York.

Davson, H. (1939). *Biochem. J.* **33**, 389.

Davson, H. (1940). *J. Cellular Comp. Physiol.* **15**, 317.

Davson, H. (1942). *J. Cellular Comp. Physiol.* **20**, 325.

Dean, R. B., Noonan, T. R., Haege, L., and Fenn, W. O. (1941). *J. Gen. Physiol.* **24**, 353.

Dick, D. A. T., and Lowenstein, L. M. (1958). *Proc. Roy. Soc.* (*London*) *Ser. B* **148**, 241.

Dill, D. B., Edwards, H. T., and Consolazio, W. V. (1937). *J. Biol. Chem.* **118**, 635.

Dingle, J. T., and Lucy, J. A. (1962). *Biochem. J.* **84**, 611.

Dische, Z. (1951). *In* "Phosphorus Metabolism" (W. D. McElroy and B. Glass, eds.), John Hopkins Press, Baltimore, Maryland.

Dische, Z., and Iglas, D. (1961). *Arch. Biochem. Biophys.* **93**, 201.
Dische, Z., Shigeura, H. T., and Landsberg, E. (1960). *Arch. Biochem. Biophys.* **89**, 123.
Doisy, E. A., and Eaton, E. P. (1921). *J. Biol. Chem.* **47**, 377.
Donnan, F. G. (1911). *Z. Elektrochem.* **17**, 572.
Donnan, F. G., and Guggenheim, E. A. (1932). *Z. physik. Chem.* **A162**, 346.
Drabkin, D. L. (1950). *J. Biol. Chem.* **185**, 231.
Dunham, E. T. (1957). *Physiologist* **1**, 23.
Dunham, E. T., and Glynn, I. M. (1961). *J. Physiol.* (*London*) **156**, 274.
Dunker, E., and Passow, H. (1953). *Arch. Ges. Physiol.* **256**, 446.
Durbin, R. P. (1960). *J. Gen. Physiol.* **44**, 315.
Durbin, R. P., Frank, H., and Solomon, A. K. (1956). *J. Gen. Physiol.* **30**, 535.
Eckel, R. E. (1958). *J. Cellular Comp. Physiol.* **51**, 81, 109.
Edelberg, R. (1952). *J. Cellular Comp. Physiol.* **40**, 529.
Edelberg, R. (1953). *J. Cellular Comp. Physiol.* **41**, 37.
Ege, R. (1922). *Biochem. Z.* **130**, 99, 116.
Euler, H. von, and Eistert, B. (1957). "Reduktone and Reduktonate." Enke, Stuttgart.
Evans, J. V., King, J. B. B., Cohen, B. L., Harris, H., and Warren, F. L. (1956). *Nature* **178**, 849.
Fahn, S., Albers, R. W., and Koval, G. J. (1963). *Federation Proc.* **22**, 213.
Fitzsimons, E. J., and Sendroy, J., Jr. (1961). *J. Biol. Chem.* **236**, 1595.
Flynn, F., and Maizels, M. (1949). *J. Physiol.* (*London*) **110**, 301.
Frazier, H. S., Dempsey, E. F., and Leaf, A. (1962). *J. Gen. Physiol.* **45**, 529.
Fricke, H., and Curtis, H. J. (1935). *J. Gen. Physiol.* **18**, 821.
Fricke, H., and Morse, S. (1926). *J. Gen. Physiol.* **9**, 153.
Gabrio, B. W., and Huennekens, F. M. (1955). *Biochem. Biophys. Acta* **18**, 585.
Gabrio, B. W., Hennessey, M., Thomasson, J., and Finch, C. A. (1955). *J. Biol. Chem.* **215**, 357.
Gàrdos, G. (1958). *Acta Physiol. Acad. Sci. Hung.* **14**, 1.
Gàrdos, G. (1959). *Acta Physiol. Acad. Sci. Hung.* **15**, 121.
Gàrdos, G. (1961). *In* "Membrane Transport and Metabolism" (A. Kleinzeller and A. Kotyk. eds.), p. 553. Academic Press, New York.
Gàrdos, G., and Straub, F. B. (1956). *Acta Physiol. Acad. Sci. Hung.* **12**, 1.
Gerlach, E., Fleckenstein, A., Gross, E., and Lübben, K. (1958). *Arch. Ges. Physiol.* **266**, 528.
Giebel, O., and Passow, H. (1960). *Arch. Ges. Physiol.* **271**, 378.
Giebel, O., and Passow, H. (1961). *Naturwissenschaften* **23**, 721.
Gierer, A., and Wirtz, K. (1953). *Z. Naturforsch.* **8a**, 532.
Glasstone, S., Laidler, K. J., and Eyring, H. (1941). "The Theory of Rate Processes." McGraw-Hill, New York and London.
Glynn, I. M. (1956). *J. Physiol.* (*London*) **134**, 278.
Glynn, I. M. (1957a). *Progr. Biophys. Biophys. Chem.* **8**, 242.
Glynn, I. M. (1957b). *J. Physiol.* (*London*) **136**, 148.
Glynn, I. M. (1962). *J. Physiol.* (*London*) **160**, 18P.
Gold, G. L., and Solomon, A. K. (1955). *J. Gen. Physiol.* **38**, 389.
Goldacre, R. J. (1952). *Intern. Rev. Cytol.* **1**, 135.
Goldman, D. E. (1943). *J. Gen. Physiol.* **27**, 37.
Goldstein, D., and Solomon, A. K. (1960). *J. Gen. Physiol.* **44**, 1.
Gourley, D. R. H. (1952). *Arch. Biochem. Biophys.* **40**, **1**, 13.
Green, J. W., and Bond, G. (1961). *Federation Proc.* **20**, 143.
Grievers, A., and Wirtz, K. (1953). *Z. Naturforsch.* **8a**, 532.

Grigarzik, H., and Passow, H. (1958). *Arch. Ges. Physiol.* **267**, 73.
Gryns, G. (1896). *Arch. Ges. Physiol.* **63**, 86.
Gruner, H., and Passow, H. (1963). *Arch. Ges. Physiol.* **278**, 2.
Guest, G. M. (1948). *Blood* **3**, 541.
Gürber, G. (1895). *Sitzsber. physik. med. Ges., Wurzburg*; cited in Gellhorn, E. (1929). "Das Permeäbilitatsproblem. Springer, Berlin.
Hahn, L., and Hevesy, G. (1941). *Acta Physiol. Scand.* **3**, 193.
Halpern, L. (1936). *J. Biol. Chem.* **114**, 747.
Hamburger, H. J. (1891). *Z. Biol.* **28**, 405.
Hamburger, H. J. (1893). *Zentr. Physiol.* **6**, 161.
Hamburger, H. J. (1893b). *Zentr. Physiol.* **7**, 758.
Hamburger, H. J. (1897). *Virchow's Arch. Pathol. Anat.* p. 489.
Hamburger, H. J. (1902). "Osmotischer Druck und Ionenlehre." Bergmann, Wiesbaden.
Harkins, H. N., and Hastings, A. B. (1931). *J. Biol. Chem.* **90**, 565.
Harris, J. E. (1941). *J. Biol. Chem.* **141**, 579.
Harris, E. J. (1954). *Symp. Soc. Exptl. Biol.* **8**, 228.
Harris, E. J., and Prankerd, T. A. (1955). *Biochem. J.* **61**, xix.
Harris, E. J., and Prankerd, T. A. (1958). *J. Gen. Physiol.* **41**, 197.
Hartridge, H., and Roughton, F. J. W. (1923). *Proc. Roy. Soc. London Ser. A* **104**, 376.
Hastings, A. B., Sendroy, J., Jr., McIntosh, J. F., and van Slyke, D. D. (1928). *J. Biol. Chem.* **79**, 193.
Heckmann, K. (1962). *In* "Funktionelle und morphologische Organisation der Zelle," Konferenz der Gesellschaft deutscher Naturforscher u. Ärzte in Rottach-Egern, p. 241. Springer, Berlin.
Hedin, S. G. (1892). *Skand. Arch. Physiol.* **2**, 134.
Hedin, S. G. (1895). *Skand. Arch. Physiol.* **5**, 207.
Hedin, S. G. (1897). *Arch. Ges. Physiol.* **68**, 229.
Hedin, S. G. (1898). *Arch. Ges. Physiol.* **70**, 525.
Heinz, E., and Hoffman, J. F. (1963). *Federation Proc.* **22**, 212.
Hendry, E. B. (1954). *Edinburgh Med. J.* **61**, 7.
Herbert, E. (1956). *J. Cellular Comp. Physiol.* **47**, 11.
Hill, A. V., and Kupalov, P. S. (1930). *Proc. Roy. Soc.* (*London*) *Ser. B* **106**, 445.
Höber, R. (1962). "Physikalische Chemie der Zellen und Gewebe," 6th ed. Engelmann, Leipzig.
Höber, R. (1910). *Arch. Ges. Physiol.* **133**, 237.
Höber, R. (1912). *Arch. Ges. Physiol.* **148**, 189.
Höber, R. (1913). *Arch. Ges. Physiol.* **150**, 15.
Hodgkin, A. L., and Keynes, R. D. (1955). *J. Physiol. London.* **128**, 61.
Hoffman, J. F. (1960). *Ciba Found. Study Group* **5**, 85.
Hoffman, J. F. (1962a). *Abstr. Commun. Biophys. Soc., Washington, D.C.*
Hoffman, J. F. (1962b). *Federation Proc.* **21**, 145.
Hoffman, J. F. (1962c). *Circulation.* **26**, 1201.
Hoffman, J. F., and Tosteson, D. C. (1956). *Abstr. Commun. 20th Intern. Physiol. Congr., Brussels*, 1956, p. 429.
Hoffman, J. F., and Tosteson, D. C. (1959). Abstr. Biophys. Soc. Pittsburgh.
Hokin, L. E., and Hokin, M. R. (1959). *Nature* **184**, 1068.
Hokin, L. E., and Hokin, M. R. (1960). *J. Gen. Physiol.* **44**, 61.
Hokin, L. E., and Hokin, M. R. (1961). *Nature* **189**, 836.
Hokin, L. E., and Hokin, M. R. (1963). *Federation Proc.* **22**, 8.
Huennekens, F. M., Nurk, E., and Gabrio, B. W. (1956). *J. Biol. Chem.* **221**, 971.

Hutchinson, E. (1952). *Arch. Biochem. Biophys.* **38**, 35.
Hutchinson, E., and Bean, K. E. (1955). *Arch. Biochem. Biophys.* **58**, 81.
Jacobs, M. H., and Stewart, D. R. (1947). *J. Cellular Comp. Physiol.* **30**, 79.
Jacobs, M. H., Glassman, H. N., and Parpart, A. K. (1936). *J. Cellular Comp. Physiol.* **8**, 403.
Järnefelt, J. (1961). *Biochim. Biophys. Acta* **48**, 111.
Järnefelt, J. (1962). *Federation Proc.* **21**, 147.
Jones, N. C., and Gardner, B. (1962). *Biochem. J.* **83**, 404.
Joyce, C. R. B., Moore, H., and Wheatherall, M. (1954). *Brit. J. Pharmacol.* **9**, 463.
Katchalsky, A. (1960). *In* "Membrane Transport and Metabolism" (A. Kleinzeller and A. Kotyk, eds.), p. 69. Academic Press, New York.
Kedem, O., and Katchalsky, A. (1961). *J. Gen. Physiol.* **45**, 143.
Koefoed-Johnson, V., and Ussing, H. H. (1953). *Acta Physiol. Scand.* **28**, 60.
Koeppe, H. (1895). *du Bois-Reymonds Arch.* **154**.
Koeppe, H. (1897). *Arch. Ges. Physiol.* **67**, 189.
Koshland, D. E., Jr., Yankeelov, J. A., Jr., and Thoma, J. A. (1962). *Federation Proc.* **21**, 1031.
Kregenow, F. M., and Hoffman, J. F. (1962). *Abstr. Communs. Biophys. Soc., Washington, D.C.*
Laris, P. C., and Letchworth, P. E. (1962). *J. Cellular Comp. Physiol.* **60**, 229.
Lassen, N. A., Munck, O., and Thayssen, J. H. (1960). *Acta Physiol. Scand.* **51**, 371.
Lehmann, C. (1894). *Arch. Ges. Physiol.* **58**, 428.
Lepke, S., and Passow, H. (1960a). *Arch. Ges. Physiol.* **271**, 389.
Lepke, S., and Passow, H. (1960b). *Arch. Ges. Physiol.* **271**, 473.
Lindemann, B., and Passow, H. (1960a). *Arch. Ges. Physiol.* **271**, 497.
Lindemann, B., and Passow, H. (1960b). *Arch. Ges. Physiol.* **271**, 488.
Lindemann, B., and Passow, H. (1960c). *Arch. Ges. Physiol.* **271**, 497.
Loewy, A., and Zuntz, N. (1894). *Arch. Ges. Physiol.* **58**, 511.
London, I. M., and Schwarz, H. (1953). *J. Clin. Invest.* **32**, 1248.
Lovelock, J. E., James, A. T., and Rowe, C. E. (1960). *Biochem. J.* **74**, 137.
Luckner, H., and Lo-Sing (1938). *Arch. Ges. Physiol.* **239**, 278.
Lundsgaard-Hansen, P. (1957). *Arch. Exptl. Pathol. Pharmacol.* **231**, 577.
Maizels, M. (1935). *Biochem. J.* **29**, 1970.
Maizels, M. (1949). *J. Physiol.* (*London*) **108**, 254.
Maizels, M. (1951). *J. Physiol.* (*London*) **112**, 59.
Meier, K. H., and Sievers, J. F. (1936). *Helv. Chim. Acta* **19**, 649, 665.
Michaelis, L., and Fugita, A. (1925). *Biochem. Z.* **161**, 47.
Michaelis, L., and Perlzweig, W. A. (1927). *J. Gen. Physiol.* **10**, 575.
Mond, R. (1927). *Arch. Ges. Physiol.* **217**, 618.
Mond, R. (1928). *Arch. Ges. Physiol.* **219**, 467.
Mond, R., and Gertz, H. (1929). *Arch. Ges. Physiol.* **221**, 623.
Mond, R., and Hoffmann, F. (1928). *Arch. Ges. Physiol.* **220**, 194.
Morris, R., and Wright, R. D. (1954). *Australian J. Exptl. Biol. Med. Sci.* **32**, 669.
Mueller, C. B., and Hastings, A. B., *J. Biol. Chem.* **189**, 869. (1951a).
Mueller, C. B., and Hastings, A. B., *J. Biol. Chem.* (1951b). **189**, 881.
Muir, H., Perrone, J. C., and Popják, G. (1951). *Biochem. J.* **48**, iv.
Mukai, G. (1921). *J. Physiol.* (*London*) **55**, 356.
Mullins, L. J., Fenn, W. O., Noonan, T. R., and Haege, L. (1941). *Am. J. Physiol.* **135**, 93.
Netter, H. (1959). "Theoretische Biochemie." Springer, Berlin.
Oertel, G. W., Kaiser, E., and Brühe, P. (1962). *Biochem. Z.* **336**, 154.
Opie, E. L. (1954)., *J. Exp. Med.* **99,** 29.

Ørskov, S. L. (1935). *Biochem. Z.* **297**, 250.
Ørskov, S. L. (1946). *Acta Physiol. Scand.* **12**, 202.
Overbeck, J. Th. G. (1956). *Progr. Biophys. Biophys. Chem.* **6**, 57.
Paganelli, C. V., and Solomon, A. K. (1957). *J. Gen. Physiol.* **41**, 259.
Pappenheimer, J. R., Renkin, E. M., and Borrero, L. M. (1951). *Am. J. Physiol.* **167**, 13.
Parpart, A. K., and Green, J. W. (1951). *J. Cellular Comp. Physiol.* **38**, 347.
Passow, H. (1960). *Ciba Found. Study Group* **5**, 48.
Passow, H. (1961). *In* "Biochemie des aktiven Transports." Colloq. Ges. Physiol. Chem., Mosbach/Baden, Springer, Berlin.
Passow, H. (1963a). *Klin. Wochschr.* **41**, 130.
Passow, H. (1963b). *In* "Cell Interface Reactions," (Brown, H. D. ed.), p. 57. Scholars Library, New York.
Passow, H., and Lepke, S. (1959). *Arch. Ges. Physiol.* **272**, 40.
Passow, H., and Schütt, L. (1956). *Arch. Ges. Physiol.* **262**, 193.
Passow, H., and Wilde, U. (1961). *Abstr. Intern. Biophys. Congr., Stockholm, 1961*, p. 175.
Passow, H., Lohmann, H., and Privat, V. (1960). *Arch. Ges. Physiol.* **272**, 40.
Passow, H., Rothstein, A., and Clarkson, T. W. (1961). *Pharmacol. Rev.* **13**, 185.
Pauly, H., and Schwan, H. P. (1958). *Moore School Elect. Eng. ONR Tech. Rept.* **28**. Philadelphia, Pennsylvania.
Pfleger, K., Rummel, W., Seifen, E., and Baldauf, J. (1961). *Med. Exptl.* **5**, 473.
Ponder, E. (1944). *J. Gen. Physiol.* **27**, 273.
Ponder, E. (1947a). *J. Gen. Physiol.* **30**, 379.
Ponder, E. (1947b). *J. Gen. Physiol.* **30**, 479.
Ponder, E. (1948). "Hemolysis and Related Phenomena." Grune & Stratton, New York.
Ponder, E. (1949). *J. Gen. Physiol.* **32**, 53.
Ponder, E. (1950a). *J. Gen. Physiol.* **33**, 177.
Ponder, E. (1950b). *J. Gen. Physiol.* **33**, 745.
Ponder, E. (1951a). *J. Gen. Physiol.* **34**, 359.
Ponder, E. (1951b). *J. Gen. Physiol.* **34**, 567.
Ponder, E. (1955). "Red Cell Structure and Its Breakdown." Springer, Berlin.
Post, R. L., Merrit, C. R., Kinsolving, C. R., and Albright, C. D. (1960). *J. Biol. Chem.* **235**, 1796.
Pragay, D. (1956). *Acta Physiol. Acad. Sci. Hung.* **12**, 9.
Raker, J. W., Taylor, I. M., Weller, J. M., and Hastings, A. B. (1950). *J. Gen. Physiol.* **33**, 691.
Rapoport, S., and Guest, G. M. (1939). *J. Biol. Chem.* **131**, 675.
Renkin, E. M. (1954). *J. Gen. Physiol.* **38**, 225.
Rinehart, R. K., and Green, J. W. (1962). *J. Cellular Comp. Physiol.* **59**, 85.
Robbins, E., and Mauro, A. (1960). *J. Gen. Physiol.* **43**, 523.
Robinson, J. R. (1953). *Biol. Rev.* **28**, 158.
Roepke, R. R., and Baldes, E. J. (1942). *J. Cellular Comp. Physiol.* **20**, 71.
Rummel, W., Seifen, E., and Baldauf, J. (1963). *Biochem. Pharmacol.* **12**, 557.
Sanui, H., Carvalho, A. P., and Pace, N. (1962). *J. Gen. Physiol.* **59**, 241.
Schatzmann, H. J. (1953). *Helv. Physiol. Pharmacol. Acta* **11**, 346.
Schatzmann, H. J. (1954). *Experientia* **10**, 189.
Schmidt-Thomé, J. (1942). *Z. Physiol. Chem.* **175**, 183.
Schwan, H. P. (1957). *Advan. Biol. Med. Phys.* **5**, 148.
Schwietzer, C. H., and Passow, H. (1953). *Arch. Ges. Physiol.* **256**, 419.
Sen, A. K., and Post, R. L. (1961). *Federation Proc.* **20**, 138.
Shaw, T. I. (1955). *J. Physiol. (London)* **129**, 464.

Sheppard, C. W., and Householder, A. S. (1951). *J. Appl. Phys.* **22**, 510.
Sheppard, C. W., and Martin, W. R. (1950). *J. Gen. Physiol.* **33**, 703.
Sheppard, C. W., Martin, W. R., and Beyl, G. (1951). *J. Gen. Physiol.* **34**, 411.
Skou, J. C. (1957). *Biochim. Biophys. Acta* **23**, 394.
Skou, J. C. (1960). *Biochim. Biophys. Acta* **42**, 6.
Skou, J. C. (1962). *Biochim. Biophys. Acta* **58**, 314.
Soldano, B. A., and Boyd, G. E. (1954). *J. Am. Chem. Soc.* **75**, 6091.
Solomon, A. K. (1952). *J. Gen. Physiol.* **36**, 57.
Solomon, A. K. (1960a). *In* "Mineral Metabolism" (C. L. Comar and F. Bronner, eds.), p. 119. Academic Press, New York.
Solomon, A. K. (1960b). *In* "Membrane Transport and Metabolism" (A. Kleinzeller and A. Kotyk, eds.), p. 94. Academic Press, New York.
Solomon, A. K., and Gold, G. L. (1955). *J. Gen. Physiol.* **38**, 371.
Staverman, A. J. (1952). *Trans. Faraday Soc.* **48**, 176.
Straub, F. B. (1953). *Acta Physiol. Acad. Sci. Hung*, 4, 235.
Streeten, D. H. P., and Solomon, A. K. (1954). *J. Gen. Physiol.* **37**, 643.
Székely, M., Mánai, S., and Straub, F. B. (1953). *Acta Physiol. Acad. Sci. Hung.* **4**, 31.
Tammann, G. (1896). *Z. Physiol. Chem.* **20**, 180.
Taylor, C. B. (1962). *Biochim. Biophys. Acta* **60**, 437.
Teorell, T. (1935). *Proc. Soc. Exptl. Biol. Med.* **33**, 282.
Teorell, T. (1951). *Z. Elektrochem.* **55**, 6.
Teorell, T. (1952). *J. Gen. Physiol.* **35**, 669.
Teorell, T. (1953). *Progr. Biophys. Biophys. Chem.* **3**, 305.
Tosteson, D. C. (1959). *Acta Physiol. Scand.* **46**, 19.
Tosteson, D. C. (1963). *Federation Proc.* **22**, 19.
Tosteson, D. C., and Hoffman, J. F. (1960). *J. Gen. Physiol.* **44**, 169.
Tosteson, D. C., Carlson, E., and Dunham, E. T. (1955). *J. Gen. Physiol.* **39**, 31.
Tosteson, D. C., Blaustein, M. P., and Moulton, R. H. (1961). *Federation Proc.* **20**, 138.
Tsuboi, K. K., and Hudson, P. B. (1957). *J. Biol. Chem.* **224**, 879.
Tsuboi, K. K., and Hudson, P. B. (1957). *J. Biol. Chem.* **224**, 889.
Turkington, R. W. (1962). *Biochim. Biophys. Acta* **65**, 386.
Ussing, H. H. (1949a). *Acta Physiol. Scand.* **19**, 43.
Ussing, H. H. (1949b). *Physiol. Rev.* **29**, 127.
Van Slyke, D. D., Wu, H., and McLean, F. C. (1923). *J. Biol. Chem.* **56**, 765.
Van Slyke, D. D., Hastings, A. B., Murray, D. C., and Sendroy, J., Jr. (1925). *J. Biol. Chem.* **65**, 701.
Vestergaard-Bogind, B., and Hesselbo, T. (1960). *Biochim. Biophys. Acta* **44**, 117.
Villegas, R., Barton, T. C., and Solomon, A. K. (1959). *J. Gen. Physiol.* **42**, 2, 355.
Vogt, W. (1957). *J. Physiol.* (*London*) **137**, 154.
Vogt, W. (1958). *Pharmacol. Rev.* **10**, 407.
von Limbeck (1895). *Arch. Exptl. Pathol. Pharmacol.* **35**, 309.
Warburg, E. J. (1922). *Biochem. J.* (*London*) **16**, 153.
Weed, R. I., and Berg, G. (1963). In press.
Weed, R. I., Eber, J., and Rothstein, A. (1962). *J. Gen. Physiol.* **45**, 395.
Weed, R. I., Reed, G., and Berg, G. G. (1963). In press.
Wheeler, K. P., and Whittam, R. (1962). *Biochem. J.* **85**, 495.
Whittam, R. (1958). *J. Physiol.* (*London*) **140**, 479.
Whittam, R. (1962). *Biochem. J.* **84**, 110.
Whittam, R., and Ager, M. F. (1962). *Biochim. Biophys. Acta* **65**, 383
Wiechmann, E. (1921). *Arch. Ges. Physiol.* **189**, 109.

Wilbrandt, W. (1937). *Trans. Faraday Soc.* **33**, 959.
Wilbrandt, W. (1940a). *Arch. Ges. Physiol.* **243**, 519.
Wilbrandt, W. (1940b). *Arch. Ges. Physiol.* **243**, 537.
Wilbrandt, W. (1941). *Arch. Ges. Physiol.* **245**, 22.
Wilbrandt, W. (1942a). *Arch. Ges. Physiol.* **246**, 274.
Wilbrandt, W. (1942b). *Arch. Ges. Physiol.* **246**, 291.
Wilbrandt, W. (1953). *Schweizer Med. Wochschr.* **83**, 1023.
Wilbrandt, W. (1963). *Ann. Rev. Physiol.* **25**, 601.
Wilbrandt, W., and Schatzmann, H. J. (1960). *Ciba Found. Study Group* **5**, 34.
Williams, T. F., Fordham, C. C., III, Hollander, W., Jr., and Welt, L. G. (1959). *J. Clin. Invest.* **38**, 1587.
Wolff, J. (1960). *Biochim. Biophys. Acta* **38**, 316.
Yoshida, H., and Fugisawa, H. (1962). *Biochim. Biophys. Acta* **60**, 443.
Zilversmit, D. B., Entenman, C., Fishler, M. C., and Chaikoff, I. L. (1943). *J. Gen. Physiol.* **26**, 333.

CHAPTER 4

Overall Red Cell Metabolism

Charles Bishop

I. Introduction[1]

The red cell has one vital reason for existence—to carry oxygen from lungs or gills to all cells of the animal and to return with the resulting carbon dioxide. The cell which ultimately becomes the mature circulating erythrocyte begins life as a complete cell with nucleus, mitochondria, and microsomes, and the ability to perform almost any metabolic reaction. In the process of becoming an erythrocyte the mammalian red cell sheds its nucleus by a process not very well understood, becoming a reticulocyte. The term reticulocyte merely indicates that these cells can be stained supravitally with brilliant cresyl blue or some similar dye to reveal a net (reticulum). Such cells almost certainly must retain some mitochondria since they respire quite actively, possess citric acid cycle activity, and have other metabolic capacities. Before the red cell becomes mature it must accumulate an amount of hemoglobin which is appropriate for the species involved (see Chapter 8). Reticulocytes circulating in the peripheral blood are known to ripen in a few days into mature erythrocytes which lack reticula, mitochondria, and nuclei, but with a proper amount of hemoglobin. By this time they are well suited to their prime function of O_2 and CO_2 carriage, but are in a metabolic straitjacket. Although it is often assumed that the reticulocytes seen in peripheral mammalian blood are red cells in the process of maturation, it is not clear as to what percentage of reticulocytes finish their maturation in the marrow and what percentage mature after reaching the circulation. It is also not clear whether the site of maturation is correlated with a normal or shortened cell life.

Mature nonmammalian red cells retain both their nuclei and their mitochondria. They obviously have a more typical metabolic potential, as evidenced by their active respiration. One function they would appear not to need is the ability to synthesize deoxyribonucleic acid (DNA) since they do not undergo

[1] Abbreviations of compounds in this chapter conform with the usage of the *Journal of Biological Chemistry*.

further mitosis. Bianco *et al.* (1962), using glycine-2-C^{14} with duck cells, agreed with Allfrey and Mirsky (1952) that turnover of DNA in avian red cells is low (nil?) when measured with isotopic glycine. They found, however, that with $NaHC^{14}O_3$ the incorporation appeared much higher. Such results are disconcerting and should be confirmed or denied. It has been shown that the chicken red cell is unable to synthesize purines *de novo* from glycine (Bishop, 1960). Curiously, reticulocytes *can* synthesize purines *de novo* from glycine or formate (Lowy *et al.*, 1961b).

Why should the red cell be energetically active? The exchange of gases is presumably due to concentration gradients and does not require energy expenditure by the cell. The red cell appears to synthesize relatively little protein or lipid after it matures and begins circulating. Its hemoglobin is completely formed and the cell need not replicate its genetic material. The circulating red cell must, however, maintain its shape, internal ionic composition, and structural integrity. It must also keep most of its hemoglobin in the reduced form. All these tasks require energy, hence the viable mature erythrocyte must produce energy. The problem of transporting ions to maintain the necessary gradients across the cell membrane is well discussed in Chapter 3. Simple relationships among glycolysis, adenosine triphosphate (ATP) levels, and Na^+ and K^+ distribution in the human red cell were reported by Konsek and Bishop (1962).

A random sample of blood drawn from a human subject or rabbit will include a small percentage of reticulocytes, some very new mature erythrocytes, some senescent erythrocytes, and all ages of cells in between. What can we say about the characteristics of such a population? In general much has been said, but for particular details the literature is often fuzzy. A reticulocyte-rich population can be obtained in a mammal by repeated bleeding, phenylhydrazine injections, or low O_2 atmosphere. Whether such stress-produced reticulocytes are similar in all respects to reticulocytes produced under normal homeostatic conditions is a moot point, but such blood samples have been extensively studied. Another way of obtaining a reticulocyte-rich population is to centrifuge cells and withdraw the top layer of red cells after the plasma and buffy coat have been removed. The rationale behind this is that reticulocytes are larger and less dense than erythrocytes. The reticulocyte is pictured as diminishing in size as it matures to an erythrocyte and this shrinking process is thought by some to continue for the life of the cell. In other words, density would be a direct function of red cell age. Some support for this continuous shrinking, or increase in density, can be mustered, but the gradual change is poorly documented. Prankerd (1958) separated cells by density but could not demonstrate size differences. He invoked differences in lipid content, especially phospholipid, to explain the differences in density. Experiments are currently in progress in the reviewer's laboratory to clarify this problem.

Another characteristic of young cells is their relative ability to resist hemolysis in hypotonic salt solutions. Osmotic fragility curves have been used to characterize the "cell age" of, for example, stored blood (*inter alia* Parpart *et al.*, 1947; Marks and Johnson, 1958) and to fractionate cell populations to remove the older cells. Murphy (1962) found that osmotic fragility increased in incubated red cells, not only if their energy sources were cut off, but also if the free cholesterol content of the incubation medium decreased. For example, when human red cells were incubated in native serum, the serum free cholesterol gradually decreased due to esterification by serum enzymes. The osmotic fragility of the red cells increased under these circumstances. Inactivation of the esterifying enzymes or addition of more free cholesterol proscribed these fragility changes. The key role of cholesterol in the integrity of the red cell membrane was shown by the fact that cholesterol added to the medium after fragility changes had occurred was of no value.

An excellent discussion of the properties of rabbit reticulocytes and the use of centrifugation for their enrichment is given by Chalfin (1956). This paper has also an electron micrograph of a reticulocyte which appears to contain a mitochondrion. Rudzinska and Trager (1959) present a photograph of a cat reticulocyte with mitochondria. The relationships of reticula, polychromatophilia, and mitochondria in red cells were discussed at some length by Key (1921), who concluded that the recognition of mitochondria in reticulocytes was quite difficult because of the large quantities of hemoglobin present. Other workers have noted the presence of mitochondria up to the reticulocyte stage (Ackerman and Bellios, 1955a,b). Rubinstein *et al.* (1956b) had evidence for a tricarboxylic acid cycle and mitochondria in reticulocytes. For rabbit reticulocytes the O_2 uptake was 250 mm.^{3}/g. moist cells/hour as against 8 mm.^{3} for orthochromatic rabbit erythrocytes (Ramsey and Warren, 1933). Thorell (1961) discussed cell structure in red cell maturation. Bertles and Beck (1962) produced reticulocytosis (30–60%) in rabbits and incubated the cells *in vitro* to allow maturation of reticulocytes. The disappearance of the RNA-rich reticulum was correlated with the appearance of low molecular weight extracellular products such as hypoxanthine, cytidine, and uracil. Yasuzumi (1960) published electron micrographic details of nucleate red cells. A method for preparing newt red cell nuclear material for electron microscopy was described by Gall (1963). From the foregoing it might be generally assumed that the citric acid cycle would operate in nucleated erythrocytes and in reticulocytes, since this cycle is intimately linked with the mitochondrion. Various aspects of this question have been investigated by Jones *et al.* (1953); Rapoport and Hofmann (1955); Rubinstein and Denstedt (1953, 1956); Mirčevová (1962c), and Engelhardt and Lyubimova (1936).

Many studies have been reported in the literature in which mammalian red cells, either with or without an enhanced reticulocyte population, have been centrifuged and "top" and "bottom" layers separately removed. These layers are inevitably designated as "new" and "old" red cells and when differences in the activities of certain enzymes are found in the two layers, the conclusion is almost inevitably reached that enzyme activity (at least of certain ones) declines as the red cell ages. The reverse is then stated, that the cell ages because enzyme activity declines. Very few studies cite comparable reticulocyte counts, although it is plain from many studies that reticulocytes are metabolically much more active than mature erythrocytes. Of course one can include both reticulocytes and less dense mature erythrocytes under the heading of "new" red cells, but with what can this mixed population be compared in any meaningful fashion? Tada *et al.* (1961) injected rabbits with acetylphenylhydrazine and assayed the blood for activity of aldolase, lactic dehydrogenase, glucose-6-phosphate dehydrogenase, and other factors. The rise and fall in activity coincided exactly with the fluctuations in reticulocyte count.

II. Fermentation versus Respiration

The foregoing simplified framework has a fascinating evolution. In 1909 Otto Warburg became intrigued by the O_2 consumption of red cells. For man and rabbit he obtained oxygen uptakes (as "percent of maximum oxygen content") of 1–3% per hour. He was also interested in the stainability of cells with methylene blue as a chemical expression of differences in oxidation ability of red cells. Goose red cells suspended in serum or salt solutions gave oxygen utilization figures of 27–60% per hour. No CO_2 was produced without O_2 uptake. He made the statement that the magnitude of oxygen utilization was parallel to the basophilia of the red cells involved, but he could not decide if only basophils respired. Young rabbits (5–20 days) gave a large percentage of basophilic anucleate red cells. Parenthetically it might be added that in performing studies of this kind one must be careful to exclude leucocytes because of their much higher rate of both respiration and glycolysis. For example, Guest *et al.* (1953) found for dogs and humans that glycolysis was 0.014–0.028 μg. glucose/hour per million erythrocytes and 4.7–13.2 μg./hour per million leucocytes. Glycolysis by platelets appeared to be insignificant.

The low oxygen consumption of normal human erythrocytes separated from leucocytes and platelets was confirmed by Harrop (1919), who later with Barron (1928) addressed himself to the problem of whether the maturing erythrocyte developed some inhibiting substance or lost "some essential link in the respiratory mechanism." By adding methylene blue (0.0005–0.005%) before incubating blood they were able to raise the oxygen consumption of nonnucleated mammalian red cells to levels approaching those of avian (goose) cells. The effect was shown not to be due to methemoglobin formation.

Carbon dioxide production was linked with oxygen utilization. The addition of cyanide had no influence on the methylene blue effect. The respiration of goose erythrocytes, from either normal or anemic geese, was stimulated by methylene blue but to a lesser extent. In this case, however, methylene blue restored some of the respiration activity that had been abolished by cyanide. Of other dyes tried, only toluylene blue was as effective. They repeated some earlier experiments of Warburg on centrifuged goose blood hemolysate and confirmed that respiration was greatly reduced and mainly confined to the bottom layer which contained remains of formed elements, but that methylene blue would increase oxygen consumption in both layers, being more marked in the upper layer which contained no "nuclear material." In a subsequent study by Barron and Harrop (1928) the relationship between lactic acid formation and glucose utilization was explored, using the "glycolytic quotient" (a value of 1 when 1 mole glucose gave rise to 2 moles lactic acid). It was found that, in contrast to mammalian blood, the glycolytic quotient of avian blood was always less than 1, indicating some oxidative fate of glucose. The addition of methylene blue to mammalian blood as well as to avian blood lowered the glycolytic quotient. In dog blood (apparently without added glucose), the rate of glycolysis was 1.20 mmoles/liter in the first hour and fell to 0.48 in the third hour. The glycolytic quotient approximated unity in each period. With added methylene blue (0.005%), glycolysis was somewhat enhanced but the glycolytic quotient was markedly depressed. Cyanide did not influence the effect of methylene blue, which suggested according to Warburg's ideas that iron was not involved in the oxidations considered here. Washing of red cells impaired glycolysis in the presence or absence of dye. Hemolysis impaired but did not stop glycolysis. In goose blood, glucose disappearance and lactate production were greater under a nitrogen atmosphere than under oxygen, methylene blue having little effect in the absence of oxygen. In trying to arrive at some interpretation of their results, the authors presciently concluded that the methylene blue acts upon the oxidation of hexose monophosphate, rendering it "more sensitive to oxidation by molecular oxygen," since added phosphate enhanced the effect. Michaelis and Salomon (1930) reported that aqueous extract of liver had an effect somewhat similar to methylene blue. The active principle or the mechanism was not demonstrated.

Warburg *et al.* (1930b) re-entered the picture, trying to tie the action of methylene blue to hemoglobin oxidation and reduction, and this in turn led to re-examination of the effect of phenylhydrazine on red cells (1931a,b). This compound increased red cell respiration and glucose oxidation, but the effect was apparently due to the splitting out of iron which then acted catalytically.

Wendel (1933) showed that, because the mammalian erythrocyte did not further metabolize pyruvate, it could be demonstrated that lactate in the presence of methylene blue and the absence of glucose was quantitatively converted to pyruvate. Attempts to account for the glucose disappearance in the presence of methylene blue revealed that an excess "appears to be oxidized not via lactate or pyruvate but by some unknown route to CO_2." Brin and Yonemoto (1958) first demonstrated that oxygen consumption increased with increasing concentration of methylene blue and then, by use of C^{14}-glucose labeled at C-1, C-2, or C-6, they were able to show that methylene blue stimulated oxidation of the upper half of the molecule and indeed that in the presence of methylene blue the intact mammalian erythrocyte carried on active glucose metabolism via the pentose shunt pathway (see Chapters 5 and 13).

Although the mammalian erythrocyte has the capacity to degrade glucose via the pentose shunt when methylene blue is present, it appears normally to metabolize virtually no glucose carbon to CO_2 in this way (Bartlett and Marlow, 1953a). Essentially no C^{14}-labeled glucose was found in the ribose-5-phosphate (Bartlett and Marlow, 1953b).

In 25 studies of 17 individuals' blood at pH 7.5, 2.10 μg. glucose/ml. blood/minute was metabolized (hematocrit 50%). The average amount through the phosphogluconic pathway was 0.23 μg./ml./minute (Murphy, 1960). The aerobic metabolism varied little with pH while the anaerobic glycolysis, when compared to the rate at pH 7.4, increased by 43% at pH 7.8 and decreased by 53% at pH 7.1. A high oxygen atmosphere favored the shunt (aerobic) pathway. Methylene blue by acting as an intermediary between NADPH (reduced nicotinamide adenine dinucleotide phosphate, formerly termed TPNH) and oxygen, markedly stimulated CO_2 production from C^{14}-glucose even when the label was in other than the C-1 position (recycling).

DeLoecker and Prankerd (1961) studied human red cells in phosphate buffer with glucose-1-C^{14}. Their cells utilized 20.6 μl. O_2/ml. cells in 3 hours and 2.05 μmoles glucose/ml. cells/hour and produced 4.4 μmoles lactate. From the CO_2 produced it was calculated that 8.5% of the glucose was metabolized via the hexose monophosphate shunt. Addition of methylene blue stimulated the shunt pathway 20-fold. The shunt pathway was not appreciably inhibited by cyanide, fluoride, or azide, but was completely blocked by iodoacetate. The blocking of glucose oxidation by iodoacetate is not ordinarily considered, since one usually associates the action by this inhibitor with glyceraldehyde-3-phosphate dehydrogenase. Moruzzi (1936), moreover, observed no effect of iodoacetate on methylene blue catalysis. Perhaps level of inhibitor is critical. Much earlier literature on the effect of iodoacetate was discussed by Runnström and Michaelis (1935). The rate of O_2 uptake by rabbit erythrocytes in the presence of methylene blue seemed to be less affected by salt concentration than by glucose concentration, pH, and temperature (Olmstead, 1962).

Thus, it appears that the mature anucleate erythrocyte has a good system for anaerobic glycolysis, deriving its energy by changing glucose to lactic acid. If supplied with a mediator for NADPH oxidation, it has the ability to oxidize some glucose-6-phosphate through the phosphogluconic acid pathway, an ability, incidentally, which is said to be blocked by phenothiazine derivatives (Carver and Roesky, 1959). It cannot oxidize pyruvate, lacking a functioning citric acid cycle (Dajani and Orten, 1958; Rubinstein and Denstedt, 1953; Mirčevová, 1962c). Nucleated erythrocytes carry on fairly typical cellular oxidation (see Schweiger, 1962). Despite this ability, the nucleated erythrocyte has many metabolic shortcomings and can hardly be considered a typical body cell.

III. Anaerobic Glycolysis

A. Hexokinase

Warburg *et al.* (1930a) and Warburg and Christian (1931b) early noted that in the presence of methylene blue and oxygen, hexose phosphate but not glucose itself, could be utilized by hemolysates. Stroma was not required (Warburg and Christian, 1931a). Obviously glucose must be "activated" (phosphorylated). Runnström and Michaelis (1935) observed the same phenomenon, i.e. hemolyzed blood plus glucose did not exhibit glycolysis. They also showed that the addition of NAD to hemolyzed blood in the presence of methylene blue increased the oxidation and the formation of hexose phosphate. Huennekens *et al.* (1957) concluded that the oxidation of glucose in intact human erythrocytes depended upon the oxidation of NADPH by either cell diaphorase or an artificially added codiaphorase such as a dye. Furthermore, the ability of hemolysates to oxidize glucose in the presence of methylene blue was restored by adding Mg^{++}, ATP, and hexokinase. Hexokinase from human red cells was found to have a pronounced optimum at pH 7.8 and a lesser one at pH 6.0 (Kashket *et al.*, 1957). Other workers report optimal pH as 7.5 (Grignani and Löhr, 1960) or 8.1 (Rapoport *et al.*, 1961). This enzyme is regarded by Kashket *et al.* (1957) and Rubinstein *et al.* (1959) to be an important factor in the gradual slowing down of glycolysis in stored blood, inasmuch as stored blood becomes gradually more acid. Hinterberger *et al.* (1961a,b) noted that the pH optimum for glycolysis and for hexokinase coincide and regard hexokinase as the rate-determining step of glycolysis. Rapoport *et al.* (1961) call hexokinase the pacemaker of anaerobic glycolysis, and point out how it decreases when the reticulocyte matures to the erythrocyte and that it seems to be present in lowest activity when compared to the other glycolytic enzymes of the red cell. Mg^{++} is said to be a cofactor for hexokinase, but this is probably consistent with the usual Mg^{++} requirement of ATP-coupled phosphorylations. The reaction of glucose with ATP under the influence of hexokinase is usually thought of as a strongly exergonic reaction, hence the equilibrium should lie well toward glucose-6-phosphate, which furthermore should be rapidly syphoned off. It is, however, inhibited by the products of the reaction. Gabrio *et al.* (1955a) say that glucose to glucose-6-phosphate is the limiting reaction in stored blood, but because of lack of ATP rather than hexokinase. They cite a personal communication from Dr. E. G. Krebs that hexokinase activity is unchanged throughout storage.

Rat erythrocyte hexokinase was examined by Christensen *et al.* (1949) in hemolysates. It acted upon glucose, fructose, and mannose in the ratio 1.0:0.77:0.36, but not upon galactose. Plasma inhibited the reaction, salts influenced it, and insulin, adrenal cortical extract, or pathological conditions had no effect. They observed that hemolysates from 1 ml. red cells caused the disappearance of 10 μmoles glucose/hour, while in rat whole blood *in vitro* glucose utilization was approximately one-third this value for a like number of red cells. One wonders if this difference is due to more ready availability of glucose or some other factitious circumstance of the hemolysate experiments, or does it suggest that hexokinase in the intact rat red cell is not the rate-limiting step? Mirčevová (1962a) noted that hemolysates in the presence of sufficient ATP and NAD glycolyzed at a normal rate, suggesting that hexokinase activity did not decrease because of hemolysis. Kildema (1960) also observed greater activity in hemolysates than in whole cells.

Eldjarn and Bremer (1962) reported experiments indicating that hexokinase activity was abolished by disulfide compounds such as $(NH_2CH_2CH_2S)_2$ (cystamine) suggesting that hexokinase contained SH groups even more susceptible than the classic glyceraldehyde-3-phosphate dehydrogenase. After addition of cystamine, human erythrocytes with methylene blue showed no O_2 uptake with glucose as substrate. With adenosine or other purine nucleoside instead of glucose their O_2 uptake was normal. The levels of ATP seemed adequate in either case, strongly suggesting the abolishment of hexokinase activity by the disulfide. Grignani and Löhr (1960) had noted that iodoacetate inhibited hexokinase, suggesting that the enzyme needed SH groups.

B. Phosphoglucomutase

It has been known for years that red cells contain glucose-1,6-diphosphate, its identity having been well demonstrated by Bartlett (1959a). If glucose-1,6-diphosphate is in fact a catalytic intermediate in the interconversion of glucose phosphates, one might postulate that large amounts of the diphosphate could arise either because there was no completely functioning phosphoglucomutase present, or because enzymes for converting glucose to glycogen appear to be absent in the red cell. Inasmuch as no glucose-1-phosphate was found in red cells by Bartlett (1959a), it would seem that glucose-1,6-diphosphate represents a metabolic cul-de-sac. Its concentration did not change in stored acid–citrate–dextrose (ACD) blood (Bartlett and Shafer, 1960).

C. *Phosphohexose Isomerase*

Marks *et al.* (1958) separated new erythrocytes from old ones by osmotic hemolysis and demonstrated that phosphohexose isomerase activity was several times higher in the new cells.

D. *Phosphofructokinase*

Mirčevová and Vosykova (1961) described an assay method for this enzyme. In experiments on pyruvate-reducing ability, Blanchaer and Weiss (1954) postulated that intact stored red cells lost their ability to convert glucose to fructose diphosphate. Hemolysates from these cells, however, were competent in this respect. Blanchaer *et al.* (1955a,b) were able to narrow the defect to phosphofructokinase which by the twenty-fifth day of storage had lost 80% of its activity, other glycolytic enzymes meanwhile having started at a lower level but not having decreased appreciably. Adenosine protected against loss of this activity in stored blood (Brownstone and Blanchaer, 1957). It could be pointed out that lack of ATP as well as lack of phosphofructokinase could preclude the conversion of fructose-1-phosphate to fructose-1,6-diphosphate.

That this enzyme might indeed be a critical point in the failure of glycolysis in the ACD stored red cell is suggested by the findings of Bartlett and Shafer (1960). When they collected blood in herapin, there was a hexose diphosphate fraction containing fructose-1,6-diphosphate and glucose-1,6-diphosphate in 4:1 ratio. In blood collected in ACD, only glucose-1,6-diphosphate was present. No fructose-1,6-diphosphate was formed during the blood storage and intermediates past this point in the anaerobic glycolysis scheme disappeared. Meanwhile the hexose monophosphate fraction increased during storage. If this represented only glucose-6-phosphate, one must conclude that hexokinase was active during storage. If this hexose monophosphate were both glucose-6-phosphate and fructose-6-phosphate, as suggested by another of Bartlett's papers (1959a), we must then assume that both hexokinase and phosphohexose isomerase are still active in ACD stored red cells, pushing the defect more toward phosphofructokinase. Perhaps another point to note is that when ACD blood was stored with inosine there was marked increase in sedoheptulose-7-phosphate, a product which arises at one stage in the shunt pathway and which might accumulate if its congener from the transketolase reaction, glyceraldehyde-3-phosphate, were siphoned off through the Embden-Meyerhof reactions rather than remaining with the sedoheptulose-7-phosphate for subsequent shunt reactions via transaldolase. Sedoheptulose-7-phosphate can be phosphorylated by exactly the enzyme whose failure we are postulating, namely, phosphofructokinase. Sedoheptulose-1,7-diphosphate was found after 4-hour incubation of heparinized (not ACD) human blood (Bucolo and Bartlett, 1960). This compound could, of course, arise alternately via action of aldolase on erythrose-4-phosphate and triose phosphate.

Mirčevová (1962b) noted that hemolysate utilized fructose-1,6-diphosphate considerably better than fructose-1-phosphate, suggesting a limiting amount of phosphofructokinase.

E. Aldolase

This enzyme, needed to split fructose-1,6-diphosphate to the triose phosphate level, was said to increase with aging of cells and decrease with aging of the individual (Bertolini *et al.*, 1961d). Schapira (1959) concludes the opposite, that aldolase decreases as red cells age *in vivo*. The enzyme is said to be low in hemolysate (Blanchaer and Weiss, 1954; Blanchaer *et al.*, 1955a). Corsini *et al.* (1959) found that aldolase activity of the stroma was about 40% that of the erythrocytes. The whole erythrocytes showed no systematic variation as the donors' age increased.

F. Glyceraldehyde-3-Phosphate Dehydrogenase

In the first oxidation step in the Embden-Meyerhof pathway, NAD^+ is reduced to NADH, which under anaerobic conditions is later reoxidized when pyruvate is reduced to lactate. The enzyme has SH groups which must be kept in reduced form. *A priori* one might think that this enzyme would be liable to inactivation by oxidation of the SH groups, and in fact Löhr and Waller (1959) observed in anucleate erythrocytes that, whereas most of the glycolytic enzymes decreased linearly with aging, glyceraldehyde-3-phosphate dehydrogenase and glucose-6-phosphate dehydrogenase decreased exponentially. This puts the cell in triple jeopardy because it cannot (1) glycolyze via the Embden-Meyerhof pathway, (2) synthesize more ribose for nucleotide synthesis, and (3) synthesize or utilize ribose phosphate for energy. On this basis, protection of the SH groups of glyceraldehyde-3-phosphate dehydrogenase would seem to be a major objective in blood storage.

If glyceraldehyde-3-phosphate dehydrogenase were the key point at which stored erythrocytes developed metabolic difficulty, added nucleosides should be of no help energetically, inasmuch as the energy-producing reactions for their utilization lie past this step. Nucleosides *are* beneficial, arguing against the crucialness of this one enzyme. More observations and reflections may temper this conclusion.

Scheuch and Rapoport (1962) note the inactivation of glyceraldehyde-3-phosphate dehydrogenase and glucose-6-phosphate dehydrogenase by various oxidizing agents. Blanchaer *et al.* (1955a) demonstrated in hemolysates of

ACD stored blood (5–22 days) the presence of glyceraldehyde-3-phosphate dehydrogenase and other enzymes close to it in anaerobic glycolysis. They could demonstrate oxidation of NADH by reversal of the phosphoglycerate kinase and glyceraldehyde-3-phosphate dehydrogenase, beginning with 3-phosphoglycerate, ATP, and NADH.

The NADH from this step in the Embden-Meyerhof pathway is normally used to reduce pyruvate to lactate, but has a major role in reducing methemoglobin via a so-called diaphorase (Scott and McGraw, 1962; see also Chapter 11). This NAD diaphorase was deficient in Alaskan Indians with hereditary methemoglobinemia (Scott, 1960) and less active in children than in adults, an explanation for the greater susceptibility of children to drug-induced methemoglobinemia (Ross, 1963).

G. *Interconversion of Di- and Monophosphoglycerates*

1,3-Diphosphoglycerate is the normal product of glycolysis at this point in the Embden-Meyerhof pathway. The red cell, however, contains large quantities of 2,3-diphosphoglycerate (Greenwald, 1925). The absence of 1,3-diphosphoglycerate is not surprising since the 1-phosphate is a high-energy phosphate and would be rapidly utilized via phosphoglycerate kinase to give 3-phosphoglyceric acid. This, under the influence of phosphoglycerate mutase, would be converted to 2-phosphoglycerate, and 2,3-diphosphoglycerate could be an intermediate seen in quantity in red cells but not to any extent in other tissues. The catalytic role of the diphosphoglycerate was shown by Sutherland *et al.* (1949) in enzyme studies. Under these circumstances 2,3-diphosphoglycerate would be metabolically active. It is active, as shown by Bartlett and Marlow (1953a) and Prankerd and Altman (1954b) among others. Furthermore, the levels of 2,3-diphosphoglycerate fall progressively in stored blood (Bartlett and Shafer, 1960) as would be expected if the subsequent glycolytic reactions continued to operate. Rapoport and Luebering (1950) claimed a diphosphoglycerate mutase that could convert 1,3-diphosphoglycerate to 2,3-diphosphoglycerate, a reaction that would be energy-wasting because of conversion of a high-energy to a low-energy phosphate. Although one cannot rule out the existence or importance of such an enzyme in red cells, the data presented do admit of other interpretations. A subsequent study by Rapoport and Luebering (1952) claimed to confirm the existence and some properties of diphosphoglycerate mutase. Much uncertainty in this whole area has resulted from the methods available, a matter discussed by Bartlett subsequently (1959b). Prankerd (1961) reiterates the suggestion that energy wasting, via conversion of 1,3-diphosphoglycerate to 2,3-diphosphoglycerate, could have some raison d'être in red cell economy, perhaps as a ready source of phosphate.

Zipursky *et al.* (1960) studied erythrocytes from both adults and newborn babies and concluded that although phosphate partitions were not greatly dissimilar when the blood was drawn, the changes on incubation were much more rapid in the newborn red cells. The difference lay mainly in the non-hydrolyzable phosphate which is thought to be mainly 2,3-diphosphoglycerate. This observation coupled with others in their paper, such as more rapid incorporation of P^{32} into adult red cells, led them to conclude that the rate of synthesis of 2,3-diphosphoglycerate in adult red cells was greater than in red cells of the newborn.

In newborn rabbits with respiratory acidosis from breathing CO_2 the 2,3-diphosphoglycerate content of erythrocytes decreased quickly, indicating the metabolic lability of this compound (Kutas and Stützel, 1958b). The diphosphoglycerate level is quite low in newborn dogs and rabbits but in weeks this reaches the adult level (Kutas and Stützel, 1958a). Rohdewald and Weber (1958) found the diphosphoglycerate level low and the ATP level high in the blood of children and explained this by the shift in the phosphoglyceric acid cycle postulated by Rapoport. Rohdewald and Weber (1959) found in the blood of ruminants little 2,3-diphosphoglycerate or fructose diphosphate, although present in calves until they were able to digest vegetable feed (Weber *et al.*, 1961).

Prankerd and Altman (1954b) found after incubation of red cells with P^{32} that 2,3-diphosphoglycerate had a higher relative specific activity than ATP, suggesting that the former was precursor of the latter. Prankerd (1961) subsequently pointed out that allowance had not been made in their earlier calculation for nonlabeled P of ATP. This would reconcile their results with those of Gerlach *et al.* (1958), who reported ATP as the precursor of 2,3-diphosphoglyceric acid. Gourley (1952) also found that in human erythrocytes incubated with P^{32} the terminal P of ATP became labeled faster than diphosphoglycerate, supporting the same conclusions. Schauer and Hillmann (1961) go beyond this controversy and cite evidence for an unknown membrane acceptor (in ghosts) which attains P^{32} activities many times as high as ATP.

In patients with hereditary spherocytosis, incubation of the red cells with P^{32} gave highest radioactivity in ATP and less in 2,3-diphosphoglyceric acid. Subsequent incubation with nonradioactive phosphate led to more rapid fall in radioactivity of ATP, suggesting a precursor relationship of ATP to 2,3-diphosphoglyceric acid. The blood of patients with hereditary spherocytosis behaved no differently than that of normal individuals (Zipursky *et al.*, 1962).

A curious finding by Rapoport (1940) and Rapoport and Guest (1941) is that vertebrates with nucleated red cells have no phosphoglycerate (mono- or di-). This is "replaced" by phytic acid (inositol hexaphosphate). The methods were of necessity somewhat crude, but the striking difference in 2,3-diphosphoglycerate content between nonnucleated and nucleated cells might be illuminated by further comparison of the metabolism of the two kinds of red cells. This substitution of phytic acid for 2,3-diphosphoglycerate was again seen in the paper chromatograms of Gerlach and Lübben (1959).

Mányai and Varady (1956) studied and purified a red cell enzyme that in the presence of $NaHSO_3$ or $Na_2S_2O_4$ split 2,3-diphosphoglycerate to pyruvate and inorganic phosphate. 3-Phosphoglycerate was not a substrate. The role of such an enzyme in red cell metabolism cannot be properly evaluated until its purity and specificity are established.

H. Enolase

Hemolysates of human erythrocytes readily convert phosphoglycerate (equal mixture of 2′ and 3′) to phosphoenol pyruvate. Mg^{++} is required, and Ca^{++} inhibits probably by competing with Mg^{++} (Boszormenyi-Nagy, 1955). Blostein and Denstedt (1962) partially purified the enzyme from human erythrocytes and studied its kinetics as influenced by Mg^{++} and substrate concentration. Maximal activity was in the pH range 6.3–7.0. Miwa *et al.* (1962) investigated enolase activity and its sensitivity to fluoride in hereditary spherocytosis. They concluded that in this condition the activity of the enzyme was not diminished nor was it more sensitive to fluoride, refuting the earlier conclusions of Tabechian *et al.* (1956).

I. Lactic Dehydrogenase

Lactic dehydrogenase (LDH) is found in the soluble portion of the red cell (Alivisatos and Denstedt, 1951). Nicotinamide should be added when hemolysates are prepared to prevent the destruction of the LDH cofactor, NAD, by stromal NADase. In the case of the rabbit erythrocyte, Ottolenghi and Denstedt (1958a,b) found that the enzyme would utilize both L- and D-lactate and that many compounds inhibited the reaction, among others oxalate and malonate. The kinetics of the activity of the enzyme were studied in order to clarify its method of action. Pyruvate was shown to be an inhibitor. The mechanism of combination of substrate, enzyme, and coenzyme was discussed. The enzyme was studied by Birkbeck and Stewart (1961) and found to have a broad pH optimum of 7.0–7.8. Their method of assay was described and could be used with blood collected in almost any anticoagulant except oxalate. Whole blood at 4°C. and dilute hemolysate frozen at −10C°. could be kept for 4 weeks without loss of LDH activity. Bertolini *et al.* (1961b) confirmed that LDH activity did not change significantly with aging of erythrocytes or persons.

The recent interest in isozymes (enzymes which are identical in function but different in their protein component) has prompted the reinvestigation of the

LDH of blood. Vesell and Bearn (1962), for example, reported on LDH isozymes in the erythrocytes of 18 vertebrates. Pappius *et al.* (1954) found that oxalate inhibited glycolysis in red cells stored at 5°C., but that this could be reversed if the oxalate were removed or precipitated fairly promptly. Expired whole blood from blood banks was shown to be a satisfactory source for certain LDH fractions and for study of purification procedures (Hills and Meacham, 1961).

IV. Penetration of the Erythrocyte by Sugars

It has been shown by many investigators in many ways that glucose penetrates the human erythrocyte easily and that hormones like insulin are not only unnecessary, but have no effect. There is much evidence to suggest that the penetration of red cells by sugars may differ considerably from one species to another, and the investigator must constantly be on his guard when extrapolating results to a new situation. As a generalization, monosaccharides (pentoses or hexoses) penetrate red cells but disaccharides such as sucrose, lactose, and maltose do not. This area has been unusually well reviewed by LeFevre (1961), who has attempted to define both substrate specificity and inhibitor specificity.

The generalization that phosphorylated compounds will not penetrate cells seems to hold for red cells. DeSandre *et al.* (1959) demonstrated that the human erythrocyte would not utilize glucose-1-phosphate, as found by Ghiotto *et al.* (1959) for both glucose-1-phosphate and fructose-1,6-diphosphate.

Lacko *et al.* (1961) criticized use of the osmotic method for determining the rate of penetration of sugars and devised a method utilizing rapid filtration. Their results and speculation with respect to galactose were given. The method was extended to studies on the carrier system for aldoses as affected by disaccharides (Lacko and Burger, 1962).

V. Utilization of Sugars Other than Glucose

Glucose, fructose, and mannose but not galactose appear to be utilized by human red cells. Pentoses and disaccharides appear not to be utilized. In our laboratory, using as a criterion of utilization of the sugar its ability to sustain ATP levels during incubation, we have shown only D-glucose and D-fructose to be utilized. D-Ribose, D-lactose, D-erythrose, D-galactose, and sedoheptulose were ineffective. Lachhein *et al.* (1961) claimed that galactose and ribose utilization was about half that of glucose. Earlier Lachhein and Matthies (1960) reported that anucleate erythrocytes could utilize D-ribose and deoxyribose but not L-arabinose, D-arabinose, L-xylose, and D-xylose. They postulated a ribokinase to mediate the phosphorylation of ribose by ATP. Presumably this would feed into the shunt. Fructose may appear as a component in certain bloods, such as the fetal blood of ungulates (Huggett and Nixon, 1961). Ribose was said to prevent the fall of ATP in incubated rabbit erythrocytes (Lachman *et al.*, 1961).

Galactosemia is presumed to be caused by lack of the enzyme uridyl transferase, which promotes the exchange of galactose-1-phosphate with the glucose on uridine diphosphoglucose. In addition to testing for the enzyme, one can also incubate hemolysates of the patient's blood with galactose-1-C^{14} and measure the amount of $C^{14}O_2$ evolved (Weinberg, 1961). One product of the reactions converting galactose to glucose is glucose-1-phosphate and one wonders if it is mainly acted upon by phosphatase to give glucose or is isomerized to glucose-6-phosphate. Inouye *et al.* (1962) did incubate erythrocytes from galactosemic patients with galactose and on fractionation found both galactose-1-phosphate and galactose-6-phosphate. Perhaps all the reactions in the utilization of galactose are somewhat feeble even in normal blood.

VI. Nucleotide Metabolism

A. General

Phosphorylated intermediates in glycolysis have already been discussed at some length. We now turn to those phosphate esters which contain a purine or pyrimidine moiety. It was early noted that many phosphate-containing compounds could be extracted from tissue, such as blood, by treatment with an acid protein-precipitant such as trichloroacetic acid. These organic phosphate compounds could be fractionated according to the solubility of their barium salts or their ease of hydrolysis in boiling 1 N H_2SO_4. Results of such studies were well reviewed by Guest and Rapoport (1941). It was apparent even then that blood contained appreciable quantities of ATP, diphosphoglycerate, and other organic phosphates in addition to inorganic phosphate. These various fractions of the acid-soluble phosphate were extensively studied in blood of different species and under various pathological conditions. The close relationship between glycolysis and phosphate ester formation was apparent in many studies. Even the influence of these two processes on red cell electrolyte equilibria was appreciated.

Free purines and pyrimidines do not occur in appreciable quantities in blood. They are almost always found in combination with ribose and phosphate as nucleotides or dinucleotides. The nature of the substituents on the phosphate gives rise to many different steric and ionization effects which can be exploited in the newer techniques of chromatographic or electrophoretic separation. Methodology and results are well described in such standard references as Block *et al.* (1958) and Chargaff and Davidson (1955).

Rohdewald and Weber (1956) studied the acid-soluble fraction of human blood by paper chromatography. In the same year Gabrio *et al.* (1956a) published chromatograms of acid extracts of whole blood fractionated on anion-exchange columns (Dowex-1-formate). The changes in nucleotide distribution in fresh blood, stored blood, or stored blood plus added nucleosides were easily seen. In 1959 three separate investigators using similar

TABLE I

PHOSPHORYLATED COMPOUNDS IN HUMAN BLOOD

Compound	Amount (micromoles per liter of red cells)			
	Bartlett (1959)[a]	Bishop *et al.* (1959)[b]	Mills and Sommers (1959)[c]	Gerlach *et al.* (1958)[d]
Inorganic phosphate	280–480	—	—	250
Weak acid phosphates	200–330	—	—	—
Adenosine diphosphate	190–245	101, 112	241, 160	300
Monophosphoglycerate	50–80	—	—	—
Glucose-1,6-diphosphate	190–235	—	—	—
Fructose-1,6-diphosphate	60–120	—	—	430
2,3-Diphosphoglycerate	3600–5010	—	4640, 4010	3710
Adenosine triphosphate	900–1233	921, 1000	1185, 1280	680
Adenosine monophosphate	10–20	13, 12	50, 22	<100
Glucose-6-phosphate	80–100	—	—	—
Fructose-6-phosphate	10–20	—	—	—
Ribose-5-phosphate	trace–30	—	—	—
Unknown ketose phosphate	30–40	—	—	—
NADP	13–16	25, 27	36, 37	—
Guanosine triphosphate	—	52, 62	—	—
NAD	—	64, 74	63, 61	—
CDPX	—	—	15, 18	—
Inosine monophosphate	—	0, 0	0, 0	—
Hexose monophosphate	—	—	, <2	—
Hexose diphosphate	—	—	325, 188	—
Triose phosphate	—	—	—	380

[a] Upper part of column based on 14 human samples, lower part on 4; in recalculating the data it was assumed that compounds were monophosphates unless obviously otherwise.

[b] First value of each pair, average of 13 samples from males; second value, average from 8 females.

[c] Individual values for each of two donors.

[d] Average of 14 samples, some incubated as long as 60 minutes.

anion-exchange columns published values for blood nucleotides and other phosphorylated compounds. These values have been recalculated to micromoles of compound per liter of red cells and are presented in Table I. Included also are values derived by paper chromatography (Gerlach *et al.*, 1958).

It is apparent that of all the nucleotides, ATP is present in largest quantity, i.e. around 1000 μmoles/liter red cells. (Paper chromatography seems to give lower values for ATP and higher values for ADP, suggesting the possibility of some breakdown of ATP when determined by this technique.) The concentration of ADP is 10–20% that of ATP, and AMP is 1–2%. In order to have a distribution like this the blood must be freshly drawn and extracted with cold trichloroacetic acid promptly, a point noted by Bishop *et al.* (1959). In fact, Bishop *et al.* (1960) extracted nucleotides from several tissues other than blood and concluded that it was virtually impossible to guarantee that the extract from "solid" tissue had a nucleotide distribution that accurately mirrored *in vivo* conditions. By enzymatic methods Overgaard-Hansen and Jørgensen (1960) found 1534 ± 33 μmoles adenine nucleotide/liter red cells, 85% of which was ATP and 14% ADP. Rohdewald and Weber (1958) found more ATP and less 2,3-diphosphoglycerate in blood of children than in that of adults. No inosine monophosphate (IMP) is normally found in fresh blood, but is formed promptly at the expense of adenine nucleotides if the blood is hemolyzed (Bishop, 1960). The only purine other than adenine found in fresh blood is guanine. This is present as guanosine triphosphate (GTP) although small amounts of GDP and GMP have been reported. Gerlach and Fikentscher (1959) identified guanine nucleotides in pigeon erythrocytes. Because of the amounts present and their position in the elution pattern from columns, GDP and GMP are difficult to measure.

Pyrimidine nucleotides have been reported. Cytidine compounds are eluted early in these column chromatograms (Bishop *et al.*, 1959; Mills and Sommers, 1959; Mills, 1960). The presence of uridine diphosphoglucose was suspected by Bishop *et al.* (1959) and Mills and Sommers (1959). The absence of creatine phosphate was reported by Gerlach *et al.* (1958), who cited a similar earlier observation by Eggleton and Eggleton (1929). The separation of acid-soluble phosphorus compounds of blood was detailed for paper chromatography (Yoshikawa *et al.*, 1959) and column chromatography (Yoshikawa *et al.*, 1960). Hashimoto and Yoshikawa (1961) and Hashimoto (1961) claimed to have found adenylyldiphosphoglyceric acid in pig blood. Hashimoto *et al.* (1961) found the same compound in human and rabbit but not cow blood. Human erythrocytes depleted of ATP and then offered 2-azaadenine or 2,6-diaminopurine incorporated these into ATP analogs (Tatibana and Yoshikawa, 1962).

Uric acid riboside has been known for many years, particularly in beef red cells (Davis *et al.*, 1922; Newton and Davis, 1922a,b).

The alteration of the nucleotide pattern under various pathological situations has been extensively reported, but results are not always credible because of the way in which blood extracts have been prepared or fractionated. Bishop (1962a) demonstrated that, in terminal nephritis, the concentration of virtually all blood nucleotides was elevated when allowance was made for the anemia present in these individuals. Gouty patients were intermediate between normal and nephritic subjects. Higher values for adenine nucleotides had been reported earlier for other anemias (Rottino *et al.*, 1952), and acid-labile phosphate was shown to be elevated in renal patients with phosphate retention (Bunch *et al.*, 1958). It has been claimed (Löhr *et al.*, 1958) that red cell ATP declines as the cell ages *in vivo*. This decline in stored blood is well recognized.

Since adenine nucleotides are by far the most plentiful purine or pyrimidine compounds in the red cell, their synthesis and breakdown will occupy much of our attention. Before launching into this discussion, however, it is pertinent to remind ourselves that ATP (and ADP) is an energy reservoir *par excellence*, and inasmuch as glycolysis is presumably the only energy-generating system in the nonnucleated red cell, there is a close relationship between glycolysis and ATP level in this cell. After incubating blood with classical inhibitors of anaerobic glycolysis, such as iodoacetate and fluoride, the ATP readily disappears and other typical degradation changes in the nucleotide pattern occur (Mills and Jones, 1961; Bishop, 1961d). Even an agent like tolbutamide, whose effect on carbohydrate metabolism *in vitro* is still less than clear, had an effect on the nucleotide pattern of incubated blood (Bishop, 1961b). During incubation or storage of blood the pH gradually falls, leading to a decrease in both glycolysis rate and ATP levels. This was shown to be due to the acidity only and not the rising lactate concentration (Bishop, 1962b), and could be ameliorated by controlling the pH (Bishop, 1962c). An explanation of this, discussed under Section III, A, is loss of hexokinase activity, but other possible explanations may also be entertained.

If we are dealing with the nucleated (avian) erythrocyte, any of the inhibitors, such as cyanide and azide, that affect the cytochrome systems will inhibit oxidative phosphorylation. Gerlach and Lübben (1959), using paper chromatography (system of Fleckenstein and Gerlach, 1953) and P^{32}-orthophosphate, showed that the ATP level of pigeon erythrocytes was quite susceptible to the action of dinitrophenol or cyanide, whereas phytic acid, the predominating organophosphate fraction of avian erythrocytes, was not affected. On the other hand human erythrocytes are not sensitive to cyanide but are markedly affected by iodoacetate. In this circumstance ATP disappears rapidly, and some but not all of the phosphorylated glycolytic intermediates also decrease. In the studies on P^{32} incorporation in pigeon erythrocytes, dinitrophenol (also thyroxine to a limited degree) or cyanide inhibited incorporation of labeled phosphate into both energy phosphates and glycolytic phosphates. In human erythrocytes, iodoacetate (and to a lesser extent triethylenemelamine) acted similarly, although glycolytic intermediates up to glyceraldehyde-3-phosphate were perhaps less affected.

Inorganic phosphate in human plasma is thought by some to go to ATP in the red cell membrane and be released inside as ATP, but some diffusion could not be ruled out (Gourley, 1952). P^{32} transfer was slower in chicken blood than in human blood even though glucose utilization was higher (Gourley, 1957). Vestergaard-Bogind and Hesselbo (1960) believe that phosphate crosses the human erythrocyte membrane passively, but cite the work of many other investigators to the contrary. Zipursky and Israels (1961) suggest that phosphate entry into the red cell is not even dependent on glycolysis. Some of these discordant results may be reconciled by the observations of Christensen and Jones (1962) that low levels of phosphate act differently than higher levels and that temperature is a critical factor.

Typical body cells can synthesize purines (and pyrimidines) *de novo* from small molecules such as glycine, glutamine, CO_2, and formate. Mature erythrocytes appear unable to do this. Lowy *et al.* (1960) incubated rabbit erythrocytes with labeled precursors, such as glycine and formate, and were unable to demonstrate incorporation of these precursors into the erythrocyte purines under conditions that allowed preformed purines to be incorporated into erythrocyte nucleotides. The blood nucleotides did, however, readily become labeled if C^{14}-glycine was administered to the rabbit. The mature erythrocyte behaved similarly (Lowy *et al.*, 1962). Bishop (1960) was similarly unsuccessful in causing incorporation of C^{14}-glycine into incubated whole blood, either human blood or chicken blood with its nucleated erythrocytes. Glycine is, however, known to participate in some metabolic reactions in the nucleated erythrocyte (Dajani and Orten, 1959). Lowy and Williams (1960) subsequently showed that the mature rabbit erythrocyte could synthesize ATP and GTP from labeled formate in the presence of 5-amino-1-ribosyl-4-imidazolecarboxamide. This placed the failure in *de novo* purine synthesis earlier in the sequence. Bertino *et al.* (1962) were able to isolate from human erythrocytes three enzymes, namely: the formate-activating enzyme; N^5,N^{10}-methylenetetrahydrofolate dehydrogenase; and serine hydroxylmethylase. The formate-activating enzyme was in higher concentration in young erythrocytes and in erythrocytes of animals with shorter red cell lifespans. Lowy *et al.* (1961b) prepared rabbits with a high reticulocyte count and could then show the *in vitro* incorporation of labeled formate or glycine into blood purines. This biosynthetic capacity is apparently lost when the reticulocyte matures. Inasmuch as mature anucleate erythrocytes cannot completely synthesize purine, and since as will be seen shortly the red cell nucleotide purines are in a constant state of metabolic turnover, it follows that other tissues must supply these preformed purines to the mature red cells.

Lajtha and Vane (1958) demonstrated that when the hepatectomized rabbit was supplied with C^{14}-formate, little label turned up in bone marrow adenine. Utilizing various controls, they concluded that in the mammal the liver was the main supplier of purines for bone marrow cells and perhaps for other tissue as well. Henderson and LePage (1959) concluded from their experiments that purines might be transported among mouse tissues by blood cells, adenine being taken up (perhaps in the red cell nucleotides) as the blood passes through the liver and later released in other tissues.

Preformed purines such as adenine, guanine, and hypoxanthine are readily incorporated into red cell nucleotides, implying that these nucleotides are building up and breaking down continuously. Based on the incubation studies of Lowy *et al.* (1960, 1961a, 1962), Lowy and Williams (1960), and Bishop (1960), one can conclude that free adenine is readily incorporated into adenine nucleotides and that free hypoxanthine, xanthine, or guanine is preferentially incorporated into guanine nucleotides (essentially GTP). *In vivo* studies in human subjects after injection of C^{14}-adenine gave results similar to the *in vitro* studies on human blood (Bishop, 1961a). As cogently discussed by Lowy *et al.* (1961a) as well as by Bishop (1960), the conversion of AMP to IMP seems to go mainly in the direction of deamination although, with chicken blood, Bishop showed that there was some of the backward reaction. Lowy *et al.* (1962) stated, "It appears probable that the mature human erythrocyte lacks either adenylosuccinic synthase or adenylosuccinase, or both." It might be concluded that these enzymes are dropped when the reticulocyte matures, since Lowy *et al.* (1961b) found in the rabbit reticulocyte that with formate or glycine the adenine of ATP became more highly labeled than the guanine of GTP. When nucleosides instead of free bases are used for incorporation studies, the results are essentially the same as with the free bases except for adenosine. This nucleoside is deaminated so quickly that it behaves like hypoxanthine or inosine. These various reactions are summarized as follows:

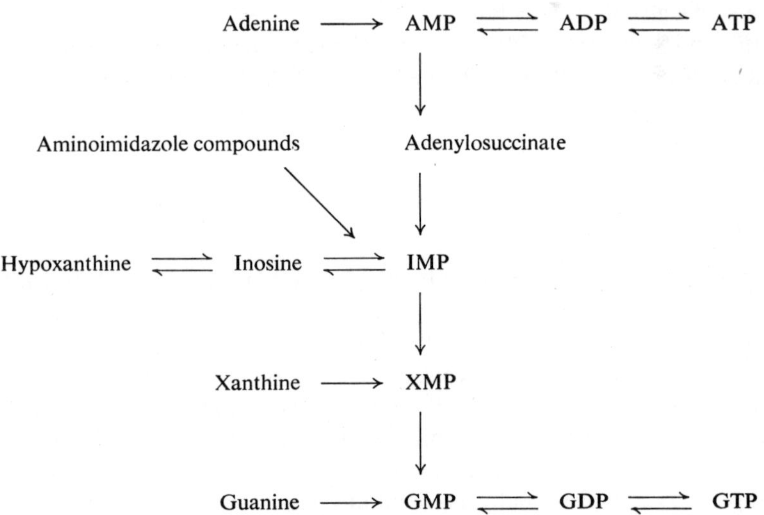

The breakdown of ATP proceeds to hypoxanthine as follows (Bishop, 1961c):

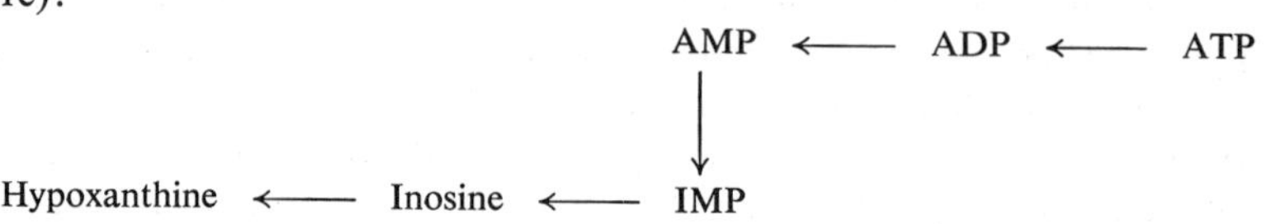

Breakdown stops at hypoxanthine, at least in human blood, because there is no xanthine oxidase present. Jørgensen (1956a) observed that the sum of the above compounds was nearly constant in stored human blood, a point confirmed in the reviewer's laboratory (Bishop, 1961c) for human blood but not for rabbit blood. The latter observation raises the question whether rabbit blood contains xanthine oxidase.

Jørgensen and his various co-workers have concerned themselves with enzymatic methodology for determining the breakdown products of ATP in blood, and then have used these methods to quantitate the changing patterns of these compounds as blood is stored (Jørgensen, 1955, 1956a, b, 1957; Jørgensen and Poulson, 1955; Chen and Jørgensen, 1956; Jørgensen and Chen, 1956, 1957; Jørgensen and Overgaard-Hansen, 1960). All papers from this group are excellent, but one is singled out because of a questionable interpretation. Jørgensen and Grove-Rasmussen (1957) passed blood through a Ca^{++}-removing resin and added aliquots of the effluent to glucose-containing phosphate buffers to establish various initial pH's. In the one aliquot to which no buffer was added, ATP rapidly broke down to oxypurine. The authors concluded that this behavior was an effect of pH. They failed to consider that the aliquot without buffer was also without glucose and hence could not continue active glycolysis very long.

Mills and Sommers (1959) followed the changes in nucleotides during *in vitro* incubation at 37°C. Parvé (1953) determined ATP in blood enzymatically after first boiling 1 minute at pH 2.5–3.

Various enzymes concerned with nucleotide interconversions will now be discussed.

B. *ATPase*

A specific ATPase is presumed to couple ATP breakdown with active Na^+ (and K^+) transport across the red cell membrane. This topic is well discussed in Chapter 3. Otherwise ATPase activity is usually considered a nuisance which the investigator tries to minimize. Inasmuch as ATP breakdown is inevitable when energy is required by the cell for any of its reactions, it is not surprising that a situation may develop in which ATP utilization exceeds ATP synthesis. Under these circumstances there is a net disappearance of ATP, but this is not what the enzymologist usually has in mind when he speaks of ATPase activity.

Caffrey *et al.* (1956) described the isolation of ATPase from hemolysates and noted that, in addition to ATP, it split ADP and ITP and to a lesser extent uridine triphosphate (UTP). Post *et al.* (1960) studied erythrocyte membrane ATPase and concluded that it quite specifically linked ATP (not ITP) breakdown to cation transport. Herbert (1956) claimed that stroma-free hemolysates had no ATPase activity and that the enzyme activity was on the outer surface of the cell. Priwitl and Schmitt (1957) found enzyme activity at the surface of the intact erythrocyte. Szekely *et al.* (1953) said there was no ATPase in the intact cell but it could be released from stroma by hemolysis produced by freezing and thawing. Laris *et al.* (1962) studied ATPase activity in stroma of human, rabbit, and beef blood and considered its role in sugar permeability.

C. Inorganic Pyrophosphatase

This enzyme splits inorganic pyrophosphate to inorganic orthophosphate and would presumably dispose of the pyrophosphate arising when ATP breaks down to AMP. Since pyrophosphate is a high-energy compound it would seem reasonable that this energy could be trapped, but this point does not appear to have been much studied. Malkin and Denstedt (1956a) studied the activity of erythrocyte pyrophosphatase and concluded it was all contained in the cytoplasm. Cysteine or glutathione prevented diminution of activity on storage of hemolysates. Fluoride and calcium inhibited it. Scheuch *et al.* (1961) reported that oxidized glutathione inactivated inorganic pyrophosphatase of rabbit erythrocytes. The evidence points strongly to the necessity of maintaining intact SH groups.

D. Adenylate Kinase (Myokinase)

Since ADP is ordinarily converted to ATP by active glycolysis, it might be conjectured that a good reason for needing adenylate kinase would be for conversion of AMP to ADP, i.e. AMP + ATP $\rightleftharpoons$ 2 ADP. The build-up of AMP is to be avoided in red cells because of the high activity of adenylic acid deaminase which would waste the adenine moiety—a molecule not easy to come by. Tatibana *et al.* (1958) noted that adenylate kinase activity was easily shown in human red cell hemolysates and that it did not decrease on storage. Kashket and Denstedt (1958) demonstrated the presence of the enzyme in hemolysates. They also added ADP to whole erythrocyte suspensions and noted an increase in glucose utilization. Since phosphorylated compounds would not normally be expected to penetrate red cells, they reasoned that ADP reacted with adenylate kinase at the cell surface which gave rise to AMP and ATP. They postulated that the products would then be discharged on the inside of the cell membrane. Cerletti and DeRitas (1960) sedimented the stromal fraction but by various washings showed that the enzyme is not a constituent of the erythrocyte membrane. Cerletti and Bucci (1960) reaffirmed this, noting also an optimal pH of 7.5 and strong activation by Mg^{++}.

E. Breakdown of AMP

Any of the following pathways could be envisioned for the breakdown of adenosine monophosphate (adenylic acid):

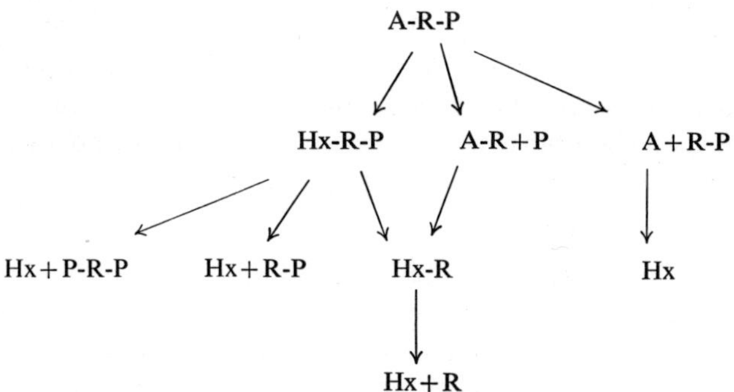

The one reaction that appears least likely is the conversion of adenine to hypoxanthine inasmuch as adenine deaminase is rarely found in tissue. In our laboratory we have often incubated or stored human blood in the presence of added adenine and have found that the adenine persists for a considerable time. Under similar conditions added adenosine would be deaminated in a few minutes.

The phosphorolysis of inosinic acid to ribose-1,5-diphosphate is pointed out by R. L. Post (personal communication) as a possible way of saving a high-energy bond if one wants to go to phosphoribosylpyrophosphate (PRPP). The presence of ribose diphosphate in the human erythrocyte was reported by Vanderheiden (1961) but he considered it an intermediate in the interconversion of ribose-1- and -5-phosphates. All the other postulated reactions appear feasible, and their enzymes, if reported, will now be discussed.

F. 5′-Adenylic Acid Deaminase

Conway and Cooke (1939b) were able to show that blood and other tissues contained both adenosine deaminase and adenylic acid deaminase, the two enzymes having somewhat different behavior. The distribution of the two in many rabbit tissues was compared. The same authors (1938) suggested that in the red cell the adenylic acid deaminase is reversibly bound to some inhibiting substance. This would be a comforting thought inasmuch as the deamination of AMP seems to be such a one-way reaction, at least in stored blood. The common statement that the ammonia content of stored blood increases (by deamination of AMP) was documented by Beal (1960).

G. Phosphatases

Valentine *et al.* (1961) studied acid phosphatase in the blood of normal subjects and in patients with various hematological disorders. Clarkson and Maizels (1952) studied the distribution of phosphatase in human erythrocytes.

H. 5′-Nucleotidase

To differentiate the activity of this enzyme from that of phosphatase, Campbell (1962) added Ni, which inhibited the nucleotidase.

VII. Utilization of Nucleosides

Many workers have suggested the addition of purine nucleosides to stored blood, adenosine and inosine having been most frequently proposed. Because of the high activity of adenosine deaminase in human blood it might be considered that the metabolism of adenosine has some identity with that of inosine, as can be seen here:

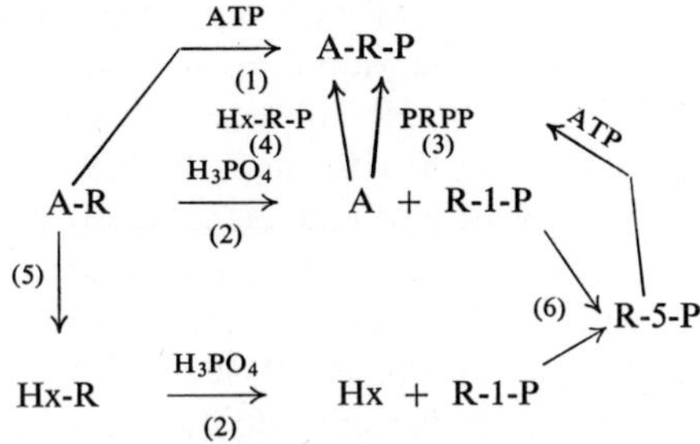

(1) Nucleoside kinase
(2) Purine nucleoside phosphorylase
(3) Nucleotide pyrophosphorylase
(4) Nucleotide transpurinase (?)
(5) Adenosine deaminase
(6) Phosphoribomutase

A. Nucleoside Kinase

Banaschak (1961) noted that when inosine was added to stroma-free hemolysate containing ATP, the rate of disappearance of ATP was markedly enhanced and considerable IMP was formed. The data suggested phosphorylation of inosine to IMP, presumably by a nucleoside kinase.

B. Purine Nucleoside Phosphorylase

On the basis of several kinds of experiment, Gabrio *et al.* (1954a, b, c) concluded that the human red cell, when stored, suffered some insult which they labeled the "storage lesion." This was presumably some intracellular alteration, since different storage media evoked similar behavior and because on return to circulation the stored cells appeared to be rejuvenated. Aging *in vitro* seemed to them to be quite different from aging *in vivo*. Stored cells gradually lost their easily hydrolyzable phosphate (chiefly ATP). Stored blood incubated with liver homogenate or some of its fractions was slightly restored, but adenosine was very effective in bringing back the easily hydrolyzable phosphate levels. Adenine and ribose were essentially ineffective. Adenosine was effective even at low temperatures such as 2°C. The explanation put forward to explain the effect of adenosine was that it entered the red cell and was cleaved by phosphate to purine base and ribose-1-phosphate, the latter participating in the shunt pathway reactions. Prankerd and Altman (1954a) had postulated the existence of nucleoside phosphorylase to explain their results with adenosine on red cell phosphate exchange. Prankerd and Altman (1954b) used adenosine and guanosine to keep up ATP and 2,3-diphosphoglycerate and the ability to incorporate P^{32}. Arsenate abolished the effect, just as arsenate did with glucose. Hence they concluded that the nucleoside, regardless of base, was utilized presumably via phosphorolysis to shunt pathway intermediates which fed into the Embden-Meyerhof pathway. These studies led naturally to the investigation of purine nucleoside phosphorylase activity in the erythrocyte (Huennekens *et al.*, 1956). Hemolysates were quite active and from them could be prepared a fraction with much higher specific activity. The purified enzyme split only inosine and guanosine (relative rates 100 and 60), whereas in earlier work (Gabrio and Huennekens, 1955) inosine, adenosine, guanosine, xanthosine, and 2,6-diaminopurine riboside were split by the crude hemolysates at the relative rates of 100, 65, 60, 40, and 25. Neither system split AMP, ATP, or the pyrimidine nucleosides thymidine, uridine, and cytidine. The authors opined that inosine and guanosine were the true enzyme substrates and that in the crude system other enzymes were present to convert other substrates to these two compounds.

Rubinstein and Denstedt (1956) incubated human blood with adenosine and noted that deamination of adenosine to inosine was the first step. The inosine was then phosphorylyzed to hypoxanthine. Whole hemolysate and stroma-free hemolysate were about equal in enzyme activity, there being little activity in the stroma. The enzyme was most active in the pH range 6.8–7.8. Since no adenine was ever produced from adenosine, the authors tended to agree with Gabrio and Huennekens (1955) that the purine nucleoside phosphorylase was not active on adenosine. Of course, such behavior would be seen if adenosine deaminase were more active than purine nucleoside phosphorylase and deaminated the adenosine before it could be phosphorylyzed. Rubinstein and Denstedt agreed with Gabrio and Huennekens that adenosine, xanthosine, inosine, and guanosine could initiate the esterification of inorganic phosphate in the red cell, and that lactate production would signify utilization of the synthesized ribose phosphate.

Sandberg *et al.* (1955) demonstrated purine nucleoside phosphorylase activity in the erythrocytes of several mammals including man. In human blood the purine nucleoside phosphorylase activity was not increased when the reticulocyte count was high, and this correlation was noted in dogs. Tsuboi and Hudson (1957a, b) describe purification and assay details for purine nucleoside phosphorylase. The enzyme was readily inactivated by trace amounts of heavy metals or by sulfhydryl reagents. Other properties were described. Lowy *et al.* (1958) showed that human erythrocytes took up and utilized purine ribosides and deoxyribosides but not pyrimidine nucleosides, suggesting the absence of pyrimidine nucleoside phosphorylase. Lactic acid was formed as a result of pentose metabolism. Incubation of red cells in saline without added phosphate gave quite different (erroneous) results. One might conclude that, in general, purine ribosides are phosphorylyzed by the red cell but pyrimidine ribosides are not. An exception is found in the enzyme nicotinamide riboside phosphorylase, discussed in Section IX of this chapter. Yamada (1961) demonstrated, in bone marrow, nucleoside phosphorylase activity toward guanosine and deoxyguanosine and also toward uridine and deoxyuridine. Red cells had essentially none of this activity.

C. *Adenosine Deaminase*

Adenosine deamination was demonstrated to take place in human plasma (Rubinstein and Denstedt, 1956), but much more rapidly in whole red cells or hemolysates. Stroma contained little of the deaminase. Adenine was not acted upon and the reaction was optimal around pH 7.0. Drury *et al.* (1938) noted that cat plasma would liberate NH_3 from adenosine. Plasma and red cells from other animals also had varying amounts of this activity. Conway and Cooke (1937) reported adenosine deaminase activity in the blood of man, fowl, frog, and lugworm. Further studies were reported later (1939a, b). Enzyme concentration was found to vary greatly among blood samples and not to correlate with tumor cases (Schaedel and Schlenk, 1948). Ababei and Rapoport (1961) noted that rabbit, human, and chicken erythrocytes have adenosine deaminase. Reticulocytes are richer in it.

D. *Phosphoribomutase*

Guarino and Sable (1955) isolated this enzyme from several sources including human blood. It converted ribose-1-phosphate to ribose-5-phosphate and was distinct from phosphoglucomutase.

VIII. Nucleosides in Blood Preservation

The addition of purine nucleosides to stored blood does restore red cell ATP to a high level. This finding is doubly exciting. On the one hand it offers the possibility of a better system of blood banking. Equally fascinating on the other hand is the question, why do red cells lose viability under blood bank conditions and what missing function is restored by the added nucleoside? Because of the volume of literature, I have elected to discuss the work of a few key groups. I shall try to summarize very succinctly their interests and point out some of their major publications.

Denstedt's group has carried on many studies on blood preservation and red cell enzymology, many of which were published in the *Canadian Journal of Biochemistry and Physiology* in the 1950's and up to the present. For example, the effects of added adenosine or inosine were reported by Rubinstein *et al.* (1956a, 1958, 1959), and Rubinstein and Denstedt (1956).

Prankerd added adenosine and later guanosine to blood and noted various biochemical effects, such as phosphate and cation exchanges and suitability for transfusion (Prankerd and Altman, 1954a; E. J. Harris and Prankerd, 1955; Prankerd, 1956a, b).

The group started by Gabrio and Finch was one of the earliest to begin systematic documentation of nucleoside effects in stored blood (see Gabrio *et al.*, 1955a, b, 1956a, b; Donohue *et al.*, 1956; Hennessey *et al.*, 1957). The joint study by Lange *et al.* (1958) suggested that red cell survival in ACD-inosine may not be as good as had been predicted earlier. A recent turn in the thinking of this group comes from work of Simon *et al.* (1962) in which adenine only, without nucleoside, was used. The implication is that the adenine moiety rather than energy is the missing factor in blood preservation.

M. Nakao's group has studied acid-soluble phosphates in stored human erythrocytes and concludes that inosine is needed for energy, and adenine for the adenine moiety (adenosine not being the equivalent because of its rapid deamination, with loss of the adenine moiety). Papers include those of Nakao *et al.* (1960a, b, d), Wada *et al.* (1960), and Motegi (1961). Nakao *et al.* (1961b) postulate that trace amounts of ATP are crucial for nucleoside efficacy since otherwise the ribose-5-phosphate from a nucleoside could not be converted to phosphoribosylpyrophosphate, which with adenine could form AMP. Recently K. Nakao *et al.* (1962) claim to have shown a direct relationship between ATP level and red cell survival, but the experimental data are too scanty for their sweeping conclusions. Perhaps one of the most exciting observations from this group was that human erythrocytes could be transformed through crenated forms to spherocytes and back to disks by inhibiting glycolysis and then freeing it (Nakao *et al.*, 1960c, 1961a).

Overgaard-Hansen reported ATP formation after the addition of inosine or adenosine (Overgaard-Hansen, 1957; Overgaard-Hansen *et al.*, 1957).

Using the elegant column chromatographic technique which he did so much to validate, Bartlett's group documented the changes in phosphorylated compounds of stored human or rabbit erythrocytes in ACD and ACD + nucleosides and purines (Bartlett and Barnett, 1960; Bartlett and Shafer, 1960, 1961; Shafer and Bartlett, 1960, 1961, 1962).

Whittam, being interested in cation transport in the red cell, has studied nucleosides as a glucose substitute for cellular energetics (1960a, b; Wiley and Whittam, 1961).

Jaffé's interest in nucleosides has related to methemoglobin reduction (Jaffé, 1959) and osmotic resistance (Jaffé *et al.*, 1958; see also Chapter 11).

Fischer (1962), Fischer *et al.* (1961), Wosegien (1962), and Wosegien *et al.* (1962) utilized incubation with P^{32} and high voltage electrophoresis to study nucleotide changes in stored ACD blood. They were impressed with the addition of inosine + adenine + guanosine, and also noted that a steroid such as prednisolone would tend to suppress hemolysis, although not affecting ATP levels.

An unusually comprehensive review by Blum (1960) details the metabolic changes in stored blood and the use of nucleosides to reverse these changes.

IX. NAD, NADP, FAD

A. General

The synthesis of NAD could presumably take place by any of the following sequences from nicotinic acid (NA), nicotinamide (NAm), ribose (R), and phosphate (P), the basic question being where amidation occurs:

```
                         glutamine
                          or NH3
NAm-R-P-P-R-A     <-------------------     NA-R-P-P-R-A
     ^                     (2)                   ^
 (1) |                                           | (3)
     |                                           |
  NAm-R-P         <- - - - - - - - - -        NA-R-P
     ^                   (R-5-P)                 ^
 (4) |   PRPP  <----------(  +  )---------> PRPP | (5)
     |                   ( ATP )                 |
    NAm           <- - - - - - - - - -          NA
                           (6)
```

Hydrolysis of NAD appears to take place at either of two places:

```
       |          |
NAm  -|- R - P -|- P - R - A
       |          |
      (7)        (8)
```

In a consecutive series of papers Preiss and Handler (1957a, b, c; 1958a, b) were able to conclude that the human red cell prefers to synthesize its NAD from nicotinic acid, first making nicotinic acid ribotide (Reaction 5), then nicotinic acid dinucleotide (Reaction 3), and finally amidating (Reaction 2). The enzymatic machinery for synthesizing nicotinamide mononucleotide (NAm-R-P) is present in the red cell, but apparently the ability to convert this to NAD is not so well developed. Nicotinamide will be utilized for NAD synthesis, but only at higher levels than nicotinic acid. In the chicken erythrocyte, however, Dietrich and Friedland (1960) found that nicotinamide and nicotinic acid were equally effective as NAD precursors. Tulpule (1958) found that of seven species of mammal, only human and guinea pig erythrocytes were able to synthesize pyridine nucleotide under his experimental conditions. He suggests that other tissues may be the active sites of NAD synthesis in the other mammals.

Kimura (1960) noted that whereas fresh human erythrocytes synthesized NAD at a good rate, in stored blood the rate of NAD synthesis was depressed, depending on the conditions. It is generally assumed that the main role of NAD in the red cell is as the common cofactor in the glyceraldehyde-3-phosphate dehydrogenase and lactic dehydrogenase reactions, one reaction reducing it and the other using the reduced form as a reducing agent. There is evidence (Strömme and Eldjarn, 1962) that methemoglobin is reduced mainly by NADH rather than NADPH. If this is true then hemoglobin will be kept in the reduced (active) form primarily by Embden-Meyerhof activity rather than by shunt activity (see Chapter 11).

B. NAD Pyrophosphorylase

Following up earlier suggestions that the enzyme for Reactions 1 and 8 was associated only with cell nuclei, Malkin and Denstedt (1956b) were able to demonstrate that hemolysate from chicken (nucleated) erythrocytes or the particulate fraction from them, but not the stroma-free hemolysate, could bring about synthesis of NAD from the two nucleotides. With rabbit reticulocytes an equivocal amount of synthesis took place, which the authors chose to ignore. With human erythrocytes NAD was neither synthesized nor phosphorylyzed.

C. NADase (NAD Nucleosidase)

Malkin and Denstedt (1956c) studied the hydrolysis of NAD at the nicotinamide-ribose bond (NADase or NAD nucleosidase) (Reaction 7). Hemolysis of rabbit blood led to disappearance of NAD, and this metabolic activation was associated with NAD nucleosidase which could be demonstrated in the stroma. This nucleosidase activity could be inhibited by nicotinamide, ADP, or adenine. The enzyme would also act on the nicotinamide mononucleotide but more slowly. Alivisatos and Denstedt (1951) had already shown that NADase (nucleosidase) was to be found in rabbit erythrocyte stroma and could be inhibited by nicotinamide. The enzyme was inactive in the intact red cell because it was on the outside of the membrane. The addition of nicotinamide to hemolysates to protect them against loss of NAD was also suggested by Blanchaer *et al.* (1952) and Alivisatos and Denstedt (1952). Hofmann (1957) and Hofmann and Rapoport (1957) were able to separate and characterize NAD- and NADP-specific nucleosidases from rabbit erythrocytes. Blum and Trepte (1961) suggested that inasmuch as the NAD-splitting ability of blood increased with storage, it might be desirable to add nicotinamide to inhibit this occurrence. Hofmann and Noll (1961) studied NAD- and NADP-specific nucleosidases in red cells of various species and during red cell maturation. A nicotinamide mononucleotide nucleotidase was reported. Nicotinamide riboside phosphorylase (Grossman and Kaplan, 1958a, b) appears to be a distinct enzyme. It is found inside the red cell and will split guanosine or inosine (although these latter reactions are atypical and may be due to contaminating enzymes). Phosphorolysis of nicotinamide riboside by this enzyme was inhibited by free nicotinamide, but this characteristic was lost when the enzyme was fractionated. A dialyzable factor, thought to be ergothionine, was apparently required as a cofactor in the exchange.

D. Flavin Nucleotides

The presence of flavin adenine dinucleotide (FAD) might not be expected in mammalian red cells inasmuch as there is neither tricarboxylic acid cycle nor cytochrome system (mitochondria) to require such a cofactor. Its absence is indicated (Bartlett, 1959a; Bishop *et al.*, 1959; Mills and Sommers, 1959). On the other hand, in both *in vivo* and *in vitro* experiments, riboflavin was said to cause FAD to increase in human red cells (Klein and Kohn, 1940). On the basis of studies on inhibition of glutathione reductase by nitrofurantoin and reactivation by FAD, Buzard and Kopko (1963) suggest the presence of FAD in rat erythrocytes.

X. Ghosts

It is possible to make from intact red cells a preparation which contains what appear microscopically to be intact red cells without their hemoglobin. These ghosts have the ability to utilize nucleosides in essentially the same way as intact red cells. The composition of the preparation would appear to be quite dependent on its method of preparation and may contain some intact erythrocytes. Such preparations have been extensively studied (Lionetti, 1955; Lionetti *et al.*, 1956, 1957, 1961; McLellan and Lionetti, 1959).

XI. Protein and Amino Acid Metabolism

It might be generally assumed that protein synthesis in anucleate red cells stops at the reticulocyte stage but that nucleated red cells continue to enjoy this ability. Most attention to protein synthesis has focused on globin (hemoglobin), this being well covered in Chapter 8.

Amino acids are assumed to penetrate red cells, but there do not seem to be enough studies to decide what sort of transport mechanisms may be involved.

XII. Lipid Metabolism

This is well discussed in Chapter 7. In general, the mature anucleate red cell appears able to exchange lipid moieties with its environment, but not to synthesize them *de novo*.

XIII. Miscellaneous Enzymes

A. Cholinesterase

Pritchard (1949) found that cholinesterase activity in rat erythrocytes was higher in the younger cells (top layer when blood was centrifuged). In stored citrated blood, erythrocyte cholinesterase disappearance seemed to coincide with onset of hemolysis (Anderson and Pethica, 1955). Carta and Vivaldi (1958) claimed that most of the cholinesterase activity of hemolyzed red cells was to be found in the stroma, which could even be lyophilized. In bovine blood, almost all the cholinesterase activity was associated with the red cells (Robbins *et al.*, 1958). Shinagawa and Ogura (1961) used electron microscopy to associate erythrocyte acetylcholinesterase with the outer layer of the cells. Another confirmation of this was by Vincent *et al.* (1961), who showed that intact erythrocytes or the corresponding hemolysates were equally active. Bertolini *et al.* (1961c) claimed that the enzyme activity declined as the cell aged. Rubin (1958) found this enzyme elevated in mental patients but Ellman and Callaway (1961) could not confirm this. Metz *et al.* (1961) inhibited red cell acetylcholinesterase with octamethylphosphoramide and noted no red cell lifespan shortening (Cr^{51} technique). They concluded that the enzyme was not essential for normal red cell lifespan. They also found that inhibition of the enzyme produced none of the features of paroxysmal nocturnal hemoglobinuria. Burman (1961) determined the enzyme in infancy and childhood, later modifying the method (1962). Greig and Holland (1949, 1950a, b, 1951) studied relationships between ionic gradients and cholinesterase, and later (Greig and Gibbons, 1955) concluded that drugs such as chlorpromazine, which prevented the removal of cholinesterase from the red cell, would prevent deterioration of the red cell in storage due to permeability changes.

B. Catalase

Catalase was said to decrease on storage of blood (Alzona and Viale, 1946), or not to decrease (Borodin and Borodina, 1959). Keilin and Wang (1947) studied two samples of horse blood that had been stored at room temperature in the dark for 24 and 42 years. The blood retained 85% of the enzymatic activity of carbonic anhydrase, catalase, glyoxalase, and cholinesterase. X-irradiation of rabbits, but not of blood hemolysates, caused a decrease in red cell catalase (Jonderko and Kosmider, 1960). Age of person had no influence on enzyme activity (DiToro *et al.*, 1961). Agents affecting liver catalase were without effect on red cell catalase (Agradi, 1961). Higashi *et al.* (1961) compared immunochemical and enzymatic assays of catalase. Methemoglobin formation *in vitro* in x-rayed blood was inversely related to catalase content (Aebi *et al.*, 1962).

C. Transaminase

Germanyuk (1961) found this enzyme in both plasma and red cell cytoplasm in cows and horses. The stroma of young human cells had higher glutamic-pyruvic transaminase activity than stroma of old cells. Glutamic-oxaloacetic transaminase activity was lower in only the older cells of older people (Bertolini *et al.*, 1961a). Increases in glutamic-oxaloacetic transaminase activity were associated with increased production of new cells as in hematological or hemorrhagic anemias (Sass and Spear, 1961a, b).

D. Aconitase

This enzyme was studied in human blood by Beutler and Yesh (1959).

E. Carbonic Anhydrase

Irradiation of the rabbit but not of hemolysates caused a decrease (Marek and Kosmider, 1960). Its activity went down about 10-fold on storage (Guminski, 1960). The kinetics of both bovine and human erythrocyte carbonic anhydrase were carefully studied by DeVoe and Kistiakowsky (1961). Photooxidative removal of histidine inactivated the enzyme (Lieflaender, 1961). Other structural features were later elucidated (Leiflaender and Stegemann, 1961). Nyman (1961) separated two forms of the enzyme from human erythrocytes. Leiner *et al.* (1962) studied the enzyme in several classes of vertebrate, showing inactivation on removal of the zinc but reactivation when small amounts of various metals were added back. Shaw *et al.* (1962) found an atypical esterase which they considered a variant of carbonic anhydrase.

F. Glyoxalase

This enzyme catalyzes reactions of the type: $CH_3COCHO \rightarrow CH_3CHOH$-$COOH$, but the importance of such reactions in red cells is obscure. Glyoxalase activity in the red cells was studied by Jowett and Quastel (1933) and Keilin and Wang (1947). The values in leucocytes, reticulocytes, and young cells may be elevated over that in mature erythrocytes (Valentine and Tanaka, 1961).

G. Others

Esterases of mouse blood were studied by Hunter and Strachan (1961). Hydrolases (phosphorylases, lipases, amylases) were determined by Cacciari *et al.* (1959). Erythrocyte arginase was purified and its kinetics studied (Cabello *et al.*, 1961). Its activity was comparable in adults and infants (Martucci *et al.*, 1961). Heparin inhibited its activity (Floch and Groisser, 1962). Human erythrocytes possess both glycyl-L-leucine dipeptidase (Haschen, 1961a) and leucine aminopeptidase (Haschen, 1961b).

XIV. General

London (1961) has given a good review of erythrocyte metabolism. Books specifically on the erythrocyte include those by Behrendt (1957), Prankerd (1961), and Harris (1963). Values for all the glycolytic enzymes for both anucleate and nucleate red cells have been recalculated from many sources and tabulated by Schweiger (1962). Löhr and Waller (1959) have studied primarily glycolytic enzymes and their alterations with aging *in vitro* and *in vivo*. Blum (1962) has tabulated the enzymes found in all human blood cells, citing nearly 400 references. Cartier and Leroux (1962) reviewed erythrocyte enzymes. Contu and Lenzerini (1960) reviewed (in Italian) physiological and pathological alterations in erythrocyte metabolism.

Much has been written about alteration of red cells in various diseases (either primarily hematological or nonhematological) and the effect of hormones, drugs, etc. on red cells either *in vivo* or *in vitro*. No conscious effort was made to include such papers in this review inasmuch as they often contribute little to our understanding of red cell metabolism. Furthermore this literature is extremely voluminous and just to list it uncritically would require considerable space.

In conclusion, the author of this chapter wishes to apologize to those many workers whose papers he has slighted, or omitted altogether. There is much literature and the reviewer must choose from the work he knows. This means he will omit important papers because he is unaware of them. Furthermore, there was a framework in this chapter, into which some good work did not easily fit. Perhaps the reader will be appreciative of the inclusions and charitable towards the omissions.

Acknowledgments

The author gratefully acknowledges support from the National Institutes of Health (Grants A-210, A-5581, and AM 06367-01 HEMA) and the Western New York Section of the Arthritis and Rheumatism Foundation during the writing of this chapter.

References

Ababei, L., and Rapoport, S. (1961). *Acta Biol. Med. Ger.* **6**, 288.
Ackerman, G. A., and Bellios, N. C. (1955a). *Blood* **10**, 3.
Ackerman, G. A., and Bellios, N. C. (1955b). *Blood* **10**, 1183.
Aebi, H., Heiniger, J. P., and Suter, H. (1962). *Experientia* **18**, 129.
Agradi, A. (1961). *Experientia* **17**, 77.
Alivisatos, S., and Denstedt, O. F. (1951). *Science* **114**, 281.
Alivisatos, S., and Denstedt, O. F. (1952). *J. Biol. Chem.* **199**, 493.
Allfrey, V. G., and Mirsky, A. E. (1952). *J. Gen. Physiol.* **35**, 841.
Alzona, L., and Viale, L. (1946). *Ric. stud. med. sper.* **16**, 129.
Anderson, P. J., and Pethica, B. A. (1955). *Biochem. Biophys. Acta* **17**, 138.
Banaschak, H. (1961). *Acta Biol. Med. Ger.* **7**, 216.
Barron, E. S. G., and Harrop, G. A., Jr. (1928). *J. Biol. Chem.* **79**, 65.
Bartlett, G. R. (1959a). *J. Biol. Chem.* **234**, 449.
Bartlett, G. R. (1959b). *J. Biol. Chem.* **234**, 469.
Bartlett, G. R., and Barnett, H. N. (1960). *J. Clin. Invest.* **39**, 56.
Bartlett, G. R., and Marlow, A. A. (1953a). *J. Lab. Clin. Med.* **42**, 178.
Bartlett, G. R., and Marlow, A. A. (1953b). *J. Lab. Clin. Med.* **42**, 188.
Bartlett, G. R., and Shafer, A. W. (1960). *J. Clin. Invest.* **39**, 62.
Bartlett, G. R., and Shafer, A. W. (1961). *J. Clin. Invest.* **40**, 1185.
Beal, R. W. (1960). *Med. J. Australia* **47**, 691.
Behrendt, H. (1957). "Chemistry of Erythrocytes." Thomas, Springfield, Illinois.
Bertino, J. R., Simmons, B., and Donohue, D. M. (1962). *J. Biol. Chem.* **237**, 1314.
Bertles, J. F., and Beck, W. S. (1962). *J. Biol. Chem.* **237**, 3770.
Bertolini, A. M., Massari, N., and Civardi, F. (1961a). *Gior. Gerontol.* **9**, 537.
Bertolini, A. M., Massari, N., and Civardi, F. (1961b). *Gior. Gerontol.* **9**, 547.
Bertolini, A. M., Massari, N., and Guardamagna, C. (1961c). *Gior. Gerontol.* **9**, 543.
Bertolini, A. M., Massari, N., Civardi, F., and Tenconi, L. (1961d). *Gior. Gerontol.* **9**, 551.
Beutler, E., and Yesh, M. K. Y. (1959). *J. Lab. Clin. Med.* **54**, 456.
Bianco, L., Giustina, G., and Lazzarini, E. (1962). *Nature* **194**, 289.
Birkbeck, J. A., and Stewart, A. G. (1961). *Can. J. Biochem. Physiol.* **39**, 257.
Bishop, C. (1960). *J. Biol. Chem.* **235**, 3228.
Bishop, C. (1961a). *J. Biol. Chem.* **236**, 1778.

Bishop, C. (1961b). *Proc. Soc. Exptl. Biol. Med.* **108**, 192.
Bishop, C. (1961c). *Transfusion* **1**, 349.
Bishop, C. (1961d). *Transfusion* **1**, 355.
Bishop, C. (1962a). *Am. J. Orthoped.* **4**, 136.
Bishop, C. (1962b). *Transfusion* **2**, 256.
Bishop, C. (1962c). *Transfusion* **2**, 408.
Bishop, C., Rankine, D. M., and Talbott, J. H. (1959). *J. Biol. Chem.* **234**, 1233.
Bishop, C., Rankine, D. M., Klein, M. B., and Talbott, J. H. (1960). *Proc. Soc. Exptl. Biol. Med.* **104**, 754.
Blanchaer, M. C., and Weiss, P. (1954). *J. Appl. Physiol.* **7**, 168.
Blanchaer, M. C., Marlatt, B., Baldwin, S., and Weiss, P. (1952). *Rev. Can. Biol.* **11**, 55.
Blanchaer, M. C., Williams, H. R., and Weiss, P. (1955a). *Am. J. Physiol.* **181**, 602.
Blanchaer, M. C., Brownstone, S., and Williams, H. R. (1955b). *Am. J. Physiol.* **183**, 95.
Block, R. J., Durrum, E. L., and Zweig, G. (1958). "A Manual of Paper Chromatography and Paper Electrophoresis." Academic Press, New York.
Blostein, R., and Denstedt, O. F. (1962). *Can. J. Biochem. Physiol.* **40**, 1005.
Blum, K. U. (1960). *Bibliotheca Haematol.* **12**, 20.
Blum, K. U. (1962). *Blut* **8**, 239.
Blum, K. U., and Trepte, G. (1961). *Klin. Wochschr.* **39**, 268.
Borodin, A. E., and Borodina, G. P. (1959). *Trudy Blagoveshch. Med. Inst.* **4**, 39.
Boszormenyi-Nagy, I. (1955). *J. Biol. Chem.* **212**, 495.
Brin, M., and Yonemoto, R. H. (1958). *J. Biol. Chem.* **230**, 307.
Brownstone, Y. S., and Blanchaer, M. C. (1957). *Am. J. Physiol.* **189**, 105.
Bucolo, G., and Bartlett, G. R. (1960). *Biochem. Biophys. Res. Commun.* **3**, 620.
Bunch, L. D., Snyder, H., and Miller, F. R. (1958). *J. Lab. Clin. Med.* **52**, 700.
Burman, D. (1961). *Arch. Disease Childhood* **36**, 362.
Burman, D. (1962). *Am. J. Clin. Pathol.* **37**, 134.
Buzard, J. A., and Kopko, F. (1963). *J. Biol. Chem.* **238**, 464.
Cabello, J., Basilio, C., and Prajoux, V. (1961). *Biochim. Biophys. Acta* **48**, 148.
Cacciari, E., Corsini, F., Manfredi, G., and Pintozzi, P. (1959). *Boll. Soc. Ital. Biol. Sper.* **35**, 395.
Caffrey, R. W., Tremblay, R., Gabrio, B. W., and Huennekens, F. M. (1956). *J. Biol. Chem.* **223**, 1.
Campbell, Diana M. (1962). *Biochem. J.* **82**, 34P.
Carta, S., and Vivaldi, G. (1958). *Boll. Soc. Ital. Biol. Sper.* **34**, 1739.
Cartier, P., and Leroux, J. P. (1962). *Ann. Biol. Clin.* (*Paris*) **20**, 273.
Carver, M. J., and Roesky, N. (1959). *Experientia* **15**, 138.
Cerletti, P., and Bucci, E. (1960). *Biochim. Biophys. Acta* **38**, 45.
Cerletti, P., and DeRitas, G. (1960). *Atti. Accad. Naz. Lincei, Rend. Classe Sci. Fis. Mat. Nat.* **29**, 81.
Chalfin, D. (1956). *J. Cellular Comp. Physiol.* **47**, 215.
Chargaff, E., and Davidson, J. N., eds. (1955). "The Nucleic Acids," Vols. I and II. Academic Press, New York.
Chen, P. S., Jr., and Jørgensen, S. (1956). *Acta Pharmacol. Toxicol.* **12**, 369.
Christensen, H. N., and Jones, J. C. (1962). *Biochim. Biophys. Acta* **59**, 355.
Christensen, W. R., Plimpton, C. H., and Ball, E. G. (1949). *J. Biol. Chem.* **180**, 791.
Clarkson, E. M., and Maizels, M. (1952). *J. Physiol.* (*London*) **116**, 112.
Contu, L., and Lenzerini, L. (1960). *Recenti Progr. Med.* **24**, 325.
Conway, E. J., and Cooke, R. (1937). *Nature* **139**, 627.
Conway, E. J., and Cooke, R. (1938). *Nature* **147**, 720.

Conway, E. J., and Cooke, R. (1939a). *Biochem. J.* **33**, 457.
Conway, E. J., and Cooke, R. (1939b). *Biochem. J.* **39**, 479.
Corsini, F., Cacciari, E., Manfredi, G., and Pintozzi, P. (1959). *Boll. Soc. Ital. Biol. Sper.* **35**, 393.
Dajani, R. M., and Orten, J. M. (1958). *J. Biol. Chem.* **231**, 913.
Dajani, R. M., and Orten, J. M. (1959). *J. Biol. Chem.* **234**, 877.
Davis, A. R., Newton, E. B., and Benedict, S. (1922). *J. Biol. Chem.* **54**, 595.
DeLoecker, W. C. J., and Prankerd, T. A. J. (1961). *Clin. Chim. Acta* **6**, 641.
DeSandre, G., Ghiotto, G., and Cortesi, S. (1959). *Arch. Sci. Med.* **108**, 778.
DeVoe, H., and Kistiakowsky, G. B. (1961). *J. Am. Chem. Soc.* **83**, 274.
Dietrich, L. S., and Friedland, I. M. (1960). *Arch. Biochem. Biophys.* **88**, 313.
DiToro, R., Miraglia, M., and Rigillo, N. (1961). *Pediatria* (*Naples*) **69**, 1048.
Donohue, D. M., Finch, C. A., and Gabrio, B. W. (1956). *J. Clin. Invest.* **35**, 562.
Drury, A. N., Lutwak-Mann, C., and Solandt, O. M. (1938). *Quart. J. Exptl. Physiol.* **27**, 215.
Eggleton, G. P., and Eggleton, P. (1929). *Brit. J. Physiol.* **68**, 193.
Eldjarn, L., and Bremer, J. (1962). *Biochem. J.* **84**, 286.
Ellman, G. L., and Callaway, E. (1961). *Nature* **192**, 1216.
Engelhardt, V. A., and Lyubimova, M. N. (1936). *Doklady Acad. Sci. U.S.S.R.* **2**, 329.
Fischer, H. (1962). *Folia. Haematol.* **78**, 356.
Fischer, H., Ferber, E., Fritzsche, W., Wosegien, F., and Spielmann, H. (1961). *Bibliotheca. Haematol.* **12**, 76.
Fleckenstein, A., and Gerlach, E. (1953). *Arch. Exptl. Pathol. Pharmakol.* **219**, 531.
Floch, M. H., and Groisser, V. W. (1962). *J. Pharmacol. Exptl. Therap.* **135**, 256.
Gabrio, B. W., and Huennekens, F. M. (1955). *Biochim. Biophys. Acta* **18**, 585.
Gabrio, B. W., Finch, C. A., Linde, W., and Rupen, A. (1954a). *J. Clin. Invest.* **33**, 242.
Gabrio, B. W., Stevens, A. R., Jr., and Finch, C. A. (1954b). *J. Clin. Invest.* **33**, 247.
Gabrio, B. W., Stevens, A. R., Jr., and Finch, C. A. (1954c). *J. Clin. Invest.* **33**, 252.
Gabrio, B. W., Hennessey, M., Thomasson, J., and Finch, C. A. (1955a). *J. Biol. Chem.* **215**, 357.
Gabrio, B. W., Donohue, D. M., and Finch, C. A. (1955b). *J. Clin. Invest.* **34**, 1509.
Gabrio, B. W., Finch, C. A., and Huennekens, F. M. (1956a). *Blood* **11**, 103.
Gabrio, B. W., Donohue, D. M., Huennekens, F. M., and Finch, C. A. (1956b). *J. Clin. Invest.* **35**, 657.
Gall, J. (1963). *Science* **139**, 120.
Gerlach, E., and Fikentscher, H. (1959). *Naturwissenschaften* **4**, 326.
Gerlach, E., and Lübben, K. (1959). *Arch. Ges. Physiol.* **269**, 520.
Gerlach, E., Fleckenstein, A., and Gross, E. (1958). *Arch. Ges. Physiol.* **266**, 528.
Germanyuk, Y. L. (1961). *Ukr. Biokhim. Zh.* **33**, 374.
Ghiotto, G., DeSandre, G., and Cortesi, S. (1959). *Arch. Sci. Med.* **108**, 789.
Gourley, D. R. (1952). *Arch. Biochem. Biophys.* **40**, 1.
Gourley, D. R. (1957). *Am. J. Physiol.* **190**, 536.
Greenwald, I. (1925). *J. Biol. Chem.* **63**, 339.
Greig, M. E., and Gibbons, A. J. (1955). *Am. J. Physiol.* **181**, 313.
Greig, M. E., and Holland, W. C. (1949). *Arch. Biochem. Biophys.* **23**, 370.
Greig, M. E., and Holland, W. C. (1950a). *Am. J. Physiol.* **162**, 610.
Greig, M. E., and Holland, W. C. (1950b). *Arch. Biochem. Biophys.* **26**, 151.
Greig, M. E., and Holland, W. C. (1951). *Am. J. Physiol.* **164**, 423.
Grignani, F., and Löhr, G. W. (1960). *Klin. Wochschr.* **38**, 796.
Grossman, L., and Kaplan, N. O. (1958a). *J. Biol. Chem.* **231**, 717.

Grossman, L., and Kaplan, N. O. (1958b). *J. Biol. Chem.* **231**, 727.
Guarino, A. J., and Sable, H. Z. (1955). *J. Biol. Chem.* **215**, 515.
Guest, G. M., and Rapoport, S. (1941). *Physiol. Rev.* **21**, 410.
Guest, G. M., Mackler, B., Graubarth, H., and Ammentorp, P. A. (1953). *Am. J. Physiol.* **172**, 295.
Guminski, T. (1960). *Polskie Arch. Med. Wewnetrznej.* **30**, 196.
Harris, E. J., and Prankerd, T. A. J. (1955). *Biochem. J.* **61**, 19.
Harris, J. W. (1963). "The Red Cell," Commonwealth Fund. Harvard Univ. Press, Cambridge, Massachusetts.
Harrop, G. A., Jr. (1919). *Arch. Internal Med.* **23**, 745.
Harrop, G. A., Jr., and Barron, E. S. G. (1928). *J. Exptl. Med.* **48**, 207.
Haschen, R. J. (1961a). *Biochem. Z.* **334**, 560.
Haschen, R. J. (1961b). *Biochem. Z.* **334**, 569.
Hashimoto, T. (1961). *J. Biochem.* (*Tokyo*) **50**, 337.
Hashimoto, T., and Yoshikawa, H. (1961). *Biochem. Biophys. Res. Commun.* **5**, 71.
Hashimoto, T., Ishii, Y., Tachibana, M., and Yoshikawa, H. (1961). *J. Biochem.* (*Tokyo*) **50**, 471.
Henderson, F. J., and LePage, G. A. (1959). *J. Biol. Chem.* **234**, 3219.
Hennessey, M., Finch, C. A., and Gabrio, B. W. (1957). *J. Clin. Invest.* **36**, 429.
Herbert, E. (1956). *J. Cellular Comp. Physiol.* **47**, 11.
Higashi, T., Yagi, M., and Hirai, H. (1961). *J. Biochem.* (*Tokyo*) **49**, 707.
Hills, B. R., and Meacham, E. J. (1961). *Ann. N.Y. Acad. Sci.* **94**, 868.
Hinterberger, U., Ockel, E., Gerischer-Mothes, W., and Rapoport, S. (1961a). *Acta Biol. Med. Ger.* **7**, 50.
Hinterberger, U., Gerischer-Mothes, W., Suckrow, D., and Rapoport, S. (1961b). *Acta Biol. Med. Ger.* **7**, 57.
Hofmann, E. C. G. (1957). *Biochem. Z.* **329**, 428.
Hofmann, E. C. G., and Noll, F. (1961). *Acta Biol. Med. Ger.* **6**, 1.
Hofmann, E. C. G., and Rapoport, S. (1957). *Biochem. Z.* **329**, 437.
Huennekens, F. M., Nurk, E., and Gabrio, B. W. (1956). *J. Biol. Chem.* **221**, 971.
Huennekens, F. M., Liu, L., Myers, H. A. P., and Gabrio, B. W. (1957). *J. Biol. Chem.* **227**, 253.
Huggett, A. St. G., and Nixon, D. A. (1961). *Nature* **190**, 1209.
Hunter, R. L., and Strachan, D. S. (1961). *Ann. N. Y. Acad. Sci.* **94**, 861.
Inouye, T., Tannebau, M., and Hsia, D. (1962). *Nature* **193**, 67.
Jaffé, E. R. (1959). *J. Clin. Invest.* **38**, 1555.
Jaffé, E. R., Vanderhoff, G. A., Lowy, B. A., and London, I. M. (1958). *J. Clin. Invest.* **37**, 1293.
Jonderko, G., and Kosmider, S. (1960). *Arch. Immunol. Terapii Doswiadczalnej* **8**, 519.
Jones, E. S., Maegraith, B. G., and Gibson, O. H. (1953). *Ann. Trop. Med. Parasitol.* **47**, 431.
Jørgensen, S. (1955). *Acta Pharm. Toxicol.* **11**, 265.
Jørgensen, S. (1956a). *Acta Chem. Scand.* **10**, 1043.
Jørgensen, S. (1956b). *Acta Pharm. Toxicol.* **12**, 294.
Jørgensen, S. (1957). *Acta Pharm. Toxicol.* **13**, 102.
Jørgensen, S., and Chen, P. S., Jr. (1956). *Scand. J. Clin. Lab. Invest.* **8**, 145.
Jørgensen, S., and Chen, P. S., Jr. (1957). *Acta Pharm. Toxicol.* **13**, 12.
Jørgensen, S., and Grove-Rasmussen, M. (1957). *Am. J. Clin. Pathol.* **28**, 579.
Jørgensen, S., and Overgaard-Hansen, K. (1960). *Scand. J. Clin. Lab. Invest.* **12**, 10.
Jørgensen, S., and Poulson, H. E. (1955). *Acta Pharm. Toxicol.* **11**, 287.

Jowett, M., and Quastel, J. (1933). *Biochem. J.* **27**, 486.

Kashket, S., and Denstedt, O. F. (1958). *Can. J. Biochem. Physiol.* **36**, 1057.

Kashket, S., Rubinstein, D., Denstedt, O. F., and Gosselin, S. M. (1957). *Can. J. Biochem. Physiol.* **35**, 827.

Keilin, D., and Wang, Y. L. (1947). *Biochem. J.* **41**, 491.

Key, J. A. (1921). *Arch. Internal Med.* **28**, 511.

Kildema, L. (1960). *Izv. Akad. Nauk. Est. SSR: Ser. Biol.* **9**, 232.

Kimura, K. (1960). *Nagoya J. Med. Sci.* **23**, 119.

Klein, J. R., and Kohn, H. (1940). *J. Biol. Chem.* **136**, 177.

Konsek, J., and Bishop, C. (1962). *Proc. Soc. Exptl. Biol. Med.* **110**, 813.

Kutas, F., and Stützel, M. (1958a). *Acta Vet. Acad. Sci. Hung.* **8**, 1.

Kutas, F., and Stützel, M. (1958b). *Acta Vet. Acad. Sci. Hung.* **8**, 401.

Lachhein, L., and Matthies, H. (1960). *Acta Biol. Med. Ger.* **4**, 403.

Lachhein, L., Grube, E., Johnigk, C., and Matthies, H. (1961). *Klin. Wochschr.* **39**, 875.

Lachman, L., Grade, K., and Matthies, H. (1961). *Acta Biol. Med. Ger.* **7**, 434.

Lacko, L., and Burger, M. (1962). *Biochem. J.* **83**, 622.

Lacko, L., Burger, M., Hejmova, L., and Rejnkova, J. (1961). *Symp. Membrane Transport Metab. Proc.* (*Prague, 1960*) p. 399.

Lajtha, L. G., and Vane, J. R. (1958). *Nature* **182**, 191.

Lange, R. D., Crosby, W. H., Donohue, D. M., Finch, C. A., Gibson, J. G., II, McManus, T. J., and Strumia, M. M. (1958). *J. Clin. Invest.* **37**, 1485.

Laris, P. C., Ewers, A., and Novinger, G. (1962). *J. Cellular Comp. Physiol.* **59**, 145.

LeFevre, P. G. (1961). *Pharm. Rev.* **13**, 39.

Leiner, M., Beck, H., and Eckert, H. (1962). *Z. Physiol. Chem.* **327**, 144.

Lieflaender, M. (1961). *Naturwissenschaften* **48**, 574.

Lieflaender, M., and Stegemann, H. (1961). *Z. Physiol. Chem.* **325**, 204.

Lionetti, F. (1955). *Biochem. Biophys. Acta* **18**, 443.

Lionetti, F., Rees, S., Healey, W., Walker, B. S., and Gibson, J. G., II, (1956). *J. Biol. Chem.* **220**, 467.

Lionetti, F. J., McLellan, W. J., Jr., and Walker, B. S. (1957). *J. Biol. Chem.* **229**, 817.

Lionetti, F. J., McLellan, W. L., Fortier, N. L., and Foster, J. M. (1961). *Arch. Biochem. Biophys.* **94**, 7.

Löhr, G. W., and Waller, H. D. (1959). *Klin. Wochschr.* **37**, 833.

Löhr, G. W., Waller, H. D., Karges, O., Schlegel, B., and Müller, A. A. (1958). *Klin. Wochschr.* **36**, 1008.

London, I. M. (1961). *Harvey Lectures, Ser.* **56**, 151.

Lowy, B. A., and Williams, M. K. (1960). *J. Biol. Chem.* **235**, 2924.

Lowy, B. A., Jaffé, E. R., Vanderhoff, G. A., Crook, L., and London, I. M. (1958). *J. Biol. Chem.* **230**, 409.

Lowy, B. A., Ramot, B., and London, I. M. (1960). *J. Biol. Chem.* **235**, 2920.

Lowy, B. A., Williams, M. K., and London, I. M. (1961a). *J. Biol. Chem.* **236**, 1439.

Lowy, B. A., Cook, J. L., and London, I. M. (1961b). *J. Biol. Chem.* **236**, 1442.

Lowy, B. A., Williams, M. K., and London, I. M. (1962). *J. Biol. Chem.* **237**, 1622.

McLellan, W. L., and Lionetti, F. J. (1959). *J. Biol. Chem.* **234**, 3243.

Malkin, A., and Denstedt, O. F. (1956a). *Can. J. Biochem. Physiol.* **34**, 121.

Malkin, A., and Denstedt, O. F. (1956b). *Can. J. Biochem. Physiol.* **34**, 130.

Malkin, A., and Denstedt, O. F. (1956c). *Can. J. Biochem. Physiol.* **34**, 141.

Mányai, S., and Varady, Z. (1956). *Biochim. Biophys. Acta* **20**, 594.

Marek, K., and Kosmider, S. (1960). *Arch. Immunol. Terapii Doswiadczalnej.* **8**, 513.

Marks, P. A., and Johnson, A. B. (1958). *J. Clin. Invest.* **37**, 1542.

Marks, P. A., Johnson, A. B., and Hirschberg, E. (1958). *Proc. Natl. Acad. Sci. U.S.* **44**, 529.
Martucci, E., Miraglia, M., and Rolando, P. (1961). *Pediatria* (*Naples*) **69**, 948.
Metz, J., Stevens, K., van Rensburg, N. J., and Hart, D. (1961). *Brit. J. Haematol.* **7**, 458.
Michaelis, L., and Salomon, K. (1930). *J. Gen. Physiol.* **13**, 683.
Mills, G. C. (1960). *Texas Rept. Biol. Med.* **18**, 43.
Mills, G. C., and Jones, R. S. (1961). *Arch. Biochem. Biophys.* **95**, 363.
Mills, G. C., and Sommers, L. B. (1959). *Arch. Biochem. Biophys.* **84**, 7.
Mirčevová, L. (1962a). *Folia Haematol.* **78**, 195.
Mirčevová, L. (1962b). *Folia Haematol.* **78**, 463.
Mirčevová, L. (1962c). *Physiol. Bohemoslov.* **11**, 30.
Mirčevová, L., and Vosykova, J. (1961). *Collection Czech. Chem. Commun.* **26**, 1469.
Miwa, S., Tanaka, K. R., and Valentine, W. N. (1962). *Nature* **195**, 613.
Moruzzi, G. (1936). *Arch. Sci. Biol.* (*Bologna*) **22**, 1.
Motegi, T. (1961). *Seikagaku* **33**, 724.
Murphy, J. R. (1960). *J. Lab. Clin. Med.* **55**, 286.
Murphy, J. R. (1962). *J. Lab. Clin. Med.* **60**, 86.
Nakao, K., Wada, T., Kamiyama, T., Nakao, M., and Nagano, K. (1962). *Nature* **194**, 877.
Nakao, M., Nakao, T., Tatibana, M., and Yoshikawa, H. (1960a). *J. Biochem.* (*Tokyo*) **47**, 661.
Nakao, M., Tachibana, M., and Yoshikawa, H. (1960b). *J. Biochem.* (*Tokyo*) **48**, 672.
Nakao, M., Nakao, T., and Yamazoe, S. (1960c). *Nature* **187**, 945.
Nakao, M., Nakao, T., Arimatsu, Y., and Yoshikawa, H. (1960d). *Proc. Japan Acad.* **36**, 43.
Nakao, M., Nakao, T., Yamazoe, S., and Yoshikawa, H. (1961a). *J. Biochem.* (*Tokyo*) **49**, 487.
Nakao, M., Motegi, T., Nakao, T., Yamazoe, S., and Yoshikawa, H. (1961b). *Nature* **191**, 283.
Newton, E. B., and Davis, A. R. (1922a). *J. Biol. Chem.* **54**, 601.
Newton, E. B., and Davis, A. R. (1922b). *J. Biol. Chem.* **54**, 603.
Nyman, P. O. (1961). *Biochim. Biophys. Acta* **52**, 1.
Olmstead, E. G. (1962). *Proc. Soc. Exptl. Biol. Med.* **109**, 196.
Ottolenghi, P., and Denstedt, O. F. (1958a). *Can. J. Biochem. Physiol.* **36**, 1085.
Ottolenghi, P., and Denstedt, O. F. (1958b). *Can. J. Biochem. Physiol.* **36**, 1093.
Overgaard-Hansen, K. (1957). *Acta. Pharm. Toxicol.* **14**, 67.
Overgaard-Hansen, K., and Jørgensen, S. (1960). *Scand. J. Clin. Lab. Invest.* **12**, 10.
Overgaard-Hansen, K., Jørgensen, S., and Praetorius, E. (1957). *Nature* **179**, 152.
Pappius, H. M., Andreae, S. R., Woodford, V. R., and Denstedt, O. F. (1954). *Can. J. Biochem. Physiol.* **32**, 338.
Parpart, A. K., Lorenz, P. B., Parpart, E. R., Gregg, J. R., and Chase, A. M. (1947). *J. Clin. Invest.* **26**, 636.
Parvé, E. P. S. (1953). *Biochim. Biophys. Acta* **10**, 121.
Post, R. L., Merritt, C. R., Kinsolving, C. R., and Albright, C. D. (1960). *J. Biol. Chem.* **235**, 1796.
Prankerd, T. A. J. (1956a). *Biochem. J.* **64**, 209.
Prankerd, T. A. J. (1956b). *Lancet* **1**, 469.
Prankerd, T. A. J. (1958). *J. Physiol.* (*London*) **143**, 325.
Prankerd, T. A. J. (1961). "The Red Cell." Thomas, Springfield, Illinois.
Prankerd, T. A. J., and Altman, K. I. (1954a). *Biochim. Biophys. Acta* **15**, 158.
Prankerd, T. A. J., and Altman, K. I. (1954b). *Biochem. J.* **58**, 622.

Preiss, J., and Handler, P. (1957a). *J. Am. Chem. Soc.* **79**, 1514.
Preiss, J., and Handler, P. (1957b). *J. Am. Chem. Soc.* **79**, 4246.
Preiss, J., and Handler, P. (1957c). *J. Biol. Chem.* **225**, 759.
Preiss, J., and Handler, P. (1958a). *J. Biol. Chem.* **233**, 488.
Preiss, J., and Handler, P. (1958b). *J. Biol. Chem.* **233**, 493.
Pritchard, J. A. (1949). *Am. J. Physiol.* **158**, 72.
Priwitl, J., and Schmitt, H. (1957). *Klin. Wochschr.* **35**, 661.
Ramsey, R., and Warren, C. O., Jr. (1933). *Quart. J. Exptl. Physiol.* **22**, 49.
Rapoport, S. (1940). *J. Biol. Chem.* **135**, 403.
Rapoport, S., and Guest, G. M. (1941). *J. Biol. Chem.* **138**, 269.
Rapoport, S., and Hofmann, E. C. G. (1955). *Biochem. Z.* **326**, 493.
Rapoport, S., and Luebering, J. (1950). *J. Biol. Chem.* **183**, 507.
Rapoport, S., and Luebering, J. (1952). *J. Biol. Chem.* **196**, 583.
Rapoport, S., Hinterberger, U., and Hofmann, E. C. G. (1961). *Naturwissenschaften* **48**, 501.
Robbins, W. E., Hopkins, T. L., and Roth, A. R. (1958). *J. Econ. Entomol.* **51**, 326.
Rohdewald, M., and Weber, M. (1956). *Z. Physiol. Chem.* **306**, 90.
Rohdewald, M., and Weber, M. (1958). *Z. Physiol. Chem.* **311**, 239.
Rohdewald, M., and Weber, M. (1959). *Z. Physiol. Chem.* **317**, 217.
Ross, J. D. (1963). *Blood* **21**, 51.
Rottino, A., Hoffman, G. T., and Albaum, H. (1952). *Blood* **7**, 836.
Rubin, L. (1958). *Science* **128**, 254.
Rubinstein, D., and Denstedt, O. F. (1953). *J. Biol. Chem.* **204**, 623.
Rubinstein, D., and Denstedt, O. F. (1956). *Can. J. Biochem. Physiol.* **34**, 927.
Rubinstein, D., Kashket, S., Denstedt, O. F., and Gosselin, S. M. (1956a). *Can. J. Biochem. Physiol.* **34**, 61.
Rubinstein, D., Ottolenghi, P., and Denstedt, O. F. (1956b). *Can. J. Biochem. Physiol.* **34**, 222.
Rubinstein, D., Kashket, S., and Denstedt, O. F. (1958). *Can. J. Biochem. Physiol.* **36**, 1269.
Rubinstein, D., Kashket, S., Blostein, R., and Denstedt, O. F. (1959). *Can. J. Biochem. Physiol.* **37**, 69.
Rudzinska, M. A., and Trager, W. (1959). *J. Biophys. Biochem. Cytol.* **6**, 103.
Runnström, J., and Michaelis, L. (1935). *J. Gen. Physiol.* **18**, 717.
Sandberg, A., Lee, G. R., Cartwright, G. E., and Wintrobe, M. M. (1955). *J. Clin. Invest.* **34**, 1823.
Sass, M. D., and Spear, P. W. (1961a). *J. Lab. Clin. Med.* **58**, 580.
Sass, M. D., and Spear, P. W. (1961b). *J. Lab. Clin. Med.* **58**, 586.
Schaedel, M. L., and Schlenk, F. (1948). *Texas Rept. Biol. Med.* **6**, 176.
Schapira, F. (1959). *Rev. Franc. Etudes Clin. Biol.* **4**, 151.
Schauer, R., and Hillmann, G. (1961). *Z. Physiol. Chem.* **325**, 9.
Scheuch, D., and Rapoport, S. (1962). *Acta Biol. Med. Ger.* **8**, 31.
Scheuch, D., Rapoport, S., and Barthel, I. (1961). *Acta Biol. Med. Ger.* **7**, 113.
Schweiger, H. G. (1962). *Intern. Rev. Cytol.* **13**, 135.
Scott, E. M. (1960). *J. Clin. Invest.* **39**, 1176.
Scott, E. M., and McGraw, J. C. (1962). *J. Biol. Chem.* **237**, 249.
Shafer, A. W., and Bartlett, G. R. (1960). *J. Clin. Invest.* **39**, 69.
Shafer, A. W., and Bartlett, G. R. (1961). *J. Clin. Invest.* **40**, 1178.
Shafer, A. W., and Bartlett, G. R. (1962). *J. Clin. Invest.* **41**, 690.
Shaw, C. R., Syner, F. N., and Tashian, R. E. (1962). *Science* **138**, 31.
Shinagawa, Y., and Ogura, M. (1961). *Kagaku (Tokyo)* **31**, 554.

Simon, E. R., Chapman, R. G., and Finch, C. A. (1962). *J. Clin. Invest.* **41**, 351.
Strömme, J. H., and Eldjarn, L. (1962). *Biochem. J.* **84**, 406.
Sutherland, E. W., Posternak, T. A., and Cori, C. F. (1949). *J. Biol. Chem.* **179**, 501.
Szekely, M., Mányai, S., and Straub, F. B. (1953). *Acta Physiol. Acad. Sci. Hung.* **4**, 31.
Tabechian, H., Altman, K. I., and Young, L. E. (1956). *Proc. Soc. Exptl. Biol. Med.* **92**, 712.
Tada, K., Watanabe, Y., and Fujiwara, T. (1961). *Tohoku J. Exptl. Med.* **75**, 384.
Tatibana, M., and Yoshikawa, H. (1962). *Biochim. Biophys. Acta* **57**, 613.
Tatibana, M., Nakao, M., and Yoshikawa, H. (1958). *J. Biochem.* (*Tokyo*) **45**, 1037.
Thorell, B. (1961). *Folia Haematol.* **78**, 275.
Tsuboi, K. K., and Hudson, P. B. (1957a). *J. Biol. Chem.* **224**, 879.
Tsuboi, K. K., and Hudson, P. B. (1957b). *J. Biol. Chem.* **224**, 889.
Tulpule, P. G. (1958). *Nature* **181**, 1804.
Valentine, W. N., and Tanaka, K. R. (1961). *Acta Haematol.* **26**, 303.
Valentine, W. N., Tanaka, K. R., and Fredericks, R. E. (1961). *Am. J. Clin. Pathol.* **36**, 328.
Vanderheiden, B. S. (1961). *Biochem. Biophys. Res. Commun.* **6**, 117.
Vesell, E. S., and Bearn, A. G. (1962). *J. Gen. Physiol.* **45**, 553.
Vestergaard-Bogind, B., and Hesselbo, T. (1960). *Biochim. Biophys. Acta* **44**, 117.
Vincent, D., Segonzac, G., and Sesque, G. (1961). *Comp. Rend. Soc. Biol.* **155**, 662.
Wada, T., Takaku, F., Nakao, K., Nakao, M., Nakao, T., and Toshikawa, H. (1960). *Proc. Japan Acad.* **36**, 618.
Warburg, O. (1909). *Z. Physiol. Chem.* **59**, 112.
Warburg, O., and Christian, W. (1931a). *Biochem. Z.* **238**, 131.
Warburg, O., and Christian, W. (1931b). *Biochem. Z.* **242**, 205.
Warburg, O., Kubowitz, F., and Christian, W. (1930a). *Biochem. Z.* **221**, 494.
Warburg, O., Kubowitz, F., and Christian, W. (1930b). *Biochem. Z.* **227**, 245.
Warburg, O., Kubowitz, F., and Christian, W. (1931a). *Biochem. Z.* **233**, 240.
Warburg, O., Kubowitz, F., and Christian, W. (1931b). *Biochem. Z.* **242**, 170.
Weber, M., Wirths, W., and Rohdewald, M. (1961). *Z. Physiol. Chem.* **324**, 219.
Weinberg, A. N. (1961). *Metab. Clin. Exptl.* **10**, 728.
Wendel, W. B. (1933). *J. Biol. Chem.* **102**, 373.
Whittam, R. (1960a). *J. Physiol.* (*London*) **154**, 608.
Whittam, R. (1960b). *J. Physiol.* (*London*) **154**, 614.
Wiley, J. S., and Whittam, R. (1961). *Biochem. J.* **78**, 27P.
Wosegien, F. (1962). *Folia Haematol.* **78**, 224.
Wosegien, F., Dose, K., and Fischer, H. (1962). *Klin. Wochschr.* **40**, 589.
Yamada, E. W. (1961). *J. Biol. Chem.* **236**, 3043.
Yasuzumi, G. (1960). *Z. Zellforsch. Mikroskop. Anat.* **51**, 325.
Yoshikawa, H., Nakao, M., Miyamoto, K., and Yanagisawa, I. (1959). *J. Biochem.* (*Tokyo*) **46**, 83.
Yoshikawa, H., Nakao, M., Miyamoto, K., and Tachibana, M. (1960). *J. Biochem.* (*Tokyo*) **47**, 635.
Zipursky, A., and Israels, L. G. (1961). *Nature* **189**, 1013.
Zipursky, A., LaRue, T., Israels, L. G., and Fairbairn, A. (1960). *Can. J. Biochem. Physiol.* **38**, 727.
Zipursky, A., Mayman, D., and Israels, L. G. (1962). *Can. J. Biochem. Physiol.* **40**, 95.

CHAPTER 5

The Pentose Phosphate Metabolism in Red Cells

Zacharias Dische

I. Introduction

Dickens (1938a) found that when glucose-6-phosphate (G-6-P) is oxidized by the G-6-P dehydrogenase in yeast extracts, an ester of a sugar is formed which gives with orcinol the characteristic reaction of pentose. He further showed (Dickens, 1938b) that ribose-5-phosphate (R-5-P) is oxidized in this yeast extract, and suggested an oxidative pathway in yeast and animal cells in which G-6-P is oxidized to R-5-P with 6-phosphogluconic and 6-phospho-2-ketogluconic as intermediates. R-5-P was assumed to be further oxidized to triose phosphate (TrP) with tetrose phosphate and phosphotetronic acid as intermediates. In 1951 it was found (Horecker *et al.*, 1951) that ribulose-5-phosphate (Ru-5-P) is the end product of the oxidation of 6-phosphogluconate and the Ru-5-P is isomerized to R-5-P. The formation of R-5-P from G-6-P in living cells gained an added significance when it was found (Dische, 1938) that human hemolysates contained an enzyme system able to phosphorylate the ribose of adenosine and convert the formed ribose phosphate to hexose phosphate and triose phosphate. The turnover in this reaction so much exceeded the rate of oxidative reactions in human red cells that it was clear that this conversion of ribose phosphate to hexose phosphate and triose phosphate is an anaerobic process. In these first experiments on human hemolysates, adenosine triphosphate (ATP) was present which was able to phosphorylate G-6-P and fructose-6-phosphate (F-6-P) to fructose-1,6-diphosphate (FDP). It was, therefore, not possible to decide what was the primary reaction product of this conversion of ribose phosphate to hexose phosphate. Waldvogel and Schlenk (1947) found that R-5-P produces G-6-P in liver homogenates. These homogenates, however, were able to dephosphorylate FDP and it was therefore not clear whether G-6-P was the primary conversion product of R-5-P. Later, however, it was reported (Dische, 1949, 1951) that when R-5-P is added to hemolysates of human red cells, from which ATP had been completely removed by prolonged dialysis in presence of NaF and which showed no phosphatase activity against either FDP or TrP, G-6-P and F-6-P were accumulated with simultaneous disappearance of R-5-P. This conversion was shown to stop after certain amounts of G-6-P and F-6-P had accumulated. After addition of ATP to the hemolysate at this moment, H-6-P (equilibrium mixture of G-6-P and F-6-P) was converted to FDP and TrP. When G-6-P or F-6-P, on the other hand, was added to the ATP-free hemolysate, the concentration of the hexose slowly decreased during about 3 hours at room temperature and this reaction came to an end when about 25% of the hexose ester had been converted to some unidentified sugar esters. When, in the calculation of the total amount of H-6-P which resulted from the conversion of R-5-P, the correction was applied for the 25% which was converted into other sugar esters, the total amount of hexose was about equivalent to the amount of ribose which disappeared. All these findings suggested the existence of a metabolic cycle in which the two-step oxidation of G-6-P results in the formation of R-5-P, which then in turn is quantitatively converted to H-6-P and TrP. The complete cycle is depicted in Fig. 1 of Chapter 6.

The molar ratio of H-6-P to TrP formed from the ribose present in the hemolysate in the form of adenosine varied in these experiments between 1.5 and 2.1. This was very nearly the value of 2 which was to be expected if all the ribose that disappeared was quantitatively converted into a mixture of H-6-P and TrP. On the basis of this stoichiometric relation, it was assumed (Dische, 1951) that the conversion of R-5-P to H-6-P and TrP proceeds in two stages. The first stage involves a transfer of the first two carbons of pentose phosphate ("activated glycolic aldehyde") to another carbon chain with formation of TrP, and the second stage the formation of H-6-P from the reaction products of the first-stage reaction, involving a transfer of three carbons to glyceraldehyde-3-phosphate (Gl-3-P) and of a 2-carbon chain to a 4-carbon intermediate. This hypothesis was supported by the observations made somewhat later (Dische and Pollaczek, 1952) that when 3 μmoles/ml. R-5-P is added

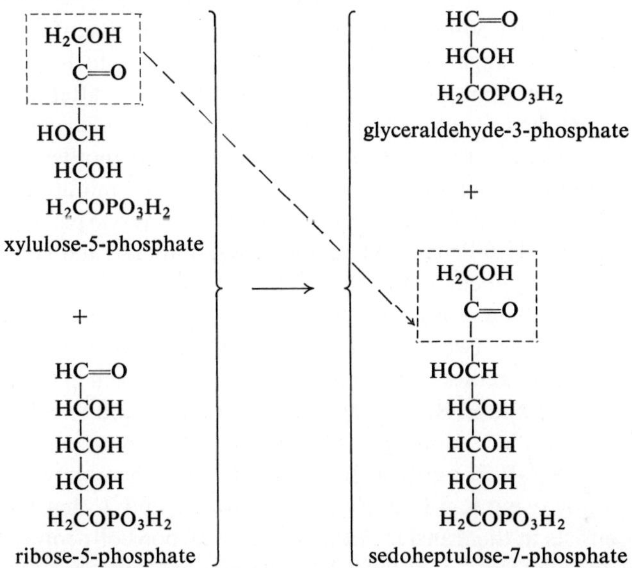

SCHEME 1. Transketolization. A "ketol" group in which the carbonyl group becomes "activated" is transferred to an aldehydic compound, the reaction representing the joining together of two adjacent carbonyl groups.

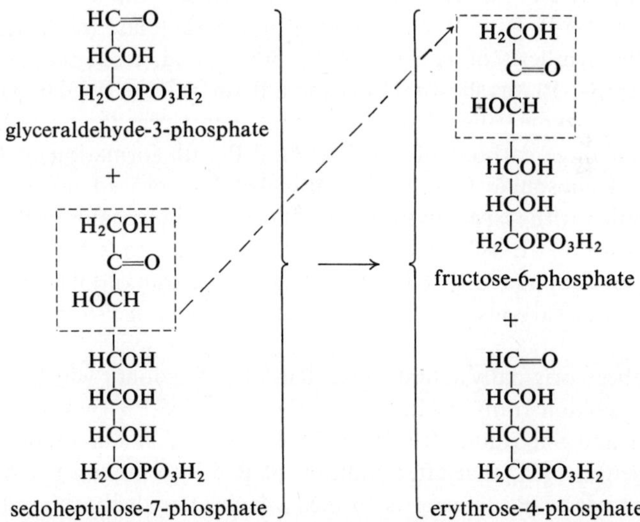

SCHEME 2. Transaldolization. The 7-carbon sugar phosphate may be thought to undergo an aldol dismutation followed by transfer and condensation of the 3-carbon unit with the glyceraldehyde-3-phosphate. In this case the original two carbonyls do not end up adjacent to each other.

to a hemolysate after 30-minute incubation at room temperature in addition to TrP an ester of a sugar is found as reaction product which, on the basis of characteristic color reactions and paper chromatography after hydrolysis was tentatively identified as sedohepulose, a 7-carbon sugar which could be formed only by transfer of 2-carbon chains from the pentose to another carbon chain. It was, furthermore, observed that in the following 60-minute time interval, the heptulose phosphate formed during the first time interval partly disappeared with formation of H-6-P. The conversion of R-5-P to TrP and H-6-P was later observed in liver (Glock, 1952; Horecker and Smyrniotis, 1952a) and yeast extracts (de la Haba and Racker, 1952).

The nature of these two types of reactions was elucidated by the work with purified enzyme preparations from liver, yeast, and spinach in the laboratories of B. L. Horecker and E. Racker. Horecker (Horecker and Smyrniotis, 1952a, b, 1953) first identified sedoheptulose phosphate as the reaction product of the conversion of R-5-P in purified liver extracts and then showed (Horecker *et al.*, 1953), by using R-5-P labeled in positions 1 and 2, that the first-stage reaction consists in the transfer of the first two carbons of pentose to a R-5-P molecule. In this reaction, carbon 1 of the pentose appeared as carbon 2 in sedoheptulose and the reaction therefore was not, as originally suggested, a transaldolization but a transketolization (see Schemes 1 and 2) and the enzyme catalyzing this reaction, therefore, was called transketolase (Racker *et al.*, 1953). The Gl-3-P was later shown to be formed from P-5-P (equilibrium mixture of R-5-P, Ru-5-P, and Xu-5-P) by transketolase (de la Haba *et al.*, 1955). The synthesis of H-6-P, on the other hand, from sedoheptulose-7-phosphate (S-7-P) was shown (Horecker and Smyrniotis, 1953) to be catalyzed by another enzyme called transaldolase, as it catalyzes the transaldolization of the first three carbons of S-7-P to Gl-3-P with formation of F-6-P and erythrose-4-phosphate (E-4-P). The transketolase proved not to be highly specific either with respect to the donor of the 2-carbon chains or the acceptor. It was shown that E-4-P can transfer carbons 1 and 2 to R-5-P in a reversible reaction and stipulated that E-4-P formed in the transaldolase reaction can accept the two carbons from Ru-5-P with formation of F-6-P (Racker *et al.*, 1954).

It had been originally assumed that Ru-5-P is the donor which in the transketolase reaction transfers the two carbons to R-5-P (Racker *et al.*, 1953; Horecker and Smyrniotis, 1953). In 1954, however, it was reported (Dische and Shigeura, 1954) that after addition of R-5-P to human hemolysates, in addition to Ru-5-P, an ester is formed which after dephosphorylation was tentatively identified by paper chromatography as xylulose phosphate. At the same time the conversion of R-5-P to xylulose phosphate was demonstrated in mouse spleen extracts by isolation of xylulose after dephosphorylation of the products of the conversion and its identification by optical rotation and as phenylosazone (Ashwell and Hickman, 1954). The authors suggested that xylulose-5-phosphate (Xu-5-P) is formed by epimerization from Ru-5-P. Soon afterwards it was shown (Srere *et al.*, 1955) that Xu-5-P is formed from Ru-5-P by a specific epimerase and that Xu-5-P is the donor of the 2-carbon chain in the transketolase reaction. The presence of epimerase in horse erythrocytes was soon afterwards demonstrated (Dickens and Williamson, 1955, 1956). The chain of reactions which leads from Xu-5-P to F-6-P and Gl-3-P is represented by the following three equations:

$$\text{Xu-5-P} + \text{R-5-P} \xrightleftharpoons{\text{transketolase}} \text{S-7-P} + \text{Gl-3-P} \quad (1)$$

$$\text{S-7-P} + \text{Gl-3-P} \xrightleftharpoons{\text{transaldolase}} \text{F-6-P} + \text{E-4-P} \quad (2)$$

$$\text{E-4-P} + \text{Xu-5-P} \xrightleftharpoons{\text{transketolase}} \text{F-6-P} + \text{Gl-3-P} \quad (3)$$

In the presence of H-6-P isomerase and TrP isomerase, the overall reaction during the conversion of P-5-P to H-6-P and TrP takes place according to the equation:

$$3\ \text{P-5-P} = 2\text{H-6-P} + 1\ \text{TrP} \quad (4)$$

as had been originally suggested from the data on the conversion of the ribose of adenosine in human hemolysates (Dische, 1951).

The biological significance of the pentose phosphate metabolism in the red cells appears to be twofold; first, it forms part of the direct oxidative pathway of glucose by the reconversion in a chain of anaerobic reactions of the reaction product of the two oxidative steps into the original substrate and TrP which can be further metabolized via the glycolytic system. In this cycle, TPN (NADP) is reduced to TPNH (NADPH). TPNH appears to be necessary for maintenance of the glutathione of red cells in reduced form and to prevent oxidation of hemoglobin to methemoglobin (Huennekens *et al.*, 1957).

On the other hand, the combined action of transketolase and transaldolase can convert G-6-P to R-5-P. Mature red cells, as well as reticulocytes, were shown to turn over their mononucleotides (Lowy *et al.*, 1961), and the level of ATP in human red cells was shown to vary reversibly in certain blood diseases and to decrease during aging of the red cells. In all these processes, synthesis of R-5-P is an essential intermediate reaction and may proceed in red cells, at least in great part, by the transketolase and transaldolase system, as shown to be the case for other living cells (Marks and Feigelson, 1957; Shuster and Golden, 1958). Although Ru-5-P is a reaction product of the direct oxidation of G-6-P, and Xu-5-P is the substrate of the transketolase-catalyzed reactions, it seems reasonable to designate for our purposes the whole reaction chain of pentose phosphate metabolism as the interconversion of G-6-P and R-5-P.

II. The Interconversion of Ribose-5-Phosphate and Glucose-6-Phosphate in Hemloysates

Although this anaerobic interconversion is completely reversible, it is more convenient, for reasons which will become apparent later, to study the whole chain of reactions in the direction from R-5-P to G-6-P. This conversion consists of four successive steps: first, the isomerization of R-5-P to Ru-5-P and epimerization of the latter to Xu-5-P. This process is catalyzed by two enzymes, P-5-P isomerase and ketopentose-5-phosphate epimerase. Then the three successive reactions take place according to Eqs. (1) to (3); reactions in Eqs. (1) and (3) are catalyzed by transketolase and in Eq. (2) by transaldolase.

The four enzymes of the red cells involved in this reaction chain have so far not been separated from each other. The demonstration and measurement of their activities can therefore be accomplished only by taking advantage of the very great differences in turnover constants between the isomerase on the one hand and the transketolase and transaldolase on the other hand, and the possibility of inactivating more than 95% of the transaldolase under conditions where no significant inactivation of the other enzymes takes place. This inactivation can be achieved by incubating dialyzed human hemolysate at 43°C. for 4 hours at pH 8.4 (inactivated hemolysate) (Dische and Shigeura, 1956, 1957). On further incubation, the rate of inactivation of the remaining transaldolase is very much less than during the first 4-hour period, due perhaps to some protective influence of the denatured enzyme on the remaining activity. To measure quantitatively the stoichiometry of the enzyme reactions, it is necessary to prevent any significant splitting of the phosphate esters by phosphatases of the hemolysate by addition of NaF. And, finally, it appears important to carry out quantitative measurements of the conversion of various substrates to end products in individual reactions at the same hemolysate concentration as was used in the experiments in which the reaction products were identified and quantitated by chromatography. Experience has shown that large differences in dilution of hemolysates or in procedures used for separation of individual enzymes may lead to significant shifts in the relation of the individual enzyme reactions. On the other hand, because of the reversibility of individual enzyme reactions, measurements of their activities can be carried out only by scaling down the reactions by enzyme dilution to such a degree that, during the accurately measurable time intervals, the turnover is small enough to eliminate the influence of the back reactions. It was possible to carry out such determinations for R-5-P isomerase and for transketolase. In human hemolysates the main bulk of the activities of these enzymes is present in solution, but a small fraction appears to be bound to the stroma, as washed stromata from cells hemolyzed by 6 parts of water were able to break down the ribose of adenosine after phosphorylation, with formation of lactic acid. This process took place with stromata at about the same rate as with intact cells (Lionetti *et al.*, 1956).

A. The Interconversion of Ribose-5-Phosphate, Ribulose-5-Phosphate, and Xylulose-5-Phosphate

1. Demonstration of Isomerase and Epimerase Activities in Human Hemolysates

When R-5-P is added to an inactive fluoridated human hemolysate, whose final volume corresponds to about a 6-fold volume of the red cells, to a final concentration of 2–11 μmoles/ml., R-5-P disappears very rapidly and at 33°C. an equilibrium is reached in which 40% of the original R-5-P is present simultaneously with its two keto isomers Ru-5-P and Xu-5-P. During this very short time interval, less than 2% of the total pentoses are converted to S-7-P and TrP.

That the conversion product of R-5-P in human hemolysates is a mixture of Xu-5-P and Ru-5-P was demonstrated (Dische and Shigeura, 1956, 1957) by incubating the hemolysate corresponding to a 6-fold dilution of red cells for 8 minutes at 33°C. with R-5-P until equilibrium between the pentose esters was reached, dephosphorylating the trichloroacetic acid (TCA) filtrate of the hemolysate with prostate phosphatase, and subjecting the resulting solution of three pentoses to paper chromatography in three different solvents. Two spots were obtained, which migrated with the R_F corresponding to the two ketopentoses and gave with the orcinol-TCA spray the colors characteristic for the two esters. Under these experimental conditions, two molecules of R-5-P were in equilibrium with three molecules of ketopentose esters (Table I).

Bruns *et al.* (1958a, b) later obtained the same result with human hemolysates diluted more than 50 times the original volume of the red cell suspension.

The ratio of the concentrations of Xu-5-P and Ru-5-P in equilibrium was determined in all these experiments on the basis of differences in development of the cysteine-carbazole-H_2SO_4 reactions between the two ketopentoses, and was found by Dische and Shigeura to be 2.65 and by Bruns *et al.* to be about 3. The conversion of R-5-P to a mixture of Ru-5-P and Xu-5-P in horse erythrocytes was demonstrated (Dickens and Williamson, 1955, 1956) with preparations of isomerase and epimerase obtained by extraction and $(NH_4)_2SO_4$ fractionation of acetone powders of erythrocytes. After equilibrium was reached at 37°C., the pentulose phosphates and, after dephosphorylation, the two pentuloses were isolated by chromatography on Dowex-1. The recovery of total pentulose corresponded to only about one-third the R-5-P used in the experiment and the ratio of Xu-5-P/Ru-5-P was only 0.1. It seems probable that a considerable destruction of Xu-5-P took place during the isolation procedure.

2. Determination of Ribose-5-Phosphate Isomerase Activities in Hemolysates

The rate of the conversion of R-5-P to Ru-5-P was determined (Bruns *et al.*, 1958a; Brownstone and Denstedt, 1961a) in hemolysates in which the original red cell suspension was diluted 2000–3000 times, and the final dilution in the assay was 6000–9000. In such dilute hemolysates the equilibrium between R-5-P and its isomers is reached at 37°C. only after several hours, and during the initial time interval of 1 hour the rate of conversion appears constant. By

TABLE I[a]

EQUILIBRIUM BETWEEN R-5-P AND ITS ISOMERS AT VARIOUS CONCENTRATIONS IN DIALYZED FLUORIDATED HEMOLYSATES

				In equilibrium			
					Ketopentose phosphate[b]		
Experiment number	R-5-P added (μmoles/ml.)	Temperature (°C.)	Time (min.)	R-5-P[b]	By cysteine-carbazole reaction	By P hydrolysis curve	pH
I	16.0	33	7	40.5	58.0	—	7.1
	16.0	33	10	33.0	62.0	—	7.1
	16.0	33	15	37.0	64.6	—	7.1
II	16.0	33	20	36.5	62.0	—	7.1
	8.0	33	8	36.2	65.0	—	7.1
	8.0	33	6	37.7			
	8.0	33	8	37.6	65.0	—	6.4
IV	8.0	33	8	37.5	—	62.0	8.4
VII	8.0	0	120	48.8	72.9	—	7.2
	8.0	33	8	36.0	61.0	—	7.2
VIII a	8.0	33	8	36.6	—	—	7.1
b	8.0	33	30	37.2	—	—	7.1
c	8.0	33	40	36.1	—	—	7.1

[a] Dische and Shigeura (1957).
[b] In % of total pentose phosphate.

this procedure Bruns *et al.* determined the activity of the R-5-P isomerase in red cells of various mammalian species at pH 7.6, at which maximum activity is reached. The results of these determinations are listed in Table II. It must be noted, however, that at this excessive dilution of hemolysates, the activity of the epimerase is apparently eliminated since, when equilibrium was reached, only 23–24% of the R-5-P was converted to its isomer. This value is almost exactly the same as the values obtained for the ratio of R-5-P to Ru-5-P in the equilibrium with purified R-5-P isomerase from liver and alfalfa, which did not contain significant amounts of epimerase (Horecker *et al.*, 1951; Axelrod and

Long, 1959). This fact, however, did not interfere with measurement of the activity of the isomerase of the hemolysate itself. K_M of the isomerase was determined to be 2.2×10^{-3} mole R-5-P/liter, Q_{10} for 30–40 minutes to be 1.6, the activation energy 8900 cal./mole.

TABLE II[a]

R 5-P ISOMERASE ACTIVITIES OF ERYTHROCYTES OF DIFFERENT SPECIES

Species	Number of samples	R-5-P isomerase activities[b] in red cells	
		Average	Range
Man	11	4.1	3.0–5.5
Cat	3	3.9	3.8–4.2
Rabbit	5	2.8	2.4–4.1
Horse	7	2.2	1.9–2.5
Hog	9	2.0	1.0–2.8
Ox	10	1.6	1.4–1.9
Mouse	6	1.6	1.5–1.6
Rat	8	1.4	1.3–1.5
Guinea pig	12	1.1	0.9–1.3
Chicken	7	0.87	0.5–1.9

[a] Bruns *et al.* (1958a).
[b] Activity = mmoles ketopentose phosphate/ml.

B. *Transketolase in Red Cells*

1. Demonstration of Transketolase Activity in Human Hemolysates with Ribose-5-Phosphate as Acceptor

To demonstrate the presence of transketolase in human hemolysates, it was necessary to demonstrate the conversion of two molecules of P-5-P into one molecule of S-7-P and one molecule of TrP. This was achieved with a hemolysate in which the initial concentration of P-5-P exceeded 10 μmoles/liter and in which the transaldolase had been inactivated to such an extent that during a certain time interval there was no significant reaction between S-7-P and TrP (Dische and Shigeura, 1956; Dische *et al.*, 1960). At this concentration of P-5-P, an inhibition of the transaldolase activity by one of the constituents of the P-5-P isomer mixture apparently takes place. In the transketolase reaction, Xu-5-P is donor of the activated 2-carbon chain and R-5-P the acceptor. It is necessary for accurate determination of P-5-P to choose as starting point of the conversion the end of the time interval necessary to achieve equilibrium between R-5-P and its isomers. When the balance of the conversion of P-5-P is calculated under these conditions during a time interval of about 200 minutes, the breakdown of P-5-P can be shown to proceed according to Eq. 1

(Table III). In calculating the decrease of P-5-P, due consideration must be paid to the fact that the Xu-5-P and Ru-5-P are unstable in solution at pH 8.4, even at room temperature (Borenfreund and Dische, 1957). It was therefore necessary to correct for the small destruction of the two ketopentose esters which, however, did not amount in this experiment to more than 10% of the total decrease of P-5-P. S-7-P in this experiment was identified by paper chromatography in three solvents, and TrP was determined as alkali-labile

TABLE III

BALANCE OF THE BREAKDOWN OF R-5-P TO S-7-P AND TRP[a]

1 Experiment number	2 pH	3 Incubation time (min.)	Ribose broken down determined as: 4 Total pentose	5 Keto-pentose	6 Sedoheptulose formed	7 Triose+FDP as triose formed	Ratio 7/6	Reaction products (in % of ribose disappearance)
II	8.4	201	3.93	4.20	1.61	1.67	1.04	84
	9.0	210	3.40	3.71	1.39	1.45	1.04	84
III	8.4	210	2.47	—	1.18	1.32	1.12	101
	7.4	210	1.82	—	0.75	0.82	1.09	—
IV	8.4	210	—	—	1.43	1.53	1.07	—
	7.4	210	—	—	0.92	0.98	1.06	—
V	8.4	210	6.1	—	2.67	2.81	1.05	90
VI	8.4	210	5.9	—	2.30	2.08	0.90	76
VII	8.4	210	3.60	3.67	1.85	1.85	1.00	103
	7.4	210	2.94	3.09	1.25	1.26	1.00	77

[a] All values in μmoles/ml. Temperature of incubation, 33°C. Initial R-5-P concentration in the hemolysate, 11.25 μmoles/ml.

phosphate and by the equilibrium constant between TrP and FDP in the reaction catalyzed by the aldolase of the hemolysate. It was not possible, however, in this experiment to determine the equilibrium between P-5-P and the reaction products of its breakdown, as the formation of H-6-P from S-7-P and TrP started before equilibrium was reached.

2. Determination of Transketolase Activity in Red Cell Hemolysates

Bruns *et al.* determined the activity of transketolase in hemolysates of a great variety of mammalian erythrocytes, of human red cells and of nucleated red cells of the chick (Bruns *et al.*, 1958b; Brownstone and Denstedt, 1961b). In these experiments only the formation of S-7-P was determined as a measure of activity. To eliminate the influence of the back reaction between S-7-P and

TrP, it was necessary to dilute the enzyme to such an extent that in the assay mixture the dilution of the hemolysate against the original cell suspension was 30-fold; under these conditions during the first hour of the experiment no more than 1% of the added substrate was converted to S-7-P, and the rate of reaction was constant during the whole 1-hour time period. Micromoles of S-7-P formed in 1 hour at 37°C. per milliliter of the original cell suspension was chosen as the unit of transketolase activity. It must be noted that no evidence is brought forward that H-6-P was not formed during the experimental period, although in the hemolysates used by the authors the transaldolase had not been

TABLE IV[a]

ACTIVITIES OF THE TRANSKETOLASE OF ERYTHROCYTES OF DIFFERENT MAMMALIAN SPECIES

Species	Number of samples	Transketolase Activity[b]	
		Average	Range
Rabbit	3	12.8	10.6–13.7
Mouse	4	11.7	10.8–12.7
Guinea pig	3	10.4	8.5–12.3
Rat	8	8.1	6.2–9.3
Man	15	4.7	2.7–6.9
Ox	7	4.6	4.1–5.4
Hog	7	4.0	3.1–5.0
Horse	4	2.9	2.7–3.5

[a] Bruns *et al.* (1958a, b).

[b] Activity in μmoles S-7-P/ml. erythrocyte suspension/hour.

inactivated. Activities of the transketolase in the hemolysates of various species reported by Bruns *et al.* are listed in Table IV. For human hemolysates, the authors reported saturation of the enzyme at a concentration of 2 μmoles of added R-5-P per ml. of hemolysate. It is not clear whether the saturation of the enzyme refers in this case to the donor or to the acceptor in the transketolase reaction.

3. The Transketolase Reaction with Erythrose-4-Phosphate as Acceptor in Human Hemolysates

In the conversion of Ru-5-P to F-6-P, the transketolase catalyzes the transfer of the activated 2-carbon chain to two different acceptors; first, to R-5-P, as was discussed in the preceding paragraph, and then, after the reaction between S-7-P and TrP catalyzed by transaldolase has taken place, the E-4-P formed in the transaldolase reaction acts as an acceptor of the activated 2-carbon chain,

TABLE V

EFFECT OF ADDITION OF R-5-P ON TURNOVER OF E-4-P[a]

Experiment number	Time of incubation (min.)	Substrate[b]	Decrease of E-4-P (in % of added amount)	Decrease of E-4-P[b] due to reaction with P-5-P	S-7-P[b] formed	G-6-P[b] formed	F-6-P[b] formed	Decrease of P-5-P[b]	
								Calculated	Found
I	2.5	(a) E-4-P (0.165)	9.4	—	—	—	—	—	—
		(b) E-4-P (0.165) + R-5-P (0.56)	39.2	0.049	0.016	—	—	—	—
	5	(a) E-4-P (0.165)	18.6	—	—	—	—	—	—
		(b) E-4-P (0.165) + R-5-P (0.56)	56.0	0.059	0.022	—	—	0.103	0.065
	5	(c) R-5-P (0.56)	—	—	0.036	—	—	—	0.067
		(d) E-4-P (0.165) + R-5-P (0.28)	38.8	0.065	0.019	—	—	0.93	0.060
	5	(e) R-5-P (0.28)	—	—	0.024	—	—	—	—
		(f) E-4-P (0.165) + R-5-P (0.14)	40.8	0.059	0.011	—	—	0.81	0.057
	5	(g) E-4-P (0.33)	17.6	—	—	—	—	—	—
		(h) E-4-P (0.33) + R-5-P (0.56)	43.6	0.096	0.027	—	0.038	0.150	0.065
		(i) R-5-P (0.56)	—	—	0.038	—	—	—	0.079
II	5	(a) E-4-P (0.33)	19.0	—	—	—	—	—	—
		(b) E-4-P (0.33) + R-5-P (0.56)	41.3	0.082	0.030	0.023	0.032	0.142	0.044
		(c) R-5-P (0.56)	—	—	0.038	—	—	—	0.079
	10	(a) E-4-P (0.33)	33.0	—	—	—	—	—	—
		(b) E-4-P (0.33) + R-5-P (0.56)	57.4	0.109	0.026	—	—	0.161	0.110
		(c) E-5-P (0.56)	—	—	0.074	—	—	—	0.135

[a] A solution of E-4-P, 0.5 ml., containing 1.25–2.5 μmoles/ml. was added to two 3-ml. samples of the hemolysate, one of which was preincubated with 0.5 ml. R-5-P (experimental sample) and the other with 0.5 ml. water (control). Both samples were incubated for various time intervals and deproteinized with TCA or $HClO_4$. A blank of 3 ml. hemolysate was simultaneously incubated with 1 ml. water (Dische and Igals, 1961).

[b] In μmole/ml.

which can be derived from either Xu-5-P or S-7-P. This reaction has been studied in inactivated human hemolysates (Dische and Igals, 1961).

When E-4-P alone is added to such hemolysates, it is immediately converted to another still unidentified ester which gives no carbohydrate reaction. In the 6-fold diluted hemolysate, this reaction comes to a standstill after about 60 minutes at 33°C., and at that time about 50% of the E-4-P appears to be in equilibrium with the conversion product. The rate of this reaction is proportional to E-4-P concentration up to about 0.33 μmole/ml. No experimental data for higher concentrations of E-4-P were obtained. If R-5-P is added together with E-4-P to the hemolysate, the disappearance of E-4-P is accelerated and at the same time H-6-P is formed. The amount of H-6-P, however, is significantly smaller than that calculated from the amount of E-4-P used up in excess of the amount which disappears when only E-4-P is added to the hemolysate. This discrepancy could be due to a side reaction between E-4-P and one of the constituents of the P-5-P isomer mixture or S-7-P simultaneously formed from P-5-P. The formation of such a side reaction is suggested by the fact that the decrease in the orcinol reaction is significantly smaller than that due to the reaction between Xu-5-P and the two acceptors P-5-P and E-4-P (Table V).

Since F-6-P is a donor of the activated 2-carbon chain (Racker *et al.*, 1954), the reaction between E-4-P and Xu-5-P is reversible. This was shown (Dische and Igals, 1961) by incubating an inactivated hemolysate with varying amounts of FDP (partly converted by aldolase to TrP) and G-6-P. Under these conditions esters are formed which give the color reactions of E-4-P, P-5-P, and S-7-P and the equilibrium is reached at 33°C. after about 90 minutes. The equilibrium is strongly in favor of F-6-P. At concentrations of TrP at which the reaction products still can be analytically determined, the latter increase with concentrations of TrP in less than a linear way. The results of a series of such experiments reported by Dische and Igals are listed in Table VI. To compare the total amounts of E-4-P and P-5-P formed in these experiments from F-6-P and Gl-3-P, it was necessary to add to the E-4-P present in solution the amount condensed by the aldolase with dihydroxyacetone (DHA) to S-1,7,-P. This value was calculated from the equilibrium constant of the condensation reaction and actual concentration of E-4-P; the amount of P-5-P converted to S-7-P and TrP had to be added to the P-5-P actually present. S-7-P was determined as total heptulose minus S-1, 7,-P.

4. Thiamine Pyrophosphate Requirement of the Transketolase of Red Cells

Transketolase preparations from spinach (Horecker and Smyrniotis, 1953) and crystalline transketolase from yeast (Racker *et al.*, 1953) were shown to require thiamine pyrophosphate (ThPP) as enzyme. The yeast preparation

TABLE VI

CONCENTRATIONS OF REACTION PRODUCTS IN THE REACTION BETWEEN F-6-P AND TRP AT VARIOUS TIME INTERVALS AND THEIR DEPENDENCE ON CONCENTRATIONS OF THE REACTANTS[a]

Experiment number	Substrate added (μmole/ml.)	Time of incubation (min.)	Reaction products formed (μmole/ml.) E-4-P	P-5-P	Sedoheptulose phosphate (S-7-P+S-1,7-P)
I	G-6-P (0.95)	90	0.112	—	—
	FDP (0.6)	180	0.112	0.087	0.06
II	(a) G-6-P (0.9)	210	0.112	0.09	—
	FDP (0.6)				
	(b) G-6-P (1.8)	210	0.142	0.13	—
	FDP (0.6)				
III	(a) G-6-P (1.8)	90	0.136	0.300	0.057
	FDP (0.6)				
	(b) G-6-P (1.8)	90	0.113	0.204	0.034
	FDP (0.3)				
	(c) G-6-P (1.8)	90	0.069	—	0.029
	FDP (0.15)				
	(d) G-6-P (1.8)	90	0.047	—	0.015
	FDP (0.075)				

[a] A solution of G-6-P, 0.5 ml., and 0.5 ml. FDP solution were incubated with 3 ml. hemolysate (experimental sample). To two control samples were added 0.5 ml. G-6-P solution plus 0.5 ml. water and 0.5 ml. FDP solution plus 0.5 ml. water, respectively. The samples were incubated simultaneously with a blank containing 3 ml. hemolysate plus 1 ml. water, deproteinized by TCA at the end of incubation, and determinations were carried out on the supernatant fractions of TCA filtrates.

becomes inactive when exhaustively dialyzed against Versene-KCl solutions. Such treatment, however, does not decrease the activity of red cell transketolase (Bruns *et al.*, 1958b). A high degree of inactivation could be achieved with the transketolase of red cells of young rats, when they were kept for more than 5 days on a thiamine-free diet. In this case the maximum inactivation was reached after 12 days and full activity could not be recovered by addition of ThPP+Mg^{++} to the hemolysate.

C. *Demonstration of Transaldolase Activity in Human Hemolysates*

The transaldolase of red cells has never been obtained separated from transketolase activity and no adequate activity measurements of this enzyme in human hemolysates seem so far to have been carried out. According to Dische *et al.* (1960), it is possible to observe in the hemolysate in which about

95% transaldolase has been inactivated the formation of H-6-P under conditions where essentially only P-5-P is the ester which disappears simultaneously with the synthesis of H-6-P, whereas the level of the intermediate S-7-P remains almost constant and only barely significant amounts of E-4-P are accumulated. By determining then the amounts of pentose which disappear and the amounts of H-6-P which are formed during that time interval and making suitable corrections for the small changes in concentration of S-7-P and E-4-P, it is possible to show that the amount of H-6-P formed is identical with that expected if H-6-P is formed first by the transaldolase reaction according to Eq. (2), and then by the reaction between E-4-P and Xu-5-P according to Eq. (3). The demonstration of transaldolase activity was thus carried out (Dische *et al.*, 1960) by incubating the inactivated hemolysate with 2.25 μmoles/ml. of R-5-P first for 210 minutes. During this time interval only insignificant amounts of H-6-P were formed. During the following time interval of 210 minutes, the formation of H-6-P took place essentially at the expense of P-5-P. That the enzyme which forms H-6-P from accumulated S-7-P and which is inactivated by incubation at 43°C. at pH 8.4 has the activity of purified transaldolase from other sources can be indirectly demonstrated by studying the stoichiometry of the formation of H-6-P by the residual transaldolase in the experiments presented in Table VII. In carrying out this calculation, it had to be considered that for every mole of E-4-P formed during the second time interval one mole of H-6-P was formed by the reaction at the expense of 2 moles of P-5-P according to Eqs. (1)+(2), and for every mole of S-7-P which disappeared during this period without formation of E-4-P two moles ofH-6-P were formed and 1 mole of P-5-P was used up, according to Eqs. (2) and (3). For 1 mole of S-7-P formed, on the other hand, 2 moles of P-5-P have to have disappeared. By subtracting from changes in amounts of P-5-P and H-6-P during this period the amounts corresponding to changes in E-4-P and S-7-P, we obtain the amounts of P-5-P which were converted to H-6-P according to Eq. (4). This equation appears satisfied within 3% by the corrected values obtained in experiments of Table VII for the P-5-P which disappeared and the H-6-P which was formed during the period between 210 and 420 minutes.

It was, furthermore, possible to show that in the fully active hemolysate, S-7-P is formed at the expense of E-4-P and H-6-P. To this end two samples of the same hemolysate, one inactivated and the other before inactivation, were incubated with H-6-P and FDP, as specified in Table VIII. The concentrations of E-4-P, H-6-P, and S-7-P at the end of the incubation period in the two samples were compared with each other. As can be seen, less E-4-P appeared and significantly more S-7-P was formed in the samples in which transaldolase was fully active than in the inactivated hemolysate. Simultaneously, a sharp decrease in H-6-P took place in the active hemolysate which did not appear in the inactivated one. That the amount of H-6-P which disappeared was

TABLE VII[a]

BALANCE OF THE BREAKDOWN OF R-5-P IN HEMOLYSATES IN SUCCESSIVE PERIODS OF INCUBATION BY COMBINED ACTION OF TRANSKETOLASE[b] AND TRANSALDOLASE

1 Experiment number	2 Time interval of incubation (min.)	3 Pentose disappeared	4 Sedoheptulose phosphate formed	5 Triose P+FDP as triose P formed	6 Hexose phosphate formed determined as		7 Tetrose phosphate formed	8 Recovery of reaction products (in % of compounds which disappeared)
					G-6-P	F-6-P		
I	(a) 10–210	1.64	0.73	—	0.058	—	0.016	93.0
	(b) 210–420	0.21	−0.01	—	0.145	—	0.018	97.0
II	(a) 10–210	1.63	0.69	0.69	0.070	—	0.025	103.0
	(b) 210–420	0.21	0.02	—	0.106	—	0.015	104.0

[a] Dische *et al.* (1960).

[b] Initial concentration of R-5-P, 2.25 μmoles/ml. All values in μmoles/ml.; pH 8.4.

greater than that equivalent to the S-7-P which was formed indicates that a side reaction takes place which may be the reaction discovered by Sie *et al.* (1959). The relation of this reaction to the pentose phosphate metabolism is not yet elucidated. The experiments of Table VIII show clearly that the enzyme which is inactivated at 43°C. at pH 8.4 forms S-7-P from E-4-P and H-6-P as does transaldolase.

TABLE VIII

FORMATION OF S-7-P FROM E-4-P AND F-6-P BY TRANSALDOLASE OF HUMAN HEMOLYSATES[a]

Experiment number	Enzyme preparation	E-4-P formed (μmole/ml.)	S-7-P formed (μmole/ml.)	H-6-P disappeared (μmole/ml.)
I	(a) Hemolysate after inactivation of transaldolase	0.165	0.005	0.050
	(b) The same before inactivation	0.059	0.109	0.320
II	(a) Hemolysate after inactivation of transaldolase	0.158	0.036	—
	(b) The same before inactivation	0.082	0.134	—

[a] Hemolysate, 3 ml., +0.5 ml. G-6-P (9 μmoles)+0.5 ml. FDP (2.7 μmoles) was incubated for 210 minutes at 33°C. (Dische, unpublished results).

III. Coordination of Reactions Simultaneously Catalyzed by Transketolase and Transaldolase in Human Hemolysates

A. *Synthesis of Ribose-5-Phosphate from Glucose-6-Phosphate by the Combined Activity of Transaldolase and Transketolase*

In the transketolase reaction between F-6-P and Gl-3-P, the equilibrium is not favorable for the formation of R-5-P, as significant amounts of this compound can only be formed in the presence of such relatively high concentrations of the two reactants as usually are not present in intact red cells or for that matter in other living cells. This situation, however, changes completely when transketolase and transaldolase in adequate concentrations are simultaneously active in the hemolysate (Dische, 1957). When G-6-P is added to a fresh, fluoridated hemolysate with no significant phosphatase activity, it is rapidly converted to other esters (Dische, 1951). These esters were tentatively determined (Dische, 1957) as sedoheptulose phosphate, TrP, and P-5-P. Sedoheptulose phosphate was tentatively identified after dephosphorylization by paper chromatography in three different solvents, the aldopentose component of P-5-P by the characteristic phloroglucinol reaction, the ketoisomers by paper chromatography using the orcinol-TCA reaction, TrP as alkali-labile phosphate. E-4-P could not be demonstrated in significant amounts and the reaction (as reported in 1951) comes to a standstill when about 25% of H-6-P is converted to the reaction products. The importance of this reaction seems to reside in the fact that it does not require the presence of even traces of priming TrP or E-4-P. This could be shown by using glucose-1-phosphate (G-1-P) as substrate (Dische, 1957, 1958), preheated with 0.2 N NaOH for up to 30 minutes at 100°C. This treatment would have completely destroyed any contaminating TrP or FDP. It did not affect at all the ability of G-1-P to form S-7-P when added to the fresh hemolysate in which it is rapidly converted to G-6-P. Somewhat later the formation of S-7-P from F-6-P was demonstrated in liver hemolysates which did not contain TrP but showed strong phosphatase activity (Bonsignore *et al.*, 1957, 1958). In these experiments no simultaneous formation of P-5-P and TrP was found in spite of the presence of transketolase. Experiments (Pontremoli *et al.*, 1960) with combinations of purified transaldolase and transketolase, however, make it very probable that at a certain ratio of concentrations of the two enzymes, the amount of TrP and E-4-P in equilibrium with the substrates and enzymes may be sufficient to prime the reaction.

$$\text{F-6-P} + \text{Gl-3-P} \xrightleftharpoons{\text{transketolase}} \text{Xu-5-P} + \text{E-4-P} \tag{5}$$

$$\text{F-6-P} + \text{E-4-P} \xrightleftharpoons{\text{transaldolase}} \text{S-7-P} + \text{Gl-3-P} \tag{6}$$

$$\text{S-7-P} + \text{Gl-3-P} \xrightleftharpoons{\text{transketolase}} \text{Xu-5-P} + \text{R-5-P} \tag{7}$$

$$\text{Xu-5-P} \xrightleftharpoons{\text{epimerase}} \text{Ru-5-P} \xrightleftharpoons{\text{isomerase}} \text{R-5-P} \tag{8}$$

It is remarkable, however, that in experiments of these authors the concentration of E-4-P necessary to achieve the observed rate of synthesis of S-7-P, when calculated from the affinity of E-4-P for transaldolase, was 1000 times greater than could be present in their enzyme solutions during the reaction. It is not possible at present to explain this discrepancy. In these experiments no time lag was observed before the maximum rate of S-7-P formation was reached. In the experiments of Dische, the addition of small amounts of E-4-P or of TrP to the hemolysate accelerated the rate of S-7-P formation during the first time interval of 30 minutes. In the hemolysate, therefore, the relative concentrations of transaldolase and transketolase apparently are not the optimal ones. A certain accumulation of minimum amounts of E-4-P and TrP by the combined action of the two enzymes in the hemolysate is necessary to achieve maximum rate of the reaction.

B. Coordination of the Transketolase Reactions with Ribose-5-Phosphate and Erythrose-4-Phosphate as Acceptors

For the economical operation of the G-6-P shunt in red cells, it is obviously essential that the P-5-P formed by the direct oxidation of G-6-P be quantitatively converted into F-6-P and TrP at the relatively very low concentrations of P-5-P found in intact red cells. This can be achieved only if the rate of the reaction according to Eq. (3) is at least as high as that of the reaction between Xu-5-P and R-5-P which leads to the formation of S-7-P and TrP used by transaldolase as substrates for the formation of E-4-P. This appears particularly important, as it has been shown that E-4-P is a powerful inhibitor of H-6-P isomerase as well as transketolase even at rather low concentration (Dische and Igals, 1961) and, therefore, any accumulation of E-4-P would tend to disrupt the continuity of the shunt pathway by significantly influencing the overall turnover of P-5-P. It is, therefore, of interest to compare the relative rates of the reactions in Eqs. (1) and (3). A determination of the true velocity of the reaction between E-4-P and Xu-5-P in the hemolysate has not so far been possible, as at a concentration of E-4-P necessary for determining the reaction rate a strong inhibition of the transketolase appears as soon as R-5-P is added to the hemolysate containing E-4-P. It has been pointed out (Dische and Igals, 1961) that this is probably due to the product of a side reaction, an unidentified ester, which gives a strong green color in Bial's orcinol reaction. It is clear, however, from experiment I of Table V that the turnover of E-4-P in the first 2.5 minutes at 33°C. is several times as high as the turnover of simultaneously added P-5-P. As the transketolase activity is lower than that of the transaldolase in the fresh hemolysate, it is clear that at very low concentrations of E-4-P, which are below the limit of our analytical procedures, the synthesis of F-6-P from E-4-P and Xu-5-P can proceed with the speed necessary to prevent any larger accumulation of E-4-P.

C. Regulatory Factors of Pentose Phosphate Metabolism in Human Red Cells

As the level of nucleotides in human red cells can undergo reversible changes in various developmental and pathological conditions, it seems reasonable to assume that the rate of synthesis and of breakdown of these cell constituents also will show significant variations. As the transketolase-transaldolase system can be assumed to play a major role in these anaerobic and metabolic processes, it appears probable that in the organized cell there will be specific regulatory mechanisms for the interconversion of P-5-P and H-6-P. One type of such regulatory factors will be concerned with the relative rate of the two competing metabolic pathways, namely, glycolysis and shunt mechanism. These two reaction chains compete for the G-6-P which can be diverted into the glycolytic pathway by being isomerized to F-6-P and then phosphorylated to FDP. It has been suggested that the intracellular pH may play a role in directing the red cell metabolism into one or the other pathway, as the pH optimum of the pentose phosphate metabolism was found to be 7.6 against 8.2 for glycolysis (Chapman *et al.*, 1960). More potent influence can be expected from the level of E-4-P which was shown strongly to inhibit the H-6-P isomerase as well as the transketolase of the hemolysate (Dische and Igals, 1961) and, on the other hand, a certain minimum level of E-4-P has been shown to be necessary to achieve maximum activity of transaldolase in the red cells (Dische, 1957). It is not possible at present, however, to decide whether the level of E-4-P necessary for such significant regulatory effects does ever materialize in erythrocytes. Another ester which may contribute to the regulation of the pentose phosphate metabolism and which is found in adequate concentration in red cells is 2,3-diphosphoglycerate. This compound has been shown to inhibit the phosphorylation of glucose by the hexokinase of red cells as well as other transphosphorylation processes in the glycolytic system (Dische, 1941). These inhibitory effects, which are very marked at physiological concentrations of the ester, represent a feedback mechanism since the ester is an intermediate in the whole chain of the glycolytic reactions but not a direct reaction product of hexokinase, the activity of which is a limiting factor for the whole chain of reactions in glycolysis. In more recent experiments (Dische and Igals, 1963), it has been found that 2,3-diphosphoglycerate at physiological concentrations also strongly inhibits the transaldolase and even more so the transketolase. It may be significant for the regulatory action of this ester that it appears to be at least partly bound to some macromolecular component of the red cell in which state it does not affect hexokinase (Solomon *et al.*, 1940; Dische, 1941). It seems probable that by releasing and binding the diphosphoglycerate within the red cell, regulatory effects on pentose phosphate metabolism as well as glycolysis may be achieved. The inhibitory effects of diphosphoglycerate on transketolase and transaldolase may be due to its nature as a pentavalent anion inasmuch as 0.1 *N* sulfate and phosphate were also shown to exert such inhibitory effects (Bonsignore *et al.*, 1960; Dische and Igals, 1963).

References

Ashwell, G., and Hickman, J. (1954). *J. Am. Chem. Soc.* **76**, 5889.

Axelrod, B., and Jang, Z. (1954). *J. Biol. Chem.* **209**, 84.

Bonsignore, A., Pontremoli, S., Forniani, G., and Grazi, E. (1957). *Italian J. Biochem.* **6**, 241.

Bonsignore, A., Pontremoli, S., and Grazi, E. (1958). *Italian J. Biochem.* **7**, 187.

Bonsignore, A., Pontremoli, S., Grazi, E., and Horecker, B. L. (1960). *J. Biol. Chem.* **235**, 1888.

Borenfreund, E., and Dische, Z. (1957). *Biochim. Biophys. Acta* **25**, 215.

Brownstone, Y. S., and Denstedt, O. F. (1961a). *Can. J. Biochem. Physiol.* **39**, 527.

Brownstone, Y. S., and Denstedt, O. F. (1961b). *Can. J. Biochem. Physiol.* **39**, 534.

Bruns, F. H., Noltmann, E., and Valhauls, E. (1958a). *Biochem. Z.* **330**, 483.

Bruns, F. H., Noltmann, E., and Valhauls, E. (1958b). *Biochem. Z.* **330**, 497.

Chapman, R. G., Huennekens, F. M., and Gabrio, B. W. (1960). *Clin. Res.* **8**, 127.

de la Haba, I. G., and Racker, E. (1952). *Federation Proc.* **11**, 201.

de la Haba, I. G., Leder, I. G., and Racker, E. (1955). *J. Biol. Chem.* **214**, 409.

Dickens, F. (1938a). *Biochem. J.* **38**, 1626.

Dickens, F. (1938b). *Biochem. J.* **38**, 1645.

Dickens, F., and Williamson, D. H. (1955). *Nature* **176**, 400.

Dickens, F., and Williamson, D. H. (1956). *Biochem. J.* **64**, 5671.

Dische, Z. (1938). *Naturwissenschaften* **26**, 252.

Dische, Z. (1941). *Bull. Soc. Chim. Biol.* **23**, 1140.

Dische, Z. (1949). *Abstr. 1st Intern. Congr. Biochem., Cambridge*, p. 572.

Dische, Z. (1951). *In* "Phosphorus Metabolism" (W. D. McElroy and B. Glass, eds.), Vol. I, p. 171. Johns Hopkins Press, Baltimore, Maryland.

Dische, Z. (1957). *Federation Proc.* **16**, 173.

Dische, Z. (1958). *Ann. N. Y. Acad. Sci.* **75**, 129.

Dische, Z., and Igals, D. (1961). *Arch. Biochem. Biophys.* **93**, 201.

Dische, Z., and Igals, D. (1963). *Arch. Biochem. Biophys.* (In press.)

Dische, Z., and Pollaczek, E. (1952). *Abstr. 2nd Intern. Congr. Biochem., Paris*, 1952, p. 289.

Dische, Z., and Shigeura, H. T. (1954). *Abstr. Meeting Carbohydrate Section Chem. Soc., 1954.*

Dische, Z., and Shigeura, H. T. (1956). *Federation Proc.* **15**, 243.

Dische, Z., and Shigeura, H. T. (1957). *Biochim. Biophys. Acta* **24**, 87.

Dische, Z., Shigeura, H. T., and Landsberg, E. (1960). *Arch. Biochem. Biophys.* **89**, 123.

Glock, G. E. (1952). *Biochem. J.* **52**, 575.

Horecker, B. L., and Smyrniotis, P. Z. (1952a). *Federation Proc.* **11**, 232.

Horecker, B. L., and Smyrniotis, P. Z. (1952b). *J. Am. Chem. Soc.* **74**, 2123.

Horecker, B. L., and Smyrniotis, P. Z. (1953). *J. Am. Chem. Soc.* **75**, 1009.

Horecker, B. L., Smyrniotis, P. Z., and Seegmiller, G. E. (1951). *J. Biol. Chem.* **193**, 383.

Horecker, B. L., Smyrniotis, P. Z., and Klenow, H. (1953). *J. Biol. Chem.* **205**, 661.

Huennekens, F. M., Caffrey, R. W., Basford, R. E., and Gabrio, B. W. (1957). *J. Biol. Chem.* **227**, 261.

Lionette, F., Rees, S. B., Healey, W. A., Walker, B. S., and Gibson, J. G. (1956). *J. Biol. Chem.* **220**, 467.

Lowy, B. A., Williams, M. K., and London, I. M. (1961). *J. Biol. Chem.* **236**, 1439.

Marks, P. A. and Feigelson, P. J. (1957). *J. Biol. Chem.* **226**, 1001.

Pontremoli, S., Bonsignore, A., Grazi, E., and Horecker, B. L. (1960). *J. Biol. Chem.* **235**, 1881.

Racker, E., de la Habe, G., and Leder, I. G. (1953). *J. Am. Chem. Soc.* **75**, 1010.

Racker, E., de la Haba, G., and Leder, I. G. (1954). *Arch. Biochem. Biophys.* **48**, 238.

Solomon, R. Z., Hald, P. M., and Peters, J. P. (1940). *J. Biol. Chem.* **132**, 723.

Shuster, L., and Golden, A. (1958). *J. Biol. Chem.* **230**, 883.

Sie, H. G., Nigam, V. N., and Fishman, W. H. (1959). *J. Am. Chem. Soc.* **81**, 6083.

Srere, P. A., Cooper, J. R., Klybas, V., and Racker, E. (1955). *Arch. Biochem. Biophys.* **59**, 535.

Waldvogel, M. J., and Schlenk, F. (1947). *Arch. Biochem. Biophys.* **14**, 484.

CHAPTER 6

Glucose-6-Phosphate Dehydrogenase: Its Properties and Role in Mature Erythrocytes

Paul A. Marks

I. Introduction[1]

Erythrocyte G-6-P dehydrogenase has been a subject of considerable interest during the past decade. This interest has been largely stimulated by the observations that a genetically determined deficiency of this enzyme is associated with an increased susceptibility of red cells to hemolysis and that there is a selective decrease in the activity of this enzyme as erythrocytes age *in vivo*.

[1] Abbreviations: G-6-P, glucose-6-phosphate; NADP (formerly TPN), nicotinamide adenine dinucleotide phosphate; NADPH (TPNH), reduced nicotinamide adenine dinucleotide phosphate; NAD (DPN), nicotinamide adenine dinucleotide; NADH (DPNH), reduced nicotinamide adenine dinucleotide; ADP, adenosine diphosphate; ATP, adenosine triphosphate; GSH, reduced glutathione.

The purpose of this chapter is to consider the role of G-6-P dehydrogenase in the erythrocyte and summarize the recent biochemical, genetic, and clinical studies of red cell G-6-P dehydrogenase.

The intensity of the work related to G-6-P dehydrogenase in recent years makes it impossible to review all aspects of this problem in the space allotted. Several reviews have appeared which deal in more detail with various aspects pertinent to red cell G-6-P dehydrogenase, among which may be cited Lemberg and Legge (1949), Szeinberg and Sheba (1958), Childs and Zinkham (1959), Dickens *et al.* (1959), Waller (1959), Larizza *et al.* (1960), London (1961), Beutler (1960), Marks (1961a), Prankerd (1961), Desforges (1962), Schapira and Rosa (1962), and Tarlov *et al.* (1962).

II. Glucose-6-Phosphate Dehydrogenase Reaction and the Pentose Phosphate Pathway

A. Reactions of the Pentose Phosphate Pathway

The pentose phosphate pathway (also referred to as the hexose monophosphate pathway or shunt) appears to be the main alternative pathway to glycolysis in the metabolism of glucose by the erythrocyte. G-6-P is the branch point for glucose utilization via glycolysis or the pentose phosphate pathway (Horecker and Hiatt, 1958; Marks and Freedman, 1962) (Fig. 1).

In the initial oxidative step of the pentose phosphate pathway, G-6-P is oxidized to 6-phosphogluconolactone by a reaction catalyzed by G-6-P dehydrogenase. After enzymatic hydrolysis of the lactone, 6-phosphogluconate is oxidized to ribulose-5-phosphate. The reactions catalyzed by G-6-P dehydrogenase and 6-phosphogluconic dehydrogenase (Reactions 1 and 3, Fig. 1) require NADP as cofactor and generate the reduced cofactor, NADPH. CO_2 is formed from the first carbon of glucose in this series of reactions. It is likely that these reactions are the only site in the mature erythrocyte for the oxidation of glucose to CO_2. This is indicated by the findings (Brin and Yonemoto, 1958; Johnson and Marks, 1958; Murphy, 1960) that mature erythrocytes oxidize glucose-1-C^{14} or glucose-2-C^{14}, but not glucose-6-C^{14}, to $C^{14}O_2$. This latter finding is consistent with the earlier observation that mature erythrocytes are deficient in certain enzymes of the tricarboxylic acid cycle (Rubinstein *et al.*, 1956). The oxidative reactions of the pentose phosphate pathway are effectively irreversible because of the essential irreversibility of the lactonase reaction.

Subsequent reactions of the pentose phosphate pathway are nonoxidative. These reactions involve the conversion of ribulose-5-phosphate to two closely related sugars, xylulose-5-phosphate and ribose-5-phosphate (Fig. 1, Reactions

4 and 5). These two pentoses may then be converted to fructose-6-phosphate via sedoheptulose-7-phosphate (Fig. 1, Reactions 6 and 7) or more directly by a reaction involving erythrose-4-phosphate (Fig. 1, Reaction 8). Recently

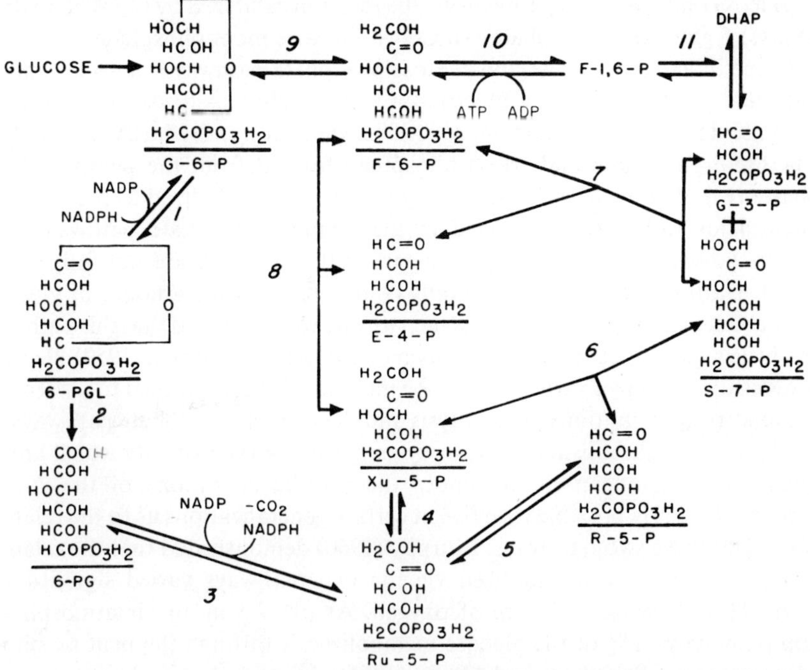

FIG. 1. Reactions of the pentose phosphate pathway.

Abbreviations: G-6-P, glucose-6-phosphate; 6-PGL, 6-phosphogluconolactone; 6-PG, 6-phosphogluconate; Ru-5-P, ribulose-5-phosphate; R-5-P, ribose-5-phosphate; Xu-5-P, xylulose-5-phosphate; S-7-P, sedoheptulose-7-phosphate; G-3-P, glyceraldehyde-3-phosphate; E-4-P, erythrose-4-phosphate; F-6-P, fructose-6-phosphate; F-1,6-P, fructose-1,6-diphosphate; DHAP, dehydroxyacetone phosphate.

Enzymes: (1) glucose-6-phosphate dehydrogenase; (2) lactonase; (3) 6-phosphogluconic dehydrogenase; (4) phosphoketopentoepimerase; (5) phosphoriboisomerase; (6) transketolase; (7) transaldolase; (8) transketolase; (9) phosphohexose isomerase; (10) phosphofructokinase; and (11) aldolase.

The conversion of fructose-6-phosphate to xylulose-5-phosphate and sedoheptulose-7-phosphate described in the text is not indicated in the above schema. Reaction 6 as indicated in the diagram is incomplete in that xylulose-5-phosphate + ribose-5-phosphate are converted to sedoheptulose-7-phosphate + glyceraldehyde-3-phosphate.

Bonsignore, Pontremoli and their co-workers (Pontremoli *et al.*, 1960 and Bonsignore *et al.*, 1962b) demonstrated the reversible interconversion of fructose-6-phosphate to xylulose-5-phosphate and sedoheptulose-7-phosphate catalyzed by transketolase and transaldolase. This latter reaction provides a mechanism for the nonoxidative formation of pentose phosphate from hexose phosphate without a requirement for triose phosphate or erythrose phosphate. The sum of all the reactions of the pentose phosphate pathway has the potential of converting one molecule of glucose to carbon dioxide for every six molecules of glucose that enter this pathway via the reaction catalyzed by G-6-P dehydrogenase: 6 glucose-6-phosphate $\rightarrow$ 6 CO_2 + 5 hexose monophosphate.

In the intact erythrocyte, the pentose phosphate pathway is a cycle. This is indicated by the fact that glucose-2-C^{14} is readily oxidized to $C^{14}O_2$ by erythrocytes (Brin and Yonemoto, 1958; Szeinberg and Marks, 1961). The fructose-6-phosphate and triose phosphate formed from the pentose phosphates (Fig. 1, Reactions 7 and 8) may be further metabolized to pyruvic and lactic acids rather than recycled in the pentose phosphate pathway. The factors governing the recycling of sugars in this pathway are not fully elucidated. Until recently, it was generally considered that the amount of glucose metabolized in the pentose phosphate pathway was small and that this pathway has little significance in the metabolism of the red cell (Altman, 1959). Several investigators, using a variety of isotope methods, have attempted to determine the relative contributions of glycolysis and the pentose phosphate pathways to total glucose metabolism by erythrocytes. Such studies give data which are of quantitative significance only under the specific conditions of the study. Nevertheless, it is possible to arrive at certain generalizations as to the relative activity of these two pathways. Murphy (1960) demonstrated that the relative amounts of glucose metabolized via the two pathways varied significantly with pH and partial pressure of oxygen. At pH 7.5 in an air atmosphere, approximately 11% of the glucose metabolized is through the pentose phosphate pathway. Szeinberg and Marks (1961) observed that in the presence of certain physiological substances, such as cysteine, ascorbic acid, or pyruvic acid, considerable increases in the percent of glucose oxidized to CO_2 occurred without an increased rate of glucose utilization or lactic acid formation. Various chemical agents, such as methylene blue, primaquine, acetylphenylhydrazine, nitrofurantoin, α- and β-naphthol, were found to cause marked increase in the percentage of total glucose metabolized via the oxidative reactions of the pentose phosphate pathway (Szeinberg and Marks, 1961; DeLoecker and Prankerd, 1961). It is not unreasonable to suggest that *in vivo* there may be considerable variation in the percentage of glucose metabolism which proceeds via one or the other pathways, depending upon a variety of factors such as the concentration of agents which can potentially cause the oxidation of NADPH.

Substances such as methylene blue, ascorbic acid, cysteine, etc., which stimulate the oxidation of glucose carbon atom 1 via the pentose phosphate pathway, also increase the rate of glucose-2-C^{14} oxidation to $C^{14}O_2$. Indeed these compounds effect a relatively greater increase in the rate of oxidation of glucose-2-C^{14} to $C^{14}O_2$ than of glucose-1-C^{14} to $C^{14}O_2$ (Brin and Yonemoto,

1958; Murphy, 1960; Szeinberg and Marks, 1961). In contrast, these substances had no detectable effect on increasing the rate of glucose-6-C^{14} oxidation to $C^{14}O_2$. These observations suggest that in mature erythrocytes the glyceraldehyde-3-phosphate, which may be formed in the reactions catalyzed by transketolase and transaldolase (Fig. 1, Reactions 6 and 7), is converted to a very limited extent, if at all, to carbon atoms 1, 2, and 3 of G-6-P. The recycling of pentose phosphate to G-6-P may proceed either by the reactions involving conversion of ribulose-5-phosphate to xylulose-5-phosphate and subsequent reaction of this pentose with erythrose-4-phosphate to form fructose-6-phosphate (Fig. 1, Reactions 4 and 8), or by the reaction of xylulose-5-phosphate with sedoheptulose-7-phosphate to form fructose-6-phosphate. It would follow from these speculations that, in the mature erythrocyte, the effective cycle in the pentose phosphate pathway involves the reactions catalyzed by transketolase and transaldolase which do not require glyceraldehyde-3-phosphate. The finding that the various substances which can markedly stimulate oxidation of glucose carbon atom 1 to $C^{14}O_2$ have a relatively greater effect on oxidation of glucose carbon atom 2 might indicate that these substances have an action at a site between ribulose-5-phosphate and glucose-6-phosphate.

B. Role of the Oxidative Reactions of the Pentose Phosphate Pathway in the Mature Erythrocyte

1. Pentose Phosphate Formation

The pentose phosphate pathway provides ribose-5-phosphate, a constituent of various substances important in erythrocytes such as pyridine nucleotides, ADP, and ATP (Preiss and Handler, 1957; Bonsignore *et al.*, 1961b). Ribose-5-phosphate may be synthesized by either of two pathways, namely, oxidation of G-6-P (Fig. 1, Reactions 1–4) or reversal of the non-oxidative reactions catalyzed by transketolase and transaldolase (Fig. 1, Reactions 5–8) (Marks and Feigelson, 1957; Hiatt, 1957; Hiatt and Lareau, 1960; Bonsignore *et al.*, 1962b). There is variation in the capabilities of adult erythrocytes of different species to synthesize nucleotides. Thus, Lowy and co-workers (1961, 1962) have demonstrated that while rabbit reticulocytes can synthesize adenosine and guanosine triphosphates, the adult erythrocytes lack the complete pathway for *de novo* purine formation and require purine and ribosyl derivatives for nucleoside triphosphate formation. On the other hand, mature human red cells can utilize preformed purines for nucleotide synthesis, but are deficient in the capacity to convert inosinic acid to adenylic acid.

2. Generation of Energy

In addition to their role as intermediates in the synthesis of nucleotides, the pentose phosphates serve as substrates in a sequence of reactions which proceed to the formation of lactic acid by the reactions catalyzed by transketolase and transaldolase and the subsequent conversion of glyceraldehyde-3-phosphate to lactic acid. For every three molecules of pentose phosphate metabolized via this series of reactions, a net of 8 molecules of ATP and none of NADH are generated. It is this sequence of reactions which presumably accounts for the effectiveness of various nucleosides, such as inosine and adenosine, in prolonging the survival of erythrocytes stored *in vitro* (Gabrio *et al.*, 1956).

3. NADPH Generation

The oxidative reactions of the pentose phosphate pathway are the only site for generation of NADPH in adult erythrocytes. There is no evidence that NADPH oxidation in mature erythrocytes may be directly involved in the production of energy (Kaplan *et al.*, 1956; Ball and Cooper, 1957). Nevertheless, NADPH serves as an essential cofactor in a number of reactions important in maintaining the integrity of the erythrocyte. NADPH appears to play a role in reducing methemoglobin in reactions mediated by a NADPH-dependent methemoglobin reductase (Huennekens *et al.*, 1958). Methemoglobin reduction to hemoglobin can be accomplished by at least two pathways in the adult red cell, one of which is NADPH-dependent and another of which is NADH-dependent (Scott, 1960) (see Chapter 11). It has been presumed that the NADH pathway is the more important under usual *in vivo* conditions. This is suggested primarily by the fact that, in patients with genetically determined deficiency of NADH-methemoglobin reductase, there is uniformly found a marked increase in methemoglobin concentration. On the other hand, in subjects with marked G-6-P dehydrogenase deficiency there is little or no evidence for increased levels of methemoglobin. This difference may not be as important as previously believed (see Section IV, D, 2, and Brewer *et al.*, 1962a) and the issue remains unresolved as to the relative importance of the two pathways of methemoglobin reduction.

NADPH appears to function in several types of reaction involved in the metabolism of drugs (Brodie *et al.*, 1958). It has not been specifically demonstrated that such reactions occur in erythrocytes. It has been shown that NADPH, which is a required cofactor in several steps in steroid biosynthesis, does function in human red cells in the transformation of estrone to 17β-estradiol in the reaction catalyzed by 17β-estradiol dehydrogenase (Migeon *et al.*, 1962). The physiological importance of this enzyme in the erythrocyte is not clear.

Of particular interest is the role of NADPH in the reduction of glutathione. Reduced glutathione is necessary to the stability of certain sulfhydryl-containing enzymes, as well as to the maintenance of the native structure of hemoglobin (Rapkine, 1938; Keilin and Hartree, 1946; Barron, 1951; Fegler, 1951;

Benesch and Benesch, 1954; Jandl and Allen, 1960; Scheuch *et al.*, 1961). It is well established that reduced glutathione is bound to at least one enzyme, glyceraldehyde-3-phosphate dehydrogenase (Krimsky and Racker, 1952). In this regard, however, it is of note that Sternschuss *et al.* (1961) observed no decrease in glyceraldehyde-3-phosphate dehydrogenase activity in erythrocytes whose GSH concentration was decreased to undetectable levels by incubation with acetylphenylhydrazine.

Mills (1957, 1959, 1960; Mills and Randall, 1958) has suggested that NADPH is important in maintaining the integrity of the red cell primarily because it is required to reduce glutathione. Reduced glutathione is a necessary substrate for the reaction involving the peroxidation of H_2O_2 to water as follows: $H_2O_2 + 2\ GSH \rightarrow 2\ H_2O + GSSG$. Mills has concluded that this reaction, catalyzed by the enzyme glutathione peroxidase rather than catalase, is the main reaction for reduction of hydrogen peroxide, thus preventing the oxidative denaturation of erythrocyte proteins. The studies of Szeinberg and Marks (1961) suggested that there may be an alternative mechanism by which NADPH serves in maintaining red cell proteins in the native state. NADP as well as NADPH were found to directly protect hemoglobin against denaturation by ascorbic acid. These data suggest that the protection afforded by pyridine nucleotides need not be mediated through GSH. It has been demonstrated that NADPH and NADP, but not GSH, are important to the stability and activity of G-6-P dehydrogenase (Marks *et al.*, 1961). GSH may not be an obligatory intermediate in all reactions involved in preventing oxidative denaturation of hemoglobin and other erythrocyte proteins. This problem is considered in further detail in Section IV, D, 6.

III. Properties of Erythrocyte Glucose-6-Phosphate Dehydrogenase

A. *Kinetic Studies of the Purified Enzyme*

G-6-P dehydrogenase has been crystallized from at least two sources, bovine mammary gland (Julian *et al.*, 1961) and yeast (Noltmann *et al.*, 1961). The enzyme from human erythrocytes has been extensively purified (Marks *et al.*, 1961; Kirkman, 1962; Marks and Tsutsui, 1963) and its properties studied. Purified G-6-P dehydrogenase from erythrocytes of human subjects with normal levels of the enzyme has a broad pH optimum of 8–9. The Michaelis constant, K_M, for G-6-P is $3.5 \times 10^{-5}\ M$, and for NADP $4 \times 10^{-6}\ M$. The specificity of the enzyme appears to be relatively high, but is not absolute. Thus if NAD is substituted for NADP, the reaction proceeds at less than 5% of the rate in the presence of NADP (Levy, 1961). No detectable reaction occurs with glucosamine-6-phosphate or with glucose. A slow rate of utilization of 2-deoxyglucose-6-phosphate and of galactose-6-phosphate by the enzyme can be detected when these sugars are substituted for G-6-P in the assay mixture. The NADP analogs, 3-acetylpyridine-NADP or thionicotinamide-NADP, do not replace NADP as cofactors for the purified red cell dehydrogenase. When 3-acetylpyridine-NADP was substituted for NADP in the standard assay procedure, a rate less than 5% of that observed with comparable concentrations of NADP was found. No detectable activity was observed when thionicotinamide-NADP was substituted for NADP. Nicotinamide, adenosine monophosphate, ADP, and ATP are all inhibitors of G-6-P dehydrogenase. This inhibition is competitive with NADP.

Red cell G-6-P dehydrogenase has a requirement for Mg^{++} for optimal activity. Ethylenediaminetetraacetate (EDTA) disodium salt concentration as high as 0.043 *M* had no detectable effect on activity of the enzyme in the absence of added magnesium. However, in the presence of 0.01 *M* magnesium, addition of sodium EDTA results in inhibition which is maximal at 0.017 *M* EDTA. At higher and lower EDTA concentration, the complex formed with the enzyme in the presence of Mg^{++} is less inhibitory.

Dehydroepiandrosterone, pregnenolone, and certain related steroids have been found to be potent inhibitors of mammalian G-6-P-dehydrogenase-catalyzed NADPH formation (Marks and Banks, 1960; McKerns and Kaleita, 1960). The action of these steroids has a specificity with regard to both dehydrogenase inhibited and structure of the inhibiting compound. Thus, G-6-P dehydrogenase of yeast and spinach and mammalian 6-phosphogluconic and isocitric dehydrogenases are not inhibited. All the steroids with an inhibitory action on erythrocyte G-6-P dehydrogenase possess a ketone group in the C-17 or C-20 position. Progesterone, corticosteroids, estrogens, and steroids with a hydroxyl rather than a ketone group at C-17 or C-20 have relatively little and generally no inhibitory effect on G-6-P dehydrogenase. On the other hand, the presence of a ketone or α- or β-hydroxyl group at C-3 or a saturated or unsaturated bond at C4-5 or C5-6 has little effect on the inhibitory action of the steroids tested. This effect of the steroids appears to be a catalytic one, since low concentrations of steroid inhibit the reduction of relatively large amounts of NADP.

B. Molecular Forms of Erythrocyte Glucose-6-Phosphate Dehydrogenase

Studies of the stability of purified preparations of erythrocyte G-6-P dehydrogenase provided evidence which first suggested that this enzyme exists in different forms varying in specific activity (Marks *et al.*, 1961). Thus, incubation of purified preparations of the erythrocyte enzyme in buffer solution was associated with an increase in its activity. Studies of the characteristics of this activation revealed that (a) it was dependent on enzyme concentration, more concentrated preparations being activated more readily than dilute preparations; (b) it was affected by the purity of the enzyme preparation; activation can readily be achieved with preparations having a specific activity of 1.3 units per ml. protein, but more purified preparations are difficult to activate; (c) maximal activation generally requires 2–4 hours and may result in as much as 10-fold increase in specific activity of the preparation; and (d) activation is temperature dependent with an optimum which varies with concentration of the enzyme and its purity (Marks *et al.*, 1961; Kirkman, 1962). Dilution of the enzyme is associated with loss in capacity to be activated. NADP or NADPH can protect the enzyme against inactivation by dilution or heat. This effect is specific in that NAD, GSH, ATP, G-6-P, and a variety of other agents are without effect.

Molecular forms of G-6-P dehydrogenase which vary in catalytic activity relative to antigenic activity and in sedimentation characteristics have been demonstrated (Tsutsui and Marks, 1962). These studies indicated that the loss of enzyme activity which occurs upon dilution of the enzyme or in the absence of NADP is associated with conversion of G-6-P dehydrogenase, in part, to a form which has lower catalytic activity per unit of antigenic activity and lower sedimentation velocity. The molecular alteration associated with removal of NADP is reversible upon reincubation of the enzyme with the pyridine nucleotide (Kirkman and Hendrickson, 1962; Tsutsui and Marks, 1962). Kirkman and Hendrickson (1962), employing such data and making the assumption that only two forms of the enzyme were present, calculated the relative molecular weights of the enzyme in the activated and subactivated states and concluded that they corresponded to a dimer and monomer, respectively.

Further evidence suggesting that NADP affects the molecular configuration of red cell G-6-P dehydrogenase was obtained by studies of the reaction between anti-human erythrocyte G-6-P dehydrogenase and enzyme (Marks and Tsutsui, 1963). The complex formed between enzyme and antibody varies with the concentration of NADP present in the reaction mixture.

NADP and NADPH appear to be strongly bound to the activated form of the enzyme (Marks *et al.*, 1961; Kirkman, 1962). Studies of the activated and subactivated states of red cell G-6-P dehydrogenase have revealed that there is no change in the affinity constants for NADP or G-6-P. The activated and subactive forms of the enzyme do differ in electrophoretic mobility (Marks, 1961a).

These data indicate that NADP is important for maintaining the configuration of human red cell G-6-P dehydrogenase optimal for catalytic activity. It seems reasonable to suggest that this enzyme exists in the erythrocyte in different molecular forms which vary in catalytic activity. These observations may have relevance to the reports by Ramot *et al.*, (1961) that an activator of G-6-P dehydrogenase exists in the stroma of normal erythrocytes, as evidenced by the finding that incubation of stroma of normal erythrocytes with hemolysates of G-6-P-deficient cells may be associated with an increase in enzyme activity (*vide infra*, Section IV, D, 5).

C. *Inactivation of Glucose-6-Phosphate Dehydrogenase by Red Cell Stroma*

The activity of G-6-P dehydrogenase decreases during incubation of hemolysates *in vitro*. The rate of decrease is temperature dependent. The stability of this enzyme in hemolysates is significantly increased if, before incubation, the stroma is removed by centrifugation (Carson *et al.*, 1959; Marks, 1961a). This is due to a factor in the stroma which inactivates the enzyme. Studies of the properties of this factor reveal that stromal inactivation of G-6-P dehydrogenase is a relatively selective phenomenon; stroma causes little or no inactivation of 6-phosphogluconic dehydrogenase, which also catalyzes NADP reduction, lactic acid dehydrogenase, an NAD-requiring enzyme, or of purine nucleoside phosphorylase. The inactivating effect of stroma on red cell G-6-P dehydrogenase can be prevented by addition of NADP, NADPH, or nicotinamide to crude hemolysates. The stromal inactivator is heat labile, nondialyzable, and destroyed by trypsin. It is associated with NADPase activity. It is possible that destruction by the stromal factor of the NADP necessary to the stability of red cell G-6-P dehydrogenase may play a role in determining the activity of this enzyme *in vivo*. These observations may have physiological significance in accounting, in part at least, for the selective decrease in activity of G-6-P dehydrogenase that occurs as erythrocytes age *in vivo* (*vide infra*, Section IV, A).

IV. Alterations in Erythrocyte Glucose-6-Phosphate Dehydrogenase under Various Biological Conditions

A. *Erythrocyte Aging in Vivo*

The major source of energy for the circulating nonnucleated erythrocyte is the metabolism of glucose (Denstedt, 1953; Bartlett, 1958). As erythrocytes age *in vivo*, the activity of several enzymes which catalyze reactions in the pathways of glucose metabolism decreases. Quantitatively, the decline in activity of G-6-P dehydrogenase and perhaps of glyceraldehyde-3-phosphate dehydrogenase appears to be more marked than that of several enzymes tested to date, including 6-phosphogluconic dehydrogenase, phosphohexose isomerase, aldolase, triose isomerase, 3-phosphoglyceric kinase, enolase, pyruvate kinase, lactic acid dehydrogenase, purine nucleoside phosphorylase and hemoglobin reductase (Marks *et al.*, 1958b; Lohr *et al.*, 1958).

The selective decrease in activity of G-6-P dehydrogenase could be an important factor in determining the lifespan of the erythrocyte. This enzyme is required in the mature red cell to generate NADPH. As might be anticipated on the basis of the changes in enzyme activity, the capacity of erythrocytes to generate NADPH declines as these cells age *in vivo* (Marks, 1962a). As indicated above (Section II, B), NADPH may be important in maintaining the integrity of certain proteins in the erythrocyte. It would follow that a deficiency in this reduced cofactor might predispose these proteins to denaturation and, as a consequence, lead to alterations in erythrocytes which make them particularly susceptible to lysis or to phagocytosis by cells of the reticuloendothelial system. The observations on alterations of enzyme activity with red cell aging *in vivo* have been made in detail with human erythrocytes. Extensive comparative studies of the activities of the several enzymes involved in carbohydrate metabolism in red cells of other animals have not been performed. The level of G-6-P dehydrogenase in rabbit reticulocytes appears to be significantly higher than in the mature erythrocyte (Tada *et al.*, 1961; Marks, unpublished observations). Studies of the level of G-6-P and 6-phosphogluconic dehydrogenases in erythrocytes of patients with reticulocytosis suggest that the activity of these enzymes is significantly higher in human reticulocytes than in mature nonreticulated cells (Marks, 1958).

An important role for G-6-P dehydrogenase in determining the survival of erythrocytes is also suggested with the genetically determined deficiency of this enzyme in man. Beutler *et al.* (1954b) demonstrated that in subjects with 6-G-P dehydrogenase deficiency, the older red cells are selectively destroyed during an acute episode of drug-induced hemolysis. The relative resistance of the younger red cells to hemolysis has been interpreted as reflecting the higher levels of G-6-P dehydrogenase in these cells which make them more resistant to destruction (Gross *et al.*, 1958). The increased susceptibility to hemolysis associated with genetically determined deficiency of G-6-P dehydrogenase may reflect the fact that the hereditary deficiency of the enzyme causes a premature senescence of red cells. Several lines of evidence are compatible with this hypothesis. Brewer *et al.* (1961) demonstrated that in subjects with genetically determined G-6-P dehydrogenase deficiency the erythrocyte lifespan is shorter than normal even in the absence of known exposure to potentially hemolytic agents. In erythrocytes of Negro subjects with genetically determined G-6-P dehydrogenase deficiency, the enzyme activity is higher in young than in old red cells and declines rapidly as the cells age (Marks and Gross, 1959). Jandl *et al* (1960) suggested that in the presence of G-6-P dehydrogenase deficiency, whether genetically determined or in normal aged cells, a similar sequence of events ensues which may result in the oxidative denaturation of hemoglobin. Recently Danon and co-workers (1961) have provided impressive electron microscope evidence that the majority of cells in subjects with the genetically determined enzyme deficiency have the same structural changes associated with normal aging of erythrocytes *in vivo*.

B. Maturation of the Subject

The activities of some enzymes in erythrocytes of premature and full-term infants differ from those of adults. Among the enzymes studied, G-6-P dehydrogenase and 6-phosphogluconic dehydrogenase activities appear to be significantly higher in premature and full-term infants than in normal adults (Gross and Hurwitz, 1958). In addition, the data of these authors suggested that G-6-P dehydrogenase activity is probably higher in red cells of premature infants than of full-term infants. The elevation in activities of the enzymes does not represent a transient state associated with birth, as it is not until well into the second six months of life that they consistently fall within the range of values for erythrocytes of normal adult subjects. The mechanism of the increased levels of these enzyme activities and their biological significance are unknown. It has been suggested that the higher levels reflect the fact that newborn infants have a red cell population with a younger mean age than adult subjects. This possibility has not been definitively evaluated experimentally. It would imply, of course, that the younger mean cell age of the population may persist through the first 8–10 months of life. Alternatively, the changes in enzyme level with maturation of the organism may be due to alteration in requirements for NADPH.

C. Blood Stored in Vitro

As erythrocytes are stored *in vitro* under usual blood bank conditions, that is, in acid-citrate-dextrose solution under sterile conditions at 4°C., there is a gradual loss in the average posttransfusion survival of cells (Gabrio *et al.*, 1956). Associated with this decrease in posttransfusion viability is a variety of biochemical changes, including decrease in glycolytic rate, decrease in potassium and increase in sodium content, increased osmotic fragility, decrease in concentration of ATP and other organic phosphates, and increase in concentration of inorganic phosphate. These striking metabolic changes occur in the absence of detectable decrease in activity of G-6-P dehydrogenase or 6-phosphogluconic dehydrogenase (Marks *et al.*, 1958a; Szeinberg *et al.*, 1958b; Marks, 1962b). These findings suggest a basic difference in the factors determining the deterioration of erythrocytes during storage *in vitro* under blood bank conditions and the aging of red cells *in vivo*. It would seem that the alterations associated with storage of red cells *in vitro* reflect primarily substrate exhaustion and accumulation of products of cell metabolism. On the other hand, the survival of cells *in vivo* appears to be limited by stability of the proteins necessary to catalyze one or more critical reactions or maintain structural integrity of the cell wall.

D. Genetically Determined Erythrocyte Glucose-6-Phosphate Dehydrogenase Deficiency

In studying the mechanism of primaquine-induced hemolytic anemia, Dern and co-workers (1954a) first provided evidence clearly indicating that the anemia caused by this drug involved an intrinsic abnormality of the erythrocyte. Further studies showed that the hemolysis induced by primaquine was self-limited and a function of the age of the cell, that is, the older cells were more susceptible to destruction (Dern *et al.*, 1954b; Beutler *et al.*, 1954a). Carson and co-workers (1956) subsequently demonstrated that the major defect in erythrocytes of subjects susceptible to primaquine-induced hemolytic anemia was a deficiency in G-6-P dehydrogenase activity. Erythrocyte G-6-P dehydrogenase deficiency was soon recognized to be a genetically determined trait of intermediate dominance, transmitted by a gene linked to the X-chromosome (Childs *et al.*, 1958; Gross *et al.*, 1958; Larizza *et al.*, 1958; Szeinberg *et al.*, 1958c). It was demonstrated that this genetically determined enzyme deficiency was the predisposing factor in the increased susceptibility to hemolysis in certain subjects upon exposure to a wide variety of drugs, ingestion of *Vicia faba*, and exposure to certain bacterial and viral infections (Table I).

TABLE I[a]

AGENTS REPORTED TO INDUCE HEMOLYTIC ANEMIA IN SUBJECTS WITH GLUCOSE-6-PHOSPHATE DEHYDROGENASE DEFICIENCY

Primaquine	Quinine
Pamaquine	Quinidine
Pentaquine	*p*-Aminosalicyclic acid
Quinocide	Antipyrine
Sulfanilamide	Probenecid
Sulfapyridine	Acetanilide
Sulfisoxazole	Phenylhydrazine
Sulfacetamide	Acetophenetidine
Sulfamethoxypyridazine	Pyramidone
Salicylazosulfapyridine	Chloroquine
Sulfones (sulfoxone)	Fava bean
Naphthalene	Viral respiratory infections
Methylene blue	Infectious hepatitis
Vitamin K	Infectious mononucleosis
Acetylsalicylic acid	Bacterial pneumonias and
Nitrofurantoin	septicemias (e.g. typhoid)
Furazoladone	Diabetic acidosis

[a] Detailed references to sources for this table are cited in Larizza *et al.* (1958); Szeinberg and Sheba (1958); Waller (1959); Marks (1961a), Kellermeyer *et al.* (1962), Tarlov *et al.* (1962).

1. Clinical Course

The characteristics of the clinical course of the hemolytic anemia following ingestion of primaquine by a Negro subject with red cell G-6-P dehydrogenase deficiency have been well characterized (Dern *et al.*, 1954b, Kellermeyer *et al.*, 1961b). In these studies primaquine, 30 mg. per day, was administered to healthy adult Negro males with G-6-P dehydrogenase deficiency. In the typical course, acute hemolysis becomes clinically detectable as a fall in hematocrit by the second to fourth day of drug administration. The hematocrit reaches its lowest level between the seventh and twelfth days of drug therapy and thereafter tends to rise toward normal values despite continued administration of the drug. During the acute hemolytic phase symptoms are uncommon but, if present, are related to the anemia. Heinz bodies appear in large numbers during the first few days of drug administration, but disappear as the acute hemolytic phase progresses. A rise in serum bilirubin with darkening of the urine may occur. It was demonstrated (Beutler *et al.*, 1954a) that it is the older erythrocytes that are destroyed during the acute hemolytic phase. If drug administration is continued during the recovery phase when the hematocrit is returning to normal levels, a marked shortening of the life-span of the cell will continue to be present. Under these circumstances, there is a "compensated" hemolytic anemia with increased rate of production and destruction of red cells. Following an acute hemolytic episode, there is a phase of relative resistance to further hemolysis upon subsequent exposure to a potentially offending agent. This resistance decreases with time and is related to the dose of offending agent administered; the higher the dose the less the apparent resistance to hemolysis. The increased resistance to hemolysis following an acute hemolytic episode has been interpreted as reflecting the fact that the surviving erythrocytes, being primarily young cells, have higher levels of G-6-P dehydrogenase and are therefore relatively more resistant to destruction (Gross *et al.*, 1958).

In contrast to the rather mild clinical picture of primaquine-induced hemolytic anemia, the acute anemia which may follow exposure of a G-6-P-dehydrogenase-deficient subject to *Vicia faba* may be quite severe (Sansone and Segni, 1957; Sansone *et al.*, 1958; Larizza *et al.*, 1958; Panizon, 1960). In a typical case a susceptible subject, a few minutes after walking through a blossoming broad bean field or a few hours after ingestion of the seeds, suddenly experiences headache, malaise, chills, nausea and vomiting, lumbar pains, dizziness; occasionally he may lose consciousness. Temperature rises to 39–40°C. and after 5–30 hours hemoglobinuria, often massive, appears and persists for 1–3 days. Icterus develops a few hours after the appearance of hemoglobinuria, with hepatosplenomegaly. The disease follows a rapid course. In less severe cases, or when transfusion therapy is promptly started, fever and symptoms subside in 2–6 days. In fatal cases, death almost invariably takes place within the first 2 days. In a series of 1211 cases (Fermi, 1905 quoted by Luisada, 1941), the death rate was 8% and entirely restricted to children. In this series the attacks had been caused by ingestion of the bean in 62% of the cases and by inhalation in 38%. The blood picture is characterized by severe anemia, with red cell counts as low as 1 million, reticulocyte counts as high as 50–60%, anisocytosis, and presence of Heinz bodies in a large proportion of cells. Leucocytosis is often seen during the acute phase.

As indicated in Table I, in addition to a variety of drugs, hemolytic anemia has been seen in association with viral and bacterial infections and certain profound disturbances in metabolic states such as diabetic acidosis (Larizza *et al.*, 1958; Marks, 1959; Szeinberg *et al.*, 1960a, b; Gant and Winks, 1961). The hemolytic effect of most agents appears to be related to dose. The presence of renal or liver disease, perhaps by affecting rate of excretion of drugs, seems to be a factor contributing to increased severity of hemolytic episodes in affected subjects.

Brewer and co-workers (1961) demonstrated that the lifespan of erythrocytes of Negro male subjects with erythrocyte G-6-P dehydrogenase deficiency may be 25% shorter than normal even in the absence of normal exposure to a potentially hemolytic agent. This increased rate of hemolysis is generally not associated with clinically detectable anemia and presumably is accompanied by an increased rate of erythropoiesis. The mean age of the erythrocyte population of these subjects is younger than normal, and the cells are reported to show an increase in mean cell size and decrease in osmotic fragility (Tarlov *et al.*, 1962).

2. Biochemical Alterations

The deficiency in G-6-P dehydrogenase (Carson *et al.*, 1956) is probably the primary manifestation of the altered gene in subjects with increased susceptibility to drug-induced hemolytic anemia. This concept is based on the fact that to date, while a great variety of biochemical alterations have been described in the red cells of these subjects, the decrease in G-6-P dehydrogenase is quantitatively the most marked deviation from normal, and genetic analysis of the transmission of this trait, employing G-6-P dehydrogenase as a marker, yields the most consistent results (Gross *et al.*, 1958; Childs and Zinkham, 1959).

The biochemical alterations found in erythrocytes of affected subjects include an impaired capacity to generate NADPH (Marks, 1962b) and an increased concentration of NADP (Schrier *et al.*, 1958a; Bonsignore *et al.*, 1961b); a decreased oxygen consumption (Johnson and Marks, 1958; Kellermeyer *et al.*, 1961a); a diminished rate of methemoglobin reduction (Dawson *et al.*, 1958; Brewer *et al.*, 1960a); a diminished pentose formation in the presence of methylene blue (Kellermeyer *et al.*, 1961a; Fornaini *et al.*, 1962);

and a decreased capacity to respond to various potentially oxidative reagents, such as methylene blue, ascorbic acid, cysteine, etc., by increasing the rate of NADPH generation (Szeinberg and Marks, 1961; Kellermeyer *et al.*, 1961a; Fornaini *et al.*, 1962).

GSH concentration in red cells of affected subjects is generally lower than that of normal persons (Beutler, 1955a; Flanagan *et al.*, 1958). Beutler *et al.* (1955b, 1957) reported that, following *in vitro* incubation with acetylphenylhydrazine, erythrocytes of affected subjects, but not of normal subjects, show marked decrease in GSH concentration. The author suggested that this reduced stability of GSH in G-6-P-dehydrogenase-deficient red cells might be used as a basis for a test to detect individuals with genetically determined G-6-P dehydrogenase deficiency. The alterations in NADPH metabolism, oxygen consumption, pentose formation, and GSH stability are presumably a consequence of G-6-P dehydrogenase deficiency.

Of particular interest with regard to the disordered NADPH metabolism of these cells are the studies of Bonsignore *et al.* (1961b) on the biosynthesis of pyridine coenzymes in erythrocytes of subjects with G-6-P dehydrogenase deficiency. These investigators found that pyridine nucleotide formation is normal or even increased in the red cells of affected subjects. This suggests that the nonoxidative reactions of the pentose phosphate pathway play a major role in pentose formation in red cells.

In addition to the biochemical changes which may be related to the decreased G-6-P dehydrogenase activity, a variety of alterations have been reported whose significance remains conjectural. The activities of glutathione reductase (Schrier *et al.*, 1958b) and aldolase (Schrier *et al.*, 1959) were reported to be increased and that of catalase decreased (Alving *et al.*, 1960). At variance with these findings, however, are reports of normal levels of catalase (Beutler *et al.*, 1955a; Szeinberg *et al.*, 1957), aldolase (Heller and Weinstein, 1959), and glutathione reductase (Bonsignore *et al.*, 1960a). Methemoglobin reductase activity was found to be markedly decreased (Bonsignore *et al.*, 1960a; Jaffé, 1963) and activities of transketolase and transaldolase increased in red cells of subjects with a history of favism (Bonsignore *et al.*, 1961a). No such elevations in transketolase or transaldolase were detected among affected Negro subjects (Kellermeyer *et al.*, 1961a). The activities of 6-phosphogluconic dehydrogenase, phosphohexo isomerase, triose isomerase, glyceraldehyde-3-phosphate dehydrogenase, isocitric dehydrogenase, malic dehydrogenase, purine nucleoside phosphorylase, lactic acid dehydrogenase, glutathione peroxidase, and acetyl cholinesterase were all found to be within normal levels (Johnson and Marks, 1958; Gross *et al.*, 1958; Schrier *et al.*, 1958b; Heller and Weinstein, 1959; Tarlov *et al.*, 1962). The mechanism of the elevation in activity of enzymes in red cells of subjects with G-6-P dehydrogenase deficiency remains to be elucidated. An increase in enzyme activity could reflect a younger than normal mean red cell age with shortened lifespan. On the other hand, these elevations in enzyme activity may indeed represent an increase in activity which is a "compensation" for the G-6-P dehydrogenase deficiency. The apparent discrepancies in findings between different groups of investigators, such as those relating to transketolase and transaldolase activities (Bonsignore *et al.*, 1961a; Kellermeyer *et al.*, 1961a) and to catalase activity (Alving *et al.*, 1960; Szeinberg *et al.*, 1957), may reflect a heterogeneity in the expression of G-6-P deficiency in different ethnic groups.

Among other metabolic defects detected in red cells of affected subjects is a decreased rate of incorporation of glycine into glutathione (Szeinberg *et al.*, 1959b). There is decreased stability of ATP upon *in vitro* incubation of the erythrocytes with phenylhydrazine (Mohler and Williams, 1961). Ascorbic acid, cysteine, pyruvic acid, and a variety of potentially hemolytic agents can markedly decrease the conversion of glucose to lactic acid, presumably with consequent decrease in ATP generation (Szeinberg and Marks, 1961). The diminished glycolytic activity in acetylphenylhydrazine-treated cells is not associated with alteration in activity of glyceraldehyde-3-phosphate dehydrogenase or lactic acid dehydrogenase (Sternschuss *et al.*, 1961).

In addition to the biochemical changes present in erythrocytes of asymptomatic affected subjects, a variety of biochemical changes have been reported which occur only during hemolytic episodes. Among these changes is a fall in catalase activity, reported to be among the first detectable changes in the erythrocyte which occur following exposure to a potentially hemolytic agent (Tarlov and Kellermeyer, 1959). A sharp drop in reduced glutathione may occur within 36 hours after the initial dose of drug and before major hemolysis takes place (Flanagan *et al.*, 1958). The methemoglobinemia occurring during the course of a hemolytic episode is generally slight and transient. Brewer *et al.* (1962a) have suggested that this is due to the fact that, though there is an increase in methemoglobin formation, it is the older cells which contain the highest concentration and these cells are quickly destroyed in the hemolytic episodes. The total lipids of G-6-P-dehydrogenase-deficient cells has been reported to be lower than normal and to decrease further during drug-induced hemolysis (Tarlov *et al.*, 1962). G-6-P dehydrogenase activity of the whole red cell population rises during the acute hemolytic episode in affected Negro subjects, reflecting the selective destruction of older cells (Marks, unpublished observations). Such increases in erythrocyte G-6-P dehydrogenase activity following acute hemolytic episodes has not been found among Sardinians (Bonsignore *et al.*, 1960b). These differences between affected Negroes and affected Caucasians are consistent with the observations that the dehydrogenase level in erythrocytes of affected Negro males, but not of affected Caucasian males, is significantly higher in young compared with old red cells (Marks and Gross, 1959).

3. Incidence

G-6-P dehydrogenase deficiency is widespread and varies markedly in incidence among different population groups (Table II). It has been estimated that more than one hundred million people carry this trait (Carson and Tarlov, 1962).

TABLE II[a]
INCIDENCE OF GLUCOSE-6-PHOSPHATE DEHYDROGENASE DEFICIENCY TRAIT

Group	Incidence
Ashkenazic Jews (males)	0.4
Sephardic Jews (males)	
Kurds	58.2
Iraq	24.8
Persia	15.1
Caucasus	28.0
Cochin	10.3
Yemen	5.3
North Africa	<1.0–4.0
Arabs	4.4
Sardinians (males)	4.0–30.0
Greeks (including Cyprus and Crete)	0.7–3.0
American Negroes	13.0
Nigerians	10·0
Bantu	20.0
Iranians	8.5
Chinese	±[c]
Malays	+[b]
Javanese	3
American Indians	
Oyana (males)	16
Carib (males)	2
Peruvian (males)	0

[a] Detailed references to sources for this table are given in Beutler (1960); Marks (1961a); Tarlov *et al.* (1962). The data on the Jews is based on a personal communication from A. Szeinberg and C. Sheba.

[b] Trait has been reported among members of this population group, but incidence figures are not available.

[c] Trait exists in this group, but may be relatively rare.

The geographic distribution of the trait corresponds roughly to that of falciparum malaria. This apparent relationship between the geographic distribution of G-6-P dehydrogenase deficiency and falciparum malaria suggested to Motulsky (1960) and to Allison and Clyde (1961) that the enzyme deficiency may represent an example of a balanced polymorphism. The detrimental effects of the mutation would be balanced by the protection it affords against the lethal effects of this type of malaria. Recently this hypothesis has been questioned by Kidson and Gorman (1962a) on the basis of the finding of a low incidence of the deficiency in large groups such as Malays, Indonesians, and Armenians and small groups such as the Tolai and Sause in Melanesia, all of whom inhabit haloendemic malarious areas. Of interest is the finding of Fletcher and Maegraith (1962) that malarial infection in monkeys caused by *Plasmodium knowlesi* is associated with striking increase in erythrocyte G-6-P dehydrogenase activity, which could not be accounted for on the basis of the development of a younger than normal erythrocyte population. The authors suggested that it might reflect the fact that the malaria organism causes activation of the inactive form of G-6-P dehydrogenase as a compensatory phenomenon for its increased needs for NADPH or pentose. The low GSH content and diminished activity of the pentose phosphate pathway of G-6-P-dehydrogenase-deficient erythrocytes may produce an environment unfavorable to intracellular survival of the malaria parasite (Trager, 1941; McKee, 1951).

It is likely that interaction of the enzyme defect with several factors, including viral and bacterial infections, dietary habits, and social customs of a particular ethnic group, as well as malaria, contributes to the present distribution of this trait. In addition to malaria, it has been specifically suggested that thalassemia may play a role in determining the incidence of G-6-P deficiency among certain population groups (Siniscalco *et al.*, 1961). Both G-6-P dehydrogenase deficiency and thalassemia may protect their carriers against malaria. Subjects with thalassemia minor have erythrocytes with a short survival time and consequently a younger than normal red cell population with relatively higher levels of G-6-P dehydrogenase. In Sardinia there is a particularly high incidence of favism. The tendency toward higher levels of red cell G-6-P dehydrogenase in subjects with thalassemia may be a factor in protecting against the hemolytic crisis associated with favism.

In certain areas there is a significant incidence of neonatal jaundice and kernicterus, unassociated with blood group incompatibility, among Negro (Gilles and Arthur, 1960) and Caucasian (Doxiadis *et al.*, 1961; Vella, 1959; DeToni, 1961; Panizon, 1960; Harley and Robin, 1962) infants having erythrocyte G-6-P dehydrogenase deficiency. In such populations mortality during the newborn period due to hyperbilirubinemia might be a factor in determining the incidence of the enzyme deficiency.

4. Mode of Inheritance

Family studies and analysis of the incidence of G-6-P dehydrogenase deficiency among Negro and Caucasian populations have suggested that this trait is due to a gene of intermediate dominance which is linked to the X-chromosome (Childs *et al.*, 1958; Gross *et al.*, 1958; Szeinberg *et al.*, 1958b; Larizza *et al.*, 1960). More definitive proof of this suggestion was obtained from various studies on the linkage relationships between G-6-P dehydrogenase and other traits believed to be due to genes on the X-chromosome. Such studies have suggested that G-6-P dehydrogenase and color blindness, of both the protan and deutan types, are closely linked with a recombination fraction of about 5% in African (Porter *et al.*, 1962) and Mediterranean people (Adam, 1961; Siniscalco *et al.*, 1961). These studies further suggested that the protan and deutan loci for color blindness may be separated and that the G-6-P dehydrogenase locus may lie between the two loci for color blindness (Kalmus. 1962). In addition, Adam and his colleagues (1962) studied the relationship between G-6-P dehydrogenase deficiency and X_g blood groups and found a recombination fraction of approximately 25%, indicating that these two factors were due to genes rather widely separated on the X-chromosome.

The relationship between gene dosage and enzyme level has been studied in a variety of laboratories. The normal XX female has no higher erythrocyte G-6-P dehydrogenase activity than the normal XY male (Marks, 1958). In affected males with a single gene for G-6-P dehydrogenase which is the mutant gene, the level of enzyme is generally very low. By contrast, similarly low levels of the enzyme are uncommon among females, probably reflecting the fact that the homozygous female is a relatively rare individual. More commonly, affected females are heterozygous and the level of enzyme in red cells is generally intermediate between that of affected males and normal levels. The level of erythrocyte G-6-P dehydrogenase in persons with 3 or 4 X-chromosomes was found not to be elevated, with a single exception (Grumbach *et al.*, 1962). The exception, a subject with a 4 X-chromosome constitution, had an elevated dehydrogenase level and the presence of a young red cell population was not excluded.

One explanation for the fact that homozygous normal females with two X-chromosomes have no more enzyme than the normal male with one X-chromosome is that only one X-chromosome per cell is genetically active during interphase (Lyon, 1962). In females heterozygous for G-6-P dehydrogenase deficiency with intermediate levels of the enzyme, Beutler *et al.* (1962) studied the *in vitro* rate of disappearance of red cell GSH in the presence of acetylphenylhydrazine. He interpreted his findings as indicating the presence of two populations of erythrocytes, one with normal levels and one with very low levels of G-6-P dehydrogenase. An alternative explanation of these findings is that each cell had two types of enzyme rather than two populations of cells, each with a different type of enzyme. Thus the data obtained by Beutler *et al.* neither support nor refute the mosaic hypothesis of Lyon. Brewer *et al.* (1962b) investigated this problem by a study of erythrocyte survival in heterozygous females and failed to demonstrate cells with a normal survival and cells with a short survival. These findings, unfortunately based on relatively few observations, would suggest that the mosaic theory does not obtain for the G-6-P dehydrogenase trait in man.

Davidson *et al.* (1963) have recently presented the first direct evidence in favor of the mosaic hypothesis. These authors developed cell clones from single cells of tissue cultures of skin biopsies from females who were normal or who were heterozygous for G-6-P dehydrogenase deficiency. Both quantitative assay of enzyme activity and qualitative evaluation of the electrophoretic mobility of the enzyme showed that there are two distinct populations of cells in females with respect to G-6-P dehydrogenase.

5. Molecular Heterogeneity of G-6-P Dehydrogenase Deficiency

Genetically determined G-6-P dehydrogenase deficiency is not a homogeneous entity. Rather, the present evidence indicates that the molecular defect associated with the decreased enzyme activity may differ in affected subjects of varying ethnic origin. It is not yet known whether this heterogeneity reflects different mutations at a single locus on the X-chromosome or mutations at different loci which determine the formation and function of the dehydrogenase.

The molecular heterogeneity in G-6-P dehydrogenase is manifest as (1) variations in severity of the decrease in enzyme activity, (2) differences in electrophoretic mobility of the enzyme, (3) differences in susceptibility of the enzyme to inactivation by erythrocyte stroma, and (4) alterations in properties of the catalytic site of the enzyme (Table III).

A molecular heterogeneity in G-6-P dehydrogenase deficiency was first suggested by the observation that significant differences existed between affected subjects of different ethnic origin with respect to the severity of enzyme deficiency in erythrocytes and in leucocytes (Marks and Gross, 1959). Affected Caucasian males predominantly of Greek and Southern Italian extraction were found to have on the average significantly lower red cell G-6-P dehydrogenase activities than affected Negro males. In addition, in affected Caucasian males the leucocyte enzyme level averaged 30% of normal, while in affected Negro males it was only slightly reduced or within the normal range. Recently a third type of G-6-P dehydrogenase deficiency was distinguished on the basis of the severity of decrease in enzyme activity. In a family in Northern Italy (Barbieri family), affected males have only 50% decrease in red cell G-6-P dehydrogenase activity and normal levels of leucocyte (Marks *et al.*, 1962). No differences have been detected among heterozygous females of these three population groups with respect to erythrocyte or leucocyte enzyme levels. Affected females generally have about 50% decrease in red cell G-6-P dehydrogenase and normal leucocyte enzyme activity (Marks and Gross, 1959). There are

TABLE III.

HETEROGENEITY IN PROPERTIES OF G-6-P DEHYDROGENASE AMONG DIFFERENT POPULATION GROUPS

Ethnic or geographic group	Enzyme activity[a] % of normal		Substrate affinities		pH Optima	Stability[b]	Electrophoretic[c] mobility
	Red cells	White cells	K_m(G6P)	K_m(TPN)			
Negro males (1)[d]	10–15	Normal or slightly decreased	Normal	Normal	Normal	Decreased	A−
Barbieri, males (2)[d] (Northern Italian)	50	Normal	Slightly increased	Increased	Normal	Normal	Fast
Sicilian (3)[d]	1–4	Decreased	Slightly increased	Increased	Normal	Decreased	Unknown
Sardinian (4)[d]	<1	Decreased	Unknown	Unknown	Unknown	Decreased markedly	Fast
CNSH (Caucasian) (5)[d]	3–9	Unknown	Increased	Increased	"Symmetrically narrow"	Decreased markedly	Unknown
CNSH (Caucasian) (3)[d]	<1	Decreased	Increased	Normal	Higher	Decreased markedly	Unknown
Sephardic Jew (6)[d]	3–6	Decreased	Slightly decreased	Slightly decreased	"Broad"	Decreased	Normal

ABBREVIATIONS: CNHS—Chronic, non-spherocytic hemolytic anemia. K_{mG6P} and K_{mTPN} are the Michaelis constants of the enzyme for G-6-P and TPN, respectively.

[a] Enzyme activity is expressed in percent of the mean normal level in red cells or white cells.

[b] Stability of G-6-P dehydrogenase during incubation of hemolysates in the presence of stroma.

[c] Electrophoretic mobility of G-6-P dehydrogenase in starch gel.

A− refers to type of G-6-P dehydrogenase and follows nomenclature of Boyer *et al.* (1962). Three electrophoretic patterns of G-6-P dehydrogenase were found in normal erythrocytes. A slow G-6-P dehydrogenase, designated A, a slightly faster component, designated B, and a broad band which seemed to represent a mixture of both and was observed only in females, designated AB. For all parameters, differences in methods employed in the several laboratories may contribute to apparent differences between the enzyme of various affected subjects.

[d] For details, reference should be made to the original papers as follows: (1) Kirkman (1959); Marks *et al.* (1959b); Marks *et al.* (1961); Boyer *et al.* (1962). (2) Marks *et al.* (1962). (3) Marks (1961a), Marks (1963). (4) Bonsignore, Fornaini, Segni, Leoncini, and Marks

females with erythrocyte and leucocyte dehydrogenase levels comparable to those of affected males and it is presumed that these women are homozygous. In addition to deficiency of the enzyme in erythrocytes and leucocytes, among affected Caucasian males it is decreased in liver (Brunetti *et al.*, 1960), saliva (Ramot *et al.*, 1960), platelets (Ramot *et al.*, 1959a), and skin (Gartler *et al.*, 1962). By contrast, among affected Negro males the level of G-6-P dehydrogenase in leucocytes and hepatic tissue is only slightly decreased or within the normal range (Marks *et al.*, 1959a). The activity of the enzyme is markedly decreased in lens tissue (Zinkham, 1960) and in platelets (Wurzel *et al.*, 1961), which are nonnucleated cells as are erythrocytes. [Deficiency of G-6-P dehydrogenase may be present in many tissues of affected Negro subjects. Thus, affected Negro subjects have a defect in steroid reduction presumably requiring NADPH (Borkofsky *et al.*, 1962), and the rate of whole body oxidation of glucose-1-C^{14} determined by measuring $C^{14}O_2$ in the expired air was markedly below normal (Tarlov *et al.*, 1962).]

Recent studies by Boyer *et al.* (1962) and Kirkman (1963) have demonstrated several electrophoretic variants of G-6-P dehydrogenase among Negro subjects with normal levels of the enzyme. A particular G-6-P dehydrogenase variant, referred to as type A, was found in all but one of 63 G-6-P-dehydrogenase-deficient Negro males (Boyer *et al.*, 1962). In contrast to these affected Negroes, Greek G-6-P-dehydrogenase-deficient subjects were found to possess a different electrophoretic type, referred to as type B. One subject with congenital nonspherocytic hemolytic anemia presented a unique electrophoretic pattern differing from either type A or B. The relevance of this latter finding to the electrophoretic variant reported by Marks *et al.* (1962) is not known.

Further indications of heterogeneity at a molecular level in G-6-P dehydrogenase deficiency are found in the studies of properties of the enzyme in various affected subjects. The enzyme in crude hemolysates from erythrocytes of affected Caucasian subjects is significantly more thermolabile than that in comparable preparations from erythrocytes of affected Negro males (Marks *et al.*, 1959b). Despite this difference in thermostability of the enzyme in crude hemolysates, no differences were detected in studies of a wide variety of properties of the catalytic site (Kirkman, 1959; Marks *et al.*, 1961) and antigenic properties (Marks and Tsutsui, 1963) of purified enzyme preparations from erythrocytes of affected Negro and Caucasian males. The differences in thermostability of G-6-P dehydrogenase in crude hemolysates are not detected upon purification of the enzyme. This suggests that this difference reflects a variation in the rate of inactivation of the enzyme by the stromal inactivator. No quantitative or qualitative difference has been detected with respect to the inactivator of G-6-P dehydrogenase in stroma prepared from erythrocytes of affected Negro and Caucasian males, compared with that prepared from erythrocytes of subjects with normal levels of the dehydrogenase (Marks and

Szeinberg, 1960; Marks, 1962b). It is likely that the enzyme in affected Negroes and Caucasians is altered so as to be more susceptible to inactivation by the stroma.

Anomalous properties have been detected in purified preparations of G-6-P dehydrogenase from erythrocytes of a patient with nonspherocytic hemolytic anemia associated with G-6-P dehydrogenase deficiency (Kirkman *et al.*, 1960). Several other patients, all Caucasians, with chronic nonspherocytic hemolytic anemia in association with marked erythrocyte G-6-P dehydrogenase deficiency have been reported (Newton and Bass, 1958; Lohr and Waller, 1958; Zinkham and Lenhard, 1959; Shahidi and Diamond, 1959; Marks, 1961a). In the patient reported by Marks (1961a), studies of enzyme properties revealed little, if any, alterations from those of the normal enzyme. A G-6-P dehydrogenase with altered properties with respect to catalytic site and electrophoretic mobility was found in affected members of the Barbieri family (Marks *et al.*, 1962).

Recently Ramot and co-workers (Rimon *et al.*, 1960; Ramot *et al.*, 1961) reported evidence which they interpreted as indicating that there is an activator of G-6-P dehydrogenase present in stroma of normal red cells and lacking in subjects with genetically determined G-6-P dehydrogenase deficiency. In an attempt to confirm these observations, data have been obtained to suggest that the results indicating an apparent stromal activator may be due, in part, to G-6-P dehydrogenase retained in stroma prepared from red cells by gradual hemolysis (Marks *et al.*, 1961). No evidence for lack of an activator could be detected in stroma prepared from red cells of affected subjects in these latter studies. Grignani *et al.* (1960) and Kidson and Gorman (1962b) presented studies similar to those of Ramot *et al.*, which they interpreted as confirming the presence of G-6-P dehydrogenase activator in normal erythrocyte stroma, which was absent in certain affected subjects. However, Kidson and Gorman (1962b) failed to demonstrate lack of an activator in the many deficient subjects studied and suggested that this reflects a possible heterogeneity among G-6-P-dehydrogenase-deficient subjects in the New Guinea population from which their affected subjects were derived. While the suggestion that G-6-P dehydrogenase deficiency may reflect the deficiency of an activator in at least certain affected subjects is a potentially exciting finding, conclusions as to its validity must await more definitive demonstration of the nature of the activator. The relationship is not clear between the activation observed in the studies by Ramot *et al.*, and the effect of NADP in activating G-6-P dehydrogenase (Marks *et al.*, 1961; Kirkman, 1962).

On the basis of studies to date it is apparent that there are several types of G-6-P dehydrogenase deficiency. It is not yet possible to describe with any precision the number or exact nature of the different types of G-6-P dehydrogenase. This may well have to await an understanding of the molecular basis for the apparent differences in the properties of the G-6-P dehydrogenases from different population groups. All affected Negro males described to date may be characterized as a rather homogeneous group with a G-6-P dehydrogenase having a mobility like that of the faster electrophoretic component normally present, a decrease in stability in the presence of stromal inactivator, roughly a 90% decrease in red cell enzyme activity, and no detectable alteration in the properties of the catalytic or antigenic sites of the enzyme (Marks, 1963; Kirkman and Hendrickson, 1963). Affected Caucasians comprise a heterogeneous group with respect to the properties of the dehydrogenase and the levels of enzyme activity in erythrocytes and other cells. Differences in the properties of the catalytic site of the enzyme and of the electrophoretic mobility have been described (Kirkman *et al.*, 1960; Marks, 1961a; Marks *et al.*, 1962; Marks, 1963; Kirkman, 1963). The degree of homogeneity among affected Caucasians could reflect a variety of structural gene mutations as the basis of the enzyme deficiency. On the other hand, the failure to detect evidence of an abnormal protein in affected Negroes and the apparent homogeneity in expression of the deficiency of this group make it attractive to speculate that a regulator gene mutation is the basis of the enzyme deficiency among these people.

6. Mechanism of Hemolysis

The mechanism by which a deficiency in G-6-P dehydrogenase, either genetically determined or normally occurring in aged cells, may predispose the erythrocyte to destruction is not defined. Some of the evidence suggesting that the enzyme deficiency leads to decrease in the reducing potential (NADPH) necessary to protect red cell proteins against oxidative denaturation has been summarized in Section II, B of this chapter.

It has been postulated or demonstrated by a number of investigators that potentially hemolytic agents, such as phenylhydrazine, and physiological substances, such as ascorbic acid and cysteine, can cause an oxidative denaturation of hemoglobin and probably other proteins (Emerson *et al.*, 1941; Heubner, 1941; Keilin and Hartree, 1943, 1946; Horecker, 1944; Lemberg and Legge, 1949; Merlini, 1952; Beaven and White, 1954; Mills and Randall, 1958; Jandl *et al.*, 1960a; Szeinberg and Marks, 1961). It has been suggested that the oxidative denaturation caused by these agents results from generation of hydrogen peroxide (Cohen and Hochstein, 1961). On the other hand, these compounds with the potential for causing hemolytic anemia may be intermediates between oxygen and hemoglobin and in the presence of oxygen each catalyze the destruction of the other (Emerson *et al.*, 1941; Lemberg and Legge, 1949; Beaven and White, 1954; Jandl *et al.*, 1960).

NADPH either directly or through the generation of GSH can protect red cells against the damaging effects of various potentially oxidative agents

(Keilin and Hartree, 1943; Fegler, 1951; Benesch and Benesch, 1954; Mills, 1957; Beutler, 1960; Szeinberg and Marks, 1961). Mills (1957) demonstrated that GSH can protect hemoglobin of bovine red cells from oxidation in the presence of the enzyme glutathione peroxidase. In studies with hemolysates of human red cells, it was found that NADP or NADPH without added GSH could protect hemoglobin against denaturation in the presence of ascorbic acid (Szeinberg and Marks, 1961). NADP or NADPH is important to the stability of proteins other than hemoglobin, specifically G-6-P dehydrogenase.

In G-6-P-dehydrogenase-deficient cells the capacity to generate NADPH is limited, as previously indicated (Section II, A). Cysteine, ascorbic acid, pyruvic acid, and agents recognized as potentially hemolytic, e.g., methylene blue, acetylphenylhydrazine, α- and β-naphthol, primaquine, and nitrofurantoin, appear to increase the rate of NADPH oxidation. It seems reasonable to suggest that, under conditions of limited NADPH generation, various substances which reoxidize NADPH could lead to an inadequate supply of reducing potential. Under such circumstances, vital enzymes or constituents of the red cell membrane may be susceptible to oxidative denaturation. It was also observed that these compounds markedly decreased the rate of conversion of glucose to lactic acid. This could be associated with decrease in the rate of ATP formation, an additional factor predisposing erythrocytes to destruction.

V. Glucose-6-Phosphate Dehydrogenase Assays

Adequate methods for quantitative estimation of G-6-P dehydrogenase in erythrocytes, leucocytes, and other tissues have been described in detail (Glock and McLean, 1954; Marks, 1958; Carson, 1961). These several methods have been critically evaluated (Carson, 1961; Marks, 1962a).

In addition to quantitative techniques for assay of G-6-P dehydrogenase, several semiquantitative tests have been developed which provide a more ready means of determining the presence of G-6-P dehydrogenase deficiency. These methods include a dye reduction test (Motulsky, personal communication) based on the principle that reduction of certain dyes may be coupled with reoxidation of NADPH. Thus, in the presence of excess G-6-P and NADP, the rate at which dye reduction occurs is proportional to the rate of NADPH formation, which in turn is in proportion to the enzyme concentration. The details of this method and critical evaluation of its indications and limitations are described elsewhere (Marks, 1962a). More recently a simple assay of G-6-P dehydrogenase has been devised, based on the principle of linking NADPH formation to methemoglobin reduction (Brewer *et al.*, 1960a; Tarlov *et al.*, 1962). Other relatively simple assays for G-6-P dehydrogenase have been described by Ells and Kirkman (1961) and Fairbanks and Beutler (1962).

ACKNOWLEDGMENTS

Studies cited in this review from the author's laboratory were supported, in part, by grants from the U.S. Public Health Service and the National Science Foundation. The author is indebted to Doctor Lucio Luzzatto for aid in preparing portions of this manuscript relating to favism.

REFERENCES

Adam, A. (1961). *Nature* **189**, 686.

Adam, A., Sheba, C., Race, R. R., and Sanger, R. (1962). *Lancet* **1**, 1188.

Allison, A. C., and Clyde, D. F. (1961). *Brit. Med. J.* **1**, 1346.

Altman, K. I. (1959). *Am. J. Med.* **27**, 936.

Alving, A. S., Tarlov, A. R., Brewer, G., Carson, P. E., Kellermeyer, R. W., and Long, W. K. (1960). *Trans. Assoc. Am. Physicians* **72**, 80.

Ball, E. G., and Cooper, O. (1957). *Proc. Natl. Acad. Sci. U.S.* **43**, 357.

Barron, E. S. G. (1951). *Adv. Enzymol.* **11**, 201.

Bartlett, G. R. (1958). *Ann. N. Y. Acad. Sci.* **75**, 110.

Beaven, G. H., and White, J. C. (1954). *Nature* **173**, 389.

Benesch, R. E., and Benesch, R. (1954). *Arch. Biochem. Biophys.* **48**, 38.

Beutler, E. (1957). *J. Lab. Clin. Med.* **49**, 84.

Beutler, E. (1960). "The Metabolic Basis of Inherited Disease," p. 1031. McGraw-Hill, New York.

Beutler, E., Yeh, M., and Fairbanks, V. F. (1962). *Proc. Natl. Acad. Sci. U.S.* **48**, 9.

Beutler, E., Dern, R. J., and Alving, A. S. (1954a). *J. Lab. Clin. Med.* **44**, 177.

Beutler, E., Dern, R. J., and Alving, A. S. (1954b). *J. Lab. Clin. Med.* **44**, 439.

Beutler, E., Dern, R. J., Flanagan, C. L., and Alving, A. S. (1955a). *J. Lab. Clin. Med.* **45**, 286.

Beutler, E., Dern, R. J., and Alving, A. S. (1955b). *J. Lab. Clin. Med.* **45**, 40.

Bonsignore, A., Pontremoli, S., and Grazi, E. (1957). *Boll. Soc. Ital. Biol. Sper.* **33**, 1768.

Bonsignore, A., Fornaini, G., Segni, G., and Fantoni, A. (1960a). *Giorn. Biochim.* **9**, 345.

Bonsignore, A., Fornaini, G., Segni, G., and Seitun, A. (1960b). *Boll. Soc. Ital. Biol. Sper.* **36**, 1215.

Bonsignore, A., Fornaini, G., Segni, G., and Seitun, A. (1961a). *Biochem. Biophys. Res. Commun.* **4**, 147.

Bonsignore, A., Fornaini, G., Segni, G., and Fantoni, A. (1961b). *Giorn. Biochim.* **10**, 213.

Bonsignore, A., Fornaini, A., Fantoni, P., Segni, P., Spanu, G., and Fancello, F. (1962b). *Boll. Soc. Ital. Biol. Sper.* **38**, 1127.

Bonsignore, A., Pontremoli, S., Mangiarotti, G., DeFlora, A., and Mangiarotti, M. (1962b). *J. Biol. Chem.* **237**, 3597.

Borkofsky, A. J., Marks, P. A., Katz, F. H., Lipman, M., and Christy, N. P. (1962). *J. Clin. Invest.* **41**, 1346.

Boyer, S. H., Porter, I. H., and Weilbacher, R. G. (1962). *Proc. Natl. Acad. Sci. U.S.* **48**, 1868.

Brewer, G. J., Tarlov, A. R., and Alving, A. S. (1960a). *Bull. World Health Organ.* **22**, 633.

Brewer, G. J., Tarlov, A. R., and Kellermeyer, R. W. (1961). *J. Lab. Clin. Med.* **58**, 217.

Brewer, G. J., Tarlov, A. R., Kellermeyer, R. W., and Alving, A. S. (1962a). *J. Lab. Clin. Med.* **59**, 905.

Brewer, G. J., Tarlov, A. R., and Powell, R. D. (1962b). *J. Clin. Invest.* **41**, 1348.

Brin, M., and Yonemoto, R. H. (1958). *J. Biol. Chem.* **230**, 307.

Brodie, B. B., Gillette, J. R., and Ladu, B. N. (1958). *Ann. Rev. Biochem.* **27**, 427.

Brunetti, P., Rosetti, R., and Broccia, G. (1960). *Rass. fisiopatol. clin. terap.* **32**, 338.
Carson, P. E. (1961). *Federation Proc.* **19**, 995.
Carson, P. E., and Tarlov, A. R. (1962). *Ann. Rev. Med.* **13**, 105.
Carson, P. E., Flanagan, C. L., Ickes, C. E., and Alving, A. S. (1956). *Science* **124**, 484.
Carson, P. E., Schrier, S. L., and Kellermeyer, R. W. (1959). *Nature* **184**, 1292.
Childs, B., and Zinkham, W. H. (1959). "Biochemistry of Human Genetics," p. 76. Little, Brown, Boston, Massachusetts.
Childs, B., Zinkham, W., Browne, E. A., Kimbro, E. L., and Torbert, J. V. (1958). *Bull. Johns Hopkins Hosp.* **102**, 21.
Cohen, G., and Hochstein, P. (1961). *Science* **134**, 1756.
Danon, D., Sheba, C., and Ramot, B. (1961). *Blood* **17**, 229.
Davidson, R. G., Nitowsky, H. M., and Childs, B. (1963). *Proc. Natl. Acad. Sci. U.S.* **50**, 481.
Dawson, J. P., Thayer, W. W., and Desforgês, J. F. (1958). *Blood* **13**, 1113.
DeLoecker, W. C. J., and Prankerd, T. A. J. (1961). *Clin. Chim. Acta* **6**, 641.
Denstedt, O. F. (1953). "Enzymology of the Erythrocyte, in Blood Cells and Plasma Proteins," p. 223. Academic Press, New York.
Dern, R. J., Weinstein, I. M., Leroy, G. V., Talmadge, D. W., and Alving, A. S. (1954a). *J. Lab. Clin. Med.* **43**, 303.
Dern, R. J., Beutler, E., and Alving, A. S. (1954b). *J. Lab. Clin. Med.* **44**, 171.
Dern, R. J., Beutler, E., and Alving, A. S. (1955). *J. Lab. Clin. Med.* **45**, 30.
Desforges, J. (1962). *Med. Clin. N. Am.* **46**, 1331.
DeToni, G. (1961). *Panminerva Medica* **3**, 499.
Dickens, F., Glock, G. E., and McLean, P. (1959). *Ciba Found. Symp. Regulation Cell Metab.* p. 150.
Doxiadis, S. A., Fessas, P. H., Valaes, T., and Mastrokalos, N. (1961). *Lancet* **1**, 297.
Ells, H. A., and Kirkman, H. N. (1961). *Proc. Soc. Exptl. Biol. Med.* **106**, 607.
Emerson, C. P., Ham, T. H., and Castle, W. B. (1941). *J. Clin. Invest.* **20**, 451.
Fairbanks, V. F., and Beutler, E. (1962). *Blood* **20**, 591.
Fegler, G. (1951). *J. Physiol.* (*London*) **115**, 123.
Flanagan, C. L., Schrier, S. L., Carson, P. E., and Alving, A. S. (1958). *J. Lab. Clin. Med.* **51**, 600.
Fletcher, K. A., and Maegraith, B. G. (1962). *Nature* **196**, 1316.
Fornaini, G., Leoncini, G., Luzzatto, L., and Segni, G. (1962). *J. Clin. Invest.* **41**, 1446.
Gabrio, B. W., Finch, C. A., and Huennekens, F. M. (1956). *Blood* **11**, 103.
Gant, F. L., and Winks, G. F., Jr. (1961). *Clin. Res.* **9**, 27.
Gartler, S. M., Gandini, E., and Ceppellini, R. (1962). *Nature* **193**, 602.
Gilles, H. M., and Arthur, L. J. H. (1960). *W. African Med. J.* **9**, 266.
Glock, G. E., and McLean, P. (1954). *Biochem. J.* **56**, 171.
Grignani, F., Cornicchi, D., and Maxia, C. (1960). *Klin. Wochschr.* **38**, 1171.
Gross, R. T., and Hurwitz, R. E. (1958). *Pediatrics* **22**, 453.
Gross, R. T., Hurwitz, R. E., and Marks, P. A. (1958). *J. Clin. Invest.* **37**, 1176.
Grumbach, M. M., Marks, P. A., and Moroshima, A. (1962). *Lancet* **1**, 1330.
Harley, J. D., and Robin, H. (1962). *Australian Ann. Med.* **11**, 148.
Heller, P., and Weinstein, H. G. (1959). *J. Lab. Clin. Med.* **54**, 824.
Heubner, W. (1941). *Klin. Wochschr.* **20**, 137.
Hiatt, H. H. (1957). *J. Biol. Chem.* **229**, 724.
Hiatt, H. H., and Lareau, J. (1960). *J. Biol. Chem.* **235**, 1241.
Horecker, B. L. (1944). *Public Health Bull.* **285**.
Horecker, B. L., and Hiatt, H. H. (1958). *New Engl. J. Med.* **258**, 177.
Huennekens, F. M., Caffrey, R. W., and Gabrio, B. W. (1958). *Ann. N.Y. Acad. Sci.* **75**, 167.

Jaffé, E. R. (1963). *Blood.* In press.
Jandl, J. H., and Allen, D. W. (1960). *J. Clin. Invest.* **39**, 1000.
Jandl, J. H., Engle, L. K., and Allen, D. W. (1960). *J. Clin. Invest.* **39**, 1818.
Johnson, A. B., and Marks, P. A. (1958). *Clin. Proc.* **6**, 187.
Julian, G. R., Wolfe, G. R., and Reithel, F. J. (1961). *J. Biol. Chem.* **236**, 754.
Kalmus, H. (1962). *Nature* **194**, 215.
Kaplan, N. D., Swartz, M. H., Frech, M. E., and Ciotti, M. M. (1956). *Proc. Natl. Acad. Sci. U.S.* **42**, 481.
Keilin, D., and Hartree, E. F. (1943). *Nature* **151**, 390.
Keilin, D., and Hartree, E. F. (1946). *Nature* **157**, 210.
Kellermeyer, R. W., Carson, P. E., Schrier, S. L., Tarlov, A. R., and Alving, A. S. (1961a). *J. Lab. Clin. Med.* **58**, 715.
Kellermeyer, R. W., Tarlov, A. R., Schrier, S. L., Carson, P. E., and Alving, A. S. (1961b). *J. Lab. Clin. Med.* **58**, 225.
Kellermeyer, R. W., Tarlov, A. R., Brewer, G. J., Carson, P. E., and Alving, A. S. (1962). *J. Am. Med. Assoc.* **180**, 388.
Kidson, C., and Gorman, J. G. (1962a). *Nature* **196**, 49.
Kidson, C., and Gorman, J. G. (1962b). *Biochem. Biophys. Res. Commun.* **7**, 268.
Kirkman, H. N. (1959). *Nature* **184**, 1291.
Kirkman, H. N. (1962). *J. Biol. Chem.* **237**, 2364.
Kirkman, H. N. (1963). *Pediat. Clin. of North Am.* **10**, 299.
Kirkman, H. N., and Hendrickson, E. M. (1962). *J. Biol. Chem.* **237**, 2371.
Kirkman, H. N., and Hendrickson, E. M. (1963). *Am. J. Human. Genet.* **15**, 241.
Kirkman, H. N., Riley, H. D., Jr., and Crowell, B. B. (1960). *Proc. Natl. Acad. Sci. U.S.* **46**, 938.
Krimsky, I., and Racker, E. (1952). *J. Biol. Chem.* **198**, 721.
Larizza, P., Brunetti, P., Grignani, F., and Ventura, S. (1958). *Haematologica* (*Pavia*) **43**, 205.
Larizza, P., Brunetti, P., and Grignani, F. (1960). *Haematologica* (*Pavia*) **45**, 129.
Lemberg, R., and Legge, J. W. (1949). "Hematin Compounds—Bile Pigments, Their Constitution, Metabolism, and Function." Wiley (Interscience), New York.
Levy, H. R. (1961). *Biochem. Biophys. Res. Commun.* **6**, 49.
Lohr, G. W., and Waller, H. D. (1958). *Klin. Wochschr.* **36**, 865.
Lohr, G. W., Waller, H. D., Karges, O., Schlegel, B., and Muller, A. A. (1958). *Klin. Wochschr.* **36**, 1008.
London, I. M. (1961). *Harvey Lectures, Ser.* **56**, 151.
Lowy, B. A., Ramot, B., and London, I. M. (1961). *J. Biol. Chem.* **235**, 2920.
Lowy, B. A., Williams, M. K., and London, I. M. (1962). *J. Biol. Chem.* **237**, 1622.
Lyon, M. F. (1962). *Ann. Human. Genet.* **25**, 423.
Luisada, A. (1941). *Medicine* **20**, 229.
McKee, R. W. (1951). "Biochemical and Metabolism of Malarial Parasite in Parasitic Infections in Man," p. 114. Columbia Univ. Press, New York.
McKerns, K. W., and Kaleita, E. (1960). *Biochem. Biophys. Res. Commun.* **2**, 344.
Marks, P. A. (1958). *Science* **127**, 1338.
Marks, P. A. (1959). *Trans. First Conf. on Genet.* p. 198. Josiah Macy, Jr. Found., New York.
Marks, P. A. (1961a). *Nouvelle Rev. Franc. Hematol.* **1**, 900.
Marks, P. A. (1961b). *Cold Spring Harbor Symp. Quant. Biol.* **26**, 343.
Marks, P. A. (1962a). *Methods Med. Res.* **9**, 24.
Marks, P. A. (1962b). "Biological Interactions in Normal and Neoplastic Growth," Henry Ford Hosp. Intern. Symposium, Little, Brown, Boston, Massachusetts.

Marks, P. A. (1963). *In* "The Genetics of Migrant and Isolate Populations" (E. Goldschmidt, ed.), p. 75. Williams and Wilkins, New York.
Marks, P. A., and Banks, J. (1960). *Proc. Natl. Acad. Sci. U.S.* **46**, 447.
Marks, P. A., and Freedman, A. D. (1962). *In* "Clinical Diabetes Mellitus" (Ellenberg and Rifkin, eds.), p. 1. McGraw-Hill, New York.
Marks, P. A., and Feigelson, P. (1957). *J. Biol. Chem.* **226**, 1001.
Marks, P. A., and Gross, R. T. (1959). *J. Clin. Invest.* **38**, 2253.
Marks, P. A., and Tsutsui, E. A. (1963). *Ann. N. Y. Acad. Sci.* **103,** 902.
Marks, P. A., and Szeinberg, A. (1960). *Federation Proc.* **19**, 193.
Marks, P. A., Johnson, A. B., DeBellis, R. H., and Banks, J. (1958a). *Federation Proc.* **17**, 269.
Marks, P. A., Johnson, A. B., and Hirschberg, E. (1958b). *Proc. Natl. Acad. Sci. U.S.* **44**, 529.
Marks, P. A., Gross, R. T., and Hurwitz, R. E. (1959a). *Nature* **183**, 1266.
Marks, P. A., Banks, J., and Gross, R. T. (1959b). *Biochem. Biophys. Res. Commun.* **1**, 199.
Marks, P. A., Szeinberg, A., and Banks, J. (1961). *J. Biol. Chem.* **236**, 10.
Marks, P. A., Banks, J., and Gross, R. T. (1962). *Nature* **194**, 454.
Merlini, D. (1952). *Omnia Med.* **30**, 251.
Migeon, C. J., Lescure, O. L., Zinkham, W. H., and Sidbury, J. B., Jr. (1962). *J. Clin. Invest.* **41**, 2025.
Mills, G. C. (1957). *J. Biol. Chem.* **229**, 189.
Mills, G. C. (1959). *J. Biol. Chem.* **234**, 502.
Mills, G. C. (1960). *Arch. Biochem.* **86**, 1.
Mills, G. C., and Randall, H. P. (1958). *J. Biol. Chem.* **232**, 589.
Mohler, D. N., and Williams, W. J. (1961). *J. Clin. Invest.* **40**, 1735.
Motulsky, A. G. (1960). *Human Biol.* **32**, 1.
Murphy, J. R. (1960). *J. Lab. Clin. Med.* **55**, 281.
Newton, W. A., Jr., and Bass, J. C. (1958). *A.M.A. J. Diseases Children* **96**, 501.
Noltmann, E. A., Gubler, C. J., and Kuby, S. A. (1961). *J. Biol. Chem.* **236**, 155.
Panizon, F. (1960). *Lancet* **2**, 1093.
Pontremoli, S., Bonsignore, A., Grazi, E., and Horecker, B. L. (1960). *J. Biol. Chem.* **235**, 1881.
Porter, I. H., Schulze, J., and McKusick, V. A. (1962). *Nature* **193**, 506.
Prankerd, T. A. J. (1961). "The Red Cell." Thomas, Springfield, Illinois.
Preiss, J., and Handler, P. (1957). *J. Am. Chem. Soc.* **79**, 1514.
Ramot, B., Szeinberg, A., Sheba, C., and Fagni, D. (1959a). *J. Clin. Invest.* **38**, 1659.
Ramot, B., Fisher, S., Szeinberg, A., Adam, A., Sheba, C., and Gafni, D. (1959b). *J. Clin. Invest.* **38**, 2234.
Ramot, B., Sheba, C., Adam, A., and Ashkenasi, I. (1960). *Nature* **185**, 931.
Ramot, B., Ashkenazi, I., Rimon, A., Adam, A., and Sheba, C. (1961). *J. Clin. Invest.* **40**, 611.
Rapkine, L. (1938). *Biochem. J.* **32**, 1729.
Rapoport, A., and Scheuch, D. (1960). *Nature* **186**, 967.
Rimon, A., Ashkenasi, I., Ramot, B., and Sheba, C. (1960). *Biochem. Biophys. Res. Commun.* **2**, 128.
Rubinstein, D., Ottolenghi, P., and Denstedt, O. F. (1956). *Can. J. Biochem. Physiol.* **34**, 222.
Sansone, G., and Segni, G. (1957). *Boll. Soc. Ital. Biol. Sper.* **33**, 1057.
Sansone, G., Segni, G., and DeCecco, C. (1958). *Boll. Soc. Ital. Biol. Sper.* **34**, 1.
Schapira, G., and Rosa, J. (1962). *Ann. Biol. Clin.* (*Paris*) **20**, 307.

Scheuch, D., Kahrig, C., Ockel, E., Wagenknecht, C., and Rapoport, S. M. (1961). *Nature* **190**, 631.

Schrier, S. L., Kellermeyer, R. W., and Alving, A. S. (1958a). *Proc. Soc. Exptl. Biol. Med.* **99**, 354.

Schrier, S. L., Kellermeyer, R. W., Carson, P. E., Ickes, C. E., and Alving, A. S. (1958b). *J. Lab. Clin. Med.* **52**, 109.

Schrier, S. L., Kellermeyer, R. W., Carson, P. E., Ickes, C. E., and Alving, A. S. (1959). *J. Lab. Clin. Med.* **54**, 232.

Scott, E. M. (1960). *J. Clin. Invest.* **39**, 1176.

Shahidi, N. T., and Diamond, L. K. (1959). *Pediatrics* **24**, 245.

Siniscalco, M., Motulsky, A. G., Latte, B., and Bernini, L. (1960). *Atti Accad. Naz. Lincei, Rend. Classe Sci. Fis., Mat. Nat.* **28**, 1.

Siniscalco, M., Bernini, L., Latte, B., and Motulsky, A. G. (1961). *Nature* **190**, 1179.

Smith, G. D., and Vella, F. (1960). *Lancet* **1**, 1133.

Sternschuss, N., Vanderhoff, G. A., Jaffe, E. R., and London, I. M. (1961). *J. Clin. Invest.* **40**, 1083.

Szeinberg, A., and Marks, P. A. (1961). *J. Clin. Invest.* **40**, 914.

Szeinberg, A., and Sheba, C. (1958). *Israel Med. J.* **17**, 158.

Szeinberg, A., Sheba, C., Hirschorn, N., and Bodonyi, E. (1957). *Blood* **12**, 603.

Szeinberg, A., Asher, Y., and Sheba, C. (1958a). *Blood* **13**, 348.

Szeinberg, A., Sheba, C., and Adam, A. (1958b). *Israel Med. J.* **17**, 11.

Szeinberg, A., Sheba, C., and Adam, A. (1958c). *Blood* **13**, 1043.

Szeinberg, A., Pros, M., Sheba, C., Adam, A., and Ramot, B. (1959a). *Israel Med. J.* **18**, 176.

Szeinberg, A., Adam, A., Ramot, B., Sheba, C., and Myers, F. (1959b). *Biochim. Biophys. Acta* **36**, 65.

Szeinberg, A., Sheba, C., Ramot, B., and Adam, A. (1960a). *Clin. Res.* **8**, 18.

Szeinberg, A., Kellerman, J., Adam, A., Sheba, C., and Ramot, B. (1960b). *Acta Haematol.* **23**, 58.

Tada, K., Watanabe, Y., and Fujiwara, T. (1961). *Tohoku J. Exptl. Med.* **75**, 384.

Tarlov, A. R., and Kellermeyer, R. W. (1959). *Federation Proc.* **18**, 156.

Tarlov, A. R., Brewer, G. J., Carson, P. E., and Alving, A. S. (1962). *Arch. Internal Med.* **109**, 209.

Trager, W. (1941). *J. Exptl. Med.* **74**, 441.

Tsutsui, E., and Marks, P. A. (1962). *Biochem. Biophys. Res. Commun.* **8**, 338.

Vella, F. (1959). *Med. J. Malaya* **13**, 298.

Vullo, C., and Panizon, F. (1959). *Acta Haematol.* **22**, 146.

Waller, H. D. (1959). *Blut* **5**, 1.

Wurzel, H., McCreary, T., Baker, L., and Gumerman, L. (1961). *Blood* **17**, 314.

Zinkham, W. H. (1960). *A.M.A. J. Diseases Children* **100**, 525.

Zinkham, W. H., and Lenhard, R. E., Jr. (1959). *J. Pediat.* **55**, 319.

CHAPTER 7

Chemical Composition and Metabolism of Lipids in Red Cells of Various Animal Species

L. L. M. van Deenen and J. de Gier

I. General Introduction

As in other living cells, lipids are essential constituents of the erythrocyte, and this class of compounds appears to form an integral part of the red cell protoplasma membrane. Inasmuch as erythrocytes at the present time, contrary to most other cells, offer the possibility of isolating a "ghost" which is believed to resemble the original protoplasma membrane rather closely, the unique opportunity is given to investigate the chemical composition of a cell membrane. Knowledge of the exact chemical structure of the members of various lipid classes as well as their quantitative proportions is a strict requirement for definite formulation of the molecular structure of biointerfaces.

Only detailed chemical studies on the membranous lipids can supply the information necessary for the better understanding of the architecture and functioning of the red cell membrane. Previous reviews on this subject (Ponder, 1948, 1955; Parpart and Ballentine, 1952; Douste-Blazy, 1959; Prankerd, 1961) have recorded the complexity of the red cell lipids and the difficulties involved in obtaining definite information on their chemical composition. Only a few years ago Douste-Blazy (1959) was prompted to draw attention to highly conflicting results reported in the literature on an ostensibly simple characteristic like the lecithin content of the human red cell. Recent progress in the chemistry of lipids has allowed a vast extension of the knowledge of red cell lipids, and various topics to be discussed in this chapter will deal with the literature of the past few years only.[1]

While the lipids of homologous membranes from various cells or cell particles are believed to show a certain resemblance among different animal species, a quite different situation was encountered in studying the red cell. Striking differences have been found in several lipid characteristics among red cells from various species, already known to differ with respect to their membrane properties. For these reasons a comparison of the available data on the red cell lipids among various species will be emphasized in this chapter.

The efforts of many investigators in this field have been directed towards the elucidation of the chemical composition of the lipids from the human erythrocyte, these combined results having given a detailed, though still incomplete, picture of the lipid pattern of this cell membrane. Considerable attention was also paid to the lipids of abnormal human red cells, e.g., in hereditary anemias.

In addition to the ultimate lipid composition of the mature red cell, the dynamic aspects of these compounds have to be envisaged. The apparent variations in lipid composition raise questions of the biosynthetic origins as well as the possible differences in function between various individual lipids in the red cell membrane. A possible dynamic role of certain lipids in the functioning of membranes is a subject of current interest. Inasmuch as the intriguing process of the termination of the life of the circulating red cell may involve primarily a breakdown of the cell membrane, catabolic aspects of red cell lipids are of importance.

A trend familiar in lipid biochemistry these days, viz., the investigation of the effects of dietary lipids, did not bypass the red cell. Actually, with the red cell again serving as a model, it appeared possible to demonstrate the influence of ingested lipids on the chemical composition of cell membranes.

[1] This review roughly covers the literature available to September 1962. The authors wish to thank Drs. D. J. Hanahan, P. Ways, and J. Farquhar for donating data prior to publication.

II. Localization and Functions of Lipids in the Red Cell

A. Abundance of Lipids in the Red Cell Ghost

The isolation of the erythrocyte membrane with maintenance of its original composition is an essential requirement for the study of its chemical properties and proved to be a challenge to many investigators (compare the review by Ponder, 1948). The colorless framework of red blood corpuscles remaining after hemolysis has been referred to as ghosts, stroma, stromata, or post-hemolytic residues. There is a trend in the literature to reserve the usage of the term ghost for post-hemolytic residues, which are to a certain extent intact cell envelopes. Among the large number of methods for the preparation of the red cell ghost, those procedures employing hemolysis in hypotonic solutions for removal of hemoglobin are most commonly used. Microscopic examinations strongly suggested that this material was identical with the plasma membrane. Although this opinion was open to criticism (Ponder, 1955), recent progress made with electron microscopy of ghosts (Bayer, 1960) favors the opinion of those investigators (Parpart and Ballentine, 1952) who believed the red cell ghost to represent as closely as possible a plasma membrane.

Confining ourselves to the lipids of the red cells, it can be stated that no reports are available denying the presence of lipids in the red cell ghosts. On the contrary, several investigators obtained ghosts which were demonstrated to contain practically the entire lipid content of the red cell.

According to Parpart (1942), the ghost of most species of mammal cannot be separated from the surrounding fluid by centrifugal force alone. Precipitation methods involving agglutination of the red cell ghost at pH 4.5–5.5 have been frequently employed. By introducing a medium saturated with carbon dioxide, Parpart was able to obtain ghosts containing no more than 0.01% of hemoglobin. The total lipid and lipid fraction content of the ghost and the entire red cell was found by this investigator to be virtually the same. Using the principles of this method, essentially identical results were obtained by the present authors.

On the other hand, lipid loss in the preparation of ghosts has been reported by several investigators (Anderson and Turner, 1960; Dawson *et al.*, 1960). Using hemolysis in water, Dawson *et al.* (1960) observed that even after high speed centrifugation (36,000–90,000 *g* for 90 minutes), 41% of the lipid phosphorus was found not to be recovered in the sediment. However, no obvious differences were found between the phospholipid distribution in these ghosts and in whole cells.

Apparently the methods used in the ghost preparation can influence the recovery of red cell lipids in this material to a notable extent. The effects of pH and ionic strength of the hemolyzing solution have been investigated recently in detail by Dodge *et al.* (1963). Conditions were found that allowed the preparation of hemoglobin-free ghosts by hemolysis in 20 ideal (i.e., theoretical) milliosmolar phosphate buffer at pH 7.4. Essentially all the red cell lipid was recovered in the ghosts, which showed up brilliantly by phase microscopy.

The information obtained independently by various authors using different methods indicates lipids to be constituents of the red cell ghost. Inasmuch as it is possible under certain conditions to remove hemoglobin completely, thereby recovering the lipids quantitatively in microscopically evident cell envelopes, the red cell lipids can be considered to act to a major extent as structurally important components of the red cell framework.

B. Molecular Organization of Lipids in the Red Cell Membrane

The abundance of lipids in the red cell ghost raises the question of how these compounds are arranged molecularly and contribute to the stability of the framework. Highly stimulating was the work of Gorter and Grendel (1925, 1926), who as a result of measurements with the monolayer technique concluded that the erythrocyte contains a sufficient amount of lipids to cover the erythrocyte surface with a bimolecular layer having a thickness of about 50 Å. Although the experimental basis and various assumptions made when formulating this concept need a new approach, using fresh information on lipid content, spreading characteristics of lipids, and red cell surface, the idea that a bimolecular lipid layer represents a fundamental part of cell membranes has been retained ever since.

The fundamental investigation of Waugh and Schmitt (1940) with the analytical leptoscope indicated that the dimensions of the lipid layer of the red cell membrane are limited indeed.

Further advance was supplied by surface tension measurements on red cells and droplets of lipid extracts, which led to the conclusion that the polar end groups of the oriented lipid molecules are outwardly directed, thereby associating with two layers of proteins (Danielli and Harvey, 1935). The molecular arrangement, as recently refined and formulated by Danielli, is reproduced in Fig. 1. The complete reasoning underlying this picture of the cell membrane is given in several reviews (Danielli, 1952, 1958; Davson and Danielli, 1952). The lipoprotein character of the red cell membrane is in agreement with various independent observations on the nature of the ghost obtained by hemolytic means (Parpart and Dziemian, 1940; Moskowitz and Calvin, 1952; Ponder, 1955).

Important conclusions about the molecular structure of cell membranes and the red cell membrane in particular were also reached by Bungenberg de Jong and co-workers, who obtained their information mainly from colloidal systems termed coacervates (Bungenberg de Jong, 1949). Guided by the idea that phospholipids take part in the structure of the cell membrane, Bungenberg de Jong *et al.* made detailed studies of the phenomenon of coacervation in systems with lipids carrying polar end groups and related substances. The properties of these artificial systems led them to propose a theory that biological interfaces are composed of one or more double layers of oriented phospholipid molecules. The stability of these lipid films could be explained by van der Waals forces between hydrocarbon chains with interposed cholesterol molecules and by the electrostatic interaction of the polar groups of the lipids (Bungenberg de Jong and Saubert, 1937). Furthermore it was envisaged that a protein colloid could be involved to furnish counter ions. Extension of these investigations led Bungenberg de Jong and his school to regard the cell membrane as a complex ternary colloidal system consisting of lipids, proteins, and cations tied together by van der Waals and Coulomb forces.

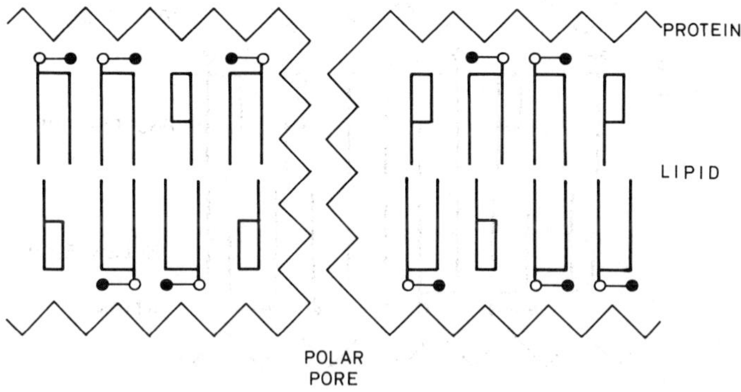

FIG. 1. Model of the structural organization of biomembranes according to the ideas of Danielli (1958).

This theory enabled Winkler and Bungenberg de Jong (1940–1941) to explain various surface properties of erythrocytes, e.g., hemolysis by hypertonic salt solution. It is noteworthy that in these considerations a monolayer of lipids was still assumed to exist in the red cell.

Results of further model experiments and their relation to cell membranes have been reviewed in detail by Booy and Bungenberg de Jong (1956) and Booy (1949). The ultimate description of the structured organization of the cell membrane as designed by Bungenberg de Jong and his school is reproduced in Fig. 2. A comparison with the proposal made by Danielli (Fig. 1) shows the resemblance of these models, both containing a bimolecular lipid leaflet surrounded by proteins. Whereas Danielli suggests the presence of hydrophilic pores to enable transport of certain molecules, Bungenberg de Jong emphasizes that a continuous mobility of the nonpolar chains of the lipids will allow passage of molecules with a more polar character.

Another theory of the arrangement of lipids in the red cell membrane (Parpart and Ballentine, 1952) will be considered later in this chapter.

Recently several investigators (Robertson, 1959; Stoeckenius, 1960) emphasized that this concept of a bimolecular lipid layer constitution is supported by results obtained through electron microscopy. As regards the red blood cell, Bayer (1960) demonstrated in erythrocytes from several animal species a triple-layered structure with a thickness of about 75 Å after $KMnO_4$ fixation. Ghosts prepared from red cells revealed, by the same techniques, a similar structure, which was lost after treatment with ether-alcohol prior to fixation. Robertson (1959) also demonstrated a triple-layered membrane structure at the red blood cell surface.

The interpretation of these structures was greatly advanced by low-angle x-ray diffraction and electron microscopy of lipid systems structurally related

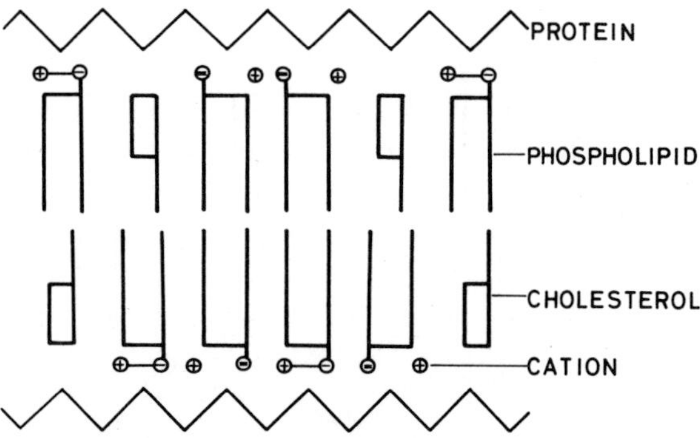

FIG. 2. Architecture of biomembranes as a complex ternary system of lipids, proteins, and cations according to proposals of Booy and Bungenberg de Jong (1956).

to the molecular configuration of the cell membrane. The evidence gained by such studies has been applied to elucidating the structure of cell membranes and is believed by most investigators to be in agreement with the presence of an oriented bimolecular lipid leaflet surrounded by protein. A discussion of the merits of these investigations is beyond the scope of this chapter, but reference can be made to a recent critical review on this subject by Elbers (1964). Although the electron microscope data strongly support the orientation of lipid molecules in the red cell membrane resembling, to a certain extent, the picture (Figs. 1 and 2) derived from earlier investigations, other arrangements cannot be ruled out completely at the present (compare Section III, E). Particularly is this true for the red cell membrane, since osmium tetroxide as contrasted with permanganate does not reveal a double membrane, but one dense band. The implications of these observations are discussed by Elbers (1964).

In any case, red cell ghosts as obtained by hemolytic means have been shown to retain a fine structure, as demonstrated by other, not readily accessible cell membranes, thus stimulating elucidation of the chemical composition of the lipids present in this membrane.

III. Chemical Composition of Red Cell Lipids

A. Lipid Content of Red Cells

Determination of the total amount of lipids present in the red cell involves complete extraction with suitable lipid solvents, followed by removal of contaminants. Information on the lipid content can then be readily obtained gravimetrically by weighing the purified lipid extract. However, the variation in results revealed between different reports indicates that this relatively simple procedure is not without pitfalls. It should be recognized, however, that in several studies having different aims, extraction and washing procedures most suitable for their final goal were employed, with incidental reporting of the amount of total extracted lipids.

Erythrocytes freed from serum and packed by means of centrifugation have been treated directly with mixtures of ethanol-ether and chloroform-methanol, respectively, at several temperatures. Some investigators preferred to suspend the erythrocytes in (hemolytic or nonhemolytic) aqueous solutions followed by treatment with methanol or ethanol. Addition of chloroform or ether has been frequently used to produce a biphasic system and to remove water-soluble compounds (including some types of lipid). After evaporation of the lipid solvents the residues have been considered either as being the final lipid extract or again extracted with nonpolar lipid solvents and filtered. Procedures used for the extraction of red cell ghosts are rather similar.

Comparison of data obtained by various investigators is somewhat hampered by the different ways of expressing the values. As has been emphasized by Erickson *et al.* (1937), measurement of lipid content per cell is most generally applicable and is to be preferred to expressing values per milliliter of packed cells.

Some differences are to be noted with respect to the lipid content of erythrocytes among various animal species (Table I). However, variations also exist among values reported by different authors. This is likewise true for the human red cell, which has attracted most investigators (Table II). It is likely that this unsatisfactory situation is brought about by various imperfections in the techniques of packing cells, extraction of lipids, removal of contaminants, and so on.

TABLE I

Total Lipid Content of Erythrocytes from Different Animal Species

Animal	Lipid (mg./ml. packed cells)	Lipid (mg. $\times 10^{-10}$/cell)	Lipid (mg. $\times 10^{-12}/\mu^2$ cell surface)
Rat[a]	6.30	3.83	4.3
Rabbit[a]	5.07	3.50	3.9
Rabbit[d]	4.8	—	—
Pig[a]	3.87	2.16	3.8
Bovine[a]	5.90	2.22	3.9
Bovine[b]	3.75	2.28	—
Sheep[a]	5.50	2.43	5.6
Sheep[b]	5.95	2.43	—
Monkey[a]	6.94	3.92	4.7
Cat[a]	5.34	2.41	4.4
Dog[a]	5.65	3.88	4.9
Dog[d]	4.9	—	—
Chicken[b]	5.50	7.26	—
Fowl[c]	5.00	—	—

[a] Parpart and Dziemian (1940).
[b] Erickson *et al.* (1938)
[c] Kates and James (1961).
[d] Prankerd (1961).

TABLE II

Total Lipid Content of Human Erythrocytes

Author	Lipid (mg./ml. packed cells)	Lipid (mg. $\times 10^{-10}$/cell)	Lipid (mg. $\times 10^{-12}/\mu^2$ cell surface)
Erickson *et al.* (1938)	4.24	3.94	—
Parpart and Dziemian (1940)	3.88	3.94	4.2
Prankerd (1961)	—	—	3.0–4.1
Reed *et al.* (1960)	6.04	4.95	—
Farquhar (1962a)	5.1	—	—
Dodge *et al.* (1963)	—	5.24	—
Ways (1964)	—	4.82	—
van Gastel *et al.* (1964)	6.13	4.80	3.65

Although red cell lipids can be recovered quantitatively from red cell ghosts, it is pointless to make a comparison of available data on their lipid content. Depending on the method used for ghost preparation, the amount of lipids can vary from 30 to 50% on the basis of dry ghost weight.

B. *Composition of Neutral Lipids*

1. Content of Neutral Lipids

According to current conventions in lipid biochemistry the designation "neutral lipids" is often reserved for a class of structurally simple lipids in distinction to the complex lipids such as glycolipids and phospholipids. The former class comprises unesterified fatty acids, glycerides (I) (mono-, di-, and triesters), cholesterol (II), and cholesterol esters (III).

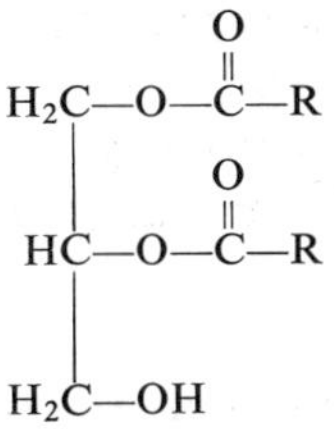

(I) α,β-Diglyceride

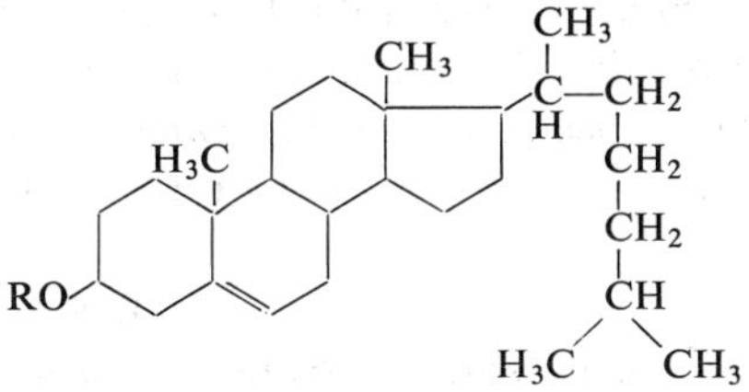

(II) Cholesterol, R = H
(III) Cholesterol ester, R = —C(=O)—R

A first approximation of the total content of neutral lipids is obtained by chromatography of crude lipid mixture on silicic acid columns (Borgström, 1952). While neutral lipids are eluted by chloroform more polar lipids, e.g. phospholipids, require solvent systems containing methanol or ethanol. Information obtained in this way on the content of neutral lipids in erythrocytes of various species is recorded in Table III, the data being in reasonable agreement with other observations (compare Douste-Blazy, 1959). Generalizing, the neutral lipid fraction always constitutes about 30% of the total lipids from

TABLE III[a]

PERCENTAGE OF NEUTRAL LIPIDS IN TOTAL LIPIDS OF ERYTHROCYTES FROM DIFFERENT ANIMAL SPECIES

Species	Neutral lipid (% of total lipid)	Cholesterol (% in neutral lipid fraction)	Ratio cholesterol:phospholipid	
			By weight	Molar[b]
Rat	28	100	0.46	0.90
Human	29	80	0.40	0.78
Rabbit	33	64	0.41	0.80
Pig	27	80	0.41	0.80
Ox	33	95	0.56	1.09
Sheep	28	96	0.45	0.88

[a] According to de Gier and van Deenen (1961).
[b] Calculated on an average molecular weight of 750 for phospholipids.

mature nonnucleated red cells of species so far investigated. Addition of the amounts of individual types of neutral lipid, determined by chromatographic techniques and/or spectrophotometric assays, provides of course another estimate of the neutral lipid content of red cells.

2. Content of Individual Neutral Lipids

a. Cholesterol and Derivatives. Cholesterol has been demonstrated to be the major compound present in the neutral lipid fraction of red cells from various animal species (Table III). This is also true for the human erythrocyte, the data obtained by various investigators being in agreement. On the one hand, studies have been conducted allowing calculation of the percentage of cholesterol in the neutral lipid fraction (Table IV); on the other hand, numerous

TABLE IV

COMPOSITION OF NEUTRAL LIPIDS FROM HUMAN ERYTHROCYTES

Neutral lipid	Douste-Blazy (1959)	Hanahan *et al.* (1960a)	Reed *et al.* (1960)	de Gier and van Deenen (1961)	Irie *et al.* (1961)
Cholesterol	74	80	92	80	83
Cholesterol esters	26	4	—	<3	4
Triglycerides	—	10	}	}	1
Free fatty acids	—	<0.5	} 8	} 17	6.5[a]
Hydrocarbon	—	5	}	}	—
"Oxycholesterol"	—	—	—	—	5

[a] May be formed during the isolation process.

reports have recorded the amount of cholesterol per volume of cells or on a cellular basis (Table V). Aside from a few exceptions within each group there is rather close agreement, particularly striking with respect to the data reproduced in Table V which was obtained over a period of 25 years. The average content of cholesterol in the human red cell appears to be rather well established.

Previous investigators (Erickson *et al.*, 1938; Parpart and Dziemian, 1940) have noted the possible significance of the considerable amount of cholesterol in the red blood corpuscle. Inasmuch as the molecular proportions of cholesterol and phospholipids in red cells of mammals tend to reach a value close to unity (Table III), speculations can be made on particular molecular associations between the two types of membranous lipids. Details of this subject will be discussed later in this chapter (Section III, E).

It is worth noting that fowl red cells show a ratio of phospholipids to cholesterol more in favor of the former (Erikson *et al.*, 1938). Kates and James (1961) suggested that an additional contribution of nucleus phospholipids may cause this difference in red cells between mammals and fowl.

In contrast to cholesterol, the acylated derivatives or cholesterol esters are present in relatively small amounts in the red cell of various species (Hanahan *et al.*, 1960a; Reed *et al.*, 1960; de Gier and Van Deenen, 1961). The more

TABLE V

CHOLESTEROL CONTENT OF HUMAN RED CELLS

Author	Cholesterol (mg./ml. packed cells)	Cholesterol (mg. × 10^{-10}/cell)
Erickson *et al.* (1938)	1.29	1.20
Brun (1939)	1.39	—
Harris *et al.* (1957)	1.76	—
Munn (1958)	1.37	—
Reed *et al.* (1960)	1.37	1.13
Fels *et al.* (1961)	1.29	—
Munn and Crosby (1961)	1.32	—
Farquhar (1962a)	1.20	—
Dodge *et al.* (1963)	—	1.42
Ways (1964)	—	1.27
van Gastel *et al.* (1964)	1.44	1.13

TABLE VI[a]

FATTY ACID COMPOSITION OF SOME NEUTRAL LIPIDS FROM HUMAN ERYTHROCYTES

Type of fatty acid	14:0[b]	16:0	16:1	18:0	18:1	18:2	20:0	20:4
Cholesterol esters	9	11	trace	4	13	63	trace	trace
Triglycerides	—	31	5	13	30	12	—	2

[a] According to Hanahan *et al.* (1960a).

[b] This shorthand designation gives the number of carbon atoms and double bonds in the fatty acid molecule; 14:0 = myristic acid, 16:0 = palmitic acid, 16:1 = palmitoleic acid, etc.

recent studies contradict previous reports, indicating a rather high level of these compounds (e.g. Williams *et al.*, 1938).

As regards the human blood cell (Table IV), the results of various investigators, obtained by independent methods, lead to the conclusion that cholesterol esters are minor constituents in this cell also. A determination of the nature of the fatty acids of cholesterol esters, by Hanahan *et al.* (1960a), notes the high content of linoleic acid in this lipid fraction (Table VI).

Studies of Irie *et al.* (1961) on the acetone-soluble lipids revealed small amounts of "oxycholesterols" in the human red cell. This nonsaponifiable fraction was divided by chromatography on alumina and cholesterol-3,5-dien-7-one, 7-ketocholesterol, and 7-hydroxycholesterol were detected.

b. Free Fatty Acids and Glycerides. In view of the considerable level of cholesterol, it is apparent that unesterified fatty acids and glycerides are present in minute amounts in the red cell. Knowledge of the composition of these lipid types in red cells of various animal species is lacking in many respects. Most detailed information is available on the human erythrocyte. In addition to the results of studies by Hanahan *et al.* (1960a) and Irie *et al.* (1961), recorded in Table IV, the report of Vacca *et al.* (1960) may be cited. The latter investigators reported the presence of mono-, di-, and triglycerides, in different proportions in red cells of man and dog. The proportions of various lipid glycerides were different from those of serum and fixed levels were observed within the red cell.

The fatty acid pattern of triglycerides, as observed in human red cell lipids by Hanahan *et al.*, is included in Table VI and, though different, does not deviate greatly from the fatty acids of plasma triglycerides.

Further studies on the composition of these minor constituents of red cells are urgently needed in connection with their possible roles as intermediates in the dynamic events of the major fatty acid-carrying lipids.

C. Composition of Glycolipids

The glycolipids present in erythrocytes reveal great variation in chemical composition. The pioneering studies of the Yamakawa and the Klenk groups on these sphingosine derivatives enable a division to be made of the erythrocyte glycolipids into several subclasses. The cerebrosides (IV), isolated from brain tissue, are known to be composed of molar equivalents of sphingosine, fatty acid, and hexose (glucose or galactose.)

$$
\begin{array}{c}
\phantom{CH_3-(CH_2)_{12}-CH=CH-CHOH-}\mathrm{R}\\
\phantom{CH_3-(CH_2)_{12}-CH=CH-CHOH-}|\\
\phantom{CH_3-(CH_2)_{12}-CH=CH-CHO}\mathrm{NH-C=O}\\
\phantom{CH_3-(CH_2)_{12}-CH=CH-CHOH-}|\\
\mathrm{CH_3-(CH_2)_{12}-CH=CH-CHOH-CH-CH_2-O-(hexose)}_n
\end{array}
$$

(IV) Cerebrosides, $n = 1$

(V) Ceramide oligohexoside, $n > 1$

Related to the cerebrosides or ceramide monohexosides are the ceramide oligohexosides (V), containing a higher number of hexose moieties. In this class of compound, found in various erythrocytes, only one nitrogen atom, supplied by sphingosine, is present. The mucolipids are distinguished from the ceramide oligohexosides by the presence of a second nitrogen-containing moiety. A second group of glycolipids is represented by those analogs containing a hexosamine. Depending on the animal species, different proportions of galactosamine (chondrosamine) or glucosamine are found to be present. A member of this sub-class, denoted as a globoside, has been isolated from ghosts of human red cells and a structure (VI) has been proposed by Yamakawa *et al.* (1956a).

$$
\begin{array}{llllll}
CH_3\text{—}(CH_2)_{12}\text{—}CH\text{=}CH\text{—} & CH\text{—} & CH\text{—}O\text{—} & \text{galactose} \\
 & | & | & | \\
 & OH & NH & \text{galactose} \\
 & & | & | \\
 & & C\text{=}O & \text{galactose} \\
 & & | & | \\
 & & C_{23}H_{47} & \text{galactosamine} \\
 & & & | \\
 & & & \text{acetyl}
\end{array}
$$

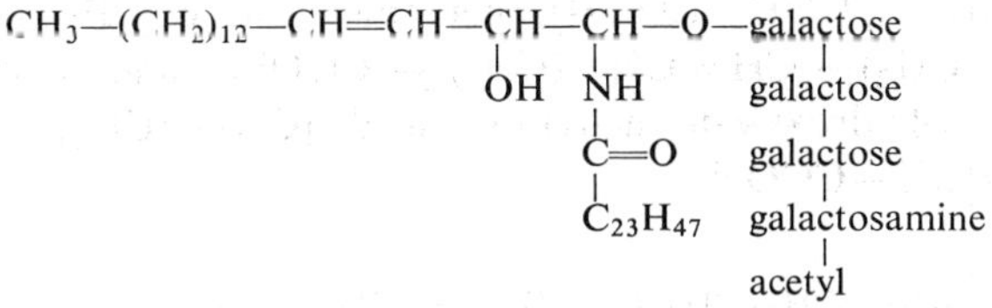

(VI) A globoside (structure proposed by Yamakawa *et al.*, 1956a).

Very recently Yamakawa *et al.* (1962) elucidated the details of this chemical structure. A third type of glycolipid occurring in red cells includes those mucolipids which contain neuraminic acid (VII) or a derivative as a second

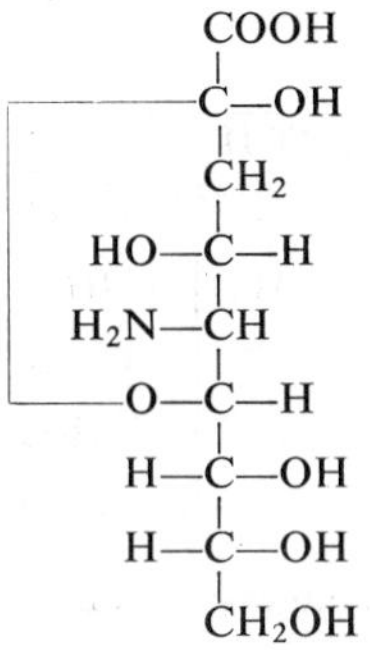

$$
\begin{array}{rcl}
 & COOH & \\
 & | & \\
\ulcorner & C\text{—}OH & \\
 & | & \\
 & CH_2 & \\
 & | & \\
HO\text{—} & C & \text{—}H \\
 & | & \\
H_2N\text{—} & CH & \\
 & | & \\
\llcorner O\text{—} & C & \text{—}H \\
 & | & \\
H\text{—} & C & \text{—}OH \\
 & | & \\
H\text{—} & C & \text{—}OH \\
 & | & \\
 & CH_2OH &
\end{array}
$$

(VII) Neuraminic acid

nitrogenous constituent in addition to sphingosine. These glycolipids, denoted as gangliosides, again show a complex composition which challenged many investigators to elucidate their exact chemical structures. Gangliosides lacking hexosamines have been encountered in erythrocytes of the horse by Yamakawa and Suzuki (1951, 1952), who proposed the name "hematoside" for compounds showing molecular proportions of sphingosine : fatty acid : hexose (galactose or glucose): neuraminic acid (*N*-glycolylneuraminic acid) of 1:1:2:1. The investigations by Klenk and Wolter (1952) confirmed the presence of hexosamine-free gangliosides in horse erythrocytes, and recently a structural formula (VIII) was given by Klenk and Padberg (1962). Gangliosides containing both neuraminic acid and hexosamines exist as well, and considerable progress has been made with regard to their chemical structure (compare Klenk and

Gielen, 1962). Several studies to be discussed below strongly suggest this type of ganglioside to be present in minute quantities in red cells of certain animal species.

The fatty acids of the glycolipids including those of red cells are very characteristic. Major fatty acids are: lignoceric acid or tetracosanoic acid [CH_3—$(CH_2)_{22}$—COOH], cerebronic acid or α-hydroxy-*n*-tetracosanoic acid [CH_3—$(CH_2)_{21}$—CHOH—COOH], nervonic acid or Δ^{15}-*n*-tetracosanoic acid [CH_3—$(CH_2)_7$—CH=CH—$(CH_2)_{13}$—COOH], and hydroxynervonic acid or Δ^{15}-α-hydroxy-*n*-tetracosanoic acid [CH_3—$(CH_2)_7$—CH=CH—$(CH_2)_{12}$—CHOH—COOH].

```
CH3—(CH2)12—CH=CH—CH—C—CH2—O—CH————┐
                   |  |         |    |
                   OH NH     H—C—OH  |
                      |         |    |
                 (CH2)22   HO—CH     O
                      |         |    |
                     CH3       HC—O—-|-——————————————CH———┐
                                |    |                |    |
                               HC————┘             HC—OH   |
                                |                     |    |
                               CH2OH      ┌——————————CH    O
                                          |           |    |
                                          O       HO—CH    |
                                          |           |    |
              OH OH                       |          HC————┘
              |  |  H  H  H               |           |
      CH2OH—C—C—C—C—C—CH2—C—COOH         CH2OH
              |  |  |  |
              H  H  |  NH
                    |  |
                    | C=O
                    |  |
                    | CH2OH
                    |          |
                    └————O————┘
```

(VIII) A ganglioside lacking hexosamines (structure proposed by Klenk and Padberg, 1962)

Distribution of Various Types of Glycolipid in Erythrocytes

Conventionally the glycolipids are extracted with warm chloroform-methanol 1:1 from dry ghosts from which neutral lipids and phospholipids have previously been removed by extraction with acetone and hexane, respectively. The crude glycolipid extract accounts for about 2% of the dry ghost weight, which corresponds to about 10% of the total lipids.

Analysis by Yamakawa and Suzuki (1953) and Yamakawa *et al.* (1956b) of crude glycolipid extracts readily showed that the composition and proportions of individual types of glycolipid vary enormously among erythrocytes of various animal species. This is demonstrated by data on the content of hexosamine and neuraminic acid and on the proportions of glucosamine and galactosamine, respectively (Table VII). Essentially these differences have been confirmed by separation of the intact compounds by means of fractional crystallization (Klenk and Lauenstein, 1952, 1953; Klenk and Wolter, 1952). The complex composition and the differences existing in this respect are also seen during attempts to separate the individual types of glycolipid from erythrocytes by chromatographic methods (Rodin, 1957; Yamakawa *et al.*, 1958, 1960; Hakomori and Jeanloz, 1961).

A short survey of some appealing facts on the occurrence of several types of glycolipid in erythrocytes of certain species will now be considered.

a. Human. Klenk and Lauenstein (1951) isolated from red blood corpuscles a glycolipid that showed some resemblance to certain gangliosides of spleen,

TABLE VII[a]

DISTRIBUTION OF NEURAMINIC ACID AND HEXOSAMINES IN THE LIPIDS FROM ERYTHROCYTES

Species	Lipid neuraminic acid (% of dry stroma)	Lipid hexosamine (% of dry stroma)	Ratio galactosamine/glucosamine
Human group O	n.d.[b]	0.18 ± 0.03	4.5
Human group A	n.d.	0.20 ± 0.05	
Human group B	n.d.	0.20 ± 0.05	
Sheep	n.d.	0.18 ± 0.05	1.3
Goat	n.d.	0.25 ± 0.05	2.3
Hog	—	0.44 ± 0.07	∞
Bovine	0.28 ± 0.07	0.15 ± 0.03	0.2
Dog	0.42 ± 0.02	0.07 ± 0.02	—
Horse	0.51 ± 0.07	0.04 ± 0.01	—
Rabbit	0.15	0.24	0
Chicken	n.d.	0.02 ± 0.01	—

[a] Data are taken from table and diagrams of Yamakawa *et al.* (1953, 1956b).
[b] Not detectable.

but upon hydrolysis no neuraminic acid was liberated. Further investigations (Klenk and Lauenstein, 1952; Yamakawa and Suzuki, 1952) revealed that lignocerylsphingosine acetylgalactosamine tri- or tetra-hexosides were involved. Chromatographic separation of these globosides by Yamakawa *et al.* (1960) indicated that seven compounds were present; the major compound was reported to correspond to a lignocerylsphingosine acetylgalactosamine trihexoside (compare VI). Furthermore, a vast amount of a ceramide oligohexoside (V) was encountered. Various minor fractions contained both hexosamine and neuraminic acid and appeared to possess blood group activity. However, Hakomori and Jeanloz (1961) reported that a fraction of glycolipids that was active in this respect did not contain neuraminic acid.

b. Horse. Studies from Yamakawa and Suzuki (1951) and Klenk's school (Klenk and Wolter, 1952; Klenk and Lauenstein, 1953; Klenk and Padberg,

1962) demonstrated a glycolipid of the ganglioside type to be abundant in horse erythrocyte. In addition to this "hematoside" (VIII), ceramide oligohexosides [viz., lignoceryl(nervonyl)sphingoside dihexosides] (compare V) have been reported to occur in these erythrocytes (Klenk and Wolter, 1952; Klenk and Lauenstein, 1953). These investigators also encountered a fraction containing both galactosamine and neuraminic acid, an observation confirmed by the chromatographic investigations of Yamakawa *et al.* (1960).

c. Bovine. Klenk and Lauenstein (1952) isolated from red cells of this species a glucosamine-containing glycolipid (VI). Furthermore, variable amounts of a neuraminic acid-carrying compound were demonstrated to be present by these investigators as well as by Yamakawa *et al.* (1960).

d. Sheep. Yamakawa *et al.* (1960) reported the presence of a major glycolipid fraction devoid of neuraminic acid and containing galactosamine: glucosamine in 4:1 ratio.

D. Composition of Phospholipids

1. Total Content

Those lipids carrying within their molecule one or more phosphate groups, termed phospholipids or phosphatides, constitute a considerable fraction of the red cell lipids. Information on the amount of phospholipids present in purified lipid extracts can be obtained from a determination of the phosphorus content. Based on an average content of 4% of phosphorus, believed to be valid for most naturally occurring phospholipids, the lipid phosphorus value permits calculation of the amount of phospholipid. A gravimetric estimation can be made by separating the phospholipids from other lipid classes by column chromatography. Separation of neutral lipids and phospholipids on silica columns by eluting with chloroform and chloroform-methanol, respectively, has been employed for determination of these lipid classes in erythrocytes.

Data obtained on the phospholipid content of human erythrocytes are compiled in Table VIII. Because of different ways of recording, a complete comparison of the data available is impossible. However, it is clear that the values reported for the absolute phospholipid content of the human erythrocyte show disagreement. More coherence is obtained by comparing values indicating the relative amount of phospholipids present in lipid extracts of red cells. Apparently the divergence of values for phospholipid content on a cellular basis results from incomplete extraction, loss of lipid during washing procedures, etc. Therefore a comparison of data on the phospholipid content of red cells in various animal species, gathered by several investigators, has been omitted. However, numerous determinations of the amount of phospholipids in lipid extracts from red cells and their ghosts indicated uniformly that the phospholipids constitute about 60% of the lipids from mammalian red cells, including those of man (compare, e.g., Hanahan *et al.*, 1960a; Reed *et al.*, 1960; de Gier and van Deenen, 1961). Fowl red cells show even a higher phospholipid content (Kates and James, 1961).

TABLE VIII

PHOSPHOLIPID CONTENT OF HUMAN ERYTHROCYTES

Author	Phospholipid [a] (mg./ml. packed cells)	Phospholipid [a] (mg. $\times 10^{-10}$/cell)
Erickson (1938)	2.44	2.27
Harris *et al.* (1957)	2.08	—
Reed *et al.* (1960)	3.43	2.88
Munn and Crosby (1961)	3.33	—
Kates *et al.* (1961)	—	1.70
Phillips and Roome (1962)	3.49	—
Farquhar (1962a)	2.98	—
Dodge *et al.* (1963)	—	3.15
Ways (1964)	—	3.15
van Gastel *et al.* (1964)	3.48	2.73

[a] Calculated from lipid phosphorus data on the assumption that in pure phospholipid the phosphorus content is 4%.

Obviously, phospholipids together with cholesterol form quantitatively the major part of the red cell lipids. The combinations of nonpolar acyl groups and polar head moieties, found in phospholipids and believed to be important in the structural organization of the cell membrane, require detailed consideration.

2. Proportions of Individual Types of Phospholipids

a. Types of Phospholipid. The class of phospholipids is recognized to consist of a great number of individual members and in this respect the phospholipids in erythrocytes are no exception. In addition to the more conventional types of phosphoglyceride like lecithin (X) and the cephalins, phosphatidylethanolamine (XI), and phosphatidylserine (XII), other types of phosphoglyceride may be present. Phosphatidic acid (IX), now known to be a key intermediate in phospholipid biosynthesis, has been found in erythrocytes also. The presence of inositol phosphatides in red cells has been reported, although it has not been established what type(s) of this complex class occurs (compare XIII and XIV). Besides the diacyl compounds, monoacyl derivatives termed lysophospholipids (XVI) have been encountered in red cells. The exact position of the fatty acid residue has not been established with certainty.

The class of phosphoglycerides is a complex one, not only because of the variable nature of the polar head groups. Differentiation is also brought about

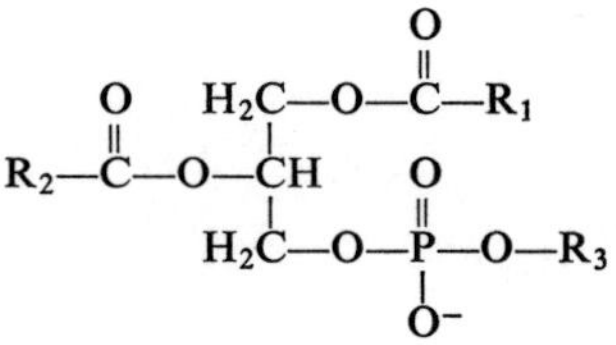

$$
\begin{array}{c}
\;\; O \quad H_2C-O-\overset{\overset{\displaystyle O}{\|}}{C}-R_1 \\
R_2-\overset{\|}{C}-O-\overset{|}{C}H \qquad \overset{\displaystyle O}{\|} \\
\qquad\quad H_2\overset{|}{C}-O-\underset{\underset{\displaystyle O^-}{|}}{P}-O-R_3
\end{array}
$$

$R_3 = H$	phosphatidic acid (IX)
$= -CH_2-CH_2-\overset{+}{N}(CH_3)_3$	phosphatidylcholine or lecithin (X)
$= -CH_2-CH_2-NH_3^+$	phosphatidylethanolamine (XI) } cephalins
$= -CH_2-\underset{\underset{\displaystyle NH_2}{\vert}}{CH}-COO^-$	phosphatidylserine (XII) } cephalins
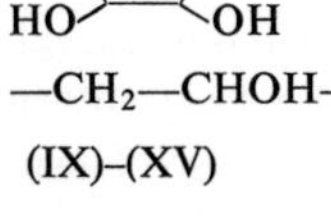 = inositol ring (HO, OH, OH, HO, OH)	phosphatidylinositol or monophosphionositide (XIII)
= inositol ring (HO, OH, OPO_3H_2, HO, OH)	diphosphoinositide (XIV)
$= -CH_2-CHOH-CH_2OH$	phosphatidylglycerol (XV)

(IX)–(XV)

by difference in chemical binding of acyl chains to the glycerol moiety. Recent progress in the chemistry of the plasmalogens has demonstrated that the

```
              O
              ||
H2C—O—C—R                          O    H2C—OH
 |                                 ||    |
HO—CH    O                      R—C—O—CH      O
 |       ||          +                   |      ||                +
H2C—O—P—O—CH2—CH2N(CH3)3           H2C—O—P—O—CH2—CH2—N(CH3)
         |                                      |
         O−                                     O−
```

(XVI) Possible structures of lysolecithin [comparable analogs of phosphatidylethanolamine (XI) and other phosphoglycerides (XII, XIII) may occur as well]

aldehydogenic unit is attached to the γ (or α') position of glycerol, while a fatty acid is esterified at the β position (XVII).

Another type of phosphoglyceride extremely important in the discussion of red cell lipids are phospholipids (XVIII) which contain saturated glyceryl ethers derived, for example, from batyl alcohol. These alkyl ether phospholipids too carry a fatty acid at the β position, although recent reports indicate that phosphoglycerides containing two saturated or unsaturated ether linkages may also occur in nature. Their existence in red cells has not been reported.

```
 O    H2C—O—CH=CH—R                O    H2C—O—CH2—CH2—R
 ||    |                           ||    |
R—C—O—CH      O                  R—C—O—CH      O
       |      ||             +           |      ||             +
      H2C—O—P—O—CH2—CH2—NH3           H2C—O—P—O—CH2—CH2—NH3
              |                                 |
              O−                                O−
```

(XVII) Phosphatidalethanolamine; an ethanolamine plasmalogen (comparable analogs, with choline and serine as head group, existing as well)

(XVIII) Glyceryl ether analog of an ethanolamine phospholipid (compare Hanahan and Watts, 1961)

Polyglycerol phospholipids have been demonstrated to be widely distributed in nature. The simplest representative of this class, viz., phosphatidylglycerol (XV), was not recognized until 1958 (Benson and Maruo, 1958), and is now known to be a major phospholipid of photosynthetic tissues. Only relatively small amounts of this phospholipid have been recovered in animal tissues and it is not established whether phosphatidylglycerol is present in the erythrocyte. This is also true with respect to cardiolipin (XIX), known to be a regular phospholipid of mitochondria. In connection with presumed specific functions of this phospholipid it seems worthwhile to ascertain whether cardiolipin does or does not constitute an erythrocyte phospholipid.

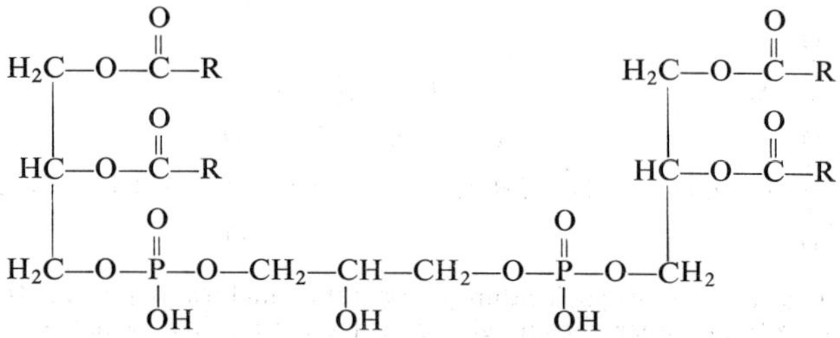

$$\begin{array}{l}
H_2C{-}O{-}\overset{\displaystyle O}{\overset{\|}{C}}{-}R \qquad\qquad\qquad\qquad\qquad\qquad\qquad H_2C{-}O{-}\overset{\displaystyle O}{\overset{\|}{C}}{-}R \\
HC{-}O{-}\overset{\displaystyle O}{\overset{\|}{C}}{-}R \qquad\qquad\qquad\qquad\qquad\qquad\qquad HC{-}O{-}\overset{\displaystyle O}{\overset{\|}{C}}{-}R \\
H_2C{-}O{-}\underset{\displaystyle OH}{\underset{|}{\overset{\displaystyle O}{\overset{\|}{P}}}}{-}O{-}CH_2{-}\underset{\displaystyle OH}{\underset{|}{CH}}{-}CH_2{-}O{-}\underset{\displaystyle OH}{\underset{|}{\overset{\displaystyle O}{\overset{\|}{P}}}}{-}O{-}CH_2
\end{array}$$

(XIX) Cardiolipin or diphosphatidylglycerol (structure according to MacFarlane, 1958)

An important phospholipid of animal tissues, occurring in considerable amounts in erythrocytes, is sphingomyelin (XX), containing the amino alcohol sphingosine.

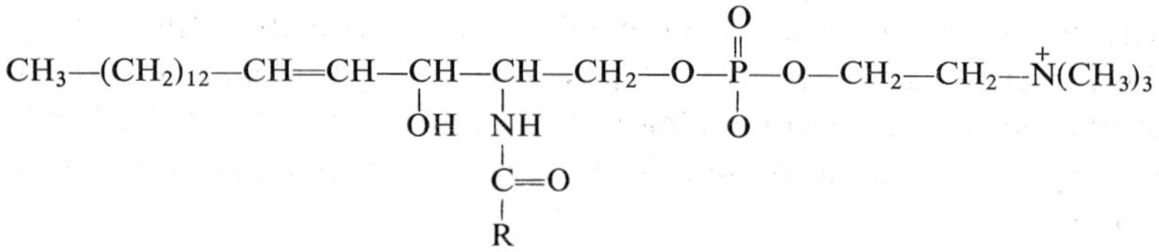

$$CH_3{-}(CH_2)_{12}{-}CH{=}CH{-}\underset{\displaystyle OH}{\underset{|}{CH}}{-}\underset{\displaystyle \underset{\displaystyle \underset{\displaystyle R}{|}}{\underset{|}{NH}{-}C{=}O}}{\underset{|}{CH}}{-}CH_2{-}O{-}\underset{\displaystyle O^-}{\underset{|}{\overset{\displaystyle O}{\overset{\|}{P}}}}{-}O{-}CH_2{-}CH_2{-}\overset{+}{N}(CH_3)_3$$

(XX) Sphingomyelin

The given classification of phospholipids is based on the types of alcohol, polar head group, and acyl-alcohol linkages present. It should be realized that a certain type of phospholipid, e.g., lecithin of biological origin, contains a great number of different long-chain constituents and that a purified lecithin preparation as obtained from red cells is not a definite compound, but consists of a large group of related but different molecules.

b. Determination of the Phospholipid Composition. The complexity of the polar as well as the nonpolar part of the phospholipid molecule has delayed the exact determination of the proportion of various types of phospholipid. Only a relatively short while ago such determinations were based merely on hydrolysis procedures combined with determinations of the water-soluble hydrolysis products. Although some of the techniques have proved to be very useful even at the present time, it can be stated that incomplete if not misleading results were obtained. The introduction of chromatographic methods in the last decade has achieved resolution of complex mixtures of phospholipid to a promising degree.

Chromatography through columns of silica and alumina with mixtures of various solvents, e.g. chloroform and methanol, gives a separation of several major classes of phospholipid. An excellent review of the possibilities and limits of these methods has recently been given by one of the pioneers in this field (Hanahan, 1960). Furthermore, paper impregnated with silica as introduced by Lea and Rhodes (1955) provides, particularly with the solvent system according to Marinetti *et al.* (1957), a rapid and convenient tool for quantitative phospholipid analysis. The wide applicability of this method has been outlined recently by Marinetti (1962). An ultramicroanalysis, giving a most striking degree of resolution, proved to be thin-layer chromatography as (re)introduced by Stahl (1957). In the recent past, the possibilities for the analysis of lipids by thin-layer chromatography have proved to be manifold (compare the review by Mangold, 1961); this method meanwhile was applied to the analysis of erythrocyte phospholipids as well. Dawson (1954) introduced a weak alkaline hydrolysis procedure removing fatty acid constituents, followed by chromatographic determination of the water-soluble phosphodiesters. This valuable method has been improved recently into a technique allowing a most impressive estimation of many if not all types of naturally occurring phospholipid (Dawson, 1960; Dawson *et al.*, 1962).

Detailed information on advantages and drawbacks of the various methods can be obtained by comparative reading of the various articles quoted above. It can be stated that a complete quantitative characterization of (erythrocyte) phospholipids, including the nature of their acyl chains, requires a combination of many techniques.

c. Phospholipid Patterns of Erythrocytes from Various Animal Species. In an attempt to correlate differences in permeability characteristics of erythrocytes with their lipid composition, Parpart and Dziemian (1940) sought to establish differences in the phospholipid composition of erythrocytes among various animal species. Because of the nonavailability of adequate methods, these pioneering investigators were unable to observe appreciable differences in red cell phospholipids of the erythrocytes studied. Using the advantages of silica paper chromatography, Turner and co-workers (1957, 1958a) demonstrated qualitatively that notable differences exist in the phospholipid patterns of erythrocytes among various animals. Most striking was the observation that in erythrocytes of certain ruminants, e.g. sheep and cow, lecithin was lacking or present in unusually low amount. Meanwhile a quantitative comparison of the phospholipid composition was carried out in several laboratories using different techniques. Dawson *et al.* (1960), de Gier (1960), Hanahan *et al.* (1960a), and de Gier and van Deenen (1961) demonstrated most significant variations in the proportions of erythrocyte phospholipids among various animal species. Some of these results and more recently published data have been compiled in Table IX, to facilitate comparison. Some variation can be noticed between the results of various investigators because of imperfections in the different methods employed. The general trend, indicating the variability in phospholipids among various species, however, is beyond doubt.

TABLE IX

DISTRIBUTION OF THE MAJOR CLASSES OF PHOSPHOLIPIDS IN ERYTHROCYTES FROM DIFFERENT ANIMAL SPECIES

Species	Lecithins	Sphingomyelins	Cephalins	Other Phospholipids
Rat[a]	56	26	18	—
Rabbit[a]	44	29	27	—
Horse[b]	43	23	23	11
Pig[a]	29	36	35	—
Pig[b]	31	16	49	4
Goat[b]	19	40	31	10
Bovine[a]	7	61	32	—
Bovine[b]	19	44	29	8
Bovine[c]	5	60	28	7
Sheep[a]	1	63	36	—
Sheep[b]	19	49	24	8
Fowl[d]	42	24	28	6

[a] De Gier and van Deenen (1961).

[b] These data are calculated from the analyses reported by Dawson *et al.* (1960) on ghosts of red cells.

[c] Hanahan *et al.* (1960a).

[d] Kates and James (1961).

Most conspicuous are the differences in the proportions of various choline-containing phospholipids in erythrocytes from different species. In the sequence of mammals recorded in Table IX there is a striking decrease of the relative amount of lecithin (X), whereas the sphingomyelin (XX) content increases in the sequence. The content of cephalins, containing various types of phospholipid (XI and XII), also reveals some differences, but as noted by various investigators the variations in lecithin content are nearly balanced by those of sphingomyelin. Hence the relative amount of phospholipids, containing choline in their polar head group, tends to reach a certain minimum value in erythrocytes of all species. These data confirm the original observation of Turner *et al.* (1957, 1958a) that the lecithin content of erythrocytes of certain ruminants is of a low order. As reported later by the latter investigator (Turner *et al.*, 1958b), this phenomenon cannot be generally ascribed to all ruminants, inasmuch as the camel was shown to have a fair amount of lecithin in the erythrocyte. (Further discussions on this subject are dealt with in Sections III, F and IV.)

The phospholipid composition of nucleated fowl cells has been shown to be closely related to those of man and rabbit (Table IX).

d. Phospholipid Pattern of the Human Erythrocyte. An attempt has been made in Table X to compile the data obtained in recent years on the phospholipid of the human red blood cell. At first glance one may be inclined to believe that a chaotic and highly conflicting situation exists. Although results indeed are at variance at certain points, this arises through the use of various analytical methods which give distinct types of information. Considering the data in detail, a fair picture of the average composition of phospholipids from the human erythrocyte can be obtained. Lysolecithin (XVI) has been observed by investigators to represent about 2–3% of the total phospholipids. The question can be raised whether the observed lysolecithin is not an artifact produced from plasmalogen lecithin (compare XVII), for example. It has been established recently that lysolecithin present in lipid extracts from serum (Newman *et al.*, 1961) and brain (Webster and Thompson, 1962) is not formed by breakdown of lecithin during the various procedures involved. In view of a possible role of lysophospholipids in the dynamic process of erythrocyte lipids (compare Section IV, B), the "native" character of red cell lysolecithin certainly needs to be ascertained.

The amount of lecithin (X) averages about 35% of total phospholipids, while 3–6% of this lipid is present in the form of plasmalogen (compare XVII). Sphingomyelin (XX) is undoubtedly an important phospholipid of the human red cell. Variation among values probably is caused by the different techniques employed. Inasmuch as lysophosphatidyl-ethanolamines (compare XVI), which may be of native origin or may arise artificially during certain analytical procedures, move on silica paper together with sphingomyelin, perhaps the values for the latter compound obtained by this method may be too high. The combined results obtained by different approaches suggest that sphingomyelin constitutes about 20% of human erythrocyte phospholipids.

The sum of all choline-containing phospholipids appears to form nearly two-thirds of the total phospholipids of the human erythrocyte. Within the class of cephalins the ethanolamine-containing compounds are predominant. The results of most investigators indicated that the ethanolamine-carrying phospholipids together represent about one-fourth of the total phospholipids. It must be appreciated that in addition to phosphatidylethanolamine (XI), a notable amount of the plasmalogen type (phosphatidalethanolamine, XVII) is present (Farquhar, 1962a). Phosphatidyl serine is a regular erythrocyte phospholipid but the values reported reveal an enormous degree of disagreement, caused partly by difficulties in the separation of this phospholipid from other types. However, the observations of various investigators indicate that phosphatidylserine is present in a non-negligible amount in the human red cell. Small amounts of phosphatidic acid have been determined by some investigators, while others recorded a phospholipid of this type to be present in small amounts without making quantitative assays. It seems of interest to elucidate

TABLE X PHOSPHOLIPID COMPOSITION OF HUMAN RED CELLS

Phospholipids	Formijne *et al.* (1957)[a]	Harris *et al.* (1957)[b]	Dawson *et al.* (1960)[b]	Dawson *et al.* (1962)[b]	Blomstrand *et al.* (1962)[b]	Phillips and Roome (1959)[c]	Hanahan *et al.* (1960,a)[c]
Lysolecithin						1.9	
Lecithin (phosphatidylcholine	41	25	36.4	33.5	36.5	32.9	
Phosphatidalcholine (plasmalogen)		—[g]	5.7	1.2	1.8		61
Sphingomyelin	28	—	16.2	20.1	28.7	22.8	
Lysocephalin							—
Phosphatidylethanolamine		9.5	17.6	17.6	11.9		
Phosphatidalethanolamine (plasmalogen)	31	—	5.6	10.4	—		28
Phosphatidylserine		5	5.1	14.3	12.4	42.5	
Phosphatidalserine (plasmalogen)		—	0.3	0	—		2
Phosphatidic acid	—	—	1.2	2.2	—		1
Phosphatidylinositol	—	—	—	0	5.6		
Other phospholipids	—	—	2.6	1.5	3.2		8

Phospholipid	Farquhar (1962a)[c]	Dodge *et al.* (1963)[c]	Ways (1964)[c, e]	Reed *et al.* (1960)[c]	de Gier and van Deenen (1961)[d]	Klibansky and Osimi (1961)[d]	Kates *et al.* (1961)[d]
Lysolecithin	—	—	—	2.5	2	2.4	3.3
Lecithin (phosphatidylcholine)	32.4	27	30	30.0	36	29.6	45.2
Phosphatidalcholine (plasmalogen)	3.6						
Sphingomyelin	21	22	23.8				
Lysocephalin	—	—	—	22.0	32	26.0	22.9
Phosphatidylethanolamine	9.7						
Phosphatidalethanolamine (plasmalogen)	19.3	27	25.7	24.9	28	24.1	27.9
Phosphatidylserine	9.2	—				14.5	—
Phosphatidalserine (plasmalogen)	0.8		15	14.9	2	—	—
Phosphatidic acid	—	18		2.0	—	—	0.7
Phosphatidylinositol	—		5.8	4.0	—	3.8	—
Other phospholipids	3	4.3[f]			—	—	—

[a] Values from choline and phosphorus analyses after acid and alkaline hydrolyses.
[b] Values from analyses after chromatographic separation of degradation products after mild alkaline hydrolyses.
[c] Values from analyses after separation of the intact phospholipids on silicic acid columns.
[d] Values from P analyses after separation of silicic acid-impregnated papers.
[e] Values from P analyses after separation on thin layers.
[f] Contained sphingomyelin and lysolecithin.
[g] Not determined.

whether related phospholipids, e.g. cardiolipin, are also present. It was observed that compounds of the phosphoinositide type (compare XIII and XIV) are present in small amounts and that several more complex phospholipids might be present in minor quantities was indicated. The studies quoted in Table X supply further insight into the phospholipid composition of the human erythrocyte. The nature of the acyl chains, constituting by weight the predominant part of the phospholipid molecule, has now to be considered.

3. Fatty Acid Constituents of Red Cell Phospholipids

a. Fatty Acid Patterns of Total Lipids. As known, the determination of fatty acid constituents was greatly advanced by gas-liquid chromatography, ingeniously invented by Martin and James. The methodology and apparatus suitable for analysis of fatty acid methyl esters have been the subject of many reviews (e.g. Burchfield and Storrs, 1962).

Confining our discussion to results obtained with gas-liquid chromatography, the reports of James and Lovelock (1957) and Kögl *et al.* (1960) should be noted on the fatty acid composition of total lipids extracted from intact erythrocytes or their ghosts in various animal species. It was demonstrated that most significant differences exist among red cells of different animals in this respect. Figure 3 represents the information obtained in the laboratory of the latter group of authors; although essentially similar to their previously published results the fatty acid patterns presented are of more recent date. Most conspicuous are the decrease of palmitic acid and arachidonic acid and the simultaneous increase of oleic acid in the given sequence of mammalian red cells. The fatty acid composition of lipids from fowl erythrocytes has been studied by Kates and James (1961).

Inasmuch as the class of phospholipids constitutes up to 80–90% of the fatty acid-carrying lipids in erythrocytes, the given patterns supply much information on the fatty acid composition of the phospholipids. The question arises as to the origin of the remarkable variation in fatty acid constituents of erythrocyte lipids among various species. Although not all details can be explained as yet, both the nature of the ingested lipids and differences in lipid metabolism among various species appear to be involved (compare Section IV,C). The data represented in Fig. 3 concern analyses of erythrocytes in subjects without a controlled or standardized diet. Results on the fatty acid composition of lipids from human erythrocytes obtained by various investigators are compared in Table XI. These data do not need extensive discussion as the general agreement is apparent. Of course several variations in percentages of certain fatty acids are evident, even when comparing the data reported by one research group on different occasions. However, it must be realized that gas-liquid chromatography is a new tool, which is making rapid progress and allowing more detailed analyses than a few years ago. The analysis under discussion concerns mostly the average of a great number of determinations. Generally, only limited differences have been found in the fatty acid composition of erythrocytes among various individuals in one study. Inasmuch as the fatty acid composition of erythrocytes is influenced by

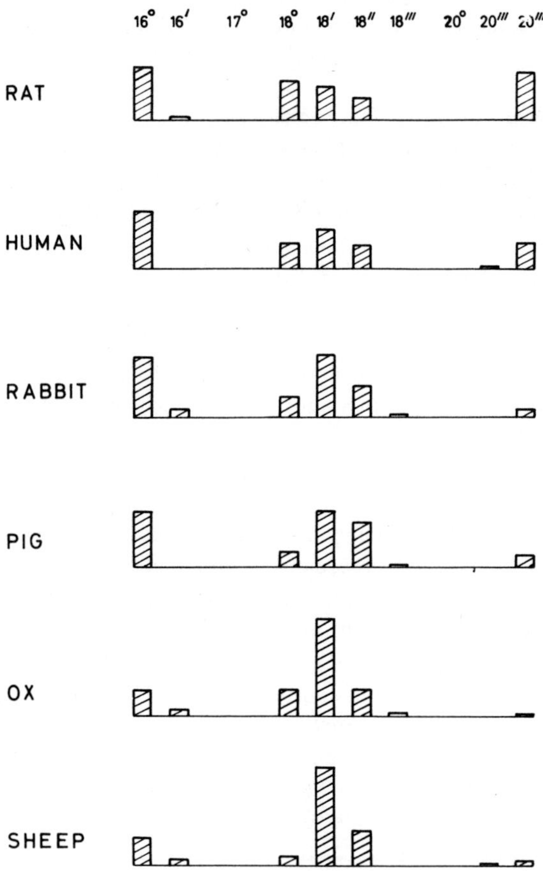

FIG. 3. Fatty acid patterns of total lipids of erythrocytes from various animal species. The blocks represent the relative amounts of individual fatty acids (as weight percentages), that are indicated by means of the number of carbon atoms and double bonds (e.g., 18″ stands for octadecadienoic acid) (Kögl *et al.*, 1960; de Gier, 1960).

certain dietary factors (Section IV), it cannot be ruled out that certain regional differences in the nature of ingested lipids are reflected in the data presented.

b. Fatty Acid Patterns of Individual Phospholipids. As outlined in the preceding sections, both the proportions of individual types of phospholipid and the fatty acid patterns of erythrocyte lipids reveal remarkable differences among various animal species. Erythrocytes of rat, rabbit, man, pig, ox, and sheep showed a gradual decrease in lecithin and increase in sphingomyelin. In nearly the same order of animals, the erythrocyte lipids showed a decrease in percentages of palmitic acid and arachidonic acid accompanied by significant augmentation of the oleic acid content. The question can be raised as to whether these simultaneously occurring shifts in the two lipid characteristics of eythrocytes are directly related. Increasing evidence indicates that a certain

TABLE XI

FATTY ACID COMPOSITION OF THE TOTAL LIPID FROM HUMAN RED CELLS

Fatty acid	James and Lovelock (1957)[b]	Kögl *et al.* (1960); de Gier *et al.* (1961a)	Kates *et al.* (1961)	Farquhar (1962a)[c]	de Gier *et al.* (1964)
12:0[a]	—	trace	0.3	—	0.3
14:0	—	trace	0.8	0.3	1.0
15:0	—	—	0.3	0.2	0.3
16:0	38.5	34.5	41.0	29.7	27.1
16:1	—	1.5	1.1	0.6	3.4
Iso-17:0	—	—	0.3	0.2	0.4
17:0	—	—	0.3	trace	0.2
18:0	20.5	14	7.9	18.1	9.4
18:1	22	24.5	18.9	19.7	19.5
18:2	15	15.5	15.3	10.5	16.5
18:3	—	2	—	trace	trace
20:0	—	—	—	trace	—
20:3	—	—	1.5	1.0	1.4
20:4	13½	8	7.9	11.5	19.5
22:? and others	—	—	4.5	8.2	—

[a] For shorthand designation see Table VI.
[b] Data calculated from the given figures.
[c] Data recalculated for weight percentages.

type of phospholipid often carries a rather specific fatty acid pattern. However, the described variations in fatty acid composition of phospholipids from erythrocytes are not to be explained directly by their apparent differences in phospholipid distribution. Analysis of the fatty acids of lecithin and cephalins separated by chromatographic procedures has been carried out recently in the author's laboratory for erythrocytes of a number of animal species. The fatty acid patterns of the class of lecithins (Fig. 4) show some evident similarities as well as differences among erythrocytes of different species. A fair amount of palmitic acid is always present, as well as C_{18} fatty acids, although the proportion of saturated mono- and di-saturated acids of this chain length differs from animal to animal. Furthermore, some differences are to be noted with respect to the content of the essential fatty acid arachidonic acid. More pronounced are the differences in fatty acid composition revealed by the cephalin fraction (ethanolamine and serine phospholipids). Of the erythrocytes studied (Fig. 5), most striking differences exist in the content of palmitic acid, oleic acid, and arachidonic acid. Although characterization of the sphingomyelin

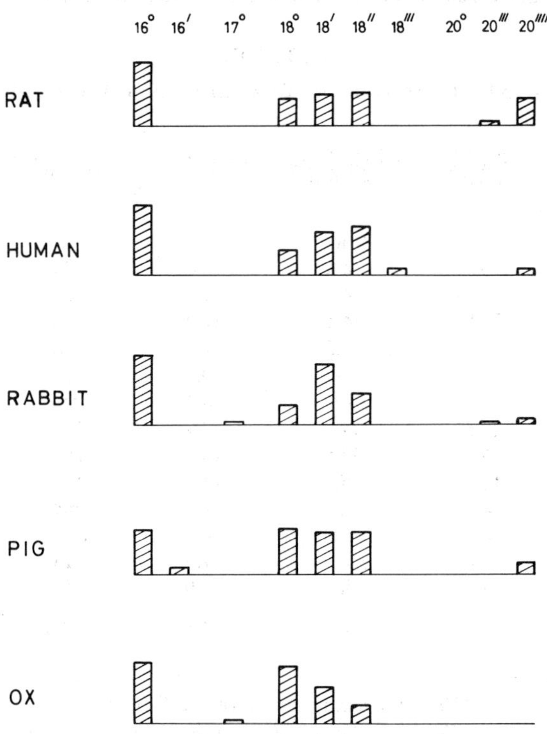

FIG. 4. Fatty acid patterns of lecithins of erythrocytes from various species of mammal. For explanation see Fig. 3 (van Deenen, 1962).

fatty acids is not yet completed, it can be concluded that the notable differences in fatty acid constituents in red cells among various species are reflected to a major extent by the cephalin fraction. It is concluded that a gradual decrease in the ratio of lecithin to sphingomyelin is accompanied by differences in the proportions of palmitic acid, oleic acid, and arachidonic acid in cephalins such as phosphatidylethanolamine. These observations on red cell lipids bear some resemblance, although not in every detail, to shifts reported to occur in phospholipid and fatty acids of human aorta in several stages of atherosclerosis (Böttcher and van Gent, 1961). Perhaps the red blood cell can serve to elucidate general relationships in lipid characteristics so far not readily recognizable.

In addition to the fatty acid patterns presented here, detailed analyses have been made on individual phospholipids in red blood cells of man (Hanahan

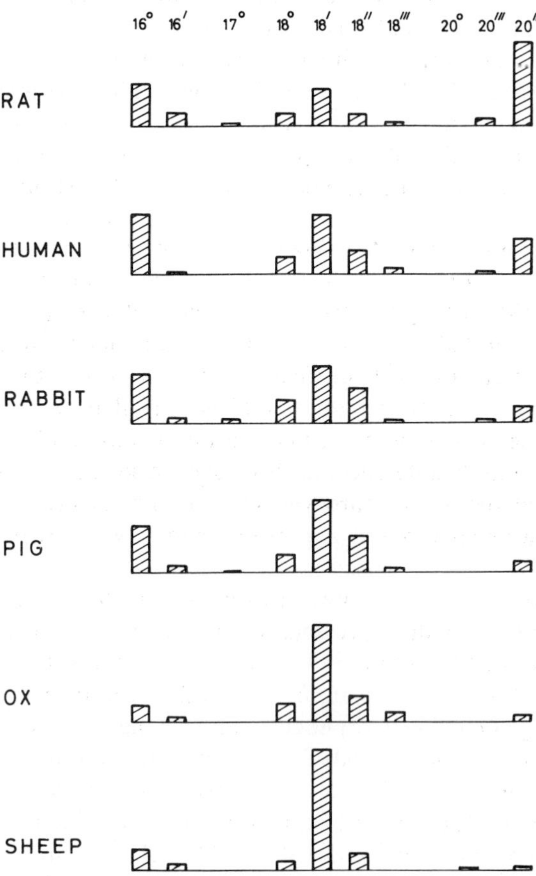

FIG. 5. Fatty acid patterns of cephalins of erythrocytes from various species of mammal. For explanation see Fig. 3 (van Deenen, 1962).

et al., 1960a; Farquhar, 1962a), cow (Hanahan *et al.*, 1960a), and fowl (Kates and James, 1961). As far as similar species and phospholipid fractions are concerned, most studies are in reasonable agreement. Confining our discussion further to the human red blood cell, it can be stated that both choline-containing phospholipids, viz. lecithin and sphingomyelin, contain a fair amount of palmitic acid. The ratio of saturated to unsaturated fatty acids in human erythrocyte lecithin is approximately 1, and through the use of snake venom phospholipase A, Hanahan *et al.* (1960a) established the unsaturated fatty acids to be located predominantly at the β position of the lecithin molecule.

Phosphatidylserine was demonstrated by Farquhar (1962a) to contain more than 40% of stearic acid. The quantitation of fatty acids in phosphatidylethanolamine demonstrated that this phospholipid, together with phosphatidylserine, was the main carrier of arachidonic acid and C_{22} polyenoic acids. The amount of stearic acid is lower than often found in phosphatidylethanolamine isolated from other sources. However, fatty acids do not constitute the whole nonpolar part of the ethanolamine-containing phospholipid in human erythrocytes, inasmuch as a considerable part exists in the plasmalogen form.

4. Fatty Aldehyde and Glyceryl Ether Constituents of Red Cell Phospholipids

a. Plasmalogens. From various studies it became clear that part of the red cell phospholipids belongs to the class of plasmalogens (XVII), known to contain an unsaturated ether linkage instead of an ester bond (Dawson *et al.*, 1960; Kates and James, 1961; de Gier and van Deenen, 1961; de Gier *et al.*, 1961d; Farquhar, 1962a). As a result of the data available in the literature and from unpublished experiments carried out in the author's laboratory, it can be stated that notable differences in this respect also exist among red cells of different animal species. Erythrocytes of man and rat proved to be rich in plasmalogen, whereas those of pig, rabbit, and cow revealed a significantly lower content.

Detailed information is at present available on the plasmalogens of the human red cell. Extending previous observations, Farquhar (1962a) conclusively established by several independent analytical methods that 67% of ethanolamine phospholipids were of the plasmalogen type, and only 8% of serine and 10% of choline phosphoglycerides belong to this class.

Gas chromatographic methods for the determination of fatty aldehyde as dimethylacetal or other derivatives have been developed by Gray (1960) and Farquhar (1962b). The complex character of the aldehyde moiety present in red cell plasmalogens is demonstrated in Table XII. A comparison of the data obtained in two laboratories, although carried out on somewhat different lipids fractions, is justified since ethanolamine plasmalogen is the major aldehyde donor in both fractions investigated. These studies demonstrated that the most abundant aldehydes in red cell phospholipids are saturated straight chains 18:0 and 16:0, a branched 17:0, the nonsaturated 18:1, and an unidentified 18:1 isomer. Determinations carried out by Farquhar on the aldehydes of individual plasmalogens showed 16:0 to be the major aldehyde of the choline class, but 18:0 for the serine and ethanolamine phosphoglycerides. The molar ratio of saturated acyl chains (fatty acids plus aldehydes) to unsaturated fatty acids appeared to be close to unity in each class. This finding is consistent and extends the previously mentioned observations of Hanahan *et al.* (1960a) that in red cell phosphoglycerides the β position is occupied mainly by an unsaturated fatty acid and the γ position by a saturated fatty acid ester or (enol) ether.

TABLE XII

Fatty Aldehyde Composition of Human Erythrocyte Plasmalogens

Fatty aldehyde	Kates *et al.* (1961)	Farquhar (1962)[b]
14:0[a]	trace	—
br. 15:0	0.8	1.6
15:0 iso or ante-iso[c]	—	0.1
15:0	0.6	0.5
Unknown	trace	0.2
cis 16:1	0.4	0.2
16:0	24.2	19.3
br. 17:?	—	0.1
br. 17:?	1.7	0.5
br. 17:0	7.5	4.4
17:0 iso or ante-iso	—	2.5
17:0	1.3	4.4
cis,cis 18:2	—	1.3
cis 18:1	6.0	8.0
18:1 isomer	2.8	12.7
18:0	42.5	44.1
Unknown	2.9	—
br. 19:0	—	0.1
20:?	3.1	—
20:?	5.6	—

[a] This shorthand designation is analogous to that used for the fatty acids (see Table VI); br. 15:0 signifies a branched saturated fatty aldehyde with 15 carbon atoms.

[b] The data reported by Farquhar are recalculated for weight percentages.

[c] Compare branched-chain fatty acids of the odd series of $CH_3CH_2CH(CH_3)(CH_2)_nCOOH$.

b. Glyceryl Ether Phospholipids. Well-known naturally occurring glyceryl ethers (XXI) are batyl alcohol with stearyl, selachyl alcohol with oleoyl, and chimyl alcohol with palmityl as the long-chain part of the molecule. The glyceryl ethers are more widespread in marine animals than in land animals. The glyceryl ethers can function as part of a glyceride as well as a phospholipid molecule. The latter compounds proved to be rather stable to treatment with acid and alkali. When investigating the phospholipids of bovine erythrocytes, Hanahan and Watts (1961) found that the phosphatidylethanolamine fraction

$$\begin{array}{l} CH_2\text{—O—R} \\ | \\ CH\text{—OH} \\ | \\ CH_2\text{—OH} \end{array}$$

(XXI)

revealed a fatty acid ester to P value notably lower than 2, while no lyso derivative or plasmalogen was present. These investigators showed the presence of an α'-glycerol ether-containing phospholipid (compare XVIII) by developing a convenient method for isolation of this type of compound. The diacyl ethanolamine was removed by rapid alkaline hydrolysis and the remaining α'-alkoxy-β-acyl-α-glyceryl-phosphorylethanolamine was obtained after chromatographic purification. The glycerol phospholipid appeared to constitute as much as 80% of the ethanolamine phospholipids. Hallgren and Larsson (1962) were unable to demonstrate glyceryl ethers in lipids from human red blood cells. Inasmuch as the percentage of plasmalogens in ethanolamine phospholipids from human erythrocytes corresponds almost to that of the glyceryl ether ethanolamine phospholipids in bovine erythrocytes, the red blood cell offers a unique opportunity for studying the possible biochemical relationships between the two types of compound.

E. Binding of Lipids to Other Red Cell Constituents

1. Linkage of Lipids to Other Cell Constituents

Direct or indirect evidence suggests that various lipid classes are mutually associated within the red cell membrane and that certain types of lipid are linked to other classes of red cell constituents. The lipoprotein character of the red cell ghost has been recognized for a long time, and is believed to be brought about mainly by interactions of the charged groups of the phospholipids with those of the structural proteins. Parpart and Ballentine (1952) were the first to emphasize that there are different sorts of combinations between lipids and protein of the plasma membrane. Using a variety of solvents, they verified the extent of binding of the various lipid types in dried ghosts of beef red cells. Treatment with dry ether removed all cholesterol and a small part of the phospholipids (mainly cephalins) and this lipid fraction was termed the "loosely bound" fraction. Solvents such as wet ether or pyridine-ether removed another part but by no means all of the cephalins and this fraction was called "weakly bound." Finally, the major part of the phospholipids containing the choline derivatives and remaining part (50%) of the cephalins was extractable only with polar solvents, e.g. alcohol-ether 3:1, and therefore considered to be "strongly bound." Experiments on this phenomenon in red cell ghosts of various species confined to determinations of loosely and strongly bound lipids were carried out by the present authors (de Gier *et al.*, 1961a; van Deenen *et al.*, 1961a, 1962b). Confirming the observations of Parpart and Ballentine, it was found that ether extracted all the cholesterol and a small but definite part of the phospholipids, being quantitatively different, however, for various animal species (Fig. 6). Binding of the major part of the phospholipids to other nonlipid constituents is apparent inasmuch as nonpolar lipid solvents fail to extract the bulk of phospholipids. The strongly bound fraction extracted once by ethanol-ether (3:1 v/v) is, after removal of solvent, readily soluble in ether. Analysis of the composition of the loosely bound

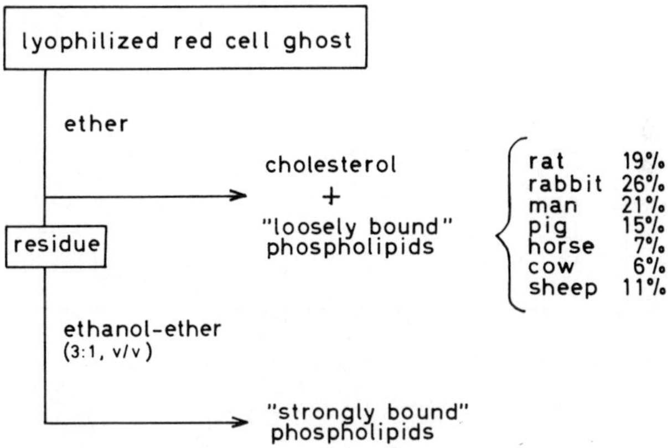

FIG. 6. Schematic representation of the distinction between "loosely bound" and "strongly bound" lipids in erythrocyte ghosts (van Deenen, 1962).

phospholipid showed cephalins to be abundant but choline phospholipids were also recovered. Although the results obtained indicated that this distinction in phospholipids is brought about by difference in extractability rather than by difference in solubility, it appears necessary, however, to establish the nature of the fatty acid constituents of the strongly and weakly bound compounds. Using mixtures of various proportions of ether-ethanol, Turner *et al.* (1958b) also observed that differences existed in the comparative liberation of phosphatides from red cell ghosts of various animal species. With these solvent systems, no differences in rates of release of the individual phospholipid components were observed.

The experimental evidence for the different sorts of binding of lipids in the red cell membrane led Parpart and Ballentine to suggest that the most numerous strongly bound phospholipid molecules are attached to the proteins, while the less numerous weakly bound and loosely bound phospholipids are attached to the corresponding fatty acid chains of the strongly bound phospholipid. Pursuing these ideas, Parpart and Ballentine (1952) proposed a model for the molecular arrangement within the red cell membrane (Fig. 7) which deviates

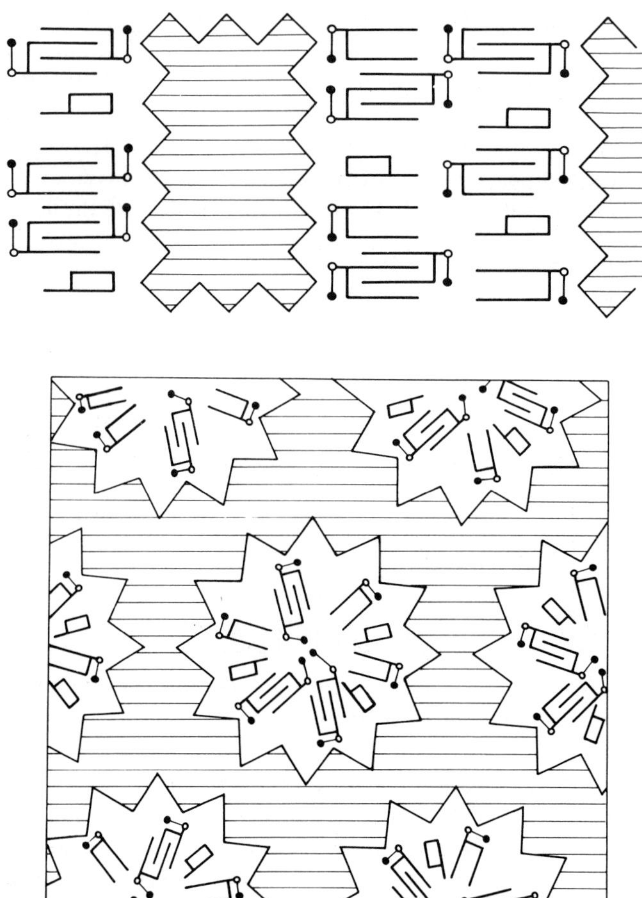

FIG. 7. Molecular orientation in the erythrocyte membrane according to suggestions of Parpart and Ballentine (1952). A: section perpendicular to the surface. B: section tangential to the surface. The lipids are represented as indicated in Figs. 1 and 2; the lined areas represent protein.

strongly from those concepts suggesting that a bimolecular lipid leaflet surrounded by protein is valid also for the red cell protoplasma membrane. For these reasons further investigations on the background of this extractability phenomenon and the exact chemical nature of phospholipids recovered in the strongly and loosely bound fractions are urgently needed. However, it will be necessary also to find out to what extent lyophilization of the ghosts affects the binding between membrane constituents. Taking into account the information available at the moment, the interpretation given by Parpart and Ballentine, viz., that the loosely bound phospholipids are not protein-bound but retained in the cell membrane by interaction of their acyl chains with those of the strongly bound class, is still attractive. On the other hand one may imagine that in a framework consisting of a bimolecular lipid leaflet, part of the phospholipid molecules, depending on their location, are attached to other membrane constituents mainly by van der Waals forces. Recently, however, support for the hypothesis of Parpart was supplied by highly interesting electron microscope observations on the surface of red cell ghost membranes by Dourmashkin *et al.* (1962), using negative staining with phosphotungstate. At certain concentrations saponin treatment caused the appearance of a hexagonal array of pits at the surface of the ghost, while digitonin prevented the formation of such pits. Identical results were obtained with other cell membranes. As discussed by Dourmashkin *et al.*, these results are in fair agreement with a mosaic arrangement of cylinders containing phospholipid and cholesterol surrounded by a protein meshwork as proposed by Parpart and Ballentine (1952) and reproduced in Fig. 7. So far it has not been possible to ascertain whether the saponin-induced pits are in fact holes through the membrane, although in transverse sections Muir (1962) observed definite discontinuities. While the use of permanganate fixation and thin-sectioning techniques in electron microscopy revealed a unit structure of cell membranes, which supports the pauci-molecular theory involving a continuous bimolecular lipid leaflet (Figs. 1 and 2), these new investigations made by negative staining after saponin treatment suggest heterogeneity in the distribution of lipids in the plane surface of the plasma membrane (Fig. 7). It is difficult to decide at present which approach is most favorable in minimizing artifacts, but chemical investigations of the amount and nature of the lipids removed by saponin from the red cell ghost pitted under the electron microscope will be helpful for the understanding of this basic problem![2]

2. Association between Lipids

In all current theories attempting to formulate the architecture of the red cell membrane, attractive forces between the nonpolar moieties of the lipid

[2] Actually, recent investigations of A. D. Bangham and co-workers (1962) showed that treatment of films of cholesterol with saponin gives rise to patterns closely resembling the electron microscope observations made by Dourmashkin *et al.* on cell membranes. Therefore Bangham *et al.* concluded that the hexagonal structure produced by adding saponin to cell membranes may represent primarily a molecular arrangement of a complex of saponin with cholesterol still attached to the membrane. Thus the pattern obtained after saponin treatment would not represent any pre-existing arrangement of lipid and protein in the cell membrane as suggested by Dourmashkin *et al.*

constituents are implicated. In this connection attention may be drawn to the fact that in ghosts of mammalian erythrocytes, cholesterol is present in an amount such as to provide a molecular ratio of cholesterol to phospholipid close to unity (Table III). It is very likely that, in addition to the van der Waals forces between fatty acyl chains of phospholipids, attractive forces between phospholipids and cholesterol are also involved in holding the lipid molecules in side-to-side aggregations.

Studies on the interaction of cholesterol and phospholipids in monomolecular layers showed a packing effect of cholesterol, resulting in reduction of the molecular area occupied by the phospholipid molecule (Dervichian, 1958; de Bernard, 1958). Recently it was shown in a study with various defined synthetic phospholipids that this effect was most pronounced when certain fatty acid constituents, e.g. oleic acid, are present in the phospholipid molecule (van Deenen *et al.*, 1962a). Model experiments on the penetration of surface tension-active hemolytic factors into films of cholesterol and phospholipids also support the view that cholesterol is involved in maintaining the stability and structure of the erythrocyte membrane (Schulman *et al.*, 1955). Although the situation in monomolecular layers at an air/water interface is remote from the red cell protoplasma boundary, it is believed likely that similar or related stabilizing effects of cholesterol may occur in biomembranes.

Of great interest is the view expressed by Finean (1953) on the molecular association between phosphatidylethanolamine and cholesterol, supported by studies on x-ray diffraction of myelin. This investigator proposed that these lipids are arranged with their nonpolar moieties approximately parallel, but with the polar head group of the phospholipid molecule curled around so as to enter into a complex with the cholesterol molecule. Further studies are required to confirm this detailed suggestion of a specific association of phospholipid and cholesterol molecules and to ascertain its validity for the red cell membrane.

F. Possible Relations between Lipid Composition and Other Characteristics of the Red Cell Membrane

The integral part occupied by lipids in the red cell membrane suggests that the chemical composition of the membranous lipids may participate in determining various properties of the limiting membrane. Inasmuch as red cells of several animal species have been known for a long time to differ in various properties (Table XIII) and recent investigations have disclosed significant distinctions in their lipid patterns, it is a matter of interest to verify whether relationships between the two characteristics have been revealed. It should be emphasized that in this respect a unique opportunity is offered by the red cell.

In the past, attempts to correlate lipid composition with other properties, e.g. permeability behavior of red cells, have been made particularly by the school of Parpart. These investigators draw attention to some existing differences in lipid data and permeability of erythrocytes of various animals (Parpart and Dziemian, 1940). Ultimately the conclusion was reached, however, that no major differences in proportions of phospholipid types existed in the red cells of vertebrates, nor was any significant correlation between lipid content and the large permeability differences of the red cells observed (compare Parpart and Ballentine, 1952). However, new analytical tools have revealed significant differences in the phospholipid distribution and composition of their fatty acid constituents among erythrocytes of different mammals. In the sequence of animals: rat, rabbit, man, pig, ox, and sheep, the content of lecithin in the erythrocytes decreases significantly while the amount of sphingomyelin increases simultaneously. As outlined before, the fatty acid patterns of the cephalin fraction from these red cells varied in nearly the same order, showing most conspicuous differences with respect to the percentages of palmitic, oleic, and arachidonic acids. For these reasons in Table XIII the erythrocytes of various species are arranged on the basis of these shifts in lipid composition and a number of heterogeneous erythrocyte characteristics have been inserted. Differences in dimension and osmotic fragility appear not to be related directly with variations in lipid composition. Probably this is true also

TABLE XIII

General Properties of Erythrocytes of Different Animal Species

Species	Dimensions		K^+ (meq./liter cells)[a]	Na^+ (meq./liter cells)[a]	Diphosphoglycerate content[b] (mg./liter cells)	Hemolysis time in isotonic solutions of			Glucose permeability[d]
	Diameter (μ)	Volume (μ^3)				Glycol[c]	Glycerol[c]	Thiourea[c]	
Rat	7.5[e]	41[e]	100	12	34.1	3.6	18.2	44.3	250
Rabbit	7.5[e]	64[e]	99	16	45.3	4.8	32.2	93	100
Man	7.9[e]	87[f]	104	10	38.0	4.2	51.4	104	—
Pig	—	58[e]	100	11	45.0	15.6	131.6	—	10
Ox	6.0[e]	48[e]	22	79	<0.7	27.4	2169	183	0
Sheep	5.2[e]	35[e]	{64, 18}	{16, 84}	<0.8	24.5	1397	—	0

[a] Prankerd (1961).

[b] Rapoport and Guest (1941).

[c] Jacobs *et al.* (1950).

[d] Increase in glucose concentration in the cell 1 hour after addition of 500 mg. glucose to 100 ml. blood. Data calculated from the figures given by Laris (1960); unit is mg. glucose/100 ml. red cell water.

[e] Ponder (1948).

[f] Albritton (1955).

with respect to the well-known differences in sodium : potassium ratio, although erythrocytes of cow and sheep, revealing a reversed ratio of these cations when compared with other recorded animal species, have been demonstrated to deviate in the lipid characteristics also. However, erythrocytes of sheep, having a low or high sodium : potassium ratio, have been shown not to differ with

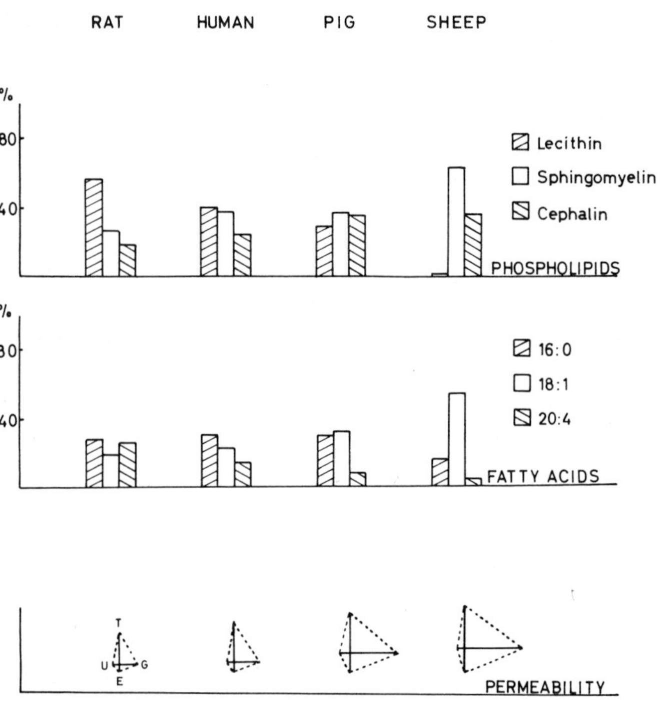

FIG. 8. Comparison between certain lipid characteristics and permeability behavior of erythrocyte membranes of various species (van Deenen *et al.*, 1962b). Data on individual types of phospholipid are expressed as percentages of the total phospholipid fraction. Fatty acids are given as percentages of the fatty acid content of total lipids (e.g., 18:1 for oleic acid and 20:4 for arachidonic acid). Figures on permeability were taken from Jacobs *et al.* (1950) and represent hemolysis times in isotonic solutions of urea (U), thiourea (T), glycol (G), and ethylene glycol (E) on four perpendicular axes in a logarithmic scale (compare also Table XIII).

respect to lecithin content (M. Oliveira and M. Vaughan, unpublished observations). Differences in content of diphosphoglycerate cannot be related in a statistically satisfactory manner with the gradual shifts in lipid composition of the erythrocytes under discussion. However, as already reported by the present authors, significant relationships exist between the differences in lipid characteristics and the variations in permeability behavior of the red cells concerned toward certain lipid-insoluble compounds (Kögl *et al.*, 1960; de Gier and van Deenen, 1961; van Deenen *et al.*, 1961a). The hemolysis time in isotonic solutions of glycol, glycerol, and thiourea, as determined by Jacobs *et al.* (1950), is related inversely to the rate of penetration and represents a fair picture of the differences in permeability of various erythrocytes to these compounds. Furthermore, Höber (1936) reported that the penetration rate of ammonium salts of fatty acids into red cells rises in the series rat, man, ox, and sheep, which is the reverse of the series found with the lipid-insoluble compounds first mentioned. Differences noted by Laris (1960) with respect to the uptake of glucose by red cells also appear to relate to some extent to variations in lipids (Table XIII).

Figure 8 summarizes the shifts in lipid composition of erythrocytes in a number of species studied and additionally demonstrates variations in permeability behavior of these red cells toward lipid-insoluble compounds. The relationship between the two characteristics of red cells as suggested by this comparison needs a great deal of further experimental proof, perhaps by inducing changes in lipid composition by dietary means and investigating the effects on the permeability characteristics of the red cell. On the other hand, it should be realized that the differences in lipids among different erythrocytes are of a complex nature, and extensive studies on the plasmalogens and glyceryl ethers still are required to complete the map of erythrocyte lipids to be compared with permeability data. Another goal is an understanding of the possible differences brought about by variation of lipid composition in the molecular orientation and fine architecture of the red cell membrane. Properties of monomolecular films of synthetic phospholipids were demonstrated to be highly dependent on the nature of fatty acid constituents (van Deenen *et al.*, 1962a).

IV. Dynamic Aspects of Red Cell Lipids

A. Relation of the Hematopoietic Bone Marrow to the Lipids

Passing on to the constitution of the required molecular orientation of the lipids in the red cell membrane, presumably a great deal of the *de novo* synthesis of these lipids proceeds in the hematopoietic bone marrow. However, relatively few studies have been made in this direction, probably because of the heterogeneous cell population of this tissue and difficulties in solving the problem of their separation. Determinations of the lipid content of bone marrow in different animal species have been reported (Dietz, 1949; Elko and Di Luzio, 1959), while in the past few years several studies have concerned the composition of these lipids. Dealing first with normal human bone marrow, Lund *et al.* (1962) showed the total extractable lipid from femur marrow to be 28–84% of tissue wet weight. These lipids belonged primarily to the class of neutral lipids and less than 3% of phospholipids appeared to be present. A similar situation was encountered in bone marrow of several other mammalian species (Elko and Di Luzio, 1959; Mulder *et al.*, 1962). However, the information available suggests that the phospholipid content does bear a relation to the hematopoietic cellularity of the tissues analyzed.

While the glyceride fraction in red cells forms only a minority, this class is dominant in bone marrow lipids. Lund *et al.* (1962) demonstrated the glycerides to account for 96–98% of the extractable lipids, their fatty acid composition being identical to that of human fat from other locations, such as adipose tissues. It has therefore been rightly argued that this marrow fat serves for the greater part as a form of lipid storage (Evans and Oppenheimer, 1955). Cholesterol, being a major red cell lipid, was, like phospholipids, recovered only in small amounts from the bone marrow, its concentration believed to be again related to the hematopoietic cellularity (Lund *et al.*, 1962). In view of the notable differences existing in phospholipid composition among red cells of various animals, it is of interest to make a comparison in this respect among the red bone marrows of the species concerned. Animal species revealing very low content of lecithin in circulating red cells, e.g. cow and sheep, have been shown in the author's laboratory to contain lecithin as a major phospholipid in unfractionated red bone marrow (Mulder *et al.*, 1962). Studies on the *in vitro* incorporation of radioactive phosphate (Mulder *et al.*, 1962) revealed an uptake mainly into lecithin or red bone marrow of several species, irrespective of the lecithin content of the red cells. Investigating the biosynthetic pathways of phospholipids of the glyceryl ether type (XXI), known to be present in unusually high amount in bovine red cells, Thompson and Hanahan (1962) reported the highest level of radioactivity to be present in lecithin after incubation of bovine hematopoietic bone marrow with labeled glucose.

The studies quoted above uniformly demonstrated that no direct quantitative relations exist between lipids of circulating red cells and lipids of whole red bone marrow. It was realized of course by the various investigators making early studies on lipids of the hematopoietic tissues, that the materials studied were of a heterogeneous nature. Further investigations on the formation of red cell lipids and their constitution in the red cell membrane will require the difficult task of isolating the cell organelles concerned from the hetamopoietic marrow.

B. *Metabolic Events of Lipids in Circulating Red Cells*

A vast number of investigations have dealt with the metabolism of lipids in circulating red cells, but conflicting opinions have been expressed. Isotopic studies carried out *in vivo* and *in vitro* frequently have been hampered by inadequate separation of different types of blood cell. Processes originally believed to occur in the mature red cell were demonstrated in further studies to be attributable to leucocytes or reticulocytes. Nevertheless, recent developments indicate that, within certain limits, lipids of mature red cells are in a dynamic state, and it is believed likely that within a few years this aspect of red cell metabolism will be established with more certainty and precision than exist at present.

1. Renewal of Cholesterol

Experiments with C^{14}-acetate revealed cholesterol in rabbit red cells to exhibit a half-life of 12–14 days (Muir *et al.*, 1951). Whether this renewal was brought about by synthesis *in situ* or uptake of plasma cholesterol remained to be established. Although experiments with C^{14}-acetate originally suggested that biosynthesis of lipids may occur in mature red cells of mammalian species (Altman, 1953), it has been shown more recently that reticulocytes (O'Donnell *et al.*, 1958) and particularly leucocytes and platelets (Marks *et al.*, 1960; Buchanan, 1960) account for most, if not all, of the lipid synthesis of blood cells.

On the other hand, evidence was put forward to support the concept that renewal of red cell cholesterol may arise by uptake of plasma cholesterol. A rapid interchange of free cholesterol between red cells and plasma from the dog was observed by Hagerman and Gould (1951). Plasma and red cells containing C^{14}-labeled cholesterol were incubated *in vitro* with their unlabeled counterparts. It was noted that equipartition of red cell and plasma unesterified cholesterol took place in about 4 hours, 50 % equilibration having been reached in 1 hour. It is of interest to note that cholesterol esters, present in only minor amount in the red cell, did not take part in the exchange phenomenon. The dynamic equilibrium between cholesterol of plasma and red cell membrane *in vivo* was demonstrated by London and Schwartz (1953) by administration of heavy water, the tracer being found equally distributed between cholesterol of blood cells and that of plasma. This approach also may be hampered somewhat by participation of leucocytes and other blood cells, but these investigators were unable to obtain evidence of incorporation of C^{14}-acetate into the red cell cholesterol. Ruyssen (1957) reported that a red cell suspension in saline containing cholesterol-4-C^{14} acquired a high specific activity, which was not released by keeping the red cells in isotonic salt solution. Summarizing, it appears that mature mammalian red cells are not capable of synthesizing cholesterol *de novo*, but interchange with plasma cholesterol may impart a dynamic feature to this important membrane constituent. Some fresh confirmation excluding any contribution of other blood cells, however, is desirable. Such an exchange reaction demonstrates the flexibility of the membranous framework, and perhaps this phenomenon may participate in supplying pores for transport across the cell boundary.

2. Biosynthesis of Fatty Acids

Several studies directed toward ascertaining whether red cells are capable of synthesizing their own fatty acid constituents have resulted in a somewhat confusing situation.

Investigating the synthesis of unfractionated blood cells, James *et al.* (1957, 1959) incubated blood with C^{14}-acetate *in vitro* and isolated blood cells and plasma lipids showing significant radioactivity in all fractions. Determination of radioactivity in the individual types of fatty acid separated by gas-liquid chromatography revealed a labeling of all common saturated and unsaturated fatty acids of a variety of chain lengths; the essential fatty acids, linoleic and arachidonic, were also reported to be labeled. Furthermore, it was reported that free interchange of phospholipids and cholesterol between red cell and plasma lipoproteins occurred, but that exchange of neutral fat from cells to plasma α-lipoprotein proceeded in only one direction. The plasma itself was shown to have no appreciable synthetic activity. It was concluded by James *et al.* (1957, 1959) that the synthesis of long-chain acids is carried out by red and possibly white cells, which incorporated these fatty acids into their lipids followed by secretion of the end products into the plasma. However, as stated by these authors the experiments had not defined the relative contributions of reticulocytes, erythrocytes, and white cells (James *et al.*, 1959).

Another report favoring a possible biosynthesis of fatty acids in red cells came from Mendelsohn (1961a,b) who observed an interrelationship between carbohydrate and lipid metabolism in the human erythrocyte *in vivo* as well as *in vitro*. Following oral ingestion of glucose, an increase in unesterified fatty acids was observed in the erythrocyte, reaching a maximum in 1–1.5 hours. This process appeared to be impaired in the diabetic human erythrocyte, but was corrected by administration of insulin. The level of free fatty acids of the plasma showed a corresponding decline, but Mendelsohn argued that the rise in red cell fatty acids could not be explained simply by uptake of these compounds from the plasma. His suggestion that the human red blood cell is able to synthesize lipid from carbohydrate was supported to some extent by *in vitro* experiments without plasma present.

Several investigators, however, emphasized that fatty acid biosynthesis is absent or of a very low level in the mature red cell. Experiments of O'Donnell *et al.* (1958) led to the conclusion that reticulocytes are able to synthesize fatty acids from labeled acetate *in vitro* but that this process no longer occurs in mature red cells of various animal species. Webb *et al.* (1960), studying *in vitro* lipid synthesis in fowl blood, showed that even nucleated fowl erythrocytes are less active than young erythrocyte preparations and much less so than leucocytes. As regards lipid synthesis in human blood cells, Marks *et al.* (1960) observed that C^{14}-acetate was incorporated into lipids by leucocytes and platelets but less into reticulocytes and only to a very limited extent, if at all, into mature erythrocytes. Lipids formed by leucocytes and platelets were demonstrated to be transferred to plasma. Buchanan (1960) also arrived at the conclusion that mature erythrocytes do not synthesize any of the labeled lipid found after incubation of blood with C^{14}-acetate, while leucocytes were extremely active and alone could account for the total amounts of synthesized lipid. An essentially similar conclusion was reached at the same time by the research group from Mill Hill (Rowe *et al.*, 1960a,b), permitting the conclusion that leucocytes and not red cells carry out the major part of the synthetic processes reported in the previously mentioned contributions from this group (James *et al.*, 1957, 1959). Studying the biosynthesis of polyenoic fatty acids in human blood, Leupold and Kremer (1961) showed that a total synthesis of linoleic acid can be precluded and additionally observed a good linearity between leucocyte count and total incorporation of labeled acetate.

When considering these recent developments the conclusion is unavoidable that biosynthesis of fatty acids in red cells is probably of a minor order, if it exists at all. This conclusion, however, does conflict with the interpretation Mendelsohn (1961a, b) put on his interesting experiments. His studies were not performed with isotopes, probably precluding a significant contribution of other cell types. As will be discussed later, red cell phospholipids have been shown, however, to be able to incorporate and probably to change fatty acids, and perhaps this process is somewhere connected with the variation brought about in free fatty acid content of red cells by administration of glucose.

3. Metabolism of Phospholipids

a. Incorporation of Radioactive Phosphate. The uptake of radioactive phosphate into the phospholipids of circulating red blood corpuscles has been demonstrated by Hevesy and Aten (1939) and Hahn and Hevesy (1939) to be of a low order. The incorporation of phosphate into phospholipids of erythrocytes incubated *in vitro* is very slight when compared with other animal cells (van Deenen *et al.*, 1961a; de Gier *et al.*, 1961b). It has been reported (Paysant-Diament and Polonovski, 1960; de Gier *et al.*, 1961b) that human erythrocytes incorporated labeled phosphate mainly into phosphatidic acid (IX). Studying the metabolism of unfractionated blood cells, Rowe (1959) observed a more uniform P^{32} labeling of the cellular phospholipids, but it is likely that these results are not to be attributed to the erythrocyte.

The determination of P^{32} distribution among phospholipids of erythrocytes of various animal species, upon incubation *in vitro*, has been the subject of studies in our laboratory, which lead to the conclusion that the significant differences existing in phospholipid composition are not clearly reflected by the radioactivity patterns. However, some of the results previously published (van Deenen *et al.*, 1961a; de Gier *et al.*, 1961b) have been shown more recently to need revision (van Deenen, 1962) without altering the substance of the previous statement. The incorporation of radiophosphate after *in vitro* incubation of relatively pure preparations of erythrocytes appeared to be of a very low order, being different for various species. Monkey, rabbit, and rat revealed, like man, a detectable incorporation into phosphatidic acid, whereas in several species, e.g. pig, ox, and sheep, the radioactivity was too low to allow determination with any reliability of the exact distribution among the several phospholipid classes. Titus *et al.* (1961) also reported sheep red cells to be uanble to incorporate radioactive phosphate. With respect to rabbit erythrocytes, Raderecht *et al.* (1962) found, in agreement with our observations, that P^{32} incorporation was almost completely limited to phosphatidic acid. Reticulocytes, however, were demonstrated by this group to exhibit the highest rates of incorporation into lecithin and cephalins. The incorporation rate of P^{32} appeared to decrease during maturation of red cells with accompanying decrease of phosphate uptake into lecithins and cephalins. These observations led Raderecht *et al.* (1962) to the conclusion that conversion of phosphatidic acid into lecithins and cephalins, as established by Kennedy's school (compare Kennedy, 1961), does not continue to function in the mature erythrocyte.

Although further studies are necessary, the studies reported so far suggest that *de novo* synthesis of quantitatively major phospholipids is probably lacking or of a low order within circulating mature red cells of mammals.

b. The Phosphatidic Acid Cycle. Phosphatidic acid can be formed by enzymatic acylation of glycerophosphate (Kornberg and Pricer, 1953), but M. R. Hokin and Hokin (1959) established in addition that phosphorylation of diglycerides, catalyzed by a diglyceride kinase can produce this compound in a great variety of tissues. Furthermore, a phosphatidic acid phosphatase, causing hydrolysis of phosphatidic acid to diglyceride, has been demonstrated. Hokin and Hokin (1960) concluded as a result of their important work that this process, termed the phosphatidic acid cycle, may function as a sodium carrier in biomembranes. Actually the enzymes involved in the phosphatidic acid cycle have been demonstrated to be present in ghosts of human erythrocytes (Hokin and Hokin, 1961). More recently these investigators (Hokin and Hokin, 1963) pointed out that in red cell ghosts, the synthesis of phosphatidic acid by the diglyceride kinase reaction (Scheme 1) is 10–40 times more active

$$\text{D-1,2-diglyceride} + \text{ATP} \xrightarrow{\text{diglyceride kinase}} \text{L-}\alpha\text{-phosphatidic acid} + \text{ADP}$$

$$\text{L-}\alpha\text{-phosphatidic acid} + H_2O \xrightarrow[\text{phosphatidic acid phosphatase}]{} \text{D-1,2-diglyceride} + H_3PO_4$$

$$\text{ATP} + H_2O \longrightarrow H_3PO_4 + \text{ADP}$$

Scheme 1. Phosphatidic acid cycle in human erythrocytes (according to Hokin and Hokin, 1961, 1963).

than synthesis of phosphatidic acid by phosphorylation of monoglycerides followed by acylation, and 2500 times more active than synthesis by acylation of α-glycero-phosphate.

The diglyceride kinase activity was as great or greater than the Na^+- and K^+-dependent ouabain-inhibitable ATPase in erythrocyte membrane. This proved to be the case also with respect to the magnesium-dependent phosphatidic acid phosphatase (Hokin *et al.*, 1963) and although no direct proof exists as yet, these findings are compatible with the idea that the phosphatidic acid cycle enzymes are components of the ATPase believed to be involved in active cation transport (Post *et al.*, 1960). The precise mechanism of the active sodium transport is still a challenge to the investigator.

The functioning of a phosphatidic cycle, found in the human red cell ghost, is in agreement with the observed incorporation of radioactive phosphate, demonstrated to proceed mainly into phosphatidic acid of intact human erythrocytes. However, it remains to be established whether the rate of this process in circulating red cells is of a sufficient order to be directly connected with the sodium pump.

c. Exchange Reactions with Plasma Phospholipids. Studies of Hahn and Hevesy (1939), exploring an *in vitro* interaction between P^{32}-labeled phospholipids of plasma and red cells, indicated that a very limited interchange (5% in 4–5 hours) may occur in rabbit blood. These authors tentatively concluded that some phospholipids exchanged fairly well and others not at all. In view of the different types of binding of phospholipids in red cell membranes it would be of interest to investigate whether the so-called loosely bound class is involved only in this exchange process (see Section III, E). In human blood an *in vivo* and *in vitro* exchange of erythrocyte and plasma phospholipid, according to an abstract by Reed (1959), appears to involve an interchange of about 10% of choline-containing phospholipids per 24 hours. As indicated previously, studies with labeled acetate (James *et al.*, 1959; Lovelock *et al.*, 1960) revealed that blood cells (white cells, reticulocytes, and platelets) synthesize lipids which are transferred during the course of incubation *in vitro* to the plasma lipoproteins. Exchanges of both unsaponifiable lipid and phospholipid between cells and plasma α- and β-lipoprotein were observed, while the glycerides were attached to plasma α-lipoprotein. Continuing these studies, Rowe (1960) reported that in spite of the phospholipid exchange between cells and plasma having a half-time of about 6 hours, large differences exist in fatty acid composition between cellular and plasma lecithin, thus limiting the exchange reactions to a fraction of the phospholipids only. Inasmuch as further studies of this group and of other investigators, discussed above, showed that leucocytes, platelets, and reticulocytes are responsible for the greater part of cellular lipid biosynthesis, it is apparent that the leucocyte phospholipids are involved in exchange with the plasma (Rowe, 1960; Rowe *et al.*, 1960a,b; Marks *et al.*,

1960). Further investigations are necessary to elucidate whether red cells depend on the lipids contributed by leucocytes to the plasma.

Taking into account the complications brought about by the presence of other types of blood cells, it is difficult to conclude from existing information whether interchange of complete phospholipid molecules between red cells and plasma proceeds to any notable extent. If this process takes place, we believe that only a limited fraction of the phospholipid molecules, located at certain sites in the membrane, is involved. To support this view it may be recalled that red cells of various animal species differ widely with respect to lecithin content, while on the other hand lecithin always represents the major phospholipid of plasma (compare, for example, Dawson *et al.*, 1960); in sheep, for instance, lecithin is practically lacking in the red cell but present as a major plasma phospholipid. Recently Jones and Gardner (1962) reported on the exchange of I^{131}-labeled lipids between red cells and plasma. Part of their results may be due to incorporation of unesterified I^{131}-fatty acids into lipids of mature red cells, a process recently established to occur (van Deenen *et al.*, 1962b) and to be later discussed.

d. Incorporation of Fatty Acids. Inasmuch as dietary studies indicate that fatty acid patterns of circulating erythrocytes are subject to change, direct incorporation of unesterified fatty acids into the complex lipids of the red cell has to be envisioned. Miras *et al.* (1961) reported on the uptake of C^{14}-palmitate into blood cells, while independent studies by Oliveira and Vaughan (1962) and van Deenen *et al.* (1962b) recently showed agreeably that fatty acids are actively incorporated into certain phospholipids of the red cell in a selective way.

As recorded in the abstract of Oliveira and Vaughan, ghosts of human red cell were able, in the presence of ATP and CoA, to incorporate C^{14}-linoleic acid mainly into lecithin, at a rate 6 times greater than that of oleic acid and palmitic acid. Sheep red cell ghosts, which contain very little lecithin, incorporated almost no C^{14}-fatty acid into phospholipid while rat red cell ghosts, known to contain more lecithin (compare Table IX) than human red cell ghosts, incorporated much more C^{14}-fatty acid. In our studies, guided originally by dietary experiments (see following section), intact erythrocytes freed from leucocytes by an ultracentrifugation technique were incubated in serum and in Krebs-Ringer solution with C^{14}-labeled fatty acids. Without addition of any cofactors, incorporation occurred to the same extent in both media and it was shown that the fatty acids were not incorporated primarily into serum lipids, but that direct utilization by the red cell was evident. Furthermore, differences were to be noted, not only with respect to rate of incorporation between saturated fatty acids of different chain length and saturated and unsaturated fatty acids, but also with regard to the types of phospholipid becoming labeled in red cells of different animal species.

As demonstrated in Fig. 9, when rabbit erythrocytes were incubated *in vitro* with C^{14}-linoleic acid, incorporation was mainly into lecithin, with some into cephalins and sometimes into phosphatidic acid. A decrease in the rate of incorporation was noted in the sequence linoleic acid, palmitic acid, and myristic acid, while lauric acid was not incorporated in any notable amount into the phospholipids of rabbit erythrocytes. This observation is in full agreement with our dietary studies showing that an elevated level of linoleic acid in the

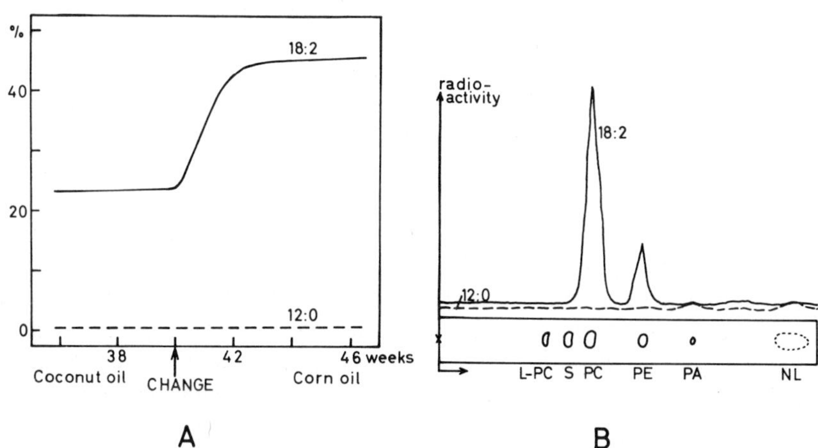

FIG. 9. Demonstration of the selective incorporation of fatty acids into phospholipids of erythrocytes (Mulder *et al.*, 1963). A: weight percentages of fatty acids in the phospholipid fraction of erythrocytes from rabbits fed a diet high in coconut oil (containing 58% lauric acid, abbreviated as 12:0) and corn oil (60% linoleic acid, 18:2), respectively. B: distribution of radioactivity on a paper chromatogram of lipids extracted from rabbit erythrocytes incubated in an equal volume of Ringer solution containing linoleic acid-1-C^{14} (18:2) and lauric acid-1-C^{14} (12:0), respectively, for 5 hours at 37°C. L-PC, lysolecithin; S, sphingomyelin; PC, phosphatidylcholine or lecithin; PE, phosphatidylethanolamine; PA, phosphatidic acid; NL, neutral lipids.

serum is reflected by increased content of this fatty acid in the red cell phospholipids, whereas increase of serum lauric acid is not followed by augmentation of this fatty acid constituent in the red cell phospholipids (Fig. 9A). This correlation between these two fundamentally different experimental approaches substantiates the physiological significance of the *in vitro* experiments on incorporation of labeled fatty acids into erythrocytes. Through the use of snake venom phospholipase A, known to release the β-fatty acid from the phosphoglyceride molecule (see Section IV, D), it was possible to ascertain that incorporated linoleic acid was located predominantly in the β position of red cell lecithin. Comparable results were obtained with red cells of other animal species having abundant red cell lecithin, although some differences were noted with respect to rate of incorporation of several fatty acids. However, bovine red cells known to have a low lecithin content (Table IX), revealed C^{14}-linoleic acid incorporation into phosphatidyl ethanolamine while the small amount of lecithin present proved to be labeled also. As regards the mechanism of incorporation of fatty acids into the red cell phospholipids, several pathways can theoretically be envisaged. Although the labeling of glycerides and phosphatidic acid was very weak after incubation, compared with lecithin, the participation of a *de novo* synthesis of phospholipids (compare Kennedy, 1961) incorporating fatty acids cannot be ruled out completely. However, P^{32} uptake (Section IV, B, a) was of a much lower order, compared with incorporation of C^{14}-fatty acids, and was restricted mainly to phosphatidic acid. Keeping in mind the small amounts of lysolecithin found in red cells, an enzymatic acylation of this compound, known to occur in the microsomal fraction of liver cells (Lands, 1960), might be involved in the process under discussion. Actually we demonstrated the ability of red cells to convert exogenous P^{32}-lysolecithin to P^{32}-lecithin (van Deenen *et al.*, 1962b); Oliveira and Vaughan (1962) also stated that incorporation of fatty acids may proceed by esterification of lysolecithin. Another problem to be elucidated in the near future is the removal of fatty acids from red cell phospholipid in order to allow incorporation of fresh acyl constituents. Dietary studies indicated that linoleic acid can displace oleic acid from red cell phosphoglycerides.

Although the precise mechanism of fatty acid renewal is not elucidated in detail as yet, this process presents a dynamic feature of the red cell membrane which may have many physiological consequences.

C. *Dietary Effects on Red Cell Lipids*

It is of great interest to determine to what extent the lipid composition of red cells is dependent on the nature of ingested lipids and other dietary factors. For correct interpretation of analytical data on normal and pathological cells, assessing the magnitude of such effects is indispensable. Furthermore, induction of changes in the lipid composition of red cells by dietary means is probably a unique tool for investigating many basic problems of the functions of lipids in membranes. Perhaps this approach furnishes the opportunity to correlate lipid composition and permeability characteristics. An improved understanding of the differences existing in lipid composition of red cells among various animal species may likewise result from dietary studies.

1. Cholesterol

The cholesterol concentration in plasma shows a high variability dependent, for example, on nutritional factors whereas the cholesterol content of red cells, appears to be rather constant. Numerous reports indicate that an elevated level of plasma cholesterol in man is not accompanied by corresponding increase within the red cell (Bürger, 1928; Brun, 1939; Olson *et al.*, 1957; Formijne *et al.*, 1957; Fels *et al.*, 1961). In animals also the amount of red cell cholesterol is not altered by dietary fat or cholesterol administration, as reported by Monsen *et al.* (1962) for rats and observed in our dietary studies on rabbits. The constancy of the cholesterol content is the more surprising because of the reports indicating a rapid exchange with plasma cholesterol (Section IV, B, 1). For these reasons one could speculate that cholesterol and phospholipids are fixed at certain defined loci within the red cell membrane, thereby limiting the number of molecules of each individual type of lipid present (compare also Olson, 1958). Fels *et al.* (1961) put forward the hypothesis that the life of the red cell is conditioned by the lipid-cholesterol content of the membrane in such a manner that when a certain cholesterol level is exceeded, the red cell may be destroyed by the reticuloendothelial system.

2. Fatty Acid Constituents

Because of limits of space our discussion of dietary effects on fatty acid patterns of the red cell will be confined to some recent reports, these references making the previous literature on the subject readily accessible.

a. Deprivation of Essential Fatty Acids. The idea that essential fatty acids, viz. linoleic and arachidonic, have a structural function stimulated investigation of the effects of deprivation of these fatty acids on lipid composition and other properties of the red cell membrane. The increased fragility of erythrocytes in fat deficiency observed by MacMillan and Sinclair (1958) demonstrates the necessity of these fatty acid constituents in the membrane framework. Recent analyses by gas-liquid chromatography showed the complex alterations in fatty acid composition in deficiencies of essential fatty acids in erythrocytes of the monkey (Greenberg and Moon, 1961) and rat (Witting *et al.*, 1961; van Deenen, 1962; van Deenen *et al.*, 1962b). Although different animals and dietary techniques were involved, the results of these studies are in good agreement with each other as well as with observations on other tissues. In general, essential fatty acid deprivation led to marked increases in the mono-unsaturated fatty acid, particularly oleic acid, and to the appearance of significant quantities of eicosatrienoic acid, while the levels of arachidonate, linoleate, and to a certain extent stearate, are decreased (compare also Fig. 10). As pointed out by Holman (1960), the ratio of trienoic to tetraenoic acids is a good index of essential fatty acid nutritional status.

Since the phospholipids are the major red cell compounds containing fatty acid constituents, the alterations in fatty acids must be localized mainly within the phospholipids. The fatty acid patterns of all major phospholipids were altered and according to expectation significant quantitative variations were noted in those compounds normally carrying essential fatty acids, e.g. cephalins (Fig. 10).

b. Effects of Feedings Excess of Certain Fatty Acids. It is important to establish to what extent an increased supply of a certain fatty acid is reflected in the fatty acid composition of the red cell. Augmentation of the ingested amount of linoleic acid was shown to be reflected in erythrocytes of man (Horwitt *et al.*, 1959; Farquhar and Ahrens, 1963), rat (Witting *et al.*, 1961; Monsen *et al.*, 1962), and rabbit (van Deenen, 1962; van Deenen *et al.*, 1962b); oleic acid behaved similarly in man (Farquhar, 1962c) and an elevated level of myristic acid in plasma was followed only partially by increase in the red cell (de Gier

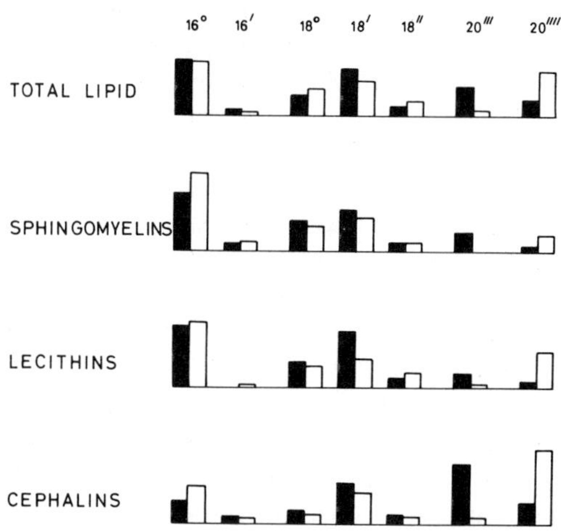

FIG. 10. Effect of low intake of essential fatty acids on the fatty acid pattern of total lipids and individual phospholipids from rabbit erythrocytes (van Deenen, 1962). Solid bars represent the relative amounts of fatty acid in animals fed a carbohydrate diet deprived of essential fatty acids; open bars indicate the data obtained in animals on a carbohydrate diet supplied with sunflower-seed oil. (For abbreviations compare Fig. 3.)

and van Deenen, unpublished), but this process failed completely with respect to uptake of lauric acid (van Deenen *et al.*, 1962b). No participation of erucic acid incorporation into red cells was observed, but this fatty acid was usually not detected in phospholipids of other tissues although it accumulated in the depot fat (Bernhard *et al.*, 1960). The conspicuous differences in uptake between various fatty acids, e.g. linoleic acid and lauric acid, focus attention on the mechanism involved in this process. Furthermore it is of interest to note that a change from oleate and linoleate can be provoked. Under a given regimen, the period necessary to reach a constant and maximal elevated level of linoleic acid in the erythrocyte appeared to be as short as 10 days in the rabbit (van Deenen *et al.*, 1962b) and 4–6 weeks in man (Farquhar and Ahrens, 1963). Inasmuch as these periods are much shorter than the normal lifespan of the erythrocytes concerned, the uptake of new acids must take place mainly by processes other than incorporation into maturing erythrocytes in the bone marrow. Many possibilities can be envisaged with respect to the question in what state the fatty acids, e.g. free or esterified as phospholipids, enter the erythrocyte envelope. Our experiments with labeled fatty acids, dealt with in the previous section, showed that erythrocytes actively incorporate unesterified

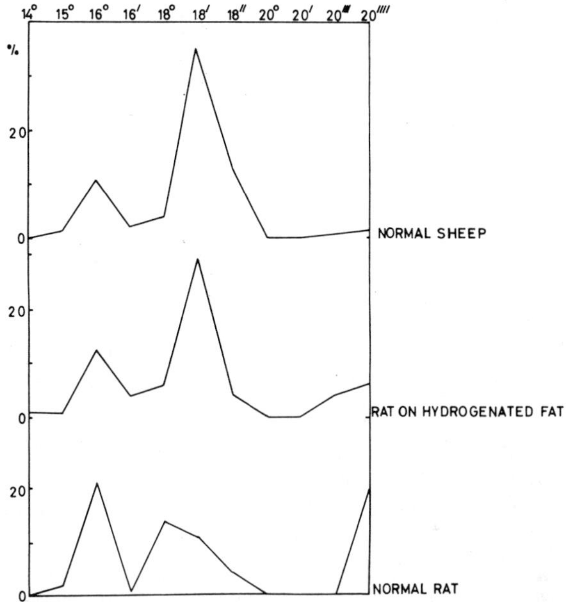

FIG. 11. Comparison of fatty acid patterns of lipids from erythrocytes of normal sheep, rat fed on a diet rich in hydrogenated fat, and normal rat; fatty acids are indicated by the number of carbon atoms and double bonds (van Deenen *et al.*, 1962b).

fatty acids into their membrane phospholipids, thereby revealing a similar selectivity to that observed during these dietary experiments (Fig. 10). For these reasons we conclude that this mechanism accounts for the greater part if not all of the alterations brought about by dietary means in fatty acid composition of phospholipids of circulating cells. The various problems concerning the exact pathways of introduction and removal of fatty acids from the red cell phospholipids have been discussed.

c. Variations in Fatty Acid Patterns of Erythrocytes among Various Animal Species. As described in Section III, significant differences exist in the fatty acid patterns of erythrocyte phospholipids among various animal species. In view of the fact that unesterified fatty acids of plasma contribute to the ultimate fatty acid composition of the circulating erythrocyte, one could expect that at least part of the aforementioned differences is to be attributed to variations in free fatty acid transported by the plasma. Variations in the nature of ingested fatty acids and differences in intestinal lipid metabolism thus could participate in effecting the significant variation in fatty acid composition of erythrocytes among different animal species, although a great deal of experimental work is needed to determine exactly the extent of these influences. But it can be stated with certainty that the aforementioned factors are indeed involved. This is illustrated by Fig. 11, showing again the notable differences existing in fatty acid patterns of erythrocytes between normal fed rat and sheep. Administration of a large amount of hydrogenated fats to rats significantly alters the fatty acid composition of these erythrocytes, and the trend of the shift occurring is clearly to alter the fatty acid pattern of rat erythrocytes in the direction of that of the sheep red cell (van Deenen *et al.*, 1962b). Actually, it has been convincingly demonstrated (compare, e.g., Ogilvie *et al.*, 1961) that differences between ruminants and nonruminants in fatty acid composition of fats arise from the hydrogenation of unsaturated dietary fats in the rumen.

3. Proportions of Individual Phospholipids

The notable effects of dietary factors on fatty acid composition of red cells raise the question whether the distribution of phospholipids, known to be characteristic but different for the red cell of each animal species, is also susceptible to dietary influences. As regards the human erythrocyte, the types and amounts of lipids were unaffected by diet-induced variations in fatty acid composition (Farquhar and Ahrens, 1963); in our experiments discussed above we observed no appreciable differences in the quantitative proportions of lipid and phospholipid classes in red cells of rat and rabbit, although in the latter a very small decrease of lecithin was observed in animals fed excess linoleic acid (van Deenen *et al.*, 1962b). Thus the fatty acid composition can be altered to a significant degree, leaving the distribution of lipid classes practically unchanged. The activity of the enzymes determining the proportions of distinct types of membranous phospholipid, apparently genetically controlled, is not greatly influenced by differences in fatty acid offered.

D. Degradation of Red Cell Lipids

When speculating that the intriguing process of the termination of the circulating erythrocyte after a life span defined for each species may involve primarily a collapse of the outer red cell region, one has to envisage a disappearance or enzymatic breakdown of the lipid constituents from the membrane. A lipolytic enzyme located at the erythrocyte membrane and (or) furnished by the reticuloendothelial system may be involved, but the question remains by what mechanism the enzyme is activated to develop its damaging action at a definite point in time. Presuming that during the process of aging the red cell membrane undergoes changes in lipid content or composition, e.g., by failure of certain fatty acid-acylating enzymes or leakage of (weakly bound) phospholipids or cholesterol (compare Section V), one could imagine that after a certain period the membranous framework becomes susceptible to a catabolic enzyme system. On the other hand, it is possible that loss of lipid from the erythrocyte leads directly to termination of the red cell existence, and in this connection it is of interest to note that surface tension-active substances have been shown to solubilize red cell cholesterol during the hemolysis process (compare Ruyssen, 1957). Speculations on possible removal or breakdown of membrane lipids as a trigger for the withdrawal of red cells from circulation provoke many questions which can be answered only by future experimental approaches. In this connection it seems of interest to review briefly some facts on the enzymes involved in catabolism of phospholipids. As indicated in Scheme 2, four types of enzyme may catalyse the hydrolysis of phosphoglycerides, some of them acting also on sphingomyelin.

```
      C           D
       ↘    O    ↙
            ‖
   H2C—O—P—O—base
    |       |
    |       OH
    |
    |         A
    |        ↙
   HC—O—C—R1
    |     ‖
    |   ↖ O
    |     B
    |    ↙
   H2C—O—C—R2
          ‖
          O
```

Scheme 2. Site of action of phospholipases on phosphoglycerides.

Phospholipase A. This enzyme, known to occur in snake venom and other animal poisons (compare Kates, 1960), has recently been demonstrated to release the fatty acid present in the β ester position only (Tattrie, 1959; Hanahan *et al.*, 1960b; de Haas *et al.*, 1960; de Haas and van Deenen, 1961). Enzymes of this type are widely distributed in nature and phospholipase A from human pancreas was recently shown to exhibit the same mode of action as the enzyme of nonmammalian origin (van Deenen *et al.*, 1963). Intact erythrocytes of many but not all mammalian species are not susceptible to the action of this enzyme, but phospholipase A-produced lysophospholipids are known to be powerful hemolytic substances. Limitations of space do not allow extensive discussion of this topic, but we want to emphasize that many misleading quotations are recorded in the literature with respect to a supposed hemolytic action of phospholipase A, which, however, is questionable. An enzyme removing fatty acid from lecithin is present in blood and may be attached to the outer surface of the red cell (van Deenen, unpublished results). The involvement of this enzyme in metabolism of red cell phospholipids, however, remains to be ascertained. Extending previous observations (e.g. Ponder, 1952) on hemolytic factors from spleen, Valdiquié *et al.* (1961) established the presence of small amounts of lysophospholipids in lipid extracts of this tissue. However, the participation of these compounds *in situ* in hemolytic processes is still doubtful inasmuch as in mixtures of lysolecithin with other lipids the hemolytic action disappears or is greatly diminished. Detectable quantities of lysolecithin are present in serum also. Although it is certainly attractive to imply a significant role of phospholipase A in the processes under discussion, conclusive evidence still is lacking.

Phospholipase B. The situation surrounding the mode of action of this type of enzyme is somewhat complicated inasmuch as at present two pathways of breakdown must be envisaged, viz., a removal of both fatty acids from the phosphoglyceride and a liberation of the fatty acid remaining in the phospholipase A-produced lysophospholipid molecule (compare Kates, 1960). As regards the latter pathway of breakdown, Marples and Thompson (1960) established that lysophospholipase activity was present in many tissues, e.g. spleen. In confirmation, we observed a breakdown of lysolecithin into glyceryl phosphorylcholine by spleen extracts, while a similar hydrolysis product was obtained from lecithin when certain negatively charged activators (e.g. phosphatidic acid) were present (van Deenen, unpublished results). The significance of these enzymatic reactions in the catabolism of red cell phospholipids is not clear.

Phospholipase C. MacFarlane and Knight (1941) established *Clostridium welchii* α toxin to be identical with phospholipase C, that catalyzes the hydrolytic cleavage of lecithin into a diglyceride and phosphoryl choline (compare also MacFarlane, 1955). Recent investigations demonstrated that during action of *C. welchii* filtrates, all major types of phospholipid present in red cells of various animal species are hydrolyzed in a comparable manner (van Deenen *et al.*, 1961b; de Gier *et al.*, 1961c). Results of MacFarlane (1950) indicated that the hemolytic action of this toxin may be due primarily to the action of this enzyme. In order to evaluate the significance of the enzyme for red cell breakdown it seems important to establish this fact by the use of pure enzyme specimens, as well as to confirm the presence of phospholipase C in animal tissues such as spleen (Fujino, 1952; Druskinina and Kritzman, 1952).

Phospholipase D. This phospholipase, discovered by Hanahan and Chaikoff (1948), is known to be widely distributed in plant material (compare Kates,

1960). So far, no convincing evidence has been presented on the occurrence of the enzyme in animal tissues.

From the foregoing it may be clear that the catabolism of red cell phospholipids still deserves considerable attention.

V. Lipids of the Human Erythrocyte under Pathological Conditions

A. Variation of Lipid Composition with Red Cell Age

A consideration of the lipids from red cells of different age may contribute to the problem as to how far alterations in these lipids are involved in the physiological breakdown of the cells. It is also indispensable for the interpretation of lipid analyses of red cells in patients with hemolytic diseases. Special attention has been paid to the younger red cells because the number of reticulocytes in the blood population can be readily enhanced by repeated bleeding, and possibilities are afforded by working with pathological or phenylhydrazine-induced anemic blood. However, it is questionable whether such samples furnish sound information with respect to normal young erythrocytes. In this connection it is noteworthy that Stohlman (1961) demonstrated that red cells, formed in response to phenylhydrazine- or bleeding-induced anemia, have a shorter life span and become smaller when the anemic state is continued. A more physiological approach is provided by making use of differences in density or osmotic fragility of cells of different age. From experiments with Fe^{59}-labeled blood it is evident that the relative cell density increases and the osmotic resistance decreases as the cell grows older (Chalfin, 1956; Hoffman, 1958; Prankerd, 1958).

Ruhenstroth-Bauer and Hermann (1950) investigated red cells of normal rabbits and of rabbits with reticulocytosis caused by repeated hemorrhage and noted great differences in amount of lipid phosphorus per cell. In red cell populations with 176 reticulocytes per 1000 the phospholipid content was twice as high as in normal populations. Raderecht *et al.* (1960) carried out similar experiments and, extrapolating their data to 100% reticulocytes, the conclusion was reached that these young cells contained 4–5 times as much phospholipid as mature red cells. The cholesterol content also was higher in reticulocytes, being 2–3 times that in the mature red cell. Analyses of ratios of the different types of phospholipid led Raderecht *et al.* to suggest that lecithin in particular leaves the cell during the process of aging. Also in several cases of human hemolytic anemias where reticulocytosis might be expected, an increase in lipid content per cell has been noted (e.g. Prankerd, 1959). Prankerd (1958) as well as Westerman *et al.* (1959) studied normal populations of red cells, separated by centrifugal force into fractions of younger and older ones.

Both investigators came to the conclusion that younger cells contained more lipid than older ones. However, Westerman *et al.* pointed out that when data on total lipid and phospholipid are related to surface area, which is known to be significantly larger in younger cells, the differences between young and old cells are no longer significant. Besides the aging process *in vivo*, the alterations of the red cell lipids *in vitro*, during storage, are of interest. Reed *et al.* (1958) studied the lipid composition of normal human red cells stored in glass in acid-citrate-dextrose at 4°C. During the first 21 days of storage a steady and equal decrease in the total lipid, lipid phosphorus, and cholesterol per cell was found. After this period no further release of lipids could be demonstrated. Raderecht and Schölzel (1960) obtained the same results and demonstrated that glycolipids in particular are released from the red cell membrane.

B. Lipids of Abnormal Human Erythrocytes

Keeping in mind the essential role of lipids in the structural organization and functioning of the red cell envelope, alterations in the lipid moiety might obviously cause abnormalities in shape, permeability characteristics, metabolic activities, and life span of the erythrocytes. From this point of view it is rather remarkable that in spite of extensive investigations, e.g., on red cells in hereditary anemias, only a few abnormalities have been noted with certainty. Furthermore, it is still questionable whether the lipid defects are primarily or secondarily involved and one must consider also that the samples studied often contain an abnormal proportion of very young cells. In several cases of hemolytic anemias an excess of all fractions of lipids was found, which may be, however, the consequence of an increased number of reticulocytes (e.g. Erickson *et al.*, 1937; Allison *et al.*, 1960; Phillips and Roome, 1962).

In 1957 Harris *et al.* reported that red cells in paroxysmal nocturnal hemoglobinuria revealed a significantly higher amount of both cholesterol and lipid nitrogen. This observation was confirmed by Formijne *et al.* (1957), who found the amount of cholesterol as well as the phospholipid content to be elevated. Studies on the ratios between different classes of phospholipids by Harris *et al.* (1957) suggested a decrease in lecithin and an increase in serine cephalin. This statement, however, was not sustained by the results of Formijne *et al.* (1957), Barry (1959), and Phillips and Roome (1962), since all these investigators found quite normal values for the different types of phospholipid.

In reports of Allison *et al.* (1960) and Kates *et al.* (1961) on the erythrocytes of two patients with hereditary spherocytosis, it was claimed that these cells in comparison to normal values showed a significant decrease of the cephalin content whereas the amount of lysocephalin was increased (Table XIV). On the other hand when lysocephalin was added to normal serum, sphering of normal red cells was observed. From the results these investigators concluded that the primary genetically controlled abnormality in hereditary spherocytosis probably is caused by a partial block in the enzyme system catalizing the conversion of lysophosphatidylethanolamine to phosphatidylethanolamine. Contrary to these findings, our analyses of erythrocyte phospholipids in several patients with hereditary spherocytosis revealed quite normal values for cephalin and lysocephalin (de Gier *et al.*, 1961d). We therefore suggested that during the analyses of Allison *et al.*, part of the cephalins (mainly of the plasmalogen type; see Section III, D) was hydrolyzed, yielding free aldehyde and lysocephalin. This point of view was recently reaffirmed by Phillips and Roome (1962) (Table XIV).

TABLE XIV

PHOSPHOLIPID COMPOSITION OF ERYTHROCYTES FROM PATIENTS WITH HEREDITARY SPHEROCYTOSIS

Phospholipid	Normal [a]	Spherocytes [a]	Normal [b]	Spherocytes [b]	Normal [c]	Spherocytes [c]
Lysolecithin	3.3	3.5	2	2	1.8	1.9
Sphingomyelin + lysophosphatidyl-ethanolamine	23	33	32	32.5	23	25.2
Lecithin	45	44	36	36	32.7	31.7
Phosphatidyl-ethanolamine	28	19	30	29.5	42.4	41.1

[a] Allison *et al.* (1960).
[b] De Gier *et al.* (1961d).
[c] Phillips and Roome (1962).

Ways *et al.* (1961) reported abnormalities in erythrocyte membrane lipids in three cases of hereditary acanthocytosis. Despite normal quantities of total red cell phospholipids, their distribution was altered, viz., the lecithin content was significantly decreased with concomitant increase of the sphingomyelin fraction. These results have been confirmed by Phillips (1962) recording the same facts in another four patients. It must be emphasized that in the plasma of the patients the amounts of all lipids were strikingly reduced, thereby revealing a similar shift in the ratio of lecithin to sphingomyelin.

In addition, attention has been directed to the red cell phospholipids of patients with pernicious anemia (Formijne *et al.*, 1957; Phillips and Roome, 1962), hereditary elliptocytosis (de Gier *et al.*, 1961d), sprue, intermediate thalassemia, sickle cell anemia, and polycythemia vera (Phillips and Roome, 1962). In all these diseases the distribution of the different classes of lipids was in keeping with values reported for normal erythrocytes. This does not preclude, however, the possibility that more detailed investigations may reveal certain differences in red cell lipids.

Besides possible alterations in lipids of abnormal red cells, one may expect a universal derangement of lipid metabolism to be reflected in erythrocyte lipids as well. This is demonstrated by the work of Balint *et al.* (1961), who reported a fall in red blood cell cephalin in a case of Niemann-Pick disease.

Various investigations have dealt with the fatty acid constituents of abnormal red cells. Munn and Crosby (1957, 1961) estimated the fatty acid patterns of red cell lipids in a great number of hemolytic diseases, using ultraviolet spectrophotometry after isomerization in alkali. Red cells of patients with paroxysmal nocturnal hemoglobinuria were found to exhibit a low concentration of oleic acid (18:1), while the content of arachidonic acid (20:4) was unusually high (Munn and Crosby, 1957). Lovelock and Prankerd (see Prankerd, 1959) were able to confirm this observation by gas-liquid chromatography. However, the data obtained by Leibetseder and Ahrens (1959) showed no clear-cut difference between fatty acid patterns of normal red cells and those in paroxysmal nocturnal hemoglobinuria. Recently Munn and Crosby (1961) published data on the fatty acid composition of a great number of patients with red cell abnormalities. Many deviating values were recorded which, however, varied individually and could not be correlated with the diseases diagnosed. However, in a number of cases these investigators found a relatively low level of polyunsaturated fatty acids e.g. linoleic acid. This deviation was considered to be a consequence of immaturity of the red cell population rather than any fault of red cell structure. Actually Munn (1958) earlier demonstrated on a patient who was being bled 2 liters per week for treatment of hemochromatosis that the unsaturated fatty acids decreased with increasing immaturity of the cell population. Recent studies from this laboratory (de Gier *et al.*, 1964) on red cells of patients with pernicious anemia, hereditary spherocytosis, hereditary elliptocytosis, and nonspherocytic hemolytic anemia point in the same direction. In a number of samples a very low linoleic acid content was evident. Perhaps an increase in the manufacture of blood cells causes a local deficiency with regard to the essential fatty acid, linoleic acid. On the other hand it will be of interest to investigate whether normal reticulocytes are lower in linoleate content than the mature red cells.

VI. Concluding Comments

The efforts of many investigators, seizing upon the advantages of recent techniques in lipid chemistry, have resulted in detailed knowledge of the lipid composition of red cells, particularly those of man. Figure 12 illustrates the average distribution of major lipid classes as an outgrowth of recent contributions. In addition to this information, an overwhelming amount of detail has been gathered concerning the nature of the acyl chain constituents from several individual lipid classes.

Studies on different animal species, although less numerous compared with investigations devoted to the human erythrocyte, unequivocally indicated intriguing differences in red cell lipids. Striking differences have been noted in glycolipids as well as in phospholipids. Variations in lecithin and sphingomyelin content among red cells of different mammals are apparent, but deserve an appropriate explanation of the genetic difference. Differences in fatty acids appear to be brought about at least in part by variation in the nature of ingested lipids or difference in intestinal or ruminal processes, but further investigations on this topic are required. This is true also with respect to the questions as to how far and in what direction variations in lipid composition contribute to other properties of the red cell. It will be unavoidable that we extend the detailed characterization of red cell lipids, including plasmalogens and glyceryl

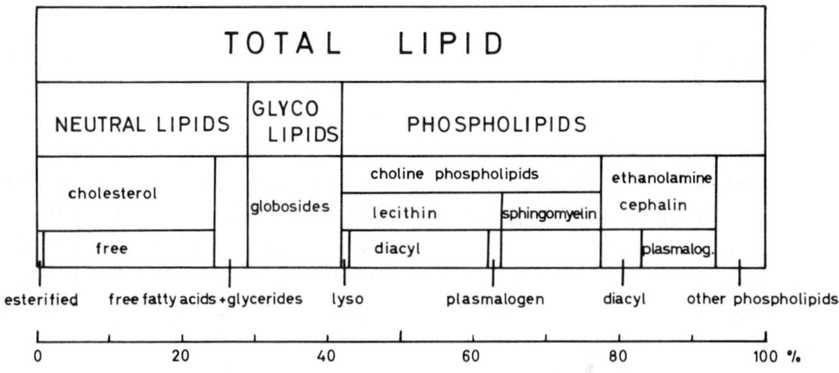

FIG. 12. Distribution of major types of lipid in the human erythrocyte.

ether phospholipids, to a great number of species in order to verify whether a relationship between lipid composition and permeability behavior of red cells does exist.

In several respects, information about the metabolic features of red cell lipids is scanty. Knowledge of the biosynthesis and introduction of lipids into the red cell membrane within the hematopoietic bone marrow is lacking. Nor is conclusive information available on the enzymatic breakdown of red cell lipids *in situ*, or with respect to the question whether such processes can initiate the termination of the red cell life span. Confusion concerning the ability of circulating mature red cells to synthesize lipids has been largely clarified. Cholesterol synthesis has been shown to be lacking in red cells, while biosynthesis of fatty acids was demonstrated to be limited, if existing at all, in mature red cells, this in contrast to leucocytes, reticulocytes, and platelets. No definite evidence has been advanced to sustain an active *de novo* synthesis of phospholipids in mature erythrocytes, but certain dynamic events in phospholipids in circulating red cells have recently become apparent. In addition to turnover of phosphatidic acid, it has been demonstrated that certain major phospholipids, e.g. lecithin, exhibit the ability to incorporate fatty acids. The latter process probably accounts normally for the renewal of certain fatty acid constituents, e.g. the essential fatty acid, linoleic acid, and participates in diet-induced alterations in fatty acid composition of red cell phospholipids. As regards an interchange with plasma lipids, a rapid exchange of red cell cholesterol has been demonstrated; fresh information on the extent of interchange of phospholipids and the nature of compounds involved in such a process is required.

Another aspiration should be a more detailed determination of possible variations in both composition and metabolic features of lipids of red cells of different age. Such information would supply a more solid basis for the interpretation of observations made on abnormal erythrocytes, e.g., in hereditary anemias.

Some information has emerged regarding the molecular organization of lipids in the red cell membrane. Binding of phospholipids to other membrane constituents, e.g. proteins, different sorts of binding of phospholipids, and interactions between phospholipids and cholesterol have been envisaged. However, the exact orientation and distribution of lipids in the membrane framework is still the subject of controversy. At present it is difficult to decide whether a continuous bimolecular lipid leaflet sandwiched between protein, and eventually containing polar pores, is present, or whether a mosaic structure consisting of a protein meshwork surrounding lipid cylinders acts as the cell envelope. Both concepts recently obtained substantial support from divergent approaches by electron microscopy. Despite this variance, it was shown that electron micrographs obtained in both ways from red cell membranes were in agreement with structures resulting from boundaries of other cell types.[3] It is therefore likely that the red cell, having its membrane so readily accessible, will continue to play an important role in the basic problem of relating chemical composition and the fine architecture of biomembranes.

References

Albritton, E. C. (1955). "Standard Values in Blood." Saunders, Philadelphia, Pennsylvania.

Allison, A. C., Kates, M., and James, A. T. (1960). *Brit. Med. J.* 1766.

Altmann, K. I. (1953). *Arch. Biochem. Biophys.* **42**, 478.

Anderson, H. M., and Turner, J. C. (1960). *J. Clin. Invest.* **39**, 1.

Balint, J. A., Nyhan, W. L., Lietman, P., and Turner, D. A. (1961). *J. Lab. Clin. Med.* **58**, 548.

Bangham, A. D., Horne, R. W., Glauert, A. M., Dingle, J. T., and Lucy, J. A. (1962). *Nature* **196**, 952, 953.

Barry, R. M. (1959). *Brit. J. Haematol.* **5**, 212.

---

[3] Compare, however, footnote 2, page 277.

Bayer, M. (1960). *Arch. Ges. Physiol.* **270**, 323.

Benson, A. A., and Maruo, B. (1958). *Biochim. Biophys. Acta* **27**, 189.

Bernard, L. de (1958). *Bull. Soc. Chim. Biol.* **40**, 161.

Bernhard, K., Lindlar, F., and Wagner, H. (1960). *Z. Ernaehrungswiss.* **1**, 48.

Blomstrand, R., Nakayama, F., and Nilsson, I. M. (1962). *J. Lab. Clin. Med.* **59**, 771.

Böttcher, C. J. F., and Gent, C. M. van (1961). *J. Atherosclerosis Res.* **1**, 36.

Booy, H. L. (1949). *Discussions Faraday Soc.* **6**, 143.

Booy, H. L., and Bungenberg, de Jong, H. G. (1956). "Biocolloids and Their Interactions," Protoplasmatologia I, 2. Springer, Vienna.

Borgström, B. (1952). *Acta Physiol. Scand.* **25**, 10.

Brun, G. C. (1939). *Acta Med. Scand. Suppl.* **1**, 99, 237.

Buchanan, A. A. (1960). *Biochem. J.* **74**, 25P.

Bürger, M. (1928). *Ergeb. Inn. Med. Kinderheilk.* **34**, 583.

Bungenberg de Jong, H. G. (1949). *In* "Colloid Science" (H. R. Kruyt, ed.), Vol. II, Chapter I, Elsevier, Amsterdam.

Bungenberg de Jong, H. G., and Saubert, G. G. P. (1937). *Koninkl. Ned. Akad. Wetensch. Proc. Ser. C.* **40**, 295.

Burchfield, H. P., and Storrs, E. E. (1962). "Biochemical Applications of Gas Chromatography." Academic Press, New York.

Chalfin, D. (1956). *J. Cellular Comp. Physiol.* **47**, 215.

Danielli, J. F. (1952). *In* "Cytology and Cellphysiology" (G. Bourne, ed.), p. 150. Oxford Univ. Press, London and New York.

Danielli, J. F. (1958). *In* "Surface Phenomena in Chemistry and Biology" (J. F. Danielli, K. G. A. Pankhurst, and A. C. Riddiford, eds.), pp. 246–265. Pergamon Press, New York.

Danielli, J. F., and Harvey, E. M. (1935). *J. Cellular Comp. Physiol.* **5**, 483.

Davson, H., and Danielli, J. F. (1952). "The Permeability of Natural Membranes." Cambridge Univ. Press, London and New York.

Dawson, R. M. C. (1954). *Biochim. Biophys. Acta* **14**, 374.

Dawson, R. M. C. (1960). *Biochem. J.* **75**, 45.

Dawson, R. M. C., Hemington, N., and Lindsay, D. B. (1960). *Biochem. J.* **77**, 226.

Dawson, R. M. C., Hemington, N., and Davenport, J. B. (1962). *Biochem. J.* **84**, 497.

Deenen, L. L. M. van (1962). *Proc. Deuel Conf. 7th Lipids, Santa Barbara, California, 1962.* In press.

Deenen, L. L. M. van, Gier, J. de, and Veerkamp, J. H. (1961a). *Biochem. Probl. Lipids, Proc. Intern. Conf. 5th, Marseille, 1960*, p. 32.

Deenen, L. L. M. van, Gier, J. de, and Haas, G. H. de (1961b). *Koninkl. Ned. Akad. Wetensch. Proc. Ser. C.* **64**, 59.

Deenen, L. L. M. van, Houtsmuller, U. T. M., Haas, G. H. de, and Mulder, E. (1962a). *J. Pharm. Pharmacol.* **14**, 429.

Deenen, L. L. M. van, Gier, J. de, Houtsmuller, U. T. M., and Mulder, E. (1962b). *Biochem. Probl. Lipids, Proc. Intern. Conf. 6th, Birmingham, 1962*, p. 413, Elsevier, Amsterdam.

Deenen, L. L. M. van, Haas, G. H. de, and Heemskerk, C. H. Th. (1963). *Biochim. Biophys. Acta.* **67**, 295.

Dervichian, D. G. (1958). *In* "Surface Phenomena in Chemistry and Biology" (J. F. Danielli, K. G. A. Pankhurst, and A. C. Riddiford, eds.), p. 70, Pergamon Press, New York.

Dietz, A. A. (1949). *Arch. Biochem. Biophys.* **23**, 211.

Dodge, J. T., Mitchell, C., and Hanahan, D. J. (1963). *Arch. Biochem. Biophys.* **180,** 119 (1963).

Dourmashkin, R. R., Daugherty, R. M., and Harris, R. J. C. (1962). *Nature* **194**, 1116.

Douste-Blazy, L. (1959). *In* "Exposés Annuels de Biochimie Médicale" (P. Boulanger, M. F. Jayle, and J. Roche, eds.), p. 187. Masson, Paris.

Druskinina, K. V., and Kritzman, M. G. (1952). *Biokhimiya* **17**, 77.

Elbers, P. F. (1964). *In* "Recent Progress in Surface Science" (J. F. Danielli, K. G. A. Pankhurst, and A. C. Riddiford, eds.) Vol. II, Academic Press, New York (in press).

Elko, E. E., and Di Luzio, N. R. (1959). *Radiation Res.* **11**, 1.

Erickson, B. N., Williams, H. H., Hummer, H. C., and Macy, I. G. (1937). *J. Biol. Chem.* **118**, 15.

Erickson, B. N., Williams, H. H., Bernstein, S. S., Arvin, I., Jones, R. L., and Macy, I. G. (1938). *J. Biol. Chem.* **122**, 515.

Evans, J. D., and Oppenheimer, M. J. (1955). *Am. J. Physiol.* **181**, 509.

Farquhar, J. W. (1962a). *Biochim. Biophys. Acta* **60**, 80.

Farquhar, J. W. (1962b). *J. Lipid Res.* **3**, 21.

Farquhar, J. W. (1962c). *Proc. Deuel Conf. 7th Lipids, Santa Barbara, California, 1962.* In press.

Farquhar, J. W., and Ahrens, E. H. (1963). *J. Clin. Invest* **42,** 675.

Fels, G., Kanabrocki, E., and Kaplan, E. (1961). *Clin. Chem.* **7**, 15.

Finean, J. B. (1953). *Experientia* **9**, 17.

Formijne, P., Poulie, N. J., Rodbard, J. A. (1957). *Clin. Chim. Acta* **2**, 25.

Fujino, Y. (1952). *J. Biochem. (Tokyo)* **39**, 35.

Gastel, C. van, Gier, J. de, and Deenen, L. L. M. van (1964). In preparation.

Gier, J. de (1960). Thesis, Univ. of Utrecht.

Gier, J. de, Deenen, L. L. M. van, Verloop, M. C. and Gastel, C. van (1964). *Brit. J. Haematol.* **10,** 246.

Gier, J. de, and Deenen, L. L. M., van (1961). *Biochim. Biophys. Acta* **49**, 286.

Gier, J. de, Mulder, I., and Deenen, L. L. M. van (1961a). *Naturwissenschaften* **48**, 54.

Gier, J. de, Mulder, E., Mulder, I., and Deenen, L. L. M. van (1961b). *Koninkl. Ned. Akad. Wetensch. Proc. Ser. B.* **64,** 274.

Gier, J. de, Haas, G. H. de, and Deenen, L. L. M. van (1961c). *Biochem. J.* **81**, 33P.

Gier, J. de, Deenen, L. L. M. van, Geerdink, R. A., Punt, K., and Verloop, M. C. (1961d). *Biochim. Biophys. Acta* **50**, 383.

Gorter, E., and Grendel, F. (1925). *J. Exptl. Med.* **41**, 439.

Gorter, E., and Grendel, F. (1926). *Koninkl. Ned. Akad. Wetensch. Proc. Ser. B.* **29**, 314.

Gray, G. M. (1960). *J. Chromatog.* **4**, 52.

Greenberg, L. D., and Moon, H. D. (1961). *Arch. Biochem. Biophys.* **94,** 405.

Haas, G. H. de, Mulder, I., and Deenen, L. L. M. van (1960). *Biochem. Biophys. Res. Commun.* **3**, 287.

Haas, G. H. de, and Deenen, L. L. M. van (1961). *Biochim. Biophys. Acta* **48**, 215.

Hagerman, J. S., and Gould, R. S. (1951). *Proc. Soc. Exptl. Biol. Med.* **78**, 329.

Hahn, L., and Hevesy, G. (1939). *Nature* **144**, 72, 204.

Hakomori, S. I., and Jeanloz, R. W. (1961). *J. Biol. Chem.* **236**, 2827.

Hallgren, B., and Larsson, S. (1962). *J. Lipid Res.* **3**, 39.

Hanahan, D. J. (1960). "Lipide Chemistry." Wiley, New York.

Hanahan, D. J., and Chaikoff, I. L. (1948). *J. Biol. Chem.* **172**, 191.

Hanahan, D. J., and Watts, R. M. (1961). *J. Biol. Chem.* **236**, PC 59.

Hanahan, D. J., Watts, R. M., and Pappajohn, D. (1960a). *J. Lipid Res.* **1**, 412.

Hanahan, D. J., Brockerhoff, H., and Barron, E. J. (1960b). *J. Biol Chem.* **235**, 1917.

Harris, I. M., Prankerd, T. A. J., and Westerman, M. P. (1957). *Brit. Med. J.*, p. 1276.

Hevesy, G., and Aten, A. H. W. (1939). *Kgl. Danske Videnskab. Selskab. Biol Medd.* **14**, 5.

Höber, R. (1936). *J. Cellular Comp. Physiol.* **7**, 367.

Hoffman, J. F. (1958). *J. Cellular Comp. Physiol.* **51**, 415.
Hokin, L. E., and Hokin, M. R. (1960). *J. Gen. Physiol.* **44**, 61.
Hokin, L. E., and Hokin, M. R. (1961). *Nature* **189**, 836.
Hokin, L. E., and Hokin, M. R. (1963). *Biochim. Biophys. Acta.* **67**, 470.
Hokin, L. E., Hokin, M. R., and Mathison, D. (1963). *Biochim. Biophys. Acta.* **67**, 485.
Hokin, M. R., and Hokin, L. E. (1959). *J. Biol. Chem.* **235**, 1796.
Holman, R. T. (1960). *J. Nutr.* **70**, 405.
Horwitt, M. K., Harvey, C. C., and Century, B. (1959). *Science* **130**, 917.
Irie, R., Iwanaga, M., and Yamakawa, T. (1961). *J. Biochem. (Tokyo)* **50**, 122.
Jacobs, M. H., Glassman, H. N., and Parpart, A. K. (1950). *J. Exptl. Zool.* **113**, 277.
James, A. T., and Lovelock, J. (1957). *In* "The Blood Lipids and the Clearing Factor." Paleis der Academiën, Brussels.
James, A. T., Lovelock, J. E., and Webb, J. P. W. (1957). *Biochem. J.* **66**, 60P.
James, A. T., Lovelock, J. E., and Webb, J. P. W. (1959). *Biochem. J.* **73**, 106.
Jones, N. C. H., and Gardner, B. (1962). *Biochem. J.* **83**, 404.
Kates, M. (1960). *In* "Lipid Metabolism" (K. Bloch, ed.), Chapter V, p. 165. Wiley, New York.
Kates, M., and James, A. T. (1961). *Biochim. Biophys. Acta* **50**, 477.
Kates, M., Allison, A. C., and James, A. T. (1961). *Biochim. Biophys. Acta* **48**, 571.
Kennedy, E. P. (1961). *Federation Proc.* **20**, 934.
Klenk, E., and Gielen, W. (1962). *Z. Physiol. Chem.* **326**, 9.
Klenk, E., and Lauenstein, K. (1951). *Z. Physiol. Chem.* **288**, 220.
Klenk, E., and Lauenstein, K. (1952). *Z. Physiol. Chem.* **291**, 249.
Klenk, E., and Lauenstein, K. (1953). *Z. Physiol. Chem.* **295**, 164.
Klenk, E., and Wolter, H. (1952). *Z. Physiol. Chem.* **291**, 259.
Klenk, E., and Padberg, G. (1962). *Z. Physiol. Chem.* **327**, 249.
Klibansky, Ch., and Osimi, Z. (1961). *Bull. Res. Council Israel Sect. D.* **9**, 143.
Kögl, F., Gier, J. de, Mulder, I., and Deenen, L. L. M. van (1960). *Biochim. Biophys. Acta* **43**, 95.
Kornberg, A., and Pricer, W. E. (1953). *J. Biol. Chem.* **204**, 345.
Lands, W. E. M. (1960). *J. Biol. Chem.* **235**, 2233.
Laris, P. C. (1960). *J. Cellular Comp. Physiol.* **51**, 273.
Lea, C. H., and Rhodes, D. N. (1955). *Biochem. J.* **60**, 353.
Leibetseder, F., and Ahrens, E. H. (1959). *Brit. J. Haematol.* **5**, 356.
Leupold, F., and Kremer, G. (1961). *Nature* **191**, 805.
London, I. M., and Schwartz, H. (1953). *J. Clin. Invest.* **32**, 1248.
Lovelock, J. E., James, A. T., and Rowe, C. E. (1960). *Biochem. J.* **74**, 137.
Lund, P. K., Abadi, D. M., and Mathies, J. C. (1962). *J. Lipid Res.* **3**, 95.
MacFarlane, M. G. (1950). *Biochem. J.* **47**, 270.
MacFarlane, M. G. (1955). *Symp. Soc. Gen. Microbiol.* **5**, 57.
MacFarlane, M. G. (1958). *Nature* **182**, 946.
MacFarlane, M. G., and Knight, B. C. J. G. (1941). *Biochem. J.* **35**, 884.
MacMillan, A. L., and Sinclair, H. M. (1958). *Proc. 4th Intern. Conf. Biochem. Problems Lipids, Oxford, 1957* p. 208.
Mangold, H. K. (1961). *J. Am. Oil Chemists' Soc.* **38**, 708.
Marinetti, G. V. (1962). *J. Lipid Res.* **3**, 1.
Marinetti, G. V., Erbland, J., and Kochem, J. (1957). *Federation Proc.* **16**, 837.
Marks, P. A., Gellhorn, A., and Kidson, C. (1960). *J. Biol. Chem.* **235**, 2579.
Marples, E. A., and Thompson, R. H. S. (1960). *Biochem. J.* **74**, 123.
Mendelsohn, D. (1961a). *S. African J. Med. Sci.* **26**, 15.

Mendelsohn, D. (1961b). *S. African J. Med. Sci.* **26**, 24.
Miras, C. J., Fillerup, D. L., and Mead, J. F. (1961). *Nature* **190**, 92.
Monsen, E. R., Okey, R., and Lyman, R. L. (1962). *Metab. Clin. Exptl.* **11**, 1113.
Moskowitz, M., and Calvin, M. (1952). *Exptl. Cell Res.* **3**, 33.
Muir, A. R. (1962). *Nature* **195**, 1023.
Muir, H. M., Perrone, J. C., and Popjak, G. (1951). *Biochem. J.* **48**, IV.
Mulder, E., Gier, J. de, and Deenen, L. L. M. van (1962). *Biochim. Biophys. Acta* **59**, 502.
Mulder, E., Gier, J. de, and Deenen, L. L. M. van (1963). *Biochem. Biophys. Acta* **70**, 94.
Munn, J. I. (1958). *Brit. J. Haematol.* **4**, 344.
Munn, J. I., and Crosby, W. H. (1957). *Proc. Soc. Exptl. Biol.* **96**, 480.
Munn, J. I., and Crosby, W. H. (1961). *Brit. J. Haematol.* **7**, 523.
Newman, H. A. I., Lui, C.-T., and Zilversmit, D. B. (1961). *J. Lipid Res.* **2**, 403.
O'Donnell, V. J., Ottolenghi, P., Malkin, A., Denstedt, O. F., and Heard, R. D. H. (1958). *Can. J. Biochem. Physiol.* **36**, 1125.
Ogilvie, B. M., McClymont, G. L., and Shorland, F. B. (1961). *Nature* **190**, 725.
Oliveira, M. M., and Vaughan, M. (1962). *Federation Proc.* **21**, 296.
Olson, R. E. (1958). *In* "Chemistry of Lipids as Related to Atherosclerosis," p. 132. Thomas, Springfield, Illinois.
Olson, R. E., Lewis, J. H., Myers, J. D., and Moran, T. J. (1957). *Trans. Assoc. Am. Physicians* **70**, 243.
Parpart, A. K. (1942). *J. Cellular Comp. Physiol.* **19**, 248.
Parpart, A. K., and Ballentine, R. (1952). *In* "Modern Trends in Physiology and Biochemistry" (E. S. G. Barron, ed.), p. 135. Academic Press, New York.
Parpart, A. K., and Dziemian, A. J. (1940). *Cold Spring Harbor Symp. Quant. Biol.* **8**, 17.
Paysant-Diament, M., and Polonovski, J. (1960). *Bull. Soc. Chim. Biol.* **42**, 337.
Phillips, G. B. (1962). *J. Lab. Clin. Med.* **59**, 357.
Phillips, G. B., and Roome, N. S. (1959). *Proc. Soc. Exptl. Biol.* **100**, 489.
Phillips, G. B., and Roome, N. S. (1962). *Proc. Soc. Exptl. Biol.* **109**, 360.
Ponder, E. (1948). "Hemolysis and Related Phenomena." Grune Stratton, New York.
Ponder, E. (1952). *J. Gen. Physiol.* **35**, 361.
Ponder, E. (1955). *In* "Red Cell Structure and its Breakdown," Protoplasmatologia X, 2 Springer, Vienna.
Post, R. L., Merritt, C. R., Kinsolving, C. R., and Albright, C. D. (1960). *J. Biol. Chem.* **235**, 1796.
Prankerd, T. A. J. (1958). *J. Physiol.* **143**, 325.
Prankerd, T. A. J. (1959). *Brit. Med. Bull.* **15**, 54.
Prankerd, T. A. J. (1961). "The Red Cell." Blackwell, Oxford.
Raderecht, H. J., and Schölzel, E. (1960). *Folia Haematol.* **78**, 345.
Raderecht, H. J., Schölzel, E., and Rapoport, S. M. (1960). *Klin. Wochschr.* **38**, 824.
Raderecht, H. J., Binnewies, S., and Schölzel, E. (1962). *Acta Biol. Med. Germ.* **8**, 199.
Rapoport, S. M., and Guest, G. M. (1941). *J. Biol. Chem.* **138**, 269.
Reed, C. F. (1959). *J. Clin. Invest.* **38**, 1032.
Reed, C. F., Eden, E. G., and Swisher, S. N. (1958). *Clin. Res.* **6**, 186.
Reed, C. F., Swisher, S. N., Marinetti, G. V., and Eden, E. G. (1960). *J. Lab. Clin. Med.* **56**, 281.
Robertson, J. D. (1959). *Biochem. Soc. Symp.* (*Cambridge, England*) **16**, 3.
Rodin, N. S. (1957). *Federation Proc.* **16**, 825.
Rowe, C. E. (1959). *Biochem. J.* **73**, 438.
Rowe, C. E. (1960). *Biochem. J.* **76**, 471.
Rowe, C. E., Allison, A. C., and Lovelock, J. E. (1960a). *Biochem. J.* **74**, 26P.

Rowe, C. E., Allison, A. C., and Lovelock, J. E. (1960b). *Biochim. Biophys. Acta* **41**, 310.
Ruhenstroth-Bauer, G., and Hermann, G. (1950). *Z. Naturforsch.* **5B**, 416.
Ruyssen, R. (1957). *Proc. Intern. Congr. Surface Activity 2nd London, 1957 IV*, p. 271.
Schulman, J. H., Pethica, B. A., Few, A. V., and Salton, M. R. J. (1955). *Progr. Biophys. Chem* **5,** 41.
Stahl, E. (1957). *Chemiker Ztg.* **82**, 323.
Stoeckenius, W. (1960). *Proc. European Reg. Conf. Electronmicroscopy, Delft, 1960,* **II,** 716.
Stohlman, F. (1961). *Proc. Soc. Exptl. Biol. Med.* **107,** 884.
Tattrie, N. H. (1959). *J. Lipid Res.* **1**, 60.
Thompson, G. A., and Hanahan, D. J. (1962). *Arch. Biochem. Biophys.* **96**, 671.
Titus, E., Nicholls, D., and Kauffer, J. (1961). *Federation Proc.* **20**, 279.
Turner, J. C. (1957). *J. Exptl. Med.* **105**, 189.
Turner, J. C., Anderson, H. M., and Gandal, C. P. (1958a). *Biochim. Biophys. Acta* **30**, 130.
Turner, J. C., Anderson, H. M., and Gandal, C. P. (1958b). *Proc. Soc. Exptl. Biol. Med.* **99**, 547.
Vacca, J. B., Waring, P. P., and Nims, R. M. (1960). *Proc. Soc. Exptl. Biol. Med.* **105**, 100.
Valdiquié, P., Blaizot, J., Douste-Blazy, L., and Souyris, J. (1961). *Compt. Rend. Soc. Biol.* **155**, 66.
Waugh, D. F., and Schmitt, F. O. (1940). *Cold Spring Harbor Symp. Quant. Biol.* **8**, 233.
Ways, P. (1964). In press.
Ways, P., Reed, C. F., and Hanahan, D. J. (1961). *J. Clin. Invest.* **40**, 1088.
Webb, J. P. W., Allison, A. C., and James, A. T. (1960). *Biochim. Biophys. Acta* **43**, 89.
Webster, G. R., and Thompson, R. H. S. (1962). *Biochim. Biophys. Acta* **63**, 38.
Westerman, M. P., Pierce, L. E., and Jensen, W. N. (1959). *J. Clin. Invest.* **38**, 1054.
Williams, H. H., Erickson, B. N., Avrin, J., Bernstein, S. S., and Macy, I. G. (1938). *J. Biol. Chem.* **123**, 111.
Winkler, K. C., and Bungenberg de Jong, H. G. (1940–1941). *Arch. Neerl. Physiol.* **25**, 431.
Witting, L. A., Harvey, C. C., Century, B., and Horwitt, M. K. (1961). *J. Lipid Res.* **2**, 412.
Yamakawa, T., and Suzuki, S. (1951). *J. Biochem.* (*Tokyo*) **38**, 199.
Yamakawa, T., and Suzuki, S. (1952). *J. Biochem.* (*Tokyo*) **39**, 393.
Yamakawa, T., and Suzuki, S. (1953). *J. Biochem.* (*Tokyo*) **40**, 1, 7.
Yamakawa, T., Matsumoto, M., Suzuki, S., and Iida, T. (1956a). *Proc. Intern. Genet. Symp., Nankodo, 1956*, p. 616.
Yamakawa, T., Matsumoto, M., and Suzuki, S. (1956b). *J. Biochem.* (*Tokyo*) **43**, 63.
Yamakawa, T., Ohta, R., Ichikawa, Y., and Ozaki, J. (1958). *Compt. Rend. Soc. Biol.* **152,** 1288.
Yamakawa, T., Irie, R., and Iwanaga, M. (1960). *J. Biochem.* (*Tokyo*) **48**, 490.
Yamakawa, T., Yokoyama, S., and Kiso, N. (1962). *J. Biochem.* (*Tokyo*) **52**, 228.

CHAPTER 8

Hemoglobin Metabolism within the Red Cell[1]

David W. Allen

I. Introduction

Most hemoglobin synthesis has occurred before the immature red blood cell is released from the bone marrow into the peripheral blood, and the remainder takes place shortly thereafter. Furthermore, the hemoglobin, once formed, is biologically a rather stable molecule, largely as a result of many biochemical defenses (Chapter 11). Hemoglobin within the mature red cell undergoes few changes that are not reversed by enzymes of the red cell during its 4-month life span, and radioactive labeling indicates that its components do not turn over. Thus, in order to study hemoglobin metabolism, attention must be focused on the birth and death of the red cell (Wintrobe, 1961; London, 1961; Schweiger, 1962; Conference on Hemoglobin, 1958).

Hemoglobin biosynthesis as demonstrated by iron uptake on radioautography starts in the most immature recognizable red cells (Lajtha and Suit, 1955). These immature red cells possess a large nucleus containing deoxyribonucleic acid (DNA) which bears the genetic information in its nucleotide sequence. The nuclear DNA is considered to direct the synthesis of cytoplasmic ribonucleic acid (RNA), thought to contain just that genetic information applicable to the red cell. This information, which results in the amino acid sequence

[1] This is publication No. 1089 of the Cancer Commission of Harvard University.

of the red cell proteins, is coded in the nucleotide sequence of the RNA. The RNA gives the cytoplasm its diffuse basophilia and is responsible for protein, specifically, hemoglobin synthesis. As the red cell precursor matures, the nucleus or DNA is lost, the cytoplasmic basophilia or RNA decreases, and the acidophilia or hemoglobin increases. The mechanism of this hemoglobin production—presumably basically the same in all stages of red cell development—will be discussed in terms of the three parts of the hemoglobin molecule: globin, protoporphyrin IX, and iron. The metabolic pathways of these components, diverse at first, meet as the completed hemoglobin molecule is assembled.

The structure of the hemoglobin molecule is now known in considerable detail from results of both amino acid sequence determinations and x-ray diffraction studies. There are four polypeptide chains—2 α chains, and 2 β chains—arranged in a tetrahedral array. The α chains and the β chains have a similar overall shape or tertiary configuration and although the amino acid sequence of the two types is not identical, it has many similarities. Each of the four heme groups is linked to each of the four polypeptide chains from the iron atom of the heme group to the imidazole ring of a particular histidine residue. Adjacent to the heme-linked histidines of the β chains are the cysteine residues bearing the reactive sulfhydryl groups of hemoglobin. The positions of further histidine, tryptophan, and proline residues account for long known properties of hemoglobin and its tertiary configuration (Perutz, 1962). Since the amino acid sequence of the polypeptide chains, together with the structure of the heme prosthetic group, bears such good promise of successfully explaining the configuration, properties, and function of hemoglobin, the mechanism of their biosynthetic determination seems a fitting object for study.

This complex molecule may conceivably be catabolized in a variety of ways, making the early steps in hemoglobin breakdown difficult to clarify. Further steps in hemoglobin catabolism are obscure because degradative changes are slight in the peripheral blood, and artificial means of increasing the rate of hemoglobin destruction have questionable application to the normal process of red cell aging. The changes in hemoglobin known to occur normally in the senescent red cell—the formation of electrophoretically fast-moving hemoglobin components and methemoglobin—will be discussed first. Further changes must occur in the hemoglobin molecule before it can be broken down into the constituent amino acids of the globin, and the iron and protoporphyrin of the heme groups. Such evidence as is available concerning these changes will be considered.

II. Hemoglobin Synthesis

Current interest in protein biosynthesis has contributed greatly to the more specific problem of hemoglobin metabolism because the immature red cell has been found such a useful experimental tool. Much investigative work on hemoglobin biosynthesis has employed the reticulocyte largely because this anucleate cell can be obtained relatively free of other cells in high concentrations in the peripheral blood. The reticulocyte is engaged in biosynthesis of a single, well-characterized, easily purified protein, and this process can be followed by incorporation of radioactive amino acids both in the intact cell (Kruh and Borsook, 1956) and in a cell-free system (Schweet *et al.*, 1958). This system, in fact, has been one of the most satisfactory for demonstrating that incorporation of the radioactive amino acids measured in cell-free protein synthesis corresponds to a limited synthesis of a specific protein (E. H. Allen and Schweet, 1962).

A. Globin Synthesis

Cell-free biosynthesis of hemoglobin has been studied most effectively in rabbit reticulocytes by Schweet and co-workers (Schweet *et al.*, 1961), using conditions of cell-free protein synthesis similar to those worked out for other cell-free mammalian systems (Zamecnik, 1960; Hoagland, 1960). Unless otherwise specified, the experiments described below will have been performed with rabbit reticulocytes; however, most of the steps in protein biosynthesis have been found similar in tissues of widely different biological origin.

1. Intracellular Accumulation of Amino Acids

Accumulation of the constituent amino acids precedes their assembly into the polypeptide chain. The mature human red cell can accumulate glycine, alanine, and glutamic acid (Christensen *et al.*, 1952) and the human reticulocyte can concentrate these amino acids to a greater extent, and can accumulate methionine, isoleucine, and leucine as well (D. W. Allen, 1960). It is of interest that the concentrative capacity of rabbit reticulocytes is inhibited by cyanide, arsenate, and dinitrophenol, unlike mature erythrocytes (T. R. Riggs *et al.*, 1952) but similar to the effect of these inhibitors at the same concentration on protein biosynthesis (Borsook *et al.*, 1952). Thus the heightened accumulative ability of the reticulocyte may be linked to its capacity to synthesize protein, and both are sensitive to inhibitors of aerobic metabolism. The mechanism of this accumulation is unknown (Christensen, 1960), but the tendency of the more immature cell to accumulate higher concentrations of amino acids is a general property of cells actively engaged in protein synthesis.

2. Activation of Amino Acids

Although Borsook and Dubnoff (1940) early recognized the endergonic nature of peptide bond synthesis, and Lipmann (1941) suggested the possibility of a phosphate carboxyl anhydride as an intermediate, it remained to demonstrate experimentally the mechanism of amino acid activation (Hoagland *et al.*,

1956). Amino acids (aa) prior to participating in protein biosynthesis become activated by reacting with adenosine triphosphate (ATP) to form aminoacyl adenylate (aa ~ AMP). The amino acid carboxyl group is linked to the phosphate of adenosine-5′-monophosphate in a mixed anhydride bond of high-energy type. Thus the amino acid carboxyl has become activated or energized

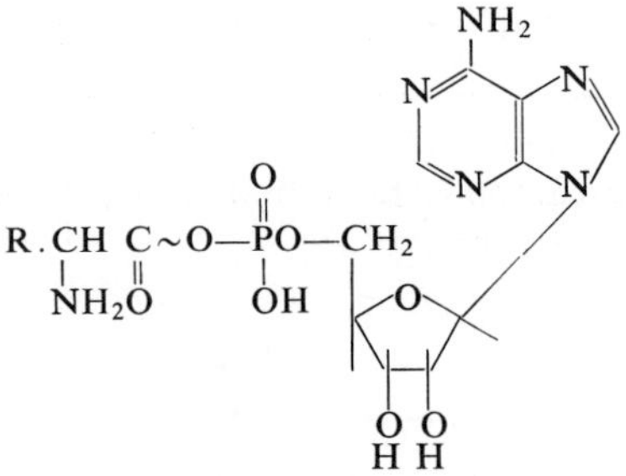

NH2 N N N N O R.CH C~O—PO—CH2 NH2O OH O O O H H

Aminoacyl ~ AMP
(I)

so it is made chemically reactive. By this means protein biosynthesis is linked to the energy-producing processes of the cell, so that the energy required for peptide bond synthesis can be supplied in the form of ATP. Each amino acid requires a specific amino acid-activating enzyme (E_I) for this step, and there has been considerable progress in the purification and characterization of these enzymes from several sources (Simpson, 1962). The activating enzymes from reticulocytes have been freed of hemoglobin and RNA (E. H. Allen and Schweet, 1962). The aminoacyl adenylates are largely enzyme-bound (aa ~AMP . . . E_I), and the concentration of these intermediates in protein biosynthesis is never high. The activation reaction (II) may be assayed by the reverse reaction, using P^{32}-labeled pyrophosphate (PP), or by using the forward reaction and trapping the activated aminoacyl group as the hydroxamate (Zamecnik, 1960; Simpson, 1962).

$$\text{aa} + \text{ATP} + E_I \rightleftharpoons \text{aa}\sim\text{AMP}\ldots E_I + \text{PP}$$
(II)

3. Transfer RNA

The next step in globin biosynthesis is the reaction of the aminoacyl adenylate enzyme complex with a specific soluble RNA or transfer RNA (TRNA) of the soluble cytoplasm to form aminoacyl transfer RNA (aa ~ TRNA) (Hoagland *et al.*, 1957; Hoagland, 1960; E. H. Allen and Schweet, 1960). Because the activating enzymes also catalyze this step in protein biosynthesis, it has been suggested that they be termed "aminoacyl RNA synthetases" (Bergmann *et al.*, 1961). The name "transfer RNA" was proposed by Schweet to describe the shuttle-like action of this compound between enzyme-bound activated amino acids and the ribosome template. There is a specific transfer RNA for each amino acid, and some of the transfer RNA's have been separated and attempts made to determine nucleotide sequence (Simpson, 1962). Each transfer RNA is used over and over in the process of hemoglobin synthesis (E. H. Allen and Schweet, 1960). Attempts to find other soluble intermediates have been unsuccessful and it is likely that aminoacyl transfer RNA is an obligatory intermediate in hemoglobin synthesis (Schweet *et al.*, 1961).

$$\text{aa}\sim\text{AMP}\ldots\text{E}_{\text{I}} + \text{TRNA} \longrightarrow \text{aa}\sim\text{TRNA} + \text{AMP} + \text{E}_{\text{I}} \qquad \text{(III)}$$

The aminoacyl residue is linked to the 2′ or 3′ position of the terminal ribosyl group of the transfer RNA, in an ester linkage (Zachau *et al.*, 1958). The terminal nucleotide sequence of all transfer RNA is identical, terminating with adenylic acid, with two cytidylate residues next in sequence internally (IV). These groups must be present, or replenished prior to amino acid uptake by the transfer RNA (Zamecnik, 1960). The uncertainty concerning the location of the aminoacyl residue is expressed as a bracket in (IV).

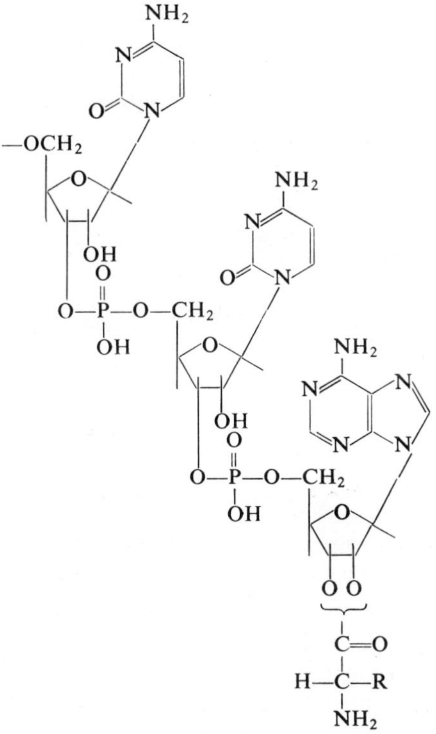

$$\text{—C—C—A}\sim\text{aa}$$

(IV)

It is of interest that Crick suspected the existence of transfer RNA on purely theoretical grounds prior to its discovery. He was unable to explain the direct recognition of amino acids by a specific sequence of nucleotide bases on the RNA template, and was forced to propose the existence of a small molecular weight "adaptor" between the activated amino acid and the ribosomal

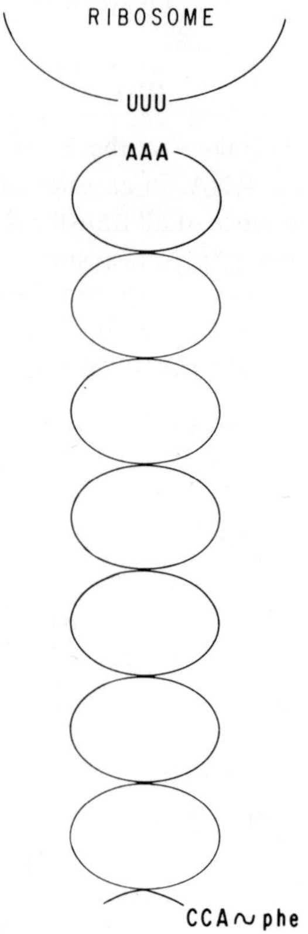

FIG. 1. Concept of the structure of phenylalanyl transfer RNA (Spencer *et al.*, 1962) A, adenine; U, uracil; C, cytosine; ∼phe, phenylalanyl residue.

RNA template (Hoagland, 1960). This role as an adaptor is carried out by the transfer RNA, which recognizes by its secondary structure its own activating enzyme and by a specific nucleotide sequence or code recognizes the positions on the ribosomal template at which its particular amino acid is required. The adaptor function of transfer RNA has recently been demonstrated experimentally. Cysteine was combined with specific cysteine transfer RNA, then converted to alanine by Raney nickel. It was demonstrated that this newly formed alanyl group when combined with cysteine transfer RNA was still considered as cysteine by an artificial template (Chapeville *et al.*, 1962).

Recent work on the physical properties of crystalline amino acid transfer RNA including x-ray diffraction studies suggests certain correlations between structure and function. Transfer RNA has a molecular weight of about 25,000, with a chain of 80 nucleotides. From x-ray diffraction evidence, the chain is folded back on itself and the two halves of the chain form a double helix by hydrogen bonding. The molecule thus resembles a twisted hairpin. The non-helical folded end of the hairpin may contain the amino acid code in its nucleotide sequence. The aminoacyl residue may be attached to a free end of the molecule (Spencer *et al.*, 1962). This present concept of the structure of TRNA is depicted in Fig. 1, which also includes current evidence for the RNA code for phenylalanine (Nirenberg and Matthaei, 1961), to be discussed further below.

This rather complex structure of transfer RNA yields as one benefit a considerable contribution to the specificity of amino acid incorporation. Thus transfer RNA must recognize the aminoacyl adenylate-activating enzyme complex, the enzyme required for transfer of the aminoacyl group to the ribosome (E_{II}), and the ribosome template itself. Some evidence even indicates that the transfer RNA can recognize the proper combination of aminoacyl adenylate and activating enzyme. Thus while isoleucine-activating enzyme will also catalyze to a limited extent the formation of valyl adenylate, only isoleucyl adenylate will be accepted by the transfer RNA from the enzyme (Bergmann *et al.*, 1961).

4. Ribosomal Stages of Hemoglobin Synthesis

It is on the ribosome that the sequence of amino acids is determined, peptide bond synthesis occurs (Littlefield *et al.*, 1955), and hemoglobin is formed (Rabinovitz and Olson, 1956). The reticulocyte ribosome is an 80S cytoplasmic ribonucleoprotein particle of about 200 Å in diameter, approximately half protein and half RNA, which is sedimentable only by ultracentrifugation. Most of the protein of the ribosome does not turn over, with only a small percent transient hemoglobin precursor (Dintzis *et al.*, 1958). There is recent evidence that ribosomes isolated from reticulocytes, like those from *Escherichia coli*, represent a heterogeneous population. Five percent of the ribosomes are more active synthetically, and more resistant to dissociation by low magnesium than the remaining 95% of the ribosomes (Lamfrom and Glowacki, 1962). A recent report explains this heterogeneity as a result of partial preparative degradation of a multiple ribosome or polysome, presumably the true *in vivo* unit in protein synthesis. Ultracentrifugal data and electron micrographs are presented which indicate that protein synthesis within the reticulocyte occurs in a multiple ribosomal structure containing 5 ribosomes. These ribosomes are strung on an RNA strand, possibly messenger RNA (Warner *et al.*, 1963).

It is probable that formation of the completed protein and its release into the soluble supernatant requires several stages. For ease of presentation a reasonable, but as yet largely unsupported, division will be made of the ribosomal stages of hemoglobin synthesis.

The first step in ribosomal protein synthesis would seem to be the attachment of aminoacyl transfer RNA to the ribosome (Hoagland and Comly, 1960) (V). The sequence of the amino acid residues in the protein is determined by the recognition by the aminoacyl transfer RNA of the code for its amino acid at a particular spot on the ribosome template.

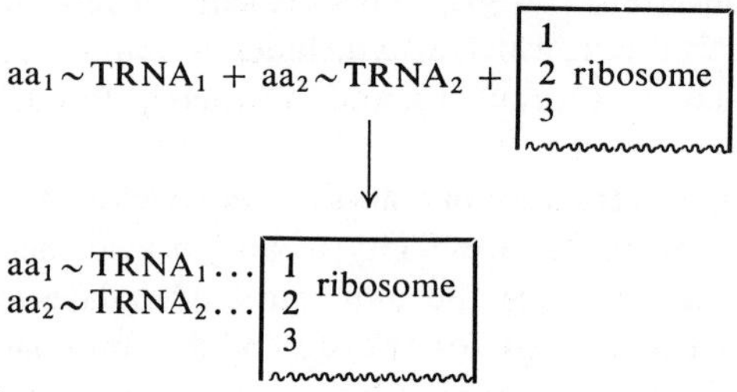

$$aa_1 \sim TRNA_1 + aa_2 \sim TRNA_2 + \boxed{\begin{matrix}1\\2 \text{ ribosome}\\3\end{matrix}}$$

$$\downarrow$$

$$\begin{matrix} aa_1 \sim TRNA_1 \ldots \\ aa_2 \sim TRNA_2 \ldots \end{matrix} \boxed{\begin{matrix}1 & \\ 2 & \text{ribosome} \\ 3 & \end{matrix}}$$

(V)

This recognition involves the ability of nucleic acid base residues to hydrogen-bond specifically with other base residues. Thus the adenine residue pairs with uracil (VI) and guanine with cytosine (VII).

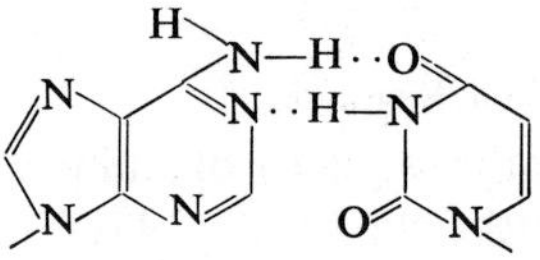

Adenine Uracil

(VI)

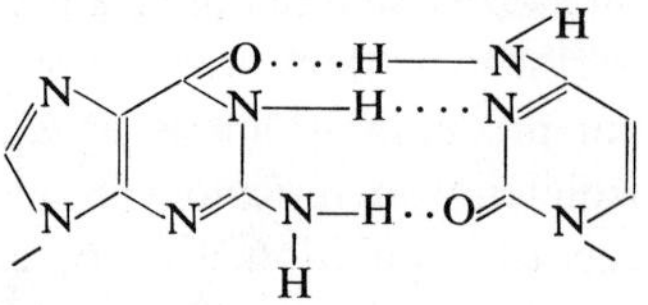

Guanine Cytosine

(VII)

There has been recent spectacular progress in identifying what combination of nucleotide bases (presumably a triplet) corresponds to a particular amino acid, by use of a system in which synthetic polynucleotides will act as templates (Nirenberg and Matthaei, 1961; Matthaei *et al.*, 1962). The sequence of nucleotides within the triplet is not known, however. From current information available, phenylalanine finds its proper place in the hemoglobin chain because three adenine residues in the nonhelical loop of the phenylalanyl transfer RNA hydrogen-bonds with three uracil residues on the ribosomal RNA of the template, as depicted in Fig. 1.

The information required for hemoglobin synthesis is apparently stored on the reticulocyte ribosome, since hemoglobin is formed from this particle regardless of the source of enzymes and transfer RNA (von Ehrenstein and Lipmann, 1961; Schweet *et al.*, 1961). Furthermore, if reticulocyte ribosomes from one animal species are mixed with soluble components from reticulocytes of another species, the hemoglobin synthesized is that of the ribosomes (Bishop *et al.*, 1961; Arnstein *et al.*, 1962).

It must be conceded that there are reports indicating an effect of the soluble supernatant as well as the ribosomes on the specificity of the hemoglobin produced (Lamfrom, 1961; Kruh *et al.*, 1961). These reports are inspired by the concept of a transient "messenger RNA" synthesized as a DNA replica and bearing the information required for protein sequence determination in the soluble supernatant, a concept derived largely from experiments with microorganisms (Jacob and Monod, 1961). While the "messenger" is considered destroyed with synthesis of the protein in microorganisms, the turnover of RNA is quite insufficient compared with the rate of synthesis of hemoglobin for this to occur in the immature red cell (Nathans *et al.*, 1962). Further, the effects of the supernatant observed by one author (Lamfrom, 1961) are slight and the experiments of the other group (Kruh *et al.*, 1961) have not been repeated (Arnstein *et al.*, 1962; D. W. Allen, unpublished observations). Recent evidence that the messenger RNA is bound to a group of 5 ribosomes, holding them together in a "polysome," has been mentioned above (Warner *et al.*, 1963).

The question of where the informational or messenger RNA for hemoglobin synthesis is located is of great importance for understanding and extending the recent observation of Weisberger (1962) on the induction of altered globin synthesis with a ribonucleoprotein. This investigator incubated normal immature red cells with sickle-cell marrow nucleoprotein and obtained a protein resembling but not identical to sickle-cell hemoglobin. It seems possible that the ribonucleoprotein introduced into the incubated cells competed successfully with the template already present.

After the aminoacyl TRNA is attached to the ribosome, with the amino acids held in proper sequence, peptide bond formation occurs (VIII). Either one or both of these steps require a soluble enzyme fraction, Mg^{++}, guanosine triphosphate (GTP), and a high-energy phosphate generating system (Nathans and Lipmann, 1961). In an *in vitro* system, the transfer RNA used with reticulocyte ribosomes may have its origin in *E. coli* (von Ehrenstein and Lipmann, 1961) or guinea pig liver (Schweet *et al.*, 1961), but apparently the transfer enzyme (E_{II}) must be of mammalian origin (Simpson, 1962). There may be a specific transfer enzyme for each amino acid (Bishop and Schweet, 1961). The role of GTP is unknown, as is the exact step in which it functions (Simpson, 1962).

Probably peptide bonds form as the activated acyl group of one aminoacyl residue attacks the amino group of the neighboring aminoacyl residue. This process starts at the N-terminal amino acid valine (Bishop *et al.*, 1960) and continues by steady sequential addition of two amino acids per second until growth terminates at the C-terminal end (Dintzis, 1961). The incomplete polypeptide chain is apparently held at its C-terminal end by the transfer RNA activating the acyl group (Hoagland and Comly, 1960) (VIII).

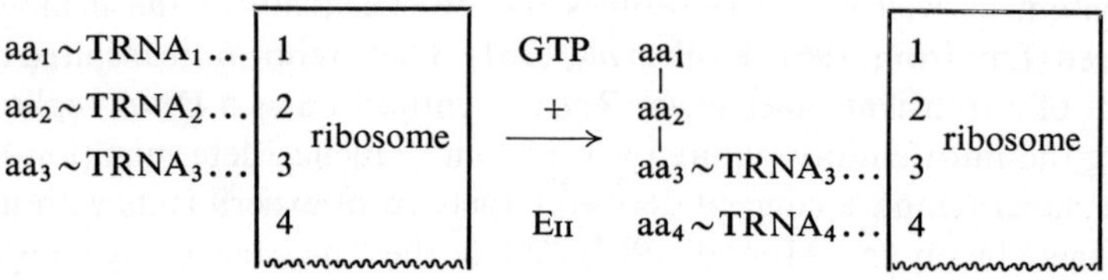

$$\begin{array}{l|l} aa_1 \sim TRNA_1 \ldots & 1 \\ aa_2 \sim TRNA_2 \ldots & 2 \quad \text{ribosome} \\ aa_3 \sim TRNA_3 \ldots & 3 \\ & 4 \end{array} \xrightarrow[E_{II}]{GTP\ +} \begin{array}{l|l} aa_1 & 1 \\ \ \mid & \\ aa_2 & 2 \quad \text{ribosome} \\ \ \mid & \\ aa_3 \sim TRNA_3 \ldots & 3 \\ aa_4 \sim TRNA_4 \ldots & 4 \end{array}$$

(VIII)

The antibiotic puromycin is a potent inhibitor of protein synthesis, in both whole cell and cell-free systems. This antibiotic apparently acts as an analog of aminoacyl transfer RNA (Yarmolinsky and de la Haba, 1959) (IX).

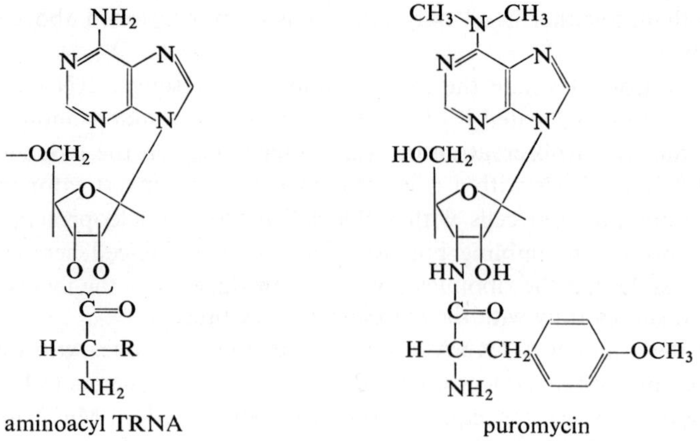

(IX)

The puromycin displaces the transfer RNA holding the nascent chain to the ribosome (Morris and Schweet, 1961; D. W. Allen and Zamecnik, 1962; Morris *et al.*, 1962) and releases polypeptide intermediates from the ribosome. In displacing the transfer RNA, the puromycin itself becomes bound to the polypeptide intermediate, probably by attachment of the amino group of the puromycin to the activated terminal acyl group of the polypeptide chain. The polypeptide intermediates are not hemoglobin but, like hemoglobin, have N-terminal valine and their tryptic digests contain peptides found in hemoglobin. Thus study of this interesting analog supports the supposition that the polypeptide chain is formed from its N-terminal end and is bound to the ribosome at its growing C-terminal end by TRNA.

The mechanism of release of the completed polypeptide chain from the ribosome is not understood. One possibility is that the chain may fall off of its own accord when there are no further bonding sites for transfer RNA on the ribosome. That the situation may be more complex than this is suggested by the observation that RNase-treated ribosomes, in which 90% of incorporation of C^{14}-amino acids is inhibited, will release preformed protein if supplied with ATP and enzymatic components of the soluble system. Since in this system amino acids cannot be incorporated, this result implies that chain completion is not responsible for this release. An enzymatic, energy-requiring step may be necessary for the release of the completed polypeptide chain (Schweet *et al.* 1961; Lamborg, 1962).

B. Porphyrin Synthesis

The precision of our knowledge of the pathway of biosynthesis of this portion of the hemoglobin molecule, its prosthetic group, contrasts favorably with knowledge of globin biosynthesis. The protoporphyrin of the heme is of a size that permits direct attack by the powerful synthetic and degradative methods of organic chemistry, so that the origin of each atom of the molecule can be investigated, and the fate of each postulated intermediate tested by synthesis and incubation. This achievement in organic and biological chemistry has been thoroughly reviewed elsewhere by those largely responsible (Shemin, 1958; Rimington, 1957; Neuberger, 1961; Granick and Mauzerall, 1961).

1. Formation of δ-Aminolevulinic Acid

Shemin's application of tracer techniques, first *in vivo* and then *in vitro* to avian erythrocytes and mammalian reticulocytes, demonstrated that the complicated protoporphyrin molecule is entirely synthesized from two simple precursors, glycine and succinate. A detailed scheme of degradation of heme has been worked out, which allows isolation of individual carbon atoms and measurement of the extent to which they are labeled (Shemin and Wittenberg,

1951). Data from these experiments led Shemin to synthesize δ-aminolevulinic acid (DAL) as a reasonable condensation product of glycine and succinate (X). Incubation of labeled DAL with hemolysates of duck erythrocytes results in the formation of heme of high specific activity and demonstrates that this compound is an intermediate in porphyrin synthesis (Shemin, 1958). The condensation of succinate and glycine occurs in the particulate matter of the cells, probably the mitochondria, and by washing away the soluble enzymes that further metabolize DAL, the condensation reaction may be studied directly. Succinate is activated as succinyl coenzyme A, pyridoxal phosphate probably is required to activate the glycine by formation of a Schiff base, and magnesium is an additional cofactor. Activation of the succinate is the means by which heme synthesis is linked to the energy-producing systems of the cell, as successive reactions are irreversible or thermodynamically favored (Granick and Mauzerall, 1961). The role of pyridoxine here is of interest as of possible significance in pyridoxine-responsive anemias.

$$\underset{\text{succinyl CoA}}{COOH{-}CH_2{-}CH_2{-}CO{-}CoA} + \underset{\text{glycine}}{\overset{\displaystyle COOH}{\overset{|}{C}}H_2{-}NH_2} + \text{pyridoxal phosphate}$$

$$\Big\downarrow \; Mg^{++} \quad \text{δ-aminolevulinic acid synthetase}$$

$$COOH{-}CH_2{-}CH_2{-}CO{-}CH_2{-}NH_2$$

δ-aminolevulinic acid (DAL)

(X)

2. Formation of Porphobilinogen

The next intermediate, porphobilinogen, was first isolated and crystallized from the urine of a patient with acute porphyria (Westall, 1952) and its structure determined later (Cookson and Rimington, 1954). It is to be noted that it is a monopyrrole of about twice the molecular weight of DAL. Enzymes capable of

$$2\ NH_2CH_2{-}CO{-}CH_2{-}CH_2{-}COOH \xrightarrow{\text{DAL dehydrase}} \text{porphobilinogen}$$

2 DAL: $NH_2CH_2{-}C{=}O$ (bearing $CH_2{-}CH_2{-}COOH$) and $O{=}C$ (bearing $CH_2{-}CH_2{-}COOH$ and $CH_2{-}NH_2$)

porphobilinogen: pyrrole ring (N–H) bearing $NH_2CH_2{-}$, $H_2C{-}COOH$ (HOOC) and $CH_2{-}CH_2{-}COOH$

(XI)

condensing two molecules of DAL to porphobilinogen are widely distributed in nature and one such has been found in hemolysates of rabbit reticulocytes and considerably purified by starch block electrophoresis (Granick and Mauzerall, 1958) (XI).

3. The Porphyrinogens and Formation of Protoporphyrin IX

Porphobilinogen is directly on the pathway of heme synthesis, four molecules being utilized stoichiometrically in this biosynthesis. The nature of the tetrapyrrole first formed by polymerization of porphobilinogen was clarified by Bogorad and Granick (1953), who demonstrated the formation of uroporphyrinogen III as the primary product (Granick and Mauzerall, 1961) (XII). Uroporphyrinogen III is a hexahydroporphyrin, and the partial saturation of the conjugated resonating ring system of the porphyrin accounts for the lack of color in this compound. The tendency of porphyrinogens to autoxidize to the porphyrins at first caused considerable confusion as to the nature of the intermediates in porphyrin synthesis. However, whereas uroporphyrin cannot be used as substrate for subsequent biochemical steps, uroporphyrinogen is readily utilized (Mauzerall and Granick, 1958).

A still unsolved problem is the mechanism by which the four monopyrrole porphobilinogen units form the unsymmetrical type III isomer. A simple linear polymerization followed by ring closure would produce the type I compound, in which the acetic and propionic side chains simply alternate around the tetrapyrrole ring (Margoliash, 1961). It has been suggested that the porphobilinogen isomerase presumed responsible for the asymmetric synthesis of the type III isomers is absent in erythropoietic or congenital porphyria to account for the large urinary excretion of uroporphyrinogen I and coproporphyrinogen I in this disease (Granick and Mauzerall, 1961).

An enzyme has been purified by starch block electrophoresis from rabbit reticulocytes which decarboxylates the acetic acid side chains on uroporphyrinogen to form coproporphyrinogen (Mauzerall and Granick, 1958) (XII).

There remains, however, the oxidation of coproporphyrinogen to protoporphyrin, and the sequence of the required steps for this conversion is not clear: two propionyl residues must be converted to vinyl groups, and the methylene bridges must be dehydrogenated. It may well be that these last steps occur within the particulate matter of the cell, since particle-free hemolysates of avian reticulocytes carry biosynthesis from porphobilinogen no further than coproporphyrinogen, while the complete hemolysate forms protoporphyrin (Dresel and Falk, 1956). Oxidation may occur from the protoporphyrinogen which is more autoxidizable than the coproporphyrinogen. It is clear, however, that the iron insertion occurs only at the level of protoporphyrin, since no iron compound of uroporphyrin or coproporphyrin is found in nature, and microorganisms requiring heme can grow with iron and protoporphyrin but not with related porphyrins (Granick and Mauzerall, 1961). The mechanism of iron insertion into heme in the immature red cell will be discussed later after the pathway of iron into the red cell is considered.

C. *Iron Incorporation*

Unlike the body of biochemical evidence concerning globin or protoporphyrin synthesis, information on iron metabolism within the red cell seems sparse and comes from a variety of disciplines. One must frequently compare data arising from such diverse sources as nutrition (Moore, 1961), or the kinetics of radioactive iron in patients (Huff and Judd, 1956), or electron microscopy (Bessis and Breton-Gorius, 1962). Thus there is need of more detailed ferrokinetic studies at an intracellular level with chemical characterization of the form of iron (Finch, 1958). Such studies are made difficult by the tendency of iron to bind chemically with a variety of groups, so that interpretation of the true form of the iron prior to fractionation of the red cell must be cautious.

1. The Red Cells' Source of Iron

Two sources of iron have been proposed for the developing erythroblast. One of the sources is transferrin, the iron-binding protein of the plasma, the other ferritin, contained in macrophages or reticulum cells of the bone marrow. At present the best available evidence favors transferrin as the immediate source of iron. The electron microscope observations on which the second possibility is based, however, have great value, as they permit quite specific identification of the ferritin molecule within the developing erythroblast.

The immature red cell readily utilizes transferrin-bound iron. Transferrin has a molecular weight of about 90,000, moves as a β_1-globulin by electrophoresis, but has solubility properties more closely resembling albumin. It binds 2 ferric ions to form a salmon-red colored complex (Surgenor *et al.*, 1949). Ionized iron is a toxic substance, and the chemistry of iron in the body reveals that it is usually rendered harmless by formation of specific chemical complexes. Transferrin represents the most labile buffer of iron in the body, and acts to prevent excessive free iron accumulation by transporting dietary or artificially administered iron to the developing normoblasts of the bone marrow or to the ferritin stores of the reticuloendothelial system (Laurell, 1960). Immature red cells can use inorganic iron as well as transferrin for hemoglobin synthesis (Walsh *et al.*, 1949). The particular virtue of transferrin lies in its iron-binding equilibrium, which enables it to release iron specifically to the immature red cell, at levels of saturation from 20–30% to about 60%, without nonspecific and possibly toxic release to other cells such as adult red cells or liver cells

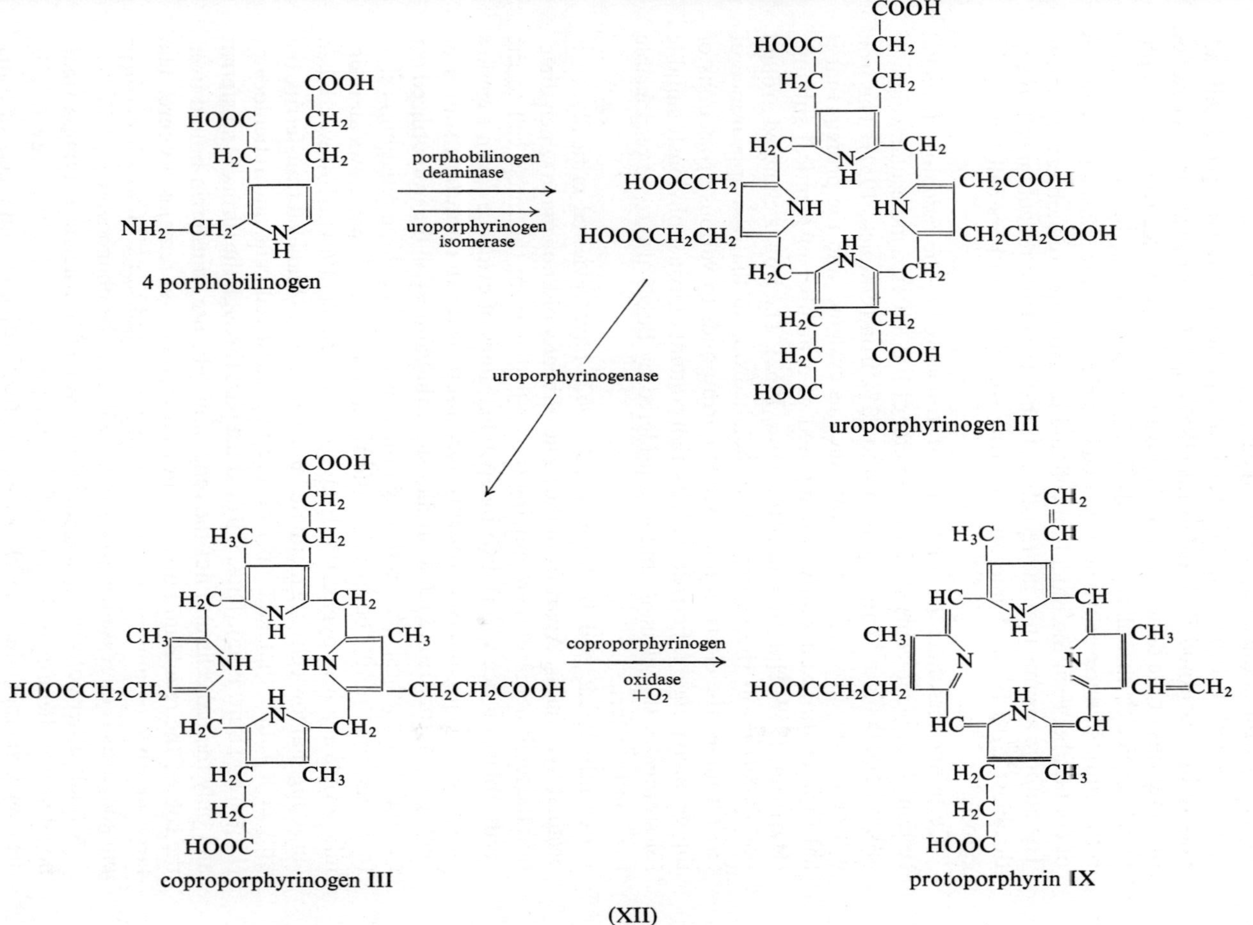
4 porphobilinogen
porphobilinogen deaminase
uroporphyrinogen isomerase
uroporphyrinogen III
uroporphyrinogenase
coproporphyrinogen III
coproporphyrinogen oxidase $+O_2$
protoporphyrin IX

(XII)

(Jandl *et al.*, 1959). Thus transferrin seems an efficient and delicate method of supplying iron to the developing red cell.

The second method proposed for iron transfer to the young red cell, advanced by Bessis and Breton-Gorius (1957), is based on electron microscope observations of the bone marrow. These authors present electron micrographs which depict erythroblastic islands in the bone marrow, in which a central reticulum cell (nurse cell) is surrounded by a ring of erythroblasts. In the region of contact between the reticulum cell and erythroblast, one observes ferritin. The authors assume that the ferritin is transferred from reticulum cell to erythroblast by a form of micropinocytosis which the authors call "rhopheocytosis."

Certainly, ferritin is the chief form of iron stored in the reticuloendothelial system. A large molecule, it has a diameter of 100–110 Å, a molecular weight of around 500,000, and can contain up to 23% iron (Granick, 1951). The iron can be removed by reducing agents such as cysteine, and the protein that is left (apoferritin) apparently is composed of a number of identical subunits (Harrison, 1959; Harrison and Hofmann, 1962). The iron is clumped around the apoferritin at the vertices of an octahedron, so that the appearance of ferritin under the electron microscope corresponds to various projections of this geometric figure. Ferritin with its high content of iron is obviously suitable for storage of this element and is considered by Bessis also to be responsible for iron transfer.

Recently Bessis and Breton-Gorius (1962) have reviewed critically their original hypothesis. Apart from the basic difficulty of knowing in which direction the ferritin granules are moving (i.e., whether from the nurse cell to the erythroblast or vice versa), two independent lines of evidence taken together imply that this mechanism probably does not provide an important source of hemoglobin iron. Iron kinetic studies show that almost all the iron utilized for hemoglobin synthesis passes through the plasma. Thus if the reticulum cell is to get its iron, it must be from transferrin as kinetic evidence shows an insignificant plasma iron bypass (Pollycove and Mortimer, 1961). However, when surviving marrow cells are incubated *in vitro* with Fe^{59}-labeled transferrin, the only cells found that take up iron are nucleated red cells and reticulocytes (Lajtha and Suit, 1955). Thus, if iron must pass through the form of transferrin and only the red cells and not the reticulum cells use transferrin-bound iron, the role of the reticulum nurse cell in iron metabolism remains obscure. The large number of nurse cells in inflammatory conditions in which erythrophagocytosis is increased suggests these cells may be phagocytes.

A final rather convincing argument in favor of transferrin playing a significant role as the principal source of iron for the erythroblast is the severe iron-deficiency anemia which developed in a patient with congenital lack of transferrin, despite adequate iron absorption (Heilmeyer *et al.*, 1961).

2. Stromal Phase of Iron

The possibility of surface receptors for iron on the reticulocyte membrane was suggested by the inability of high molar ratios of ethylenediaminetetra-acetic acid to abolish transfer of Fe^{59} from transferrin to the reticulocytes. Thus there was little unbound iron for this chelating agent to trap, in the transfer process from transferrin to the red cell. Further evidence for receptors was obtained when reticulocytes were incubated with as little as 0.01 mg./ml. of trypsin, with resulting 85% suppression of Fe^{59} uptake and no effect on oxygen consumption or lactate production (Jandl *et al.*, 1959).

Iron, after entering the immature red cell, is associated with the cell stroma: that material, including the red cell membrane, that is separated from the rest of the hemolysate by low speed centrifugation (Walsh *et al.*, 1949). The stromal iron reaches peak activity in 2 minutes, then declines over a 6–8 minute period, while the remainder of the cytoplasm and, in particular, hemoglobin increase in total radioactivity (D. W. Allen and Jandl, 1960). A preliminary report (Mazur *et al.*, 1962) indicates that this stromal iron may be ferritin, which in hematopoietic cells is especially labile and has the role of iron carrier or heme precursor rather than a storage form. Thus the turnover of ferritin in bone marrow or reticulocytes is much faster than in the liver or spleen, and red cell stroma ferritin appears as an active intermediate in the pathway of iron into hemoglobin.

This stromal ferritin iron represents in all probability the "labile erythropoietic iron pool" of iron kinetics. It is derived from transferrin and may be released back to the plasma or utilized for hemoglobin synthesis (Pollycove and Mortimer, 1961; Pollycove and Maqsood, 1962).

It was noted above that ferritin had been identified in erythroblasts and reticulocytes by the electron microscope. Fascinating observations by this same technique in the hypersideremic anemias, including thalassemia, hypochromic hypersideremic anemias, and lead poisoning, demonstrate erythroblasts loaded with iron as ferritin in apparently distinctive patterns (Bessis and Breton-Gorius, 1962). Lead poisoning represents a defect investigated both by this technique and by study of distribution of Fe^{59} (D. W. Allen and Jandl, 1960). By each approach marked accumulation of iron in the stromal phase is observed.

3. Nonheme Iron in the Soluble Phase

The iron next is transferred from the stroma to the site of heme synthesis. A possible intermediate in this intracellular iron transport is the nonheme iron bound to a soluble protein (D. W. Allen and Jandl, 1960). The kinetic evidence is consistent with its being an intermediate between stromal and hemoglobin iron (Greenough *et al.*, 1962), but is insufficient as yet to prove this assumption.

Further, the tendency of iron to be protein-bound, both as an artifact as well as naturally, complicates the interpretation of these experiments.

D. *Assembly of the Completed Hemoglobin Molecule*

The mode of assembly of the components of hemoglobin to form the finished molecule is of obvious importance but the evidence for the mechanism is incomplete. The biosynthesis of the globin has been traced to the release of this protein from the ribosome. When it is released, an appreciable fraction —80%—has the chromatographic and electrophoretic properties of hemoglobin. Hence iron, protoporphyrin, and enzymes are available for completing the molecule. Similarly, the path of porphyrin synthesis has been traced until the formation of protoporphyrin—a step noted to occur in the particulate matter of the cell. Iron too finds its way to the ribosomes although the percentage accumulation of iron on the ribosomes is always small. Rabinovitz and Olson (1958) found that ribosomes prepared from rabbit reticulocytes were able to incorporate iron into hemoglobin. Circumstantial evidence suggests, then, assembly of the hemoglobin on the ribosome.

The enzyme heme synthetase is also important in the assembly of the molecule, as it is responsible for iron incorporation into heme (Schwartz *et al.*, 1961). The enzyme, purified several hundred-fold from an acetone powder of chicken erythrocyte hemolysate, forms hemoglobin starting with iron, protoporphyrin IX, and globin. The type of hemoglobin produced depends on the type of globin supplied. It is of interest that synthesis occurs maximally at the correct ratio of heme to globin of 4:1. Other enzyme-like properties include a linear dependence of heme synthesis on enzyme concentration, heat inactivation, and pH optimum in the physiological range. The enzyme appears to be associated with the particulate matter of the cell, but has not been specifically located on the ribosome.

A speculative summary of hemoglobin synthesis is shown in Fig. 2. Glycine is afforded particular emphasis, since as a precursor of both heme and globin it has been frequently used to measure their relative rates of synthesis. The possibility of different intracellular pools for glycine intermediates in heme and globin synthesis, which would invalidate these determinations, is suggested by the diagram.

Since the mature red cell has a high concentration of hemoglobin and only negligible amounts of excess heme or globin, it seems clear that in the development of the red cell the correct final ratio of heme to globin has been attained. Reports that globin synthesis precedes heme synthesis in the life of the red cell suffer from the equating of total cell protein with globin (Lagerlöf *et al.*, 1956; Nathan *et al.*, 1961). It is reasonable to suppose that the immature erythroblast contains relatively more nonhemoglobin protein than the mature cell, and this protein of immature cells especially must not be considered to be all globin. Other evidence based on glycine incorporation indicates that although globin and heme synthesis declines, as the erythroblast matures to the reticulocyte, the ratio of heme to globin synthesis is maintained at approximately 4:1 (Morell *et al.*, 1958).

Various possible explanations exist for this regulation of heme and globin synthesis. Globin stimulates heme production by heme synthetase (Schwartz

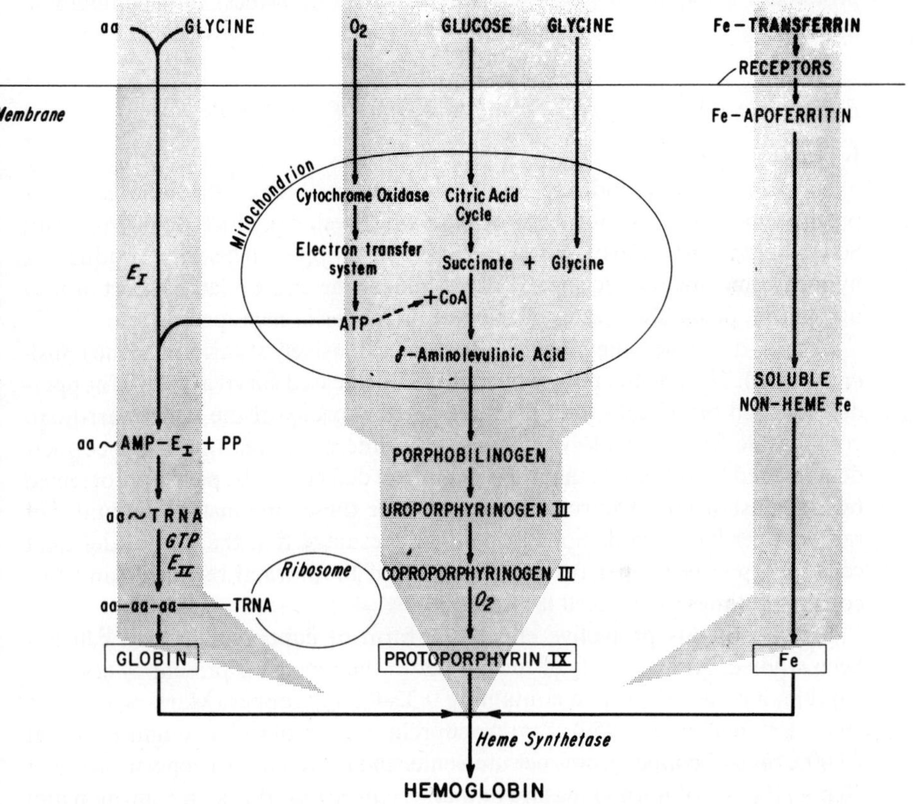

FIG. 2. Speculative summary of hemoglobin synthesis.

et al., 1961), iron stimulates globin formation (Kruh and Borsook, 1956), and iron enhances both DAL formation from glycine, and heme synthesis from protoporphyrin (Vogel *et al.*, 1960) Thus accumulation of one of the three components of hemoglobin may be avoided under normal circumstances by stimulation of synthesis of the other components. Other mechanisms undoubtedly may exist, such as inhibition of the early steps of heme or globin synthesis by the products formed.

Of related interest is the means by which hemoglobin synthesis is suppressed as the red cell matures. Perhaps this is secondary to loss of ribosomes, as cytoplasmic RNA and hemoglobin synthetic activity correlate closely with percent of reticulocytes (Holloway and Ripley, 1952). There is evidence from incubation studies of reticulocytes that stromal or nonhemoglobin protein is utilized for hemoglobin production (Schweiger, 1962). Thus the final stages of reticulocyte maturation may involve in part a conversion of parts of the machinery for producing hemoglobin (e.g., ribosomal protein, enzymes) into hemoglobin itself.

E. Possible Role of Copper, Cobalt, and Other Trace Metals

1. Copper

Nutritional studies indicate copper to be essential for erythropoiesis, but its precise function in this regard is not known (Elvehjem, 1935; Schultze, 1940; Scheinberg, 1961; Cartwright *et al.*, 1958). Copper deficiency produces a hypochromic, microcytic anemia in rats and swine and a related defect in iron utilization, probably a result of the role of copper in hemopoiesis.

Copper-deficiency anemia has been most extensively studied in swine (Bush *et al.*, 1956). The anemia results both from a decreased survival time of copper-deficient red blood cells, and from a limited capacity of the bone marrow to compensate for this hemolytic anemia. An interesting feature of the copper-deficient red blood cells is that their hemolytic defect may be partially corrected by transfusion into a normal animal. Under these circumstances uptake of radiocopper has been demonstrated. It is presumed that the copper-deficient cells incorporate copper from the plasma of the normal recipient, and this copper prolongs the red cell life span.

Because of this protective effect, the form of copper in the red cell has been studied. At least 80% of the copper in the red cell is present as erythrocuprein, a colorless protein containing 0.32–0.36% copper (Markowitz *et al.*, 1959; Kimmel *et al.*, 1959). Erythrocuprein has a molecular weight of about 35,000, binds 2 copper atoms per molecule, and is present in a concentration of 30 mg./100 ml. of normal mature human erythrocytes. It is a glycoprotein and in addition to amino acids contains hexose, hexosamine, and sialic acid. Whether this copper protein is the biologically active form of copper which prolongs the red cell life span, however, remains unknown.

The inability of the copper-deficient marrow to respond maximally to the hemolytic anemia suggests a role of copper in erythropoiesis. Copper is apparently a constituent of cytochrome oxidase (Wainio *et al.*, 1959), an enzyme essential for the mitochondrial oxidative metabolism that supplies not only DAL but also the energy for heme and globin synthesis. A correlation between copper content and cytochrome oxidase activity in copper deficiency exists (Cohen and Elvehjem, 1934). In rats, correction of the copper deficiency stimulates the cytochrome oxidase activity of the bone marrow and results in erythropoiesis (Schultze, 1941). It is tempting, then, to suspect that the erythropoietic defect of copper deficiency may be due to its role in some enzyme such as cytochrome oxidase, but there is no evidence as to which is the rate-limiting enzyme in copper deficiency. DAL dehydrase does not now appear to be related to copper-deficiency anemia (Margoliash, 1961).

2. Cobalt, Zinc, and Magnesium

Cobalt deficiency produces a progressive wasting disease in ruminants with failure of appetite and severe macrocytic anemia. Cobalt is an essential constituent of the vitamin B_{12} normally synthesized in these animals by the bacteria in the rumen. Nonruminant herbivores pastured in the same location remain healthy, possibly because their requirement for vitamin B_{12} is less than in ruminants. Thus cobalt deficiency in the special case of ruminants produces a vitamin B_{12} deficiency pattern not unlike pernicious anemia in humans (Marston, 1952), but the role of B_{12} in erythropoiesis is not fully understood.

Zinc in the red cell is present almost entirely as carbonic anhydrase (Vallee *et al.*, 1949), an enzyme important in respiratory physiology. Magnesium is so frequently cast in the role of an enzyme cofactor that it seems inappropriate to claim a special function for it in the red cell (Vallee, 1960).

III. Hemoglobin Changes within the Aging Erythrocyte

Although hemoglobin on sterile incubation *in vitro* at physiological temperatures becomes denatured and precipitates in a few days, it survives virtually intact for 4 months in the circulating red cell. During this life span of the normal red cell in the peripheral blood, irreversible changes occur in only a small percentage of the hemoglobin. This is an advantage to the organism as the essential function of oxygen transport is not compromised by the presence of hemoglobin molecules which cannot combine properly with oxygen. Perhaps the normal red cell is provided with a mechanism whereby it is eliminated before the accumulation of defective hemoglobin (except sulfhemoglobin and in congenital methemoglobinemia—see Chapter 11). However, the ability of the body to destroy red cells prior to formation of appreciable quantities of changed hemoglobin presents a problem in understanding the actual sequence of events in hemoglobin catabolism.

A. Formation of Electrophoretically Fast-Moving Hemoglobins

Evidence has been accumulated by a variety of techniques indicating the heterogeneous metabolism of both rabbit and human hemoglobin (Schapira *et al.*, 1958). Kunkel and Wallenius (1957) observed a fast-moving component of hemoglobin on electrophoresis in barbital buffer at pH 8.6 with ionic strength of 0.05. A key to this component's possible role in hemoglobin metabolism was obtained after Fe^{59} was administered to experimental subjects and specific activities of the various hemoglobin fractions were analyzed at certain times thereafter. It was found that this fast-moving fraction had a low specific activity compared to the main component shortly after administration of the label, and that the specific activity of the fast-moving fraction subsequently rose gradually (Kunkel, 1958). This observation has been confirmed in patients with sickle trait and extended to rabbits (Ranney and Kono, 1959). Thus the fast-moving hemoglobin may be formed from the main component by *in vivo* aging under stresses present in the blood stream.

Fast-moving components are also observed on column chromatography on IRC (Morrison and Cook, 1955; Prins and Huisman, 1956) and have been found to be heterogeneous (D. W. Allen *et al.*, 1958). The front-running chromatographic fraction is separated in this way more completely from the main component and comprises about 10% of the total hemoglobin. When this component undergoes electrophoresis it has the mobility of the fast-moving electrophoretic fraction.

An attempt to understand the significance of these fast-moving components has focused on their production *in vitro* by treatment of hemoglobin with various means, such as sterile incubation as oxyhemoglobin *in vitro*, oxidizing agents as ferricyanide (especially at high pH where the sulfhydryl groups are more reactive), and such drugs as phenylhydrazine that produce destruction of hemoglobin by coupled oxidation with atmospheric oxygen (Jandl *et al.*, 1960). The initial site of this oxidant attack appeared to be the two reactive sulfhydryl groups of native hemoglobin. After these groups had been either oxidized or combined with sulfhydryl-binding agents as *p*-chloromercuribenzoate, the molecule became more susceptible to further denaturation and precipitation (D. W. Allen and Jandl, 1961). The reactive sulfhydryl groups, adjacent to the heme-linked histidine residues of the β chains, are located where the two chains of the half-molecules are contiguous (Perutz *et al.*, 1960), and their oxidation or binding is known to disrupt heme-heme interactions in the oxygen equilibrium curve (A. F. Riggs, 1952). It would seem reasonable to suppose that this alteration in heme-heme interaction implies a change in configuration of the molecule, perhaps an opening up of the chains rendering them more susceptible to oxidative attack. The changes observed by Riggs in oxygen dissociation were reversible; further changes probably result in the irreversibly altered fast-moving components. These components bind more glutathione than does the main component in mixed disulfide bonds (D. W. Allen and Jandl, 1961). The increased electrophoretic mobility may result from exposure of more charged groups, the bulk being negatively charged at the alkaline pH at which hemoglobin is usually studied.

B. Methemoglobin

Although the heme group of the fast-moving components is unaltered, the globin portion of the molecule is denatured. Conversely, oxidation of the heme iron produces methemoglobin, in which the heme is changed and the globin unaltered. Methemoglobin is always formed when hemoglobin undergoes oxidative destruction *in vitro* from sterile incubation or from the action of certain drugs (Jandl *et al.*, 1960; Harley and Mauer, 1960, 1961). However, drug-induced methemoglobin *in vivo* may be transient if the methemoglobin reductase system is intact. Since certain drugs differ strikingly in their tendency to produce methemoglobin and other products of the denaturation of hemoglobin, and methemoglobinemia is not necessarily associated with a shortened red cell life span, doubt has been raised whether methemoglobin is an obligatory precursor of the oxidative destruction of hemoglobin (Beutler and Baluda, 1962).

There is, however, good evidence that methemoglobin is increased in aged erythrocytes. An increase in methemoglobin content of transfused red cells was observed from 1% immediately after transfusion to 8% after 80 days (Waller *et al.*, 1959). The authors correlated this increase in methemoglobin with the general enzymatic decline of the aging red cell, in particular the diphosphopyridine nucleotide reducing system, which is coupled to methemoglobin reductase. Methemoglobin metabolism is discussed at length in Chapter 11.

C. Further Changes in Hemoglobin

There is no change in the heme of the fast-moving components. The heme iron of methemoglobin has been oxidized from the ferrous to the ferric condition but the change is reversible. There is, however, a large group of poorly characterized brown-green to green oxidation products of hemoglobin with limited solubility, in which the protoporphyrin of the heme is altered irreversibly. These oxidized hemoglobins are not present in detectable quantities in red cells except by the action of oxidant drugs or the combined action of hydrogen peroxide and the catalase inhibitor, azide (Lemberg and Legge, 1949; Mills and Randall, 1958). Thus acceptance of these compounds as intermediates in hemoglobin catabolism has less validity than those components which have definitely been found increased in aged cells—methemoglobin and the fast-moving components, but until further direct evidence is available they provide an experimental approach to hemoglobin catabolism.

1. Choleglobin

Perhaps the best characterized of these substances is the choleglobin of Lemberg. This compound is produced by coupled oxidation of hemoglobin with ascorbic acid and hydrogen peroxide, in which methemoglobin is an intermediate. The lack of a Soret band, the mode of preparation, and the fact that iron can be detached by acetic acid treatment suggest that the prosthetic group of choleglobin may have a methine bridge of heme replaced by a labile oxygen bridge (Lemberg and Legge, 1949). As the iron is released the prosthetic group is converted into the open chain biliverdin, the first of the bile pigments.

It is likely that the process of the destruction of heme passes through some such intermediate as choleglobin with the protoporphyrin residue oxidized and the iron still present, whether or not the altered heme group is still attached to globin or to some other protein. Heme is readily converted to bile pigments while hematoporphyrin or protoporphyrin are not. Thus the presence of divalent or trivalent iron may be necessary for cleavage of the protoporphyrin ring (Schmid, 1960).

Many other green or brown pigments, denatured products of hemoglobin produced under a great variety of conditions, are known (Lemberg and Legge, 1949). It would seem reasonable to expect such a variety of partially denatured, partially oxidized products of hemoglobin when the complexity of the molecule is considered.

2. Heinz Bodies

After hemoglobin has become sufficiently denatured to lose its normally high solubility, it precipitates in the form of spherical particulate matter, whether within the red cell or in stroma-free solution. The precipitate is apparently identical with the intracellular inclusions, Heinz bodies, found in oxidant drug-induced hemolytic anemias (Beaven and White, 1954; Jandl *et al.*, 1960). The pathogenesis of Heinz body anemia has been reviewed elsewhere (Beutler, 1959) and some of the contributions this study has made to the knowledge of red cell metabolism are discussed in Chapter 6.

It seems unlikely that much hemoglobin passes through the stage of Heinz bodies before being catabolized. Although Heinz bodies have been reported in splenectomized patients (Selwyn, 1955), these inclusions are not uniformly present in splenic agenesis or after splenectomy (Buch and Ainger, 1955). Moreover, descriptions of phase contrast microscope studies of erythrophagocytosis by reticulum cells do not mention inclusions in the red cells phagocytized (Bessis and Breton-Gorius, 1962). Although red cells containing Heinz bodies are removed *in toto* by the spleen (Rothberg *et al.*, 1959), there is no detectable increase in life span of red cells after splenectomy (Berlin *et al.*, 1959), as would be expected if Heinz bodies were the normal cause of red cell death.

Thus, it is likely in normal aging of the red cell that insoluble hemoglobin does not accumulate sufficiently to allow for Heinz body formation. Before the hemoglobin can precipitate, the red cell is destroyed in the reticuloendothelial system by phagocytosis, perhaps secondary to some alteration of the red cell membrane (Jacob and Jandl, 1962) or after fragmentation of the cell (Wintrobe, 1961).

D. *Fate of the Components of Hemoglobin*

The site of further catabolism of hemoglobin is the reticuloendothelial system (extravascular hemolysis). The alternate, intravascular hemolysis, with release of hemoglobin into the plasma, usually is a minor pathway, although this may be increased in certain hemolytic anemias (Dacie, 1960).

After phagocytic destruction of the erythrocyte, the iron is stored as ferritin. Ferritin granules are observed to form around the phagocytized red cell as it is undergoing digestion (Bessis and Breton-Gorius, 1962). The iron is then released as transferrin and is reutilized for hemoglobin formation (Noyes *et al.*, 1960). The body normally conserves iron very successfully, for while 20–25 mg. iron is available daily from the destruction of erythrocytes, only about 1 mg. is excreted (Moore, 1961).

The fate of the globin residue is known with less certainty. It is likely that the globin is hydrolyzed to its constituent amino acids, which are released to the plasma and are available for protein synthesis or deamination and energy-yielding catabolism.

While the iron and amino acids are conserved, the protoporphyrin part of the hemoglobin molecule is catabolized and excreted. The biliverdin formed in the reticuloendothelial cell is converted to bilirubin and then released into the blood stream. This protein-bound water-insoluble bilirubin is removed from the blood by the liver and conjugated with glucuronic acid. The bilirubin glucuronide, which is water-soluble, is excreted in the bile into the intestine where it is further degraded into a variety of products (Watson, 1957; Schmid, 1960).

IV. Conclusion

Although the metabolism of a particular protein, in a single highly specialized cell, has been described, it is likely that this account will be found to apply to many proteins, in a number of cells. The steps in globin synthesis are similar to protein synthesis in the rat liver or the pea seedling or *E. coli* (Zamecnik, 1960). Heme is found in the cytochromes of every aerobic organism, and a magnesium porphyrin, chlorophyll, in every green plant. Protoporphyrin synthesis identical to that in the mammalian reticulocyte is found in many other cells studied and, indeed, the initial pathway is the same in chlorophyll synthesis by *Chlorella* (Granick and Mauzerall, 1961). The problem of iron uptake from the cellular environment in a utilizable but nontoxic form is faced as well by microorganisms (Neilands, 1957). The changes that occur in the hemoglobin of the aging red cell appear similar to senescent changes in the protein of the lens of the eye (Jandl *et al.*, 1960). Thus the truism that biochemical mechanisms are frequently repeated in nature finds no exception here. The study of hemoglobin metabolism within the red cell may aid understanding of processes far outside the limits of that erythrocyte membrane which circumscribed the subject matter of this chapter.

Acknowledgments

The author was supported by grants CRTY 5018 from the National Cancer Institute, U.S. Public Health Service, through 30 June, 1962 and E-277 from the American Cancer Society, Inc., from 1 July, 1962.

The author is indebted to Dr. Mehran Goulian for reviewing the manuscript.

References

Allen, D. W. (1960). *Blood* **16**, 1564.
Allen, D. W., and Jandl, J. H. (1960). *Blood* **15**, 71.
Allen, D. W., and Jandl, J. H. (1961). *J. Clin. Invest.* **40**, 454.
Allen, D. W., and Zamecnik, P. C. (1962). *Biochim. Biophys. Acta* **55**, 865.
Allen, D. W., Schroeder, W. A., and Balog, J. (1958). *J. Am. Chem. Soc.* **80**, 1628.
Allen, E. H., and Schweet, R. S. (1960). *Biochim. Biophys. Acta* **39**, 185.
Allen, E. H., and Schweet, R. S. (1962). *J. Biol. Chem.* **237**, 760.
Arnstein, H. R. V., Cox, R. A., and Hunt, J. A. (1962). *Nature* **194**, 1042.
Beaven, G. H., and White, J. C. (1954). *Nature* **173**, 389.
Bergmann, F. H., Berg, P., and Dieckmann, M. (1961). *J. Biol. Chem.* **236**, 1735.
Berlin, N. I., Waldmann, T. A., and Weissman, S. M. (1959). *Physiol. Rev.* **39**, 577.
Bessis, M. C., and Breton-Gorius, J. (1957). *J. Biophys. Biochem. Cytol.* **3**, 503.
Bessis, M. C., and Breton-Gorius, J. (1962). *Blood* **19**, 635.
Beutler, E. (1959). *Blood* **14**, 103.
Beutler, E., and Baluda, M. C. (1962). *Acta Haematol.* **27**, 321.
Bishop, J. O., and Schweet, R. S. (1961). *Biochim. Biophys. Acta* **54**, 617.
Bishop, J., Leahy, J., and Schweet, R. (1960). *Proc. Natl. Acad. Sci. U.S.* **46**, 1030.
Bishop, J., Favelukes, G., Schweet, R., and Russell, E. (1961). *Nature* **191**, 1365.
Bogorad, L., and Granick, S. (1953). *Proc. Natl. Acad. Sci. U.S.* **39**, 1176.
Borsook, H., and Dubnoff, J. W. (1940). *J. Biol. Chem.* **132**, 307.
Borsook, H., Deasy, C. L., Haagen-Smit, A. J., Keighley, G., and Lowy, P. H. (1952). *J. Biol. Chem.* **196**, 669.
Bush, J. A., and Ainger, L. E. (1955). *Pediatrics* **15**, 93.
Bush, J. A., Jensen, W. N., Athens, J. W., Ashenbrucker, H., Cartwright, G. E., and Wintrobe, M. M. (1956). *J. Exptl. Med.* **103**, 701.
Cartwright, G. E., Gubler, C. J., and Wintrobe, M. M. (1958). *In* "Conference on Hemoglobin, 2–3 May, 1957," Natl. Acad. Sci.—Natl. Res. Council, Publ. No. 557, pp. 100–110. Washington, D.C.

Chapeville, F., Lipmann, F., von Ehrenstein, G., Weisblum, B., Ray, W. J., Jr., and Benzer, S. (1962). *Proc. Natl. Acad. Sci. U.S.* **48**, 1086.

Christensen, H. N. (1960). *Advanc. Protein Chem.* **15**, 239.

Christensen, H. N., Riggs, T. R., and Ray, N. E. (1952). *J. Biol. Chem.* **194**, 41.

Cohen, E., and Elvehjem, C. A. (1934). *J. Biol. Chem.* **107**, 97.

"Conference on Hemoglobin." (1958). 2–3 May, 1957. Natl. Acad. Sci.—Natl. Res. Council, Publ. No. 557. Washington, D.C.

Cookson, G. H., and Rimington, C. (1954). *Biochem. J.* **57**, 476.

Dacie, J. V. (1960). "The Haemolytic Anaemias, Congenital and Acquired." Grune & Stratton, New York.

Dintzis, H. M. (1961). *Proc. Natl. Acad. Sci. U.S.* **47**, 247.

Dintzis, H. M., Borsook, H., and Vinograd, J. (1958). *In* "Microsomal Particles and Protein Synthesis" (R. B. Roberts, ed.), pp. 95–99. Pergamon Press, New York.

Dresel, E. I. B., and Falk, J. E. (1956). *Biochem. J.* **63**, 80.

Elvehjem, C. A. (1935). *Physiol. Rev.* **15**, 471.

Finch, C. A. (1958). *In* "Conference on Hemoglobin, 2–3 May, 1957," Natl. Acad. Sci.—Natl. Res. Council, Publ. No. 557, pp. 95–99. Washington, D.C.

Granick, S. (1951). *Physiol. Rev.* **31**, 489.

Granick, S., and Mauzerall, D. (1958). *J. Biol. Chem.* **232**, 1119.

Granick, S., and Mauzerall, D. (1961). *In* "Metabolic Pathways" (D. M. Greenberg, ed.), Vol. II, pp. 525–616. Academic Press, New York.

Greenough, W. B., III, Peters, T., Jr., and Thomas, E. D. (1962). *J. Clin. Invest.* **41**, 1116.

Harley, J. D., and Mauer, A. M. (1960). *Blood* **16**, 1722.

Harley, J. D., and Mauer, A. M. (1961). *Blood* **17**, 418.

Harrison, P. M. (1959). *J. Mol. Biol.* **1**, 69.

Harrison, P. M., and Hofmann, T. (1962). *J. Mol. Biol.* **4**, 239.

Heilmeyer, L., Keller, W., Vivell, O., Keiderling, W., Betke, K., Wöhler, F., and Schultze, H. E. (1961). *Deut. Med. Wochschr.* **86**, 1745.

Hoagland, M. B. (1960). *In* "Nucleic Acids" (E. Chargaff and J. N. Davidson, eds.), Vol. III, pp. 349–408. Academic Press, New York.

Hoagland, M. B., and Comly, L. T. (1960). *Proc. Natl. Acad. Sci. U.S.* **46**, 1554.

Hoagland, M. B., Keller, E. B., and Zamecnik, P. C. (1956). *J. Biol. Chem.* **218**, 345.

Hoagland, M. B., Zamecnik, P. C., and Stephenson, M. L. (1957). *Biochim. Biophys. Acta* **24**, 215.

Holloway, B. W., and Ripley, S. H. (1952). *J. Biol. Chem.* **196**, 695.

Huff, R. L., and Judd, O. J. (1956). *Adv. Biol. Med. Phys.* **4**, 223–237.

Jacob, F., and Monod, J. (1961). *J. Mol. Biol.* **3**, 318.

Jacob, H. S., and Jandl, J. H. (1962). *J. Clin. Invest.* **41**, 1514.

Jandl, J. H., Inman, J. K., Simmons, R. L., and Allen, D. W. (1959). *J. Clin. Invest.* **38**, 161.

Jandl, J. H., Engle, L. K., and Allen, D. W. (1960). *J. Clin. Invest.* **39**, 1818.

Kimmel, J. R., Markowitz, H., and Brown, D. M. (1959). *J. Biol. Chem.* **234**, 46.

Kruh, J., and Borsook, H. (1956). *J. Biol. Chem.* **220**, 905.

Kruh, J., Rosa, J., Dreyfus, J.-C., and Schapira, G. (1961). *Biochim. Biophys. Acta* **49**, 509.

Kunkel, H. G. (1958). *In* "Conference on Hemoglobin, 2–3 May, 1957," Natl. Acad. Sci.—Natl. Res. Council, Publ. No. 557, pp. 157–162. Washington, D.C.

Kunkel, H. G., and Wallenius, G. (1957). *Science* **122**, 288.

Lagerlöf, B., Thorell, B., and Åkerman, L. (1956). *Exptl. Cell Res.* **10**, 752.

Lajtha, L. G., and Suit, H. D. (1955). *Brit. J. Haematol.* **1**, 55.

Lamborg, M. R. (1962). *Biochim. Biophys. Acta* **55**, 719.

Lamfrom, H. (1961). *J. Mol. Biol.* **3**, 241.

Lamfrom, H., and Glowacki, E. R. (1962). *J. Mol. Biol.* **5**, 97.

Laurell, C. B. (1960). *In* "The Plasma Proteins" (F. W. Putnam, ed.), Vol. 1, pp. 349–378. Academic Press, New York.

Lemberg, R., and Legge, J. W. (1949). "Hematin Compounds and Bile Pigments." Wiley (Interscience), New York.

Lipmann, F. (1941). *Advanc. Enzymol.* **1**, 99.

Littlefield, J. W., Keller, E. B., Gross, J., and Zamecnik, P. C. (1955). *J. Biol. Chem.* **217**, **111**.

London, I. M. (1961). *Harvey Lectures, Ser.* **56** (1960–1961), 151.

Margoliash, E. (1961). *Ann. Rev. Biochem.* **30**, 549.

Markowitz, H., Cartwright, G. E., and Wintrobe, M. M. (1959). *J. Biol. Chem.* **234**, 40.

Marston, H. R. (1952). *Physiol Rev.* **32**, 66.

Matthaei, J. H., Jones, O. W., Martin, R. G., and Nirenberg, M. W. (1962). *Proc. Natl. Acad. Sci. U.S.* **48**, 666.

Mauzerall, D., and Granick, S. (1958). *J. Biol. Chem.* **232**, 1141.

Mazur, A., Carleton, A., and Carlsen, A. (1962). *Federation Proc.* **21**, 70.

Mills, G. C., and Randall, H. P. (1958). *J. Biol. Chem.* **232**, 589.

Moore, C. V. (1961). *Harvey Lectures, Ser.* **55** (1959–1960), 67.

Morell, H., Savoie, J. C., and London, I. M. (1958). *J. Biol. Chem.* **233**, 923.

Morris, A. J., and Schweet, R. S. (1961). *Biochim. Biophys. Acta* **47**, 415.

Morris, A., Favelukes, S., Arlinghaus, R., and Schweet, R. (1962). *Biochem. Biophys. Res. Commun.* **7**, 326.

Morrison, M., and Cook, J. L. (1955). *Science* **122**, 920.

Nathan, D. G., Piomelli, G., and Gardner, F. H. (1961). *J. Clin. Invest.* **40**, 940.

Nathans, D., and Lipmann, F. (1961). *Proc. Natl. Acad. Sci. U.S.* **47**, 497.

Nathans, D., von Ehrenstein, G., Monro, R., and Lipmann, F. (1962). *Federation Proc.* **21**, 127.

Neilands, J. B. (1957). *Bacteriol. Rev.* **21**, 101.

Neuberger, A. (1961). *Biochem. J.* **78**, 1.

Nirenberg, M. W., and Matthaei, J. H. (1961). *Proc. Natl. Acad. Sci. U.S.* **47**, 1588.

Noyes, W. D., Bothwell, T. H., and Finch, C. A. (1960). *Brit. J. Haematol.* **6**, 43.

Perutz, M. F. (1962). *Nature* **194**, 914.

Perutz, M. F., Rossmann, M. G., Cullis, A. F., Muirhead, H., Will, G., and North, A. C. T. (1960). *Nature* **185**, 416.

Pollycove, M., and Maqsood, M. (1962). *Nature* **194**, 152.

Pollycove, M., and Mortimer, R. (1961). *J. Clin. Invest.* **40**, 753.

Prins, H. K., and Huisman, T. H. J. (1956). *Nature* **177**, 840.

Rabinovitz, M., and Olson, M. E. (1956). *Exptl. Cell Res.* **10**, 747.

Rabinovitz, M., and Olson, M. E. (1958). *Nature* **181**, 1665.

Ranney, H. M., and Kono, P. (1959). *J. Clin. Invest.* **38**, 508.

Riggs, A. F. (1952). *J. Gen. Physiol.* **36**, 1.

Riggs, T. R., Christensen, H. N., and Palatine, I. M. (1952). *J. Biol. Chem.* **194**, 53.

Rimington, C. (1957). *Ann. Rev. Biochem.* **26**, 561.

Rothberg, H., Corallo, L. A., and Crosby, W. H. (1959). *Blood* **14**, 1180.

Schapira, G., Dreyfus, J.-C., and Kruh, J. (1958). *In* "Conference on Hemoglobin, 2–3 May, 1957," Natl. Acad. Sci.—Natl. Res. Council, Publ. No. 557, pp. 201–211. Washington, D.C.

Scheinberg, I. H. (1961). *Federation Proc.* **20**, 179.

Schmid, R. (1960). *In* "The Metabolic Basis of Inherited Disease," (J B. Stanbury, J. B. Wyngaarden, and D. S. Fredrickson, eds.) pp. 226–270. McGraw-Hill, New York.

Schultze, M. O. (1940). *Physiol. Rev.* **20**, 37.
Schultze, M. O. (1941). *J. Biol. Chem.* **138**, 219.
Schwartz, H. C., Goudsmit, R., Hill, R. L., Cartwright, G. E., and Wintrobe, M. M. (1961). *J. Clin. Invest.* **40**, 188.
Schweet, R., Lamfrom, H., and Allen, E. (1958). *Proc. Natl. Acad. Sci. U.S.* **44**, 1029.
Schweet, R., Bishop, J., and Morris, A. (1961). *Lab. Invest.* **10**, 992.
Schweiger, H. G. (1962). *Intern. Rev. Cytol.* **13**, 135.
Selwyn, J. G. (1955). *Brit. J. Haematol.* **1**, 173.
Shemin, D. (1958). *In* "Conference on Hemoglobin, 2–3 May, 1957," Natl. Acad. Sci.—Natl. Res. Council, Publ. No. 557, pp. 66–73. Washington, D.C.
Shemin, D., and Wittenberg, J. (1951). *J. Biol. Chem.* **192**, 315.
Simpson, M. V. (1962). *Ann. Rev. Biochem.* **31**, 333.
Spencer, M., Fuller, W., Wilkins, M. H. F., and Brown, G. L. (1962). *Nature* **194**, 1014.
Surgenor, D. M., Koechlin, B. A., and Strong, L. E. (1949). *J. Clin. Invest.* **28**, 73.
Vallee, B. L. (1960). *In* "The Enzymes" (P. D. Boyer, H. Lardy, and K. Myrbäck, eds.), 2nd ed. Vol. 3, pp. 225–276. Academic Press, New York.
Vallee, B. L., Lewis, H. D., Altschule, M. D., and Gibson, J. G., II. (1949). *Blood* **4**, 467.
Vogel, W., Richert, D. A., Pixley, B. Q., and Schulman, M. P. (1960). *J. Biol. Chem.* **235**, 1769.
von Ehrenstein, G., and Lipmann, F. (1961). *Proc. Natl. Acad. Sci. U.S.* **47**, 941.
Wainio, W. W., Vander Wende, C., and Shimp, N. F. (1959). *J. Biol. Chem.* **234**, 2433.
Waller, H. D., Schlegel, B., Müller, A. A., and Löhr, G. W. (1959). *Klin. Wochschr.* **37**, 898.
Walsh, R. J., Thomas, E. D., Chow, S. K., Fluharty, R. G., and Finch, C. A. (1949). *Science* **110**, 396.
Warner, J. R., Knopf, P. M., and Rich, A. (1963). *Proc. Natl. Acad. Sci. U.S.* **49**, 122.
Watson, C. J. (1957). *Ann. Internal Med.* **47**, 611.
Weisberger, A. S. (1962). *Proc. Natl. Acad. Sci. U.S.* **48**, 68.
Westall, R. G. (1952). *Nature* **170**, 614.
Wintrobe, M. M. (1961). "Clinical Hematology," 5th ed. Lea & Febiger, Philadelphia, Pennsylvania.
Yarmolinsky, M. B., and de la Haba, G. L. (1959). *Proc. Natl. Acad. Sci. U.S.* **45**, 1721.
Zachau, H. G., Acs, G., and Lipmann, F. (1958). *Proc. Natl. Acad. Sci. U.S.* **44**, 885.
Zamecnik, P. C. (1960). *Harvey Lectures, Ser.* **54** (1958–1959), 256.

CHAPTER 9

Transport of Oxygen and Carbon Dioxide

Douglas M. Surgenor

The linked reciprocating transport of the respiratory gases is without doubt the *raison d'être* of the erythrocyte. This is the function for which the adult cell was formed and fashioned. From the vantage point of teleological retrospect we can see that many, if not all, of the features of the cell contribute to this property—indeed, there is an economy of utilization of parts, and everywhere evidence of the oft observed parsimony of nature. The size and shape of the adult cell are important to its suspension stability, and therefore to its accessibility to all parts of the vascular network; and they provide desirable ratios of surface area to volume, so important to gaseous transfer. The nucleus and much of the other biochemical machinery of the parent erythroblast cell have been cast off in the adult cell to make room, as it were, for more hemoglobin. Discarded also in this process have been the whole complement of protein synthesizing elements, and with them most of the usual energy-producing mechanisms needed for synthesis. Only the barest minimum of enzymatic complement is retained in the adult cell, apparently for the prime purpose of maintaining the shape and integrity of the cell. In few other cases have we such eloquent evidence of the bringing together of chemical parts into a cellular structure whose function is so clear.

Central in any consideration of the respiratory function of the erythrocyte is hemoglobin. Here our understanding has been greatly aided by the many properties of hemoglobin which make it unique among all the proteins. These include the ease of handling, exemplified by its small size; its solubility and crystallizability; the ease of analytical access, exemplified by the iron content, the color, and the simple stoichiometry of its reactivity. Moreover, the ease of access to structural information, culminating in the recent work on its tertiary structure, was greatly facilitated by the twofold symmetry and the two pairs of identical peptide chains which make up the chemical backbone of hemoglobin (Perutz *et al.*, 1960). Even here, the mounting evidence that the α and β chains are related underlines what a choice protein hemoglobin is (Braunitzer *et al.*, 1961). Hemoglobin and its simpler congener, myoglobin, are leading the way into new knowledge of protein structure and function.

Nor is it enough to consider hemoglobin alone; it is necessary to consider hemoglobin within the intraerythrocytic environment of pH, ionic strength, dielectric strength, protein concentration, and temperature. For we begin to know that the environment can have a profound effect on how a protein behaves, whether this behavior be the activity of an enzyme, the interaction of a protein with a metallic cation, or the solubility of a protein in an aqueous medium.

I. Oxygen Transport

W. B. Cannon once remarked (1932) about the close dependence of the cells of the body upon oxygen, a dependence more absolute than for any other substance in the outside world. In the long evolutionary span of transition from an infinite and constant aqueous environment—the sea—to a small, circulating extracellular fluid, the composition of which is under steady-state control through a host of complex physiological and biochemical mechanisms, the red cell and hemoglobin are prime components. The importance of the oxygen-binding function is often illustrated by comparing the oxygen-carrying power of blood with that of an oxygen-saturated salt solution. According to one such calculation of Barcroft, 6 liters of blood can carry the volume of oxygen normally found dissolved in 350 liters of a salt solution.

A. Hemoglobin Interactions

Almost a hundred years ago, in 1865, Hoppe-Seyler published his classic work on hemoglobins; this included methods for isolation and estimation of hemoglobin, as well as accurate observations of the oxygen interaction and the iron content. By the turn of the century, Bohr had a remarkably accurate understanding of the oxygen equilibrium. In 1904 with Hasselbalch and Krogh, he published a paper which described not only the oxygen interaction, but also the effect of carbon dioxide upon the oxygen interaction. The work is illustrated by the data in Fig. 1, taken directly from the 1904 paper. The effect of carbon dioxide on oxygen binding, particularly at low oxygen pressures, has since become known as the Bohr effect.

These early data also clearly reveal a second fundamental property of hemoglobin. The oxygen saturation curve has a characteristic sigmoid shape, reflecting the existence of inter-heme interactions within the hemoglobin molecule. The net effect of these heme-heme interactions is to alter the affinity of the hemes reacting with successive oxygens. The Bohr effect and heme-heme interactions are, as we shall see, cardinal properties of hemoglobin. Their understanding has been the object of much search; even now with the flood

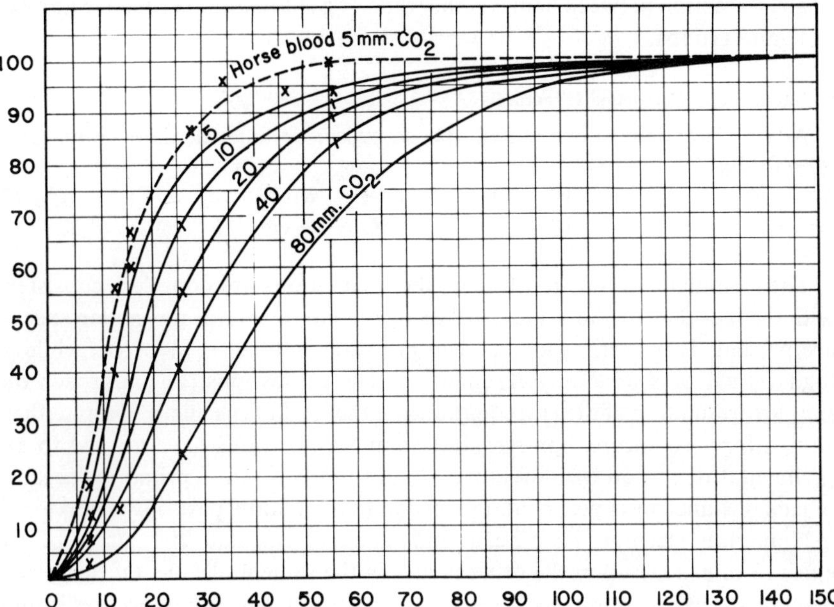

FIG. 1. Oxygen saturation curve of whole blood. Ordinate: per cent saturation. Abscissa: pO_2 in mm. pressure. (From Bohr *et al.*, 1904.)

of new molecular knowledge of hemoglobin, we do not understand these phenomena completely.

1. Hill Equation

The problem of understanding the oxygen saturation curve of hemoglobin has occupied a great deal of attention. In 1910, before the molecular weight of iron content of hemoglobin was known, A. V. Hill, working on the equation:

$$\text{Hb} + n\text{O}_2 \rightleftarrows \text{Hb}(\text{O}_2)n \tag{1}$$

formulated the physicochemical expression now known, in one form or other, as the *Hill equation*:

$$y = \frac{100Kp^n}{1 + Kp^n} \tag{2}$$

where y is the percent saturation with oxygen, K the equilibrium constant, and p the partial pressure. This equation gives a reasonably good fit with experimental data over the middle range of the curve when $n = 2.5–2.8$. However, the meaning of the Hill equation is altered by the knowledge of the molecular weight of hemoglobin and the presence of four hemes per molecule. Under these circumstances n should equal unity (there is one oxygen bound per heme group), and deviation from unity of the experimental values of n is indicative of an interaction between hemes rather than of a change in the effective number of ligand groups.

Intermediate Compound Hypothesis

Adair (1925) first formulated the stepwise, or intermediate compound, hypothesis.

$$Hb + O_2 \rightleftarrows HbO_2 \quad K_1 \tag{3}$$

$$HbO_2 + O_2 \rightleftarrows Hb(O_2)_2 \quad K_2 \text{ etc.} \tag{4}$$

The formulations that result from these equations are complex, consistent with the fact that in the middle range of the curve several molecular species are present. However, at low oxygen pressures only K_1 is involved, while at high oxygen pressures only K_4 enters in. The expressions thus approach the simple formulation of the Hill equation at either end of the curve. Despite their straightforward nature, however, the Adair formulations have not led to experimental definition of individual equilibrium constants, primarily because of lack of sufficient experimental precision in the middle part of the curve.

Numerous attempts have been made since to elucidate the nature of the effect of one heme upon the other hemes in the same molecule. Of these, two deserve special mention because of the important place they occupy in our knowledge of hemoglobin. These are contained in the papers of Pauling (1935) and of Wyman (1948).

3. Heme-Heme Interactions

Pauling (1935) considered the present state of knowledge of hemoglobin, and in characteristic fashion offered some startlingly accurate speculations about the interaction with oxygen. These are remarkable in the way they have survived, even into the era of detailed knowledge of the tertiary structure of hemoglobin. Based upon simple postulates that the four hemes are identical, that each heme is "connected" with other hemes, and that the interactions for connected pairs are equivalent, Pauling concluded with a very clear picture, now classical in its simplicity. According to this picture, the four hemes were conceived as being located at the corners of a square, so that each heme is "connected" with two others, and gives rise to an interaction energy between pairs of hemes.

In the light of recent developments on hemoglobin structure, it is especially noteworthy that Pauling considered the possibility that the four heme groups are located at the corners of a tetrahedron. This gave good agreement between predicted and actual oxygen saturation curves, but it was rejected primarily because Pauling thought the hemes would be separated by too great a distance to give the required interaction energy. These calculations were based upon a spherical model with the further assumption that the hemes were located on the surface. In this same treatment, Pauling accounted for the Bohr effect on the basis of an interaction between the oxygen sites and some unknown acid group associated with each heme.

Wyman's review, written in 1948, had the advantage of time and of considerably more experimental data upon which to test new hypotheses. Wyman's own titration data (Wyman, 1939a) had suggested that the heme was linked to the globin by a histidine group. It had also been demonstrated that the heat of reaction was the same for each step in the oxygenation process (Wyman, 1939b). This led to the conclusion that the four hemes were indeed linked in identical fashion, confirming Pauling's assumption on this point. Since it was already known that the four hemes were themselves identical, several simplifying assumptions could be made. Studies of the effect of pH on oxygen saturation revealed that the curves were all superimposable by appropriate displacement of the logarithmic scale of pressure, i.e. by movement of the curves horizontally. This suggested that at any pH, successive oxygens produced equal displacement of protons, and from this it could be concluded that all four sites of oxygen interaction were equivalent.

In 1948 there was still some question concerning the symmetry of the oxygen dissociation curve. This became an important point in any theoretical consideration. At the time, Wyman concluded that the curve was not symmetrical, a conclusion which weighed against the Pauling hypothesis. Later however, Allen *et al.* (1950) restudied the problem and produced very careful data with freshly prepared hemoglobin which showed without further question that the curve is indeed symmetrical. The conclusion was thus inescapable that the four oxygen-binding centers were equivalent. Furthermore, the data once again suggested an equivalence in spatial relationships.[1]

With regard to the nature of the heme-heme interaction, Wyman brought in new data on the oxygen interaction of hemoglobin dissolved in strong urea solution, in which the hemoglobin is dissociated into half-molecules. Here again the curves are symmetrical and, of even greater interest, the value of n in the Hill equation lies very close to the maximum value of 2, indicative of a high interaction as in the parent undissociated hemoglobin. From this kind of data Wyman concluded that the four hemes must occur in two identical pairs,

[1] It is noteworthy that recrystallized hemoglobin, several days in preparation, gave an asymmetric oxygen curve displaced in the direction of reduced affinity for oxygen (higher $p_{1/2}$).

with strong interaction between members of the same pair and weaker interactions between pairs. He suggested replacing the square model of Pauling with a rectangular model having two sets of interactions. Within each half-molecule the heme-heme interactions are large, while the interactions between hemes in different half-molecules are small.

In every case where the hemes are separated, as by dissociation in urea solution, the affinity for oxygen is *increased.* This and other data lead to the conclusion that the heme-heme interactions, whatever their nature, are stronger when neither heme has an oxygen. The interaction with oxygen is a "facilitating" interaction, i.e. oxygenation of the first heme facilitates interaction of the second, third, and fourth oxygens (Manwell, 1960). In physiological terms the effect is that the second oxygen goes on with a higher affinity than the first, the third higher than the second, and so on. In these terms, n in the Hill equation is a measure of the degree of interaction between hemes; for no interaction, $n = 1$, while for maximum interaction $n = 4$. We shall return to the molecular basis of the Bohr effect and the heme-heme interactions in a later section.

II. Carbon Dioxide Transport

A. Chemical Species Involved

The transport of carbon dioxide differs from oxygen transport in that a complex series of reactions are substituted for the relatively straightforward reactions of oxygen and hemoglobin. As is true of oxygen, very little carbon dioxide is carried in simple solution. The concentration of dissolved carbon dioxide depends upon its partial pressure according to Henry's law:

$$(CO_2) = K_h \cdot pCO_2 \tag{5}$$

Carbon dioxide is hydrated in solution by a reaction whose velocity is relatively slow in physiological terms. The hydration product, carbonic acid, is a weak acid which can dissociate:

$$H_2O + CO_2 \rightleftarrows H_2CO_3 \rightleftarrows H^+ + HCO_3^- \tag{6}$$

Bicarbonate can only be formed by the above reaction at the cost of simultaneously liberating a proton. Because of this, the amount of bicarbonate arising in the blood from simple dissociation is extremely small.

Bicarbonate is readily formed, however, when carbonic acid reacts with a Brönsted base, as:

$$H_2CO_3 + A^- \rightleftarrows HCO_3^- + HA \tag{7}$$

For this reaction to proceed in the direction of bicarbonate formation, K_{HA} should be small with respect to the equilibrium constant for Eq. (6). Because it does proceed, this reaction, by its reversible operation, provides the basis of a very efficient transport mechanism for carbon dioxide. The efficiency of this mechanism depends mainly upon two features of hemoglobin. These are, first, its great buffer capacity in the physiological range; second, the change in its acidity which accompanies oxygenation and deoxygenation.

B. Buffering by Hemoglobin

The physiological buffer capacity of hemoglobin derives from functional groups which can associate or dissociate protons at neutral pH.[2] These are principally the imidazolyl side chains of histidyl residues, of which there are 35 per mole of human hemoglobin containing 574 total residues. The plasma proteins also contain histidyl groups, but because of the molar preponderance of hemoglobin over the plasma proteins, hemoglobin accounts for over 80% of the total Brönsted basic groups in blood which are capable of accepting protons from carbonic acid in the physiological pH range. Bicarbonate formation by this process:

$$H_2CO_3 + Hb \rightleftharpoons HCO_3^- + HHb^+ \tag{8}$$

is accompanied by a pH change, albeit a small one, since the ratio Hb/HHb is reduced during bicarbonate formation. The amount of bicarbonate formed by this reaction in whole blood under physiological conditions must be very small, since the pH shift within the erythrocyte during the respiratory cycle is of the order of only 0.01 pH unit.

C. Bohr Effect

When an oxygen molecule approaches the heme group and is bound in the coordination sphere of the iron, the resulting effect on the tertiary structure of the protein in the vicinity of the heme is to increase the acid strength of an imidazolyl group (*vide infra*). This group shifts in pK from 7.93 in reduced horse hemoglobin to 6.68 in oxyhemoglobin (Wyman, 1948), but although this reflects a 20-fold increase in acid strength, it will be noted that it does not mean a stoichiometric reaction. Only about 0.7 equivalent of protons is dissociated for each mole of oxygen bound at physiological pH.

[2] Steinhardt (1962) has pointed out that the basic function of about twenty-two histidyl groups appears to be obscured in native horse hemoglobin derivatives. Nevertheless, hemoglobin has a reasonably good buffer capacity at physiological reaction, being approximately 2.6 meq./mmole hemoglobin per pH unit.

This situation can be illustrated with the following equations:

$$\begin{array}{cccccc} & HHb + O_2 & \rightleftarrows & HHbO_2 & \\ pK\,7.93 & \upharpoonleft\downharpoonright & & \upharpoonleft\downharpoonright & pK\,6.68 \\ & Hb + O_2 & \rightleftarrows & HbO_2 & \\ & + & & + & \\ & H^+ & & H^+ & \end{array} \tag{9}$$

in which the H in HHb or $HHbO_2$ represents that proton of the dissociable group in hemoglobin whose strength is altered by oxygenation. In this scheme dissociation is represented by the vertical reactions, oxygenation by the horizontal reactions. At physiological pH, the tendency is to oscillate on the diagonal according to the following nonstoichiometric equation:

$$HHb + O_2 \rightleftarrows H^+ + HbO_2 \tag{10}$$

This is precisely in phase with the needs for carbon dioxide transport, in that the proton produced by oxygenation can react with an equivalent amount of bicarbonate, thus liberating carbon dioxide:

$$\begin{array}{l} HHb + O_2 \rightleftarrows H^+ + HbO_2 \\ \qquad\qquad\quad + \\ \qquad\qquad\quad HCO_3^- \\ \qquad\qquad\quad \upharpoonleft\downharpoonright \\ \qquad\qquad\quad H_2CO_3 \\ \qquad\qquad\quad \upharpoonleft\downharpoonright \\ \qquad\qquad\quad CO_2 + H_2O \end{array} \tag{11}$$

The driving force for this reaction can be considered to be the high partial pressure of oxygen in the alveoli of the lungs. Similarly, in the peripheral tissues where the pO_2 is low and the pCO_2 is high, the reactions are reversed, liberating oxygen to the tissues and causing the conversion of carbon dioxide to bicarbonate. Unlike the previous mechanism—buffering by hemoglobin—in which a pH change accompanied the conversion of carbon dioxide to bicarbonate during transport, no pH change accompanies the oxygen-linked transport mechanism. Furthermore, the proton which tends to be bound by hemoglobin when deoxygenation occurs, reduces the net negative charge of hemoglobin, in effect "making room" for the bicarbonate ion within the erythrocyte without a net shift of cation. The proportion of the total carbon dioxide transport accounted for by this mechanism depends upon the hemoglobin concentration, as well as upon the magnitude of the arterial-venous difference in oxygen saturation and in carbon dioxide pressure. Usually about 60–70% of the net carbon dioxide transport is accounted for by this mechanism.

D. Carbamino Compounds

The remarkable observations of Christian Bohr at the turn of the century (1905) led him to suggest that there was a direct combination between carbon dioxide and hemoglobin. Indeed, he presumed that the site of combination was the same as the oxygen-combining site. Out of this came two important discoveries: the existence of carbamino compounds of hemoglobin and of the enzyme carbonic anhydrase (Meldrum and Roughton, 1933a, b). Carbonic anhydrase catalyzes the reversible hydration of carbon dioxide. It is a zinc-containing enzyme, localized in the erythrocyte—never in the plasma. It is relatively stable and is inhibited by certain compounds including carbon monoxide, cyanic acid, and Diamox (acetazolamide). Roughton has estimated that the carbonic anhydrase present in normal red cells can catalyze a rate of hydration of carbon dioxide approximately 5000-fold that which obtains in the absence of the enzyme. These features impart to the red cell a key role in the hydration and dehydration of the respiratory carbon dioxide; they have deep-seated implications for the dynamic aspects of respiration.

From the early experiments of Henriques (1928) there had long been the suggestion that part of the carbon dioxide within the erythrocyte is complexed with hemoglobin. Consistent with this, Henriques found that a part (but not all) of the carbon dioxide goes off from blood at low pressures much more rapidly than from aqueous solution of bicarbonate and carbon dioxide. Later the elegant gasometric techniques for measuring carbon dioxide revealed that the carbon dioxide content of the erythrocyte is higher than would be predicted from the Donnan ratio for anions. In other words, a part of the carbon dioxide of the red cell is difficult to account for in terms of the bicarbonate system.

This situation was greatly clarified by the classic work of Meldrum and Roughton (1933b) on the state of carbon dioxide in the blood. They showed that hemoglobin is able to form true carbamino compounds, analogous to the reactions of ammonia and amines with carbon dioxide:

$$RNH_2 + CO_2 \rightleftharpoons RNHCOOH \rightleftharpoons RNHCOO^- + H^+ \qquad (12)$$

Carbamic acids are fairly strong acids with pK's of 6 or below; thus a proton is formed for each carbamate derivative formed at neutral pH. Roughton has shown that at constant pCO_2 the extent of carbamate formation is strongly dependent upon pH, formation being favored at alkaline reaction. In blood, an increase in pCO_2 results in a corresponding decrease in pH so that carbamate formation becomes almost independent of pCO_2 (Roughton, 1944). Carbamino compounds have a high heat of formation and are thus most stable at low temperatures. For this reason it has been suggested that carbamates may be much more important in the physiology of poikilothermic animals (Meldrum and Roughton, 1933b).

The relative independence of carbamino formation of the pCO_2 might seem to exclude a role for carbamino compounds in the net transport of carbon dioxide. This would be so were it not for the observation, first reported by Meldrum and Roughton (1933b), that hemoglobin binds more carbon dioxide as carbamino compound than does oxyhemoglobin. Ferguson (1936) has concluded that as much as 29% of the expired carbon dioxide at an RQ (respiratory quotient) of 0.8 is transported by the oscillation in carbamino carbon dioxide between hemoglobin and oxyhemoglobin.

What are the groups in hemoglobin that might participate in carbamino formation? Only the N-terminal amino groups—four valine amino groups

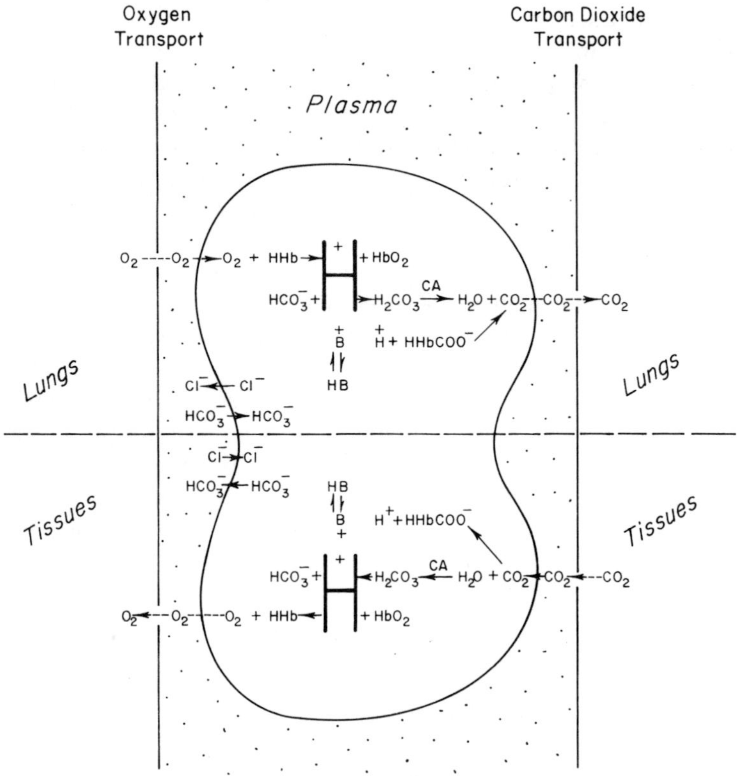

FIG. 2. Summary of reactions involved in carbon dioxide transport. CA, carbonic anhydrase; B, buffer (primarily hemoglobin).

per mole—appear to fit the requirements for an uncharged amino group outlined above. Assuming for the moment a reasonable *pK* of 7.4, then half of these groups would be free to form carbamino derivatives with carbon dioxide. Since blood contains on the order of 2 mmoles of hemoglobin per liter, 4 mmoles of carbon dioxide could be combined in this way. This is already 3–4 times the amount of carbon dioxide normally ascribed to the carbamino compartment.

If carbamino compound formation is primarily dependent upon the state of oxygenation of hemoglobin, as Meldrum and Roughton (1933b) contend, then the question is raised about the relationship of this phenomenon to the Bohr effect. This led Roughton (1944) to postulate that it is the N-terminal groups of valine which undergo the shift in *pK* from 7.93 to 6.68 on oxygenation, rather than the imidazole groups originally postulated by Wyman. At the present time this possibility, interesting though it may be, seems very unlikely in view of new evidence discussed below.

The reactions of oxygen and carbon dioxide transport are summarized schematically in Fig. 2. By this means the transport of carbon dioxide by buffering is distinguished from the oxygen-linked transport of carbon dioxide, both, of course, involving bicarbonate formation. The diagram also illustrates an important contrast between carbon dioxide and oxygen transport. The latter takes place almost exclusively *within* the erythrocyte. Similarly, the important steps of hydration of carbon dioxide and bicarbonate formation also occur almost exclusively within the erythrocyte, *but in contrast to oxygen transport*, the bicarbonate once formed has access to the total extracellular fluid space of the body (the "chloride shift"). For these and other reasons, impaired red cell transport function, from whatever cause, is usually felt more acutely in terms of oxygen transport functions than of carbon dioxide. For treatment of the acid-base aspects of carbon dioxide transport, the reader is referred to Davenport (1950) or to a physiology textbook.

III. Molecular Aspects of Hemoglobin Roles

It is tantalizing to contemplate how rapidly knowledge is accruing concerning the hemoglobin molecule, yet how much of the basic secret remains to be unlocked. We have the structure of horse hemoglobin at a resolution of 5.5 Å from the work of Perutz and his collaborators in Cambridge (1960). We have the amino acid sequences of the α and β chains of human hemoglobin from the chemical studies of the Braunitzer group in Munich (1961). In addition, important new knowledge is coming from the study of the genetic variants of hemoglobin as well as from the study of the hemoglobins of lower animals. The large body of classic knowledge about oxygen and carbon dioxide transport provides a functional framework into which all of the newer facts must be fitted. But so far the gulf remains, and we can only attempt to see where the bridges are going to be built—very little more than that.

A. Oxygen-Linked Acid Groups

We have already referred to the four dissociable groups in hemoglobin—one per heme—whose acid strength is altered from *pK* 7.93 to *pK* 6.68 on oxygenation (Wyman, 1948). A great deal of interest has focused on the nature of these groups. From a study of the heats of ionization Wyman identified the groups as being, in all likelihood, imidazole groups of histidine (1939a). Prior to this there had been considerable discussion about the possible linkage of the heme groups to globin and, among other suggestions, Conant (1933) had considered an iron-imidazole bond. It was logical, therefore, for Wyman to suggest that the oxygen-linked imidazole groups were also the groups through which the heme-globin linkage was achieved. Coryell and Pauling (1940) promptly suggested a number of possible resonating structures for such a constellation of groups. In this view, which is still current in some textbooks, the approach of the oxygen molecule so alters the electronic configuration about the iron atom as to produce the observed increased acidity of the histidyl groups. Later, however, Wyman and Allen (1951) abandoned the latter view, having concluded that the oxygen-linked changes in acidity were caused by changes in the tertiary structure of the protein. They also pointed out the incompatibility of the earlier view with species variations of the Bohr effect and indeed with the absence of a Bohr effect in myoglobin.

It should be noted here that the postulated linkage of the heme via imidazole was not impugned by these later developments; it would appear that this basic feature of the heme-globin linkage has been amply corroborated by modern physical and chemical investigations (Perutz *et al.*, 1960; Goldstein *et al.*, 1961; Keilin, 1960).

The concept that the oxygen-linked groups are imidazoles has been challenged, first, as we have seen, by Roughton (1944) who suggested amino groups instead and, second, by Riggs (1959) who found that "the magnitude of the Bohr effect appears to be directly proportional to the number of sulfhydryl groups" and concluded, therefore, that sulfhydryl—not imidazole—groups were involved. Neither of these challenges has been confirmed, but the latter, in particular, served to focus intense scrutiny upon the sulfhydryl groups of hemoglobin and has led to the considerable further illumination of the molecular basis of the Bohr effect.

Benesch and Benesch (1961), through their beautiful chemical studies on the action of the sulfhydryl-blocking reagent, *N*-ethyl maleimide, on hemoglobin, have brought the imidazole hypothesis back into the forefront, reaffirmed and strengthened. This work depended first upon the understanding of the primary and secondary reactions of *N*-ethyl maleimide and simple sulfhydryl com-

$$\mathrm{RSH} + \begin{array}{l} \mathrm{CH{-}C({=}O)} \\ \| \qquad\quad \searrow \mathrm{N{-}Et} \\ \mathrm{CH{-}C({=}O)} \nearrow \end{array} \longrightarrow \begin{array}{l} \mathrm{R{-}S{-}CH{-}C({=}O)} \\ \qquad\quad | \qquad\quad \searrow \mathrm{N{-}Et} \\ \qquad \mathrm{CH_2{-}C({=}O)} \nearrow \end{array} \qquad (13)$$

N-ethyl maleimide — substituted *N*-ethyl succinimide

pounds. The primary reaction involves addition across the double bond, Eq. (13). The product, a succinimide, is unstable, tending to hydrolyze to yield an *N*-ethyl succinic acid derivative, Eq. (14). This latter reaction, the opening of the succinimide ring, happens to be catalyzed by the undissociated form of imidazole, as has been amply demonstrated by studies in simple model systems.

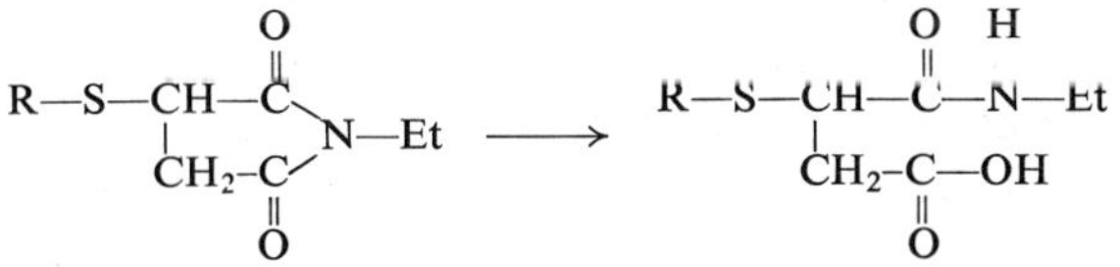

$$\mathrm{R{-}S{-}\underset{\displaystyle CH_2{-}\overset{\displaystyle O}{\overset{\|}{C}}\diagup}{CH}{-}\overset{\displaystyle O}{\overset{\|}{C}}\diagdown N{-}Et} \longrightarrow \mathrm{R{-}S{-}\underset{\displaystyle CH_2{-}\underset{\displaystyle O}{\underset{\|}{C}}{-}OH}{CH}{-}\overset{\displaystyle O}{\overset{\|}{C}}{-}\overset{\displaystyle H}{N}{-}Et} \qquad (14)$$

Normal adult hemoglobin has two reactive ("free") sulfhydryl groups. Benesch and Benesch showed that the simple addition reaction of *N*-ethyl maleimide and hemoglobin, analogous to Eq. (13), did not alter the Bohr

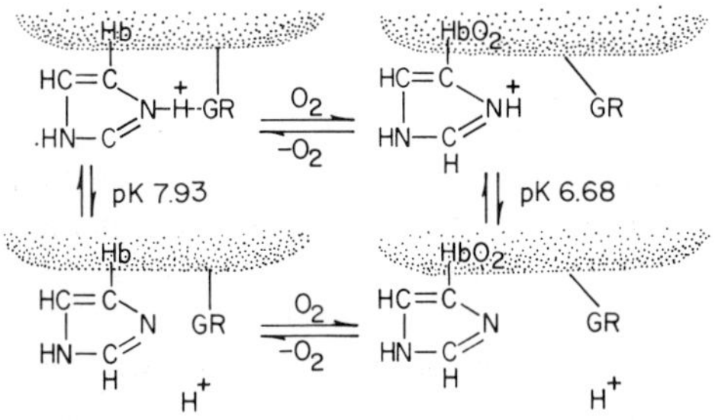

FIG. 3. Schematic representation of mechanism involved in Bohr effect. Unknown group G is attached through unknown region R to globin (After Benesch and Benesch, 1961.)

effect. Next they found that there was a secondary reaction of the addition product, whose rate without added catalyst was directly dependent upon the degree of oxygenation of the hemoglobin. When this secondary reaction occurred, the Bohr effect was inhibited. The authors concluded that the secondary reaction involved the dissociated form of the oxygen-linked groups. They attributed it to a ring opening, analogous to Eq. (14), catalyzed *intramolecularly* by an imidazole group located so close to the reactive sulfhydryl group in the hemoglobin molecule that its intramolecular catalytic potential could be realized. This work at once invalidated the suggestion that the oxygen-linked group was a sulfhydryl group and simultaneously added a significant block of support to the imidazole theory. A decrease in solubility accompanies the secondary reaction with *N*-ethyl maleimide; this tends to support the involvement of the oxygen-linked groups, because oxygenation of almost every species of hemoglobin is accompanied by a solubility change. The scheme in Fig. 3 is an attempt to show how such configurational change between hemoglobin and oxyhemoglobin could lead to the shift in acid strength of an imidazole nitrogen, in accord with the suggestions of Wyman and Allen (1951) and of Benesch and Benesch (1961). The nature of the group G which participates in the postulated hydrogen bond is unknown, but Benesch and Benesch have suggested it could be either a carboxyl ion or another imidazole group. Presumably this question will be soon answered as additional chemical and physical pressure can now be applied to this problem.

It is important to call attention to the fact that the notion of any stoichiometry, i.e. one proton dissociated per oxygen molecule bound, in connection with the Bohr effect, has long since been abandoned. Riggs has repeatedly drawn attention to a relationship between the size of a mammal and the Bohr effect of its hemoglobin; the smaller the mammal, the larger the sensitivity of its hemoglobin to oxygen-linked pH changes (Riggs, 1961). This concept is completely compatible with the view that a configurational change underlies the Bohr effect.

B. Heme-Heme Interactions

Some selected data from hemoglobin and other heme proteins are tabulated in Table I. Viewed in terms of the Bohr effect and heme-heme interactions,

TABLE I

SOME PERTINENT PROPERTIES OF CERTAIN HEME PROTEINS

Property	Myoglobin	Hemoglobin			
		A	H	Bullfrog tadpole[a]	Lamprey[b]
Number of chains	1	4	4	(4)	(1)
Peptide designations	Mb	$\alpha_2^A \beta_2^A$	β_4^A		
SH groups/mole					
Total	0	6	8		
Free	0	2	8		
Bohr effect	−	+	−	−	+
Heme-heme interactions	−	+	−	+	−

[a] Molecular weight = 68,000 (Riggs, 1951).
[b] Molecular weight = 17,000 (Wald and Riggs, 1951).

these and many other available data make it abundantly clear that we are dealing with a broad spectrum of combinations and permutations. Human hemoglobin H is particularly interesting in this regard. Unlike normal adult hemoglobin, it contains four β chains. Benesch and co-workers (1961) have found that hemoglobin H lacks both the Bohr effect and also heme-heme interactions, while it has two reactive sulfhydryl groups for each β chain, or eight per molecule. Yet the oxygen affinity of hemoglobin H is high, being approximately 10 times normal. The lack of Bohr effect in such a protein rules out for good any need to consider further a change in electronic configuration of the iron as being involved.

Of even greater interest, however, is the necessity to conclude that interactions between α and β chains in normal hemoglobin contribute to the Bohr effect, i.e. produce the configurational alterations in the four regions of the molecule that result in the acidity change. A similar explanation must be sought for the basis of the heme-heme interactions, present in adult hemoglobin and absent in H. Moreover, we must presume that the two phenomena—the Bohr effect and heme-heme interactions—are distinct and separate. This is suggested by the contrast between tadpole and lamprey hemoglobin shown in Table I, as well as by other evidence. Thus, deep-seated configurational and conformational changes in hemoglobin must lie at the heart of both the Bohr effect and of the facilitating interactions between heme groups.

Muirhead and Perutz have found that the two β chains in reduced human hemoglobin are moved apart by 7 Å. compared to oxyhemoglobin of the horse (all other differences between the two proteins being minor in comparison). Hemoglobin H, in contrast, proved to undergo no corresponding change on oxygenation (Perutz and Mazzarella, 1963). Assuming that the difference between horse oxyhemoglobin and human reduced hemoglobin is attributable to oxygenation rather than to species differences, Perutz has tentatively concluded that the structural changes result from altered heme-heme interactions (which are absent in hemoglobin H); however, it is not yet clear on what this depends. On the other hand, the Bohr effect may result from the altered environment of dissociable groups in the β chains which would affect the pK's of many groups.

C. *Environmental Determinants*

The tertiary structure of proteins is affected by intrinsic and extrinsic determinants, some of which we have already alluded to. The amino acid sequence, the secondary structural features such as the presence of helical and non-helical regions in the peptide chain, the nature of the side-chain functional groups, and, as we have seen, the presence or absence of oxygen, represent unique intrinsic determinants of structure. In addition, however, the structure and state of globular proteins are very greatly affected by the physicochemical conditions of the environment in which they exist. These conditions include such important factors as pH, ionic strength, dielectric constant, and temperature of the medium. The effect of the extrinsic factors of environment upon the interaction of hemoglobin with oxygen has received only occasional attention in the past, but is now coming under more intense scrutiny as the evidence mounts regarding the importance of tertiary structure. As early as 1909, Barcroft and Camis found that the shape of the oxygen dissociation curve is influenced by the presence of certain salts in the medium. Barcroft and Roberts (1909) showed further that the dissociation curve reverted to a rectangular hyperbola in the absence of salt. Somewhat later Sidwell and coworkers (1938) showed that increased salt concentrations depress the amount of oxygen bound to hemoglobin, but they did not distinguish between a possible effect on oxygen affinity and on heme-heme interactions. Recently Rossi-Fanelli and collaborators (1961) observed quite large effects upon oxygen affinity and lesser effects upon heme-heme interactions, when the ionic strength, dielectric constant, and salt composition were varied over relatively narrow ranges. This is illustrated by the accompanying figures taken from their work. The affinity for oxygen increases as the ionic strength decreases, and simultaneously the shape of the curve changes in the direction of decreased heme-heme interactions (Fig. 4). The data in Fig. 5 are of particular interest in that they illustrate the effects of specific ions within narrow concentration ranges, and they include the effect of a dipolar ion, glycine. In this latter series, it will be noted that the effects are primarily upon the oxygen affinity, the shape of the curves remaining relatively constant. In the most recent study in this series, the same workers joined by Jeffries Wyman (Antonini *et al.*, 1962) have shown that the magnitude of the Bohr effect decreases as the ionic strength increases to very high ranges. These data are all quite consistent with the probability that the Bohr effect and the facilitating interactions between hemes are functions of the tertiary structure of the hemoglobin. However, there is not yet sufficient theoretical basis on which to interpret these data in terms of their specific effect or effects upon tertiary structure. It must be noted that these effects, especially those illustrated in Figs. 4 and 5, are observed over a narrow range where other gross physicochemical parameters such as viscosity, light scattering, and sedimentation constant are not affected. Valtis and Kennedy (1954) described a storage lesion in preserved red cells characterized by a leftward displacement of the oxygen dissociation curve and an altered Bohr effect. It is tempting to speculate that this might reflect an altered intra-erythrocyte environment as the result of preservation (cf. J. L. Tullis, Chapter 15).

We come finally to the problem of difference in oxygen-binding properties between free hemoglobin solutions and suspended red blood cells. This brings us also into the area of the hemoglobin variants. Here striking differences between hemoglobins have long been reported. Textbooks, for example, carry the information that fetal blood has a higher oxygen affinity than maternal blood. Yet despite this and other reports concerning blood from sickle cell anemia and other abnormal states, it appears that the differences may be largely attributable to the extrinsic factors of environment within the red cell rather than to the hemoglobin per se. Allen *et al.* (1953) showed that fetal and adult hemoglobins have the same oxygen affinity ($p_{1/2}$) and *n* value when freshly laked red cells are dialyzed against the same outside solution. Similarly, Schruefer *et al.* (1962) have recently confirmed this finding and extended it to

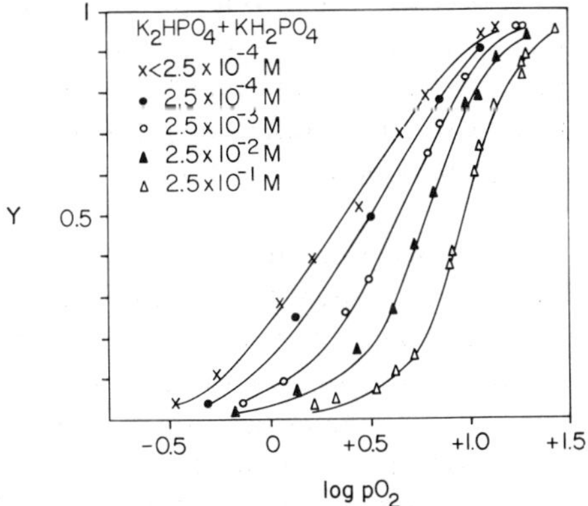

FIG. 4. Effect of buffer concentration on oxygen binding by human hemoglobin at pH 7.0. Ordinate: degree of saturation (Y). Abscissa: log pO_2. (From Rossi-Fanelli *et al.*, 1961.)

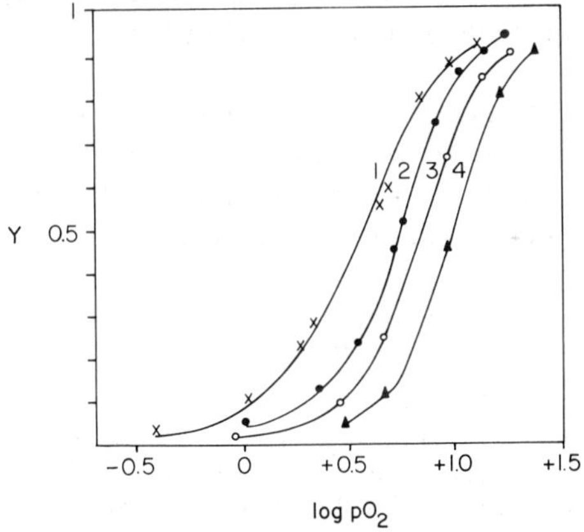

FIG. 5. Effect of electrolytes on oxygen binding at pH 7.0: curve 1, 0.2 *M* glycine; curve 2, 0.2 *M* tris; curve 3, 0.4 *M* NaCl; curve 4, 0.1 *M* citrate. Ordinate: degree of saturation (Y). Abscissa: log pO_2. (From Rossi-Fanelli *et al.*, 1961.)

include the Bohr effect. They also found that sickle hemoglobin (in contrast to sickle cell anemia cells) has the same oxygen affinity as normal adult hemoglobin.

We have here then a last and most important function of the red cell, that of providing the proper environment for the hemoglobin molecule. Within this special environment of the red cell the tertiary structure of the hemoglobin molecule receives its final adjustments, and the red cell sallies forth prepared to perform those unique roles of transport which are characterized by the proper terms, Bohr effect, heme-heme interactions, and oxygen affinity. What are the parameters of this environment that the hemoglobin molecule finds itself in? This is covered elsewhere in this book. Suffice it to say that it is an unusual environment, in its cation and anion composition, in its very high protein composition, and in many other respects as well. We know, for example, that there are unique conditions of oxidation-reduction potential that must hold.

One interesting facet of this problem concerns the state of hemoglobin within the red cell. Under such high conditions of protein concentration, protein-protein interactions would be maximal. In view of the origin and life history of the red cell, one must also ask the question whether there is any intracellular organization. One interesting point is raised by the common observation that red cell stroma, no matter how carefully prepared or how often washed, still contains hemoglobin. Anderson and Turner (1960), for example, have found that red cell membrane preparations contain about 50% by weight of hemoglobin, corresponding to about 3% of the total hemoglobin of the red cell. They conclude that this hemoglobin is somehow bound to the membrane in highly undissociable form. Clearly there is still much room for inquiry and experiment.

One obvious question concerns what differences there are between populations of red cells other than oxygen interacting characteristics. Here, too, there is a paucity of data, but one is immediately reminded of the factors which alter the resistance of sickle cells to the malaria parasite.

References

Adair, G. S. (1925). *J. Biol. Chem.* **63**, 529.

Allen, D. W., Guthe, K. F., and Wyman, J., Jr. (1950). *J. Biol. Chem.* **187**, 393.

Allen, D. W., Wyman, J., Jr., and Smith, C. A. (1953). *J. Biol. Chem.* **203**, 81.

Anderson, H. M., and Turner, J. C. (1960). *J. Clin. Invest.* **39**, 1.

Antonini, E., Wyman, J., Jr., Rossi-Fanelli, A., and Caputo, A. (1962). *J. Biol. Chem.* **237**, 2773.

Barcroft, J., and Camis, M. (1909). *J. Physiol. (London)* **39**, 118.

Barcroft, J., and Roberts, F. (1909). *J. Physiol. (London)* **39**, 143.

Benesch, R., and Benesch, R. E. (1961). *J. Biol. Chem.* **236**, 405.

Benesch, R. E., Ranney, H. M., Benesch, R., and Smith, G. M. (1961). *J. Biol. Chem.* **236**, 2926.

Bohr, C. (1905). *In* "Handbuch der Physiologie des Menschen" (W. Nagel, ed.), Vol. I, p. 54. Vieweg, Braunschweig.

Bohr, C., Hasselbalch, K., and Krogh, A. (1904). *Skand. Arch. Physiol.* **16**, 402.

Braunitzer, G., Hilschmann, N., and Wittman-Liebold, B. (1961). *Z. Physiol. Chem.* **325**, 94.

Cannon, W. B. (1932). "The Wisdom of the Body." Norton, New York.
Conant, J. B. (1933). *Harvey Lectures, Ser.* **28**, 159.
Coryell, C. D., and Pauling, L. (1940). *J. Biol. Chem.* **132**, 769.
Davenport, H. W. (1950). "The ABC of Acid-base Chemistry," 3rd ed. Univ. of Chicago Press, Chicago, Illinois.
Ferguson, J. K. W. (1936). *Am. J. Physiol.* **116**, 48.
Goldstein, J., Guidotti, G., Konigsberg, W., and Hill, R. J. (1961). *J. Biol. Chem.* **236**, PC 77.
Henriques, O. M. (1928). *Biochem. Z.* **200**, 1.
Hill, A. V. (1910). *J. Physiol.* (*London*) **40**, 4P.
Hoppe-Seyler, F. (1865). *In* "Handbuch der physiologisch- und pathologisch-chemischen Analyse" (A. Hirschwald, ed.), 2nd ed., p. 203. Springer, Berlin.
Keilin, J. (1960). *Nature* **187**, 365.
Manwell, C. (1960). *Arch. Biochem. Biophys.* **89**, 194.
Meldrum, N. U., and Roughton, F. J. W. (1933a). *J. Physiol* (*London*) **80**, 113.
Meldrum, N. U., and Roughton, F. J. W. (1933b). *J. Physiol.* (*London*) **80**, 143.
Muirhead, H., and Perutz, M. F. (1963). *Nature* **199**, 633.
Pauling, L. (1935). *Proc. Natl. Acad. Sci. U.S.* **21**, 186.
Perutz, M. F., and Mazzarella, L. (1963). *Nature* **199**, 639.
Perutz, M. F., Rossman, M. G., Cullis, A. F., Muirhead, H., Will, G., and North, A. C. T. (1960). *Nature* **185**, 416.
Riggs, A. (1951). *J. Gen. Physiol.* **35**, 23.
Riggs, A. (1959). *Nature* **183**, 1037.
Riggs, A. (1961). *Nature* **190**, 94.
Rossi-Fanelli, A., Antonini, E., and Caputo, A. (1961). *J. Biol. Chem.* **236**, 397.
Roughton, F. J. W. (1944). *Harvey Lectures, Ser.* **39**, 96.
Schruefer, J. J. P., Heller, C. J., Battaglia, F. C., and Hellegers, A. E. (1962). *Nature* **196**, 550.
Sidwell, A. E., Jr., Munch, R. H., Barron, E. S. G., and Hogness, T. R. (1938). *J. Biol. Chem.* **123**, 335.
Steinhardt, J., Remedios, O., and Beychok, S. (1962). *Biochemistry* **1**, 29.
Valtis, D. J. and Kennedy, A. C. (1954). *Lancet* **1**, 119.
Wald, G., and Riggs, A. (1951). *J. Gen. Physiol.* **35**, 45.
Wyman, J., Jr. (1939a). *J. Biol. Chem.* **127**, 1.
Wyman, J., Jr. (1939b). *J. Biol. Chem.* **127**, 581.
Wyman, J., Jr. (1948). *Advances in Protein Chem.* **4**, 407.
Wyman, J., Jr., and Allen, D. W. (1951). *J. Polymer Sci.* **7**, 499.

CHAPTER 10

Blood-Group Substances: Their Nature and Genetics

Winifred M. Watkins

I. Introduction

Blood-group divisions within each species arise from the presence of antigenic substances on the red cells of certain members of the species which are absent from the cells of other members of the same species. The antigenic substances are detected by means of serum antibodies which cause the red cells to agglutinate. These antibodies may be derived from the same species as that in which the antigen is demonstrated or from a different species. Blood-group specific agglutinins also occur in certain plant seeds (cf. Bird, 1959).

The blood-group characters of the red cells are, with minor exceptions, constant throughout life and are inherited according to Mendelian laws. A knowledge of human blood groups is essential for the safe practice of blood transfusion and, in addition, the blood groups have repercussions outside clinical medicine, since the apparently simple manner of inheritance of the characters makes them of outstanding value in fundamental genetical (cf. Race and Sanger, 1962) and anthropological (cf. Mourant, 1954) studies. Blood-group divisions have been established in nearly all mammalian species in which systematic investigations have been made (cf. Joysey, 1959). Advances in the serology and genetics of blood groups, however, have far outstripped advances in an understanding of the chemical basis of blood-group specificity. Very little chemical work has been carried out on the animal blood-group substances except for those occurring in a water-soluble form which are related in specificity to human blood-group antigens (cf. Kabat, 1956). In man, fourteen independent genetical systems have been defined, involving more than 60 different blood-group antigens (cf. Race and Sanger, 1962), but information on the chemistry of the substances is at present almost entirely limited to four blood-group systems, namely, the ABO, Lewis, MN, and P systems. This chapter will be confined to a consideration of the substances with blood-group specificities related to these four systems. Before discussing the chemical nature of the substances, the genetical and serological backgrounds of the ABO, Lewis, MN, and P systems will be briefly outlined, but for a detailed account of these and all the known human blood-group systems and their manner of inheritance, the reader is referred to Race and Sanger (1962). For reviews on the chemical basis of blood-group specificity see Kabat (1956) and Morgan (1960).

Great interest centers on the Rhesus (Rh) blood-group system because of its role in the etiology of hemolytic disease of the newborn (cf. Roberts, 1959), but the chemical nature of the Rh antigens is not yet clarified. Recently (cf. Boyd, 1962) attempts have been made to determine the nature of the serologically active groupings in Rh antigens by the method of hemagglutination inhibition with low molecular weight inhibitors (see Section V,A,1.) A clue to the structures involved in Rh specificity may eventually be found in some of the results obtained, but so many compounds of diverse chemical nature have been implicated by different investigators that it is felt that a consideration of these findings would not be informative at the present stage of the work.

A. ABO and Lewis Groups

The earliest observations on differences between the blood of normal individuals belonging to the same species were made by Landsteiner (1900). He cross-tested the red cells and sera of workers in his laboratory and found that in some instances agglutination occurred, whereas in others there was no reaction. On the basis of these tests, Landsteiner (1901) was able to divide individuals into three groups and, with the discovery by von Decastello and Sturli (1902) of a fourth group, the foundation was laid of what is now known as the ABO blood-group system. The classification is based on the presence or absence of two antigens designated A and B, on the red cell surface, and two antibodies, anti-A and anti-B, which always occur in the serum or plasma when the corresponding antigen is missing. The relationships between the antigens on the red cell and the antibodies in the serum are shown in Table I.

TABLE I

THE ABO BLOOD-GROUP SYSTEM

Blood group	Antigen on the red cell	Antibody in the serum
A	A	Anti-B (β)
B	B	Anti-A (α)
AB	A and B	—
O	—	Anti-A and anti-B

The blood-group characters are inherited according to Mendelian laws (Epstein and Ottenberg, 1908; von Dungern and Hirszfeld, 1910). Several different theories were advanced to explain the exact mechanism of inheritance, but the one generally accepted today is that put forward by Bernstein (1924), according to which the blood group of an individual depends on the presence of two of the three allelic genes *A*, *B*, and *O*. This scheme was later extended to include the subgroups A_1 and A_2 (Thomsen *et al.*, 1930). A child receives from each parent one of the four genes A_1, A_2, *B*, or *O*, which give rise to ten possible genotypes, A_1A_1, A_1A_2, A_1O, A_1B, A_2A_2, A_2O, A_2B, *BB*, *BO*, and *OO*.

The blood-group antigens are not confined to the red cell; group specific substances corresponding to the ABO group of the individual are found in the cells of almost all the organs of the body (cf. Wiener, 1943; Glynn and Holborow, 1959; Szulman, 1960, 1962). In addition, in many individuals, substances which specifically combine with anti-A or anti-B agglutinins, and thus inhibit the agglutination of A or B cells, respectively, occur in water-soluble form in secretions. Yamakami (1926) first demonstrated the presence of A and B substances in spermatic fluid and saliva, and Lehrs (1930) and Putkonen (1930) recognized that the character was dimorphic and that individuals can be divided into secretors and nonsecretors. The ability to secrete A and B substances is inherited as a Mendelian dominant character (Schiff and Sasaki, 1932). The gene *Se*, when present in single or double dose, gives rise to secretion; the gene *se* in double dose results in nonsecretion of the group substances in tissue fluids and secretions, but does not influence the appearance of the A and B characters on the red cells.

Many reagents of human, animal, and plant origin that react preferentially with O cells have been described (cf. Watkins and Morgan, 1955a) and the agglutination of O cells by these reagents can frequently be inhibited by the saliva from group O individuals. However, there are several reasons for believing that the so-called anti-O reagents are not detecting the product of the *O* gene, the most cogent one being that many individuals of group AB, who cannot on Bernstein's hypothesis possess an *O* gene, secrete the so-called O substance in addition to A and B substances. To avoid confusion, it was suggested that the serologically active substance in the secretions of group O persons should be called H substance to indicate its heterogenetic origin (Morgan and Watkins, 1948). This nomenclature is now widely accepted and will be used throughout this chapter. The ability to secrete H substance is controlled by the secretor gene *Se*. According to current ideas, H substance is a product of a gene system independent of the *ABO* system, but is considered to be the substrate which is modified under the influence of the *A* and *B* genes (see Section VI.A).

The Lewis blood-group Le^a character belongs to a genetic system which is inherited independently of the *ABO* genes, but in its phenotypic effects the Lewis system is interrelated with the ABO system. The antibody anti-Le^a, discovered by Mourant (1946), agglutinates the red cells of 22% of Europeans; Grubb (1948) observed that all persons whose red cells were Le(a+) were nonsecretors of A, B, or H substances and that moreover these individuals secreted a substance which neutralized anti-Le^a serum. Thus all individuals whose red cells are Le(a+) secrete Le^a substance. In addition, Le^a substance is secreted by most ABH secretors, although in smaller amounts than in ABH nonsecretors. An antibody which agglutinated nearly all the red cells not agglutinated by anti-Le^a sera was described by Andresen (1948) and, in the belief that it was identifying an antigen produced by an allele of the gene giving rise to Le^a reactivity, the antibody was called anti-Le^b. A substance which neutralized this antibody occurred in the saliva of about 90% of all secretors of A, B, or H substances, but was not found in the saliva of nonsecretors of A, B, or H substances. Further studies (cf. Race and Sanger, 1962) showed that anti-Le^b could not be detecting the product of an allele of Le^a, and the relationship of Le^b to the ABO and Le^a groups is still not entirely clear.

About 1% of all individuals fail to secrete A, B, H, Le^a, or Le^b substances, but these persons nevertheless have in their secretions a substance which, chemically, is very closely related to the A, B, H, and Le^a substances (see Section IV, A, 2). On the basis of their red cell phenotype and ability to secrete A, B, H, Le^a, and Le^b substances in saliva, individuals can be divided into the six groups shown in Table II. Groups 5 and 6 correspond to the very rare "Bombay" phenotype who lack A, B, and H reactivity both in their secretions and on their red cells (cf. Bhende *et al.*, 1952; Race and Sanger, 1962).

TABLE II[a]

THE RELATIONSHIP BETWEEN THE RED CELL PHENOTYPE AND THE A, B, H, Le^a AND Le^b SUBSTANCES PRESENT IN SECRETIONS

Group	Antigens on red cells			Substances in secretions		
	ABH	Le^a	Le^b	ABH	Le^a	Le^b
1	+	−	+	+	+	+
2	+	+	−	−	+	−
3	+	−	−	+	−	−
4	+	−	−	−	−	−
5	−	+	−	−	+	−
6	−	−	−	−	−	−

[a] Based on the observations of Grubb (1951), Ceppellini (1955), and Bhende *et al.* (1952).

B. *MN and P Groups*

The basis of the MN and P blood-group systems was laid down in a series of experiments carried out by Landsteiner and Levine (1927a,b). Rabbits were immunized with human red cells and the resultant sera were absorbed with red cells from certain individuals without regard to their ABO group. By this method, a few sera were obtained which gave a sharp differentiation of individual bloods within the ABO groups and revealed three additional properties designated M, N, and P. A relationship between the two factors M and N was recognized and it was found that human bloods could be divided into three types, M, N, and MN. It was suggested that two allelic genes, *M* and *N*, determine the presence of the equivalent antigen on the red cell and that there are thus three genotypes, *MM*, *MN*, and *NN* (Landsteiner and Levine, 1928b). This theory is now universally accepted, although further subgroups and antigens related to the MN system have been added in the intervening years (cf. Race and Sanger, 1962).

The P system was for many years considered as a monofactorial system and bloods were differentiated simply into P+ or P− according to whether they reacted, or failed to react, with an anti-P serum. The realization by Sanger (1955) that antigen Tj^a, discovered by Levine *et al.*, (1951) was part of the P system, however, led to a revision of this idea. Two antigens are now recognized, P and P_1, which give rise to three phenotypes, P_1, P_2, and p (Table III). The antibody formerly called anti-P is now known as anti-P_1, and the antibody once called anti-Tj^a is a mixture of anti-P plus anti-P_1 (cf. Race and Sanger, 1962).

TABLE III[a]

THE P BLOOD-GROUP SYSTEM

Red cell phenotype	Antigens on red cells	Antibodies in serum
P_1	$P+P_1$	—
P_2	P	Sometimes anti-P_1
p	—	Always anti-P+anti-P_1

[a] After Race and Sanger (1962).

II. Sources of Blood-Group Substances

A. *A, B, H, Le^a, and Le^b Substances*

Red cells are the most obvious source from which to attempt to isolate blood-group substances for chemical studies, but the earlier workers encountered considerable difficulties in obtaining any quantity of active material from this source and the reports on the chemical nature of the isolated substances were conflicting (cf. Kabat, 1956). Following the demonstration in secretions of water-soluble substances with the same specificity as the A and B antigens on the red cell, attention was largely turned to these materials as a source of group specific substances. In the last few years the problem of the nature of the A and B substances on the red cell has been re-examined and, by taking advantage of the modern techniques of extraction and chromatography, red cell preparations are now being obtained in sufficient quantity for detailed chemical study. It is still true to say, however, that insight into the chemical structures associated with A, B, H, Le^a, and Le^b specificities has been obtained largely through a study of the secreted substances or of materials from animal sources which are serologically related to human A, B, and H substances. Therefore, although the substances in secretions technically fall outside the scope of this book, they will be considered in some detail because of the contribution they have made to an understanding of the basis of the specificity of the red cell antigens.

Early investigations showed that, of the normal secretions of the body, saliva, gastric juice, seminal fluid, and urine were the most potent sources of blood-group specific substances (cf. Wiener, 1943; Kabat, 1956). Yosida (1928) reported blood-group activity in the pathological fluid from ovarian cysts, and

Morgan and van Heyningen (1944) found that these fluids frequently were very rich in blood-group A, B, and H substances. Human ovarian cyst fluids are also a convenient and potent source of Le^a and Le^b active substances (Grubb and Morgan, 1949). Meconium, the first stool of the newborn, is another rich source of A, B, and H substances (Yosida, 1928; Rapoport and Buchanan, 1950).

Substances with serological specificities closely related to A, B, and H are widely distributed in nature and are found in many animal species (cf. Kabat, 1956) and in microorganisms and certain plants (cf. Springer, 1958).

B. M, N, and P_1 Substances

Earlier workers (Zacho, 1932; Boyd and Boyd, 1934) failed to demonstrate M and N substances in normal tissues or secretions, but Kosjakov and Tribulev (1939), using a modified method for detection of the substances, found M and N activity in tissue cells. Activity could be demonstrated in liver and kidney cells, and to a lesser extent, in muscle and brain cells. These results were confirmed by Boorman and Dodd (1943), who also found M and N activity in saliva, although the amount was very small in comparison with the activity of the A and B substances in secretor individuals. Substances with serological specificities related to M and N do not seem to occur frequently in nature, but M and N antigens are found in chimpanzees (cf. Mourant, 1954), and Levine *et al.* (1955) described an N-like receptor on horse red cells.

Blood-group P_1 substance has not been demonstrated in saliva (Wiener, 1943) or human tissues (Pettenkofer, 1955). A water-soluble source of P_1 active substance became available, however, when Cameron and Staveley (1957) found that the fluid from hydatid cysts of sheep liver inhibited anti-P_1 serum. The origin of the P_1 substance in the cyst fluid is not entirely clear, but as activity was observed only when the cyst contained live scolices, or tapeworms (*Echinococcus granulosis*), one must assume that the P_1 specific substance is a product of the tapeworm and not of the host animal. Hydatid cyst fluids from man (Levine *et al.*, 1958) or pigs (Prokop and Oesterle, 1958) also show P_1 activity.

III. Isolation of Blood-Group Substances

A. Mucosal Linings, Tissue Fluids, and Secretions

1. A, B, H, and Le^a Substances

The methods devised in various laboratories for the isolation of human A, B, H, and Le^a substances from glandular tissues, saliva, amniotic fluid, ovarian cyst fluids, and meconium, and of substances having A, B, or H specificity from animal sources, such as hog or horse gastric mucosa, have been reviewed in detail by Kabat (1956); only a few general points will therefore be considered here.

The A, B, H, and Le^a substances as they occur in tissue fluids and secretions are chemically very similar and the same procedures can be used for the isolation of any one of these specific substances. The use of high temperatures or strongly acid or alkaline reagents must be avoided during the isolation in order to reduce to a minimum the possibility of producing irreversible changes in the labile blood-group active substances. The method which has found most general application is extraction of the freeze-dried tissue fluid or secretion with cold 90% phenol (Morgan and King, 1943). When this procedure is applied to dried ovarian cyst fluids, a phenol-insoluble residue is obtained which possesses most of the specific activity of the original secretion and is largely free from the accompanying unspecific protein and other impurities in the native cyst. Further purification can then be achieved by high speed centrifugation or fractionation from water or certain organic solvents (cf. Gibbons *et al.*, 1955; Pusztai and Morgan, 1961b). The phenol method can also be applied directly to obtain blood-group specific materials from meconium (Buchanan and Rapoport, 1951), but in the preparation of blood-group substances from mucosal linings autolysis, or enzymatic hydrolysis with added pepsin, is an essential first step in order to obtain the active substances in water-soluble form. Pepsin treatment influences the solubility of the substances in phenol in such a way that, after treatment, the blood-group activity is distributed between the phenol-insoluble residue and a phenol-soluble fraction (Morgan and King, 1943; Bendich *et al.*, 1946).

2. P_1 Substance

Recently the blood-group P_1 active substance has been isolated from sheep hydatid cyst fluid by the phenol extraction method (Morgan and Watkins, 1962). The phenol-insoluble residue is highly active as an inhibitor of P_1 agglutination and further purification can be achieved by fractionation with ethanol of an aqueous solution of the extracted material.

B. *Red Cells*

1. A and B Substances

The blood-group substances on the human red cell surface, with the possible exception of the Lewis antigens (cf. Sneath and Sneath, 1959), form an integral part of the red cell and cannot be extracted with water or salt solutions. The first A and B blood-group active preparations from human red cells (Schiff and Adelsberger, 1924; Landsteiner and van der Scheer, 1925; Hallauer, 1934) were isolated by extraction of red cells with alcohol. Since blood-group active substances could be removed from red cells by extraction with this solvent, the term "alcohol-soluble" was introduced to describe the A and B antigens on the red cells in contrast to the "water-soluble" substances isolated from secretions and tissue fluids.

The approach to the isolation of A and B substances from the red cell, which is being pursued today, began with the isolation from equine blood stroma of a new kind of glycolipid (Yamakawa and Suzuki, 1951) which, in many ways, resembled the gangliosides obtained earlier from brain and spleen tissues (Klenk, 1941). By extraction of human red cells with methanol-ether at room temperature, Yamakawa and Suzuki (1952) obtained a similar material which they called "globoside" and this substance was later shown to have A, B, or O blood-group activity corresponding to the group of the red cells from which the substance was obtained (Yamakawa and Iida, 1953; Yamakawa *et al.*, 1956). Radin (1957) chromatographed the lipids extracted from whole dry red cells with a hot methanol-chloroform mixture on a cellulose column and found that the major peak, presumed to be globoside, was sometimes partially resolved into two peaks. Blood-group activity did not coincide with the main peak, thus suggesting that globoside was not a homogeneous entity. Following this observation, Yamakawa, *et al.* (1958, 1960) studied the application of silicic acid chromatography to mammalian erythrocyte glycolipids and reported the separation of globoside into many fractions. Two minor fractions had blood-group activity but these were not regarded as homogeneous.

Koscielak and Zakrzewski (1959, 1960) extracted human A and B red cells with 96% ethanol and obtained material which had group A or B activity. The material was further purified by extraction with organic solvents to remove contaminating lipids followed by fractionation on a cellulose column, but fractional solubility tests showed the blood-group active fraction to be non-homogeneous. The activity of the group A preparation was equivalent to about 25% of the activity of a purified specimen of ovarian cyst A substance. Preparations obtained by Hakomori and Jeanloz (1961) by extraction of group A and B stromata with hot chloroform-methanol, followed by extraction with organic solvents and adsorption chromatography on activated silica gel and partition chromatography on cellulose columns, were also very low in hemagglutination-inhibiting activity, and indeed the final products were considerably less active than the starting materials. Despite this fact, the authors considered that they were handling the substances responsible for blood-group A and B activities on the red cell because all the other fractions were completely inactive. They were also confident that the methods used in the preparation of these fractions excluded the possibility of contamination with the type of A and B substances found in secretions and tissue fluids. It was suggested that the low solubility of the products in water and the tendency for lipid materials to form aggregates might explain the low blood-group activity.

The possibility that the state of aggregation influences the activity of blood-group materials from the red cells is supported by an interesting observation of Koscielak (1962). He found that chromatography of blood-group active material obtained from group A red cell stromata on a cellulose column gave two fractions. One fraction was inactive when tested by either the usual hemagglutination-inhibition method or by the precipitin method with a specific rabbit anti-A precipitating serum. The second fraction was only weakly active when tested in the hemagglutination-inhibition test, but was more active than the starting material in precipitating antibody from the anti-A serum. Moreover, combination of the two fractions restored the hemagglutination-inhibitory activity to its original value. It was suggested that the inactive fraction served as a "carrier" material which produces a favorable surface configuration for the reactive groupings in the second fraction to exert maximum specific activity when competing with the antigen on the intact red cell for combination with specific antibody sites. These results indicate that a fall in specific activity during the course of purification of the blood-group substances from the red cell may arise from a reduction in macromolecular size and/or a change in molecular conformation, rather than from a loss or inactivation of the chemical structures responsible for blood-group specificity.

2. M and N Substances

The method which has been most widely and successfully used for the isolation of M and N active substances from red cells or red cell stromata is a modification of the hot phenol-water method introduced by Westphal *et al.* (1952) for the isolation of the specific lipopolysaccharides from gram-negative bacteria. Red cells or stromata suspended in saline are mixed with an equal volume of liquid 90% phenol and the mixture is kept at 65° for 30 minutes. On cooling, the phenol and water phases separate and the M and N active material is found in the aqueous layer. This method, first applied to red cells for the isolation of M and N substances by Hohorst (1954), was used, with minor modifications, by Baranowski *et al.* (1956), Stalder and Springer (1960), and Klenk and Uhlenbruck (1960).

Ethanol extraction of red cells was reported by Stalder and Springer (1960, 1961) to yield materials with M and N properties, but the activity of these preparations was less, based on units per weight, than the material obtained by the phenol-saline method.

M and N receptors on the erythrocyte surface are inactivated by certain proteolytic enzymes (Morton and Pickles, 1951; Rosenfield and Vogel, 1951) and, on the assumption that inactivation results from the liberation of M and N active fragments, Klenk and Uhlenbruck (1960) and Uhlenbruck (1961a) investigated the use of proteolytic enzymes to isolate M and N substances from the red cell. Nondialyzable materials which could be recovered by phenol extraction of the cell-free supernatant were obtained after incubation of red cells with trypsin, ficin, bromelin, and papain. The materials recovered by this procedure were, however, less active than those obtained by the phenol-saline method (Uhlenbruck, 1961a).

The M and N active materials isolated by Baranowski *et al.* (1959) separated into two polydisperse fractions in the ultracentrifuge and, in free electrophoresis experiments, were nonhomogeneous at acid pH values. Further purification was attempted by paper and glass paper electrophoresis and by adsorption chromatography on a cellulose column, but no effective purification was achieved by these methods.

Stalder and Springer (1961) purified M and N substances obtained by the phenol-saline or ethanol extraction method through fractional centrifugation at 2000 *g*, 32,700 *g*, and 105,400 *g*. The phenol-saline extracted material sedimenting at 105,400 *g* showed the highest M activity. The N active material isolated by the ethanol procedure remained in the supernatant at 105,400 *g*. No evidence for the homogeneity of these materials was given.

IV. Chemical Nature and Properties of Blood-Group Substances

A. A, B, H, and Le^a Substances from Tissue Fluids and Secretions

1. Criteria for Homogeneity

One of the most difficult problems encountered in the study of the blood-group substances, and of related materials, is that of establishing the homogeneity of the isolated product. Morgan (1960) suggests that the isolated blood-group substances should be subjected to physical (electrophoresis and ultracentrifugation), chemical (fractional solubility tests), and serological (specific precipitation and inhibition of hemagglutination) examination, and only when the materials are free from demonstrable heterogeneity by any of these methods should they be used for chemical studies. With the development of new techniques for the separation of macromolecules, however, preparations which obey these criteria can sometimes be further subdivided (cf. Pusztai and Morgan, 1961b).

Immunochemical methods have been developed by Kabat and his co-workers (cf. Kabat, 1956) both for the characterization of the blood-group substances and to obtain data on the purity and homogeneity of the isolated products. The method involving the analysis of specific precipitates for distinctive constituents of the blood-group substances (Bendich *et al.*, 1946) provided the first good evidence that a substantial portion of the weight of the various preparations of blood-group substances actually combines with antibody, and hence that blood-group activity is not associated with trace contaminants of unknown nature in the materials isolated. Complete precipitation of a blood-group active preparation by a specific antiserum gives information, however, only on the immunological homogeneity of the preparation and not on its chemical or physical homogeneity.

2. Composition of the Substances

The discovery (Morgan and van Heyningen, 1944) that ovarian cyst fluids are a rich source of human blood-group substances provided a means of obtaining relatively large quantities of active substance from a single individual. Highly purified specimens of blood-group A (Aminoff *et al.*, 1950), B (Gibbons and Morgan, 1954), H (Annison and Morgan, 1952b), and Le^a (Annison and Morgan, 1952a) substances, irrespective of their blood-group specificity, had the same qualitative composition. They each contained the four sugar components L-fucose, D-galactose, *N*-acetylglucosamine, and *N*-acetylgalactosamine. The same eleven amino acids, lysine, aspartic acid, glutamic acid, glycine, serine, alanine, threonine, proline, valine, leucine, and isoleucine, were detected by paper chromatographic methods in each substance. Quantitative amino acid analysis by the method of Moore and Stein (1954) has since revealed the presence of small amounts of methionine, tyrosine, phenylalanine, and histidine in highly purified preparations of cyst substances and shown that in each substance the hydroxyamino acids threonine and serine, together with proline make up about half the total amino acids which comprise about 15% of the weight of the substance (Pusztai and Morgan, 1963). It is now recognized that sialic acid is frequently a component of the blood-group active preparation isolated from cyst fluids (Gibbons *et al.*, 1955; Pusztai and Morgan, 1961a).

Typical analytical values for human blood-group substances isolated from ovarian cysts are given in Table IV. The values for any one component of the substances show slight variations between different preparations with the same specificity, and therefore differences in composition between specimens of differing blood-group activity can be regarded as significant only if they fall outside this range. The A, B, H, and Le^a substances are very similar in quantitative composition, but the fucose content of Le^a substances is invariably lower than that of human A, B, or H substances. In addition, the galactose content is relatively greater in B substances than in A, H, or Le^a substances and the galactosamine content is greater in A than in B, H, or Le^a substances. The sialic acid content of cyst preparations of the same specificity is variable and can be as low as 0.3% or as high as 18% (Morgan, 1963). The preparation in Table IV described as "inactive substance, Fl" was isolated from an ovarian cyst obtained from an individual who was a nonsecretor of A, B, H, Le^a, or Le^b substances and therefore belonged to secretor type 4 (Table II). A series of purified blood-group active substances isolated from human ovarian cysts in a different laboratory were reported (Hiyama, 1962) to have essentially similar analytical figures to those given in Table IV. Preparations from human saliva (Baer *et al.*, 1950; Leskowitz and Kabat, 1954; Hiyama, 1962) and A, B, and H substances from animal sources (cf. Kabat, 1956) closely resemble the cyst substances in general composition and properties.

TABLE IV[a]

TYPICAL ANALYTICAL VALUES FOR PREPARATIONS OF HUMAN BLOOD-GROUP SUBSTANCES

Substance	Nitrogen (%)	Fucose (%)	Acetyl (%)	Hexosamine (%)	Reduction (%)
A	5.4	19	9.0	29	54
H	5.3	18	8.6	28	50
Le^a	5.0	14	9.9	32	56
B	5.6	16	7.0	24	52
AB	5.6	17	—	26	54
"Inactive substance, Fl"	5.4	1.6	—	28	49

[a] From Morgan (1960).

Physical examination of the blood-group substances isolated from ovarian cyst fluids has shown that they are macromolecules with average particle weights ranging from 200×10^3 to 1×10^6 (Kekwick, 1950, 1952a,b; Caspary, 1954). The preparations usually show a moderate degree of polydispersity. The behavior on electrophoresis and ultracentrifugation, and the general properties of the materials, are compatible with the view that the carbohydrate and amino acid moieties are linked together by primary valency bonds. The substances have been classified as mucopolysaccharides (cf. Kent and Whitehouse, 1955).

3. Immunological Aspects

Blood-group substances, isolated from hog gastric mucin, human saliva, and human stomach by peptic digestion, cross-react with horse anti-type XIV pneumococcus serum (Kabat *et al.*, 1948). Human blood-group A, B, or H substances isolated from ovarian cyst fluids frequently do not precipitate to any appreciable extent in the type XIV system but, after treatment with weak acid (Aminoff *et al.*, 1948) or certain specific enzymes (cf. Watkins, 1953), all the substances have the capacity to cross-react with type XIV antiserum. Le^a specific preparations usually cross-react even in the undegraded state and even more marked is the capacity of the "inactive substance, Fl" (Table IV) to precipitate with the type XIV anti-pneumococcus serum (Watkins and Morgan, 1959). All the blood-group preparations therefore possess common, or closely related, chemical structures which confer on them the capacity to cross-react in the type XIV system.

Highly purified preparations of blood-group A substance from both human and animal sources have, in addition to their A properties, the so-called Forssman property, that is, they inhibit the hemolysis of sheep cells by a rabbit immune anti-A serum in the presence of complement (cf. Kabat, 1956). All attempts to separate these two properties have failed and the Forssman character is now considered to be an integral part of the A active molecule. B, H, and Le^a substances do not show this property.

4. Multiple Specificities of Molecules

In secretions, more than one blood-group specificity can frequently be demonstrated (see Table II) and, owing to the close physical and chemical similarity of the A, B, H, and Le^a substances, it is usually not possible to separate them by chemical fractionation procedures or by electrophoretic and ultracentrifugal methods. By means of serological precipitation tests with selected monospecific antisera, however, it is possible to show that the macromolecules frequently carry more than one specificity (Morgan and Watkins, 1956; Watkins and Morgan, 1957a; Watkins, 1958; Brown *et al.*, 1959). The jointly carried specificities can arise from the activity of allelic genes such as *A* and *B*, or from the activity of genes belonging to independent genetic systems such as *A* and Le^a.

B. P_1 Substance from Hydatid Cyst Fluid

1. Chemical Composition

The most active blood-group P_1 substance as yet obtained from sheep hydatid cyst fluid showed two components when examined in the ultracentrifuge at pH 4. Further purification to obtain a P_1 substance free from heterogeneity is required before the composition of the active substance can be accurately determined. Preliminary results indicate, however, that the P_1 substance in sheep hydatid cyst fluid is a mucopolysaccharide resembling in many respects the water-soluble A, B, H, and Le^a substances. The most active preparation contained 3.4% N, 23% hexosamine, and 56% reducing sugar. Two sugars, galactose and a hexosamine, most probably glucosamine, and a number of amino acids were detected chromatographically (Morgan and Watkins, 1962).

2. Immunological Properties

The P_1 substance was completely inactive in hemagglutination-inhibition tests with anti-A, B, H, Le^a, M, N, or Rh (D) sera and did not cross-react in precipitin tests with anti-A, B, or H sera. It did, however, precipitate to a certain extent with horse anti-type XIV pneumococcus serum. When coupled with the conjugated protein of *Shigella shigae*, the P_1 substance gave rise to powerful anti-P_1 agglutinins and precipitins in rabbits (Watkins and Morgan, 1962b).

C. A and B Substances from Red Cells

1. Chemical Composition

None of the preparations of A and B substances from red cells which has been described so far can be regarded as homogeneous. However, the evidence which has accumulated from work carried out in a number of different laboratories strongly indicates that A and B blood-group activity is associated with glycolipid material, that is, with compounds which contain a carbohydrate moiety joined through sphingosine to fatty acids. Amino acids have not been detected in these materials. The A and B blood-group substances from red cells and from secretions are thus associated with macromolecular entities of different general composition.

The blood-group active glycolipid from red cells designated as globoside was characterized as a lignoceryl-sphingosine acetylgalactosamine trihexoside (Yamakawa and Suzuki, 1952). No traces of amino acids, glucosamine, or fucose were detected. Subsequent fractionation of this material on silicic acid acid columns (Yamakawa *et al.*, 1960) revealed that the blood-group activity was located in a minor fraction which contained in the carbohydrate moiety both *N*-acetylglucosamine and sialic acid in addition to galactose, glucose, and *N*-acetylgalactosamine. Analytical values for the main inactive glycolipid fraction and the blood-group active fraction are given in Table V. The activity of the preparations obtained by the Japanese workers has not been given in terms of a standard purified mucopolysaccharide blood-group substance having the same specificity, and therefore it is not possible to assess how much apparent purification has been achieved.

The most active material isolated by Koscielak and Zakrzewski (1959, 1960) from group A red cells had about 25% of the activity of a purified mucopolysaccharide preparation of A substance. This material was a glycolipid containing fatty acids, sphingosine, glucose, galactose, glucosamine, galactosamine, and a small amount of fucose. The more highly purified material obtained from group A red cell stromata by Koscielak (1962) contained in addition sialic acid.

The analytical data on the glycolipid preparations isolated from group A and B cells by Hakomori and Jeanloz (1961) are given in Table V. The blood-group activity of these preparations was very small and, although it is possible that the activity could be increased by the addition of a "carrier" lipid, as described by Koscielak (1962), in the absence of such a test the results on these materials have only limited significance. The failure to detect sialic acid, or

TABLE V

DATA ON GLYCOLIPIDS ISOLATED FROM HUMAN GROUP A AND B RED CELLS

Data	Yamakawa *et al.* (1960)		Koscielak (1962)	Hakamori and Jeanloz (1961)	
	Main inactive peak	A active fraction	A active fraction	A active fraction	B active fraction
Melting point	—	—	—	215–225	220–230
Rotation, $[\alpha]_D$	+19.5° (in pyridine)	—	—	−6° (in water)	+38° (in water)
C%	59–61	—	—	59	59
H%	9.5–10.2	—	—	9.35	9.41
N%	2.23		1.90	1.80	1.89
Hexosamine %	17.5	14.5	9.2	8	8
Sialic acid %	0	2.1	4.1	0	0
Hexose %	50	41	—	48	42
Total reducing sugars %	62–68	—	43	44	40
Fatty acids and sphingosine %	—	—	—	53	56
Component sugars	Glucose, galactose, galactosamine	Glucose, galactose, galactosamine, glucosamine, sialic acid	Glucose, galactose, galactosamine, glucosamine, sialic acid, traces of fucose	Glucose, galactose, galactosamine, traces of glucosamine,	Glucose, galactose, galactosamine, traces of glucosamine
Blood-group activity[a]					
(1) Hemagglutination inhibition	–	–	20	<1	<1
(2) Precipitation	–	–	60	–	–

[a] In % of standard mucopolysaccharide blood-group substance.

appreciable quantities of glucosamine, may indicate that the preparations of Hakomori and Jeanloz (1961) are still contaminated with large quantities of inactive glycolipid material.

It will be apparent from this brief account of the blood-group A and B substances isolated from the red cells that although considerable progress has been made, it cannot yet be considered that the nature of these materials is conclusively established.

2. Immunological Properties

The A and B active preparations obtained by Koscielak and Zakrzewski (1959, 1960) did not contain H, Rh, M, N, or P factors and exhibited no virus hemagglutination-inhibition activity. The failure of the preparation to show H activity is of interest, especially as material obtained from group O cells by the same method also failed to inhibit anti-H sera.

D. M and N Substances from Red Cells

1. Chemical Composition

The M and N active substances isolated from red cells by the phenol-saline method contain carbohydrate and amino acid constituents and are free from lipid. Their general behavior indicates that they are mucopolysaccharides in which the carbohydrate and amino acid components are bound together by primary valency bonds. No significant differences were found in the composition of substances isolated from M and from N cells. The preparations contained galactose, glucosamine, galactosamine, mannose, fucose, sialic acid (*N*-acetylneuraminic acid), and fourteen amino acids (Baranowski *et al.*, 1959; Klenk and Uhlenbruck, 1960). The recognized nonhomogeneity of the preparations, however, limits the significance which can be attached to any of the components shown to be present. Typical analytical values for M and N preparations isolated in different laboratories are given in Table VI.

TABLE VI

COMPOSITION OF M AND N ACTIVE SUBSTANCES FROM RED CELLS

Component	Preparation		
	MN active [a]	MN active [b]	M active [c]
N%	7.5	7.5	8.9
Hexose %	10	15	—
Hexosamine %	6.5	5.8	—
Sialic acid %	20	14	21.4

[a] Baranowski *et al.* (1959).
[b] Klenk and Uhlenbruck (1960)
[c] Nagai and Springer (1962).

2. Immunological Properties

In addition to specific properties for M and N blood groups, the materials isolated from red cells by the phenol-saline method are potent inhibitors of influenza virus hemagglutination (Romanowska, 1959b, 1960; Klenk and Uhlenbruck, 1960; Stalder and Springer, 1961). The M and N preparations isolated by treatment of red cells with proteolytic enzymes do not, however, have this additional property (Uhlenbruck, 1961a).

Earlier observations on the ease with which anti-N reagents are absorbed with group M cells suggested the presence of a small amount of N active substance in the M cells (Landsteiner and Levine, 1928a; Levine *et al.*, 1955; Hirsch *et al.*, 1957). In agreement with this finding, Uhlenbruck (1961b) found that the substances isolated from group M cells had small amounts of N activity, whereas the substances isolated from group N cells were free from M activity. From the results of precipitation experiments with a rabbit anti-M precipitating serum, Uhlenbruck (1961b) concluded that M and N activities probably occur on the same molecule whether they are derived from MM or MN cells. The influenza virus receptor also appeared to be bound to the same molecule.

V. Structural Studies on Blood-Group Substances

A. *Water-Soluble A, B, H, and Le^a Substances from Tissue Fluids and Secretions*

The structural information gained so far from the application to the blood-group specific mucopolysaccharides of standard chemical procedures, such as oxidation with periodate (Aminoff and Morgan, 1951; Ruszkiewicz, 1958; Schiffman *et al.*, 1962b), oxidation with hypoiodite (Rondle, 1954), methylation (Bray *et al.*, 1946), and degradation with dilute alkali (Knox and Morgan, 1954), is limited by the difficulties encountered in interpreting results obtained on such complex and labile materials. The four methods which will be mentioned here are ones that have given more precise structural information.

1. Inhibition of Blood-Group Specific Serological Reactions by Simple Sugars of Known Structure

The chemical similarity of the A, B, H, and Le^a substances, and the rapidity with which the serological activity is destroyed by procedures which bring about only minor changes in the macromolecule, suggested that the blood-group specific structures form only part of the complete mucopolysaccharide molecules. The possibility therefore existed of learning something of the nature of the serologically active groupings before the complete structure of the molecule was elucidated.

Simple substances which are structurally related to, or identical with, the immunologically determinant group of an antigen combine specifically with antibody and thereby competitively inhibit the reactions between antigen and antibody (Landsteiner, 1920). Application of this inhibition technique to the blood-group mucopolysaccharides yielded the first indication that their serological activity was associated with the carbohydrate rather than the peptide moeity of the molecules, and that one component sugar was more closely involved in specificity than were the others. L-Fucose alone of the sugars present in H substance specifically inhibited the agglutination of human group O cells by a specific anti-H reagent from the eel *Anguilla anguilla* (Watkins and Morgan, 1952). Subsequently inhibition experiments were done with an anti-H reagent from seeds of the plant *Lotus tetragonolobus*, and again the results indicated a specific role for an α-L-fucopyranosyl structure in H specificity (Morgan and Watkins, 1953).

Evidence that *N*-acetylgalactosamine is an important part of the chemical structure responsible for A specificity came from inhibition experiments in which this sugar was shown to inhibit specifically the agglutination of group A cells by the plant anti-A reagents from *Vicia cracca* seeds and Lima beans (Morgan and Watkins, 1953); α-methyl-*N*-acetylgalactosaminide was an even more effective inhibitor, thus suggesting that an α-*N*-acetylgalactosaminoyl grouping was implicated in A specificity. Human or rabbit anti-H or anti-A reagents were not inhibited by L-fucose or *N*-acetylgalactosamine, respectively, or by any of a large number of monosaccharides tested for inhibition by the hemagglutination method. Kabat and Leskowitz (1955), however, demonstrated that *N*-acetylgalactosamine inhibited the precipitation of A substance by a human anti-A reagent.

The precipitation-inhibition experiments of Kabat and Leskowitz (1955) first indicated the role of an α-D-galactosyl group in B specificity. Recently, the examination of a series of α-linked digalactosides has shown that *O*-α-D-galactosyl-(1→3)-D-galactose is the most powerful inhibitor so far tested in the B-anti-B system, (Morgan, 1959; Watkins and Morgan, 1962a; Kabat and Schiffman, 1962). (See footnote, p. 384.)

The inhibition results showed that despite the overall similarity in the qualitative and quantitative composition of A, B, and H substances, a different sugar could in each instance be implicated as the terminal nonreducing unit in the serologically specific grouping. Further information on the nature of the determinant structures in A and B substances has been obtained from examination by the inhibition method of fragments isolated directly from partial acid hydrolysis products of the substances (Section V,A,4). Evidence that more than one terminal sugar is important for H specificity has been obtained from inhibition experiments with the anti-H reagents from seeds of the plants *Laburnum alpinum* and *Cytisus sessilifolius*. These agglutinins are inhibited in

TABLE VII

STRUCTURE OF OLIGOSACCHARIDES FROM MILK

Compound number	Trivial name	Structure [a]	Reference
1	Lacto-*N*-tetraose	Gal $\xrightarrow{\beta(1\to3)}$ *N*-AcGluc $\xrightarrow{\beta(1\to3)}$ Gal $\xrightarrow{\beta(1\to4)}$ Gluc	Kuhn and Baer (1956)
2	Lacto-*N*-fucopentaose I	Gal $\xrightarrow{\beta(1\to3)}$ *N*-AcGluc $\xrightarrow{\beta(1\to3)}$ Gal $\xrightarrow{\beta(1\to4)}$ Gluc Fuc $\xrightarrow{\alpha(1\to2)}$ Gal	Kuhn *et al.* (1956)
3	Lacto-*N*-fucopentaose II	Gal $\xrightarrow{\beta(1\to3)}$ *N*-AcGluc $\xrightarrow{\beta(1\to3)}$ Gal $\xrightarrow{\beta(1\to4)}$ Gluc Fuc $\xrightarrow{\alpha(1\to4)}$ *N*-AcGluc	Kuhn *et al.* (1958)
4	Lacto-*N*-difucohexaose I	Gal $\xrightarrow{\beta(1\to3)}$ *N*-AcGluc $\xrightarrow{\beta(1\to3)}$ Gal $\xrightarrow{\beta(1\to4)}$ Gluc Fuc $\xrightarrow{\alpha(1\to2)}$ Gal; Fuc $\xrightarrow{\alpha(1\to4)}$ *N*-AcGluc	Kuhn and Gauhe (1960)
5	Lacto-*N*-difucohexaose II	Gal $\xrightarrow{\beta(1\to3)}$ *N*-AcGluc $\xrightarrow{\beta(1\to3)}$ Gal $\xrightarrow{\beta(1\to4)}$ Gluc Fuc $\xrightarrow{\alpha(1\to4)}$ *N*-AcGluc; Fuc $\xrightarrow{\alpha(1\to3)}$ Gluc	Kuhn and Gauhe (1960)
6	Lacto-difucotetraose	Gal $\xrightarrow{\beta(1\to4)}$ Gluc Fuc $\xrightarrow{\alpha(1\to2)}$ Gal; Fuc $\xrightarrow{\alpha(1\to3)}$ Gluc	Kuhn and Gauhe (1958)

[a] Gal = D-galactopyranosyl; Gluc = D-glucose; Fuc = L-fucopyranosyl; *N*-AcGluc = *N*-acetyl-D-glucosaminopyranosyl.

their action on O cells by H substances of human or animal origin, but are not inhibited by L-fucose (Morgan and Watkins, 1953). Recently a β-(1→4)-linked di-*N*-acetylglucosaminide, *N*,*N'*-diacetylchitobiose, was shown to inhibit both *Cytisus* and *Laburnum* reagents (Watkins and Morgan, 1962a), and this result indicates that a β-*N*-acetylglucosaminoyl structure is a serological determinant unit in H substance, in addition to an α-L-fucosyl structure.

The agglutination of Le(a+) red cells by human or rabbit anti-Le[a] sera is not detectably inhibited by L-fucose or by any other component sugar of the blood-group substances. When a number of oligosaccharides which contained L-fucose were tested for antibody inhibition, however, it became clear that an α-L-fucopyranosyl structure was concerned in Le[a] specificity (Watkins and Morgan, 1957b). The compounds tested were the oligosaccharides isolated from human milk by Professor Kuhn and his colleagues (cf. Kuhn, 1957), and were of great value because the structure of each was precisely known. The constitutions of five of these compounds are given in Table VII. Lacto-*N*-fucopentaose II (No. 3) and lacto-*N*-difucohexaose II (No. 5) were powerful inhibitors in the Le[a] system, whereas lacto-*N*-fucopentaose I (No. 2) and lacto-*N*-difucohexaose I (No. 4), which differ only in the disposition of the fucosyl residues, were inactive. Lacto-*N*-fucopentaose II and lacto-*N*-difucohexaose II both contain the same terminal branched trisaccharide grouping:

O-β-D-galactosyl-(1→3)↘
N-acetyl-D-glucosaminoyl-
O-α-L-fucosyl-(1→4)↗

and it is suggested that such a structure corresponds closely to the specific reactive grouping in Le[a] substance (Watkins and Morgan, 1957b, 1962a).

The compounds lacto-difucotetraose (No. 6) and lacto-*N*-difucohexaose I (No. 4) give weak but definite inhibition in the Le[b] system (Watkins and Morgan, 1957b, 1962a), whereas the compounds containing only one fucose residue are inactive. These results are compatible with the idea that two α-L-fucopyranosyl residues attached to each of two adjacent sugars are concerned in Le[b] specificity.

One other property of the blood-group mucopolysaccharides, which have been examined by the inhibition method, is the cross-precipitability of the substances with type XIV pneumococcus antiserum. A β-D-galactosyl unit most probably joined by a (1→4) linkage to *N*-acetyl-D-glucosamine has been implicated (Watkins and Morgan, 1956; Allen and Kabat, 1958).

2. Inhibition of Enzymatic Inactivation of Blood-Group Substances

Additional and independent evidence for the part played by L-fucose in H and Le[a] specificity and of *N*-acetylgalactosamine and D-galactose in A and B specificity, respectively, was obtained from the results of enzyme inhibition experiments with these sugars (Watkins and Morgan, 1955b, 1957b). Inactivation of A substance by enzyme preparations from *Clostridium welchii* or *Trichomonas foetus* was inhibited by *N*-acetylgalactosamine and not by any of the other sugar components of the blood-group substances, whereas inactivation of B substance was inhibited by D-galactose and of H substance by L-fucose. Inactivation of Le[a] substance by enzymes from *T. foetus* was also inhibited by L-fucose. Since the enzymatic hydrolysis of each substance was inhibited by the sugar that had been shown to be important for specificity, it seemed reasonable to assume that the sugars which bring about the specific inhibition are those released by the action of the enzyme destroying the particular blood-group character.

3. Changes in Blood-Group Substances Induced by Enzymes

Enzymes which destroy the serological activity of the blood-group substances are found in a variety of sources, notably in extracts of liver and digestive organs of different snail species and in extracts and culture filtrates of microorganisms (cf. Kabat, 1956). Earlier experiments designed to correlate loss of blood-group activity with chemical changes in the molecule yielded only limited structural information, because interpretation of the results was complicated by the presence of many enzymatic activities in the preparations used. In recent years, three approaches have been followed to obtain enzymatic reagents more suitable for attacking the problem of the nature of the serologically specific structures in the blood-group substances: (1) soil bacteria have been isolated and examined for the production of enzymes specific for one blood-group specificity, (2) attempts have been made to purify and identify the individual enzymes present in a crude extract from a microorganism, and (3) the action on blood-group substances of purified enzymes of known specificity has been examined. The first approach has been developed largely by Iseki and his colleagues in Japan. A bacterium, *Clostridium tertium*, producing a specific A enzyme (Iseki and Okada, 1951), two producing B enzymes, *Bacillus cereus* (Iseki and Ikeda, 1956) and *Clostridium maebashi* (Iseki *et al.*, 1959a), and one producing an H-decomposing enzyme, *Bacillus fulminans* (Iseki and Tsunoda, 1952), have been described. The absence of an H-decomposing enzyme in the *C. tertium* preparation enabled Iseki and Masaki (1953) to make the important observation that loss of A activity is accompanied by the development of H activity.

The second approach, the separation of individual enzymes from a mixture, has been applied to the enzymes produced by the protozoan flagellate *T. foetus*. Crude extracts of this organism rapidly destroy the serological activity of the A, B, H, and Le[a] blood-group substances (Watkins, 1953). Purification procedures have been directed towards the elimination of glycosidases likely to cause secondary enzymatic changes in the group substances as well as towards the separation from each other of the specific enzymes which destroy the blood-group serological activity. A preparation of H-decomposing enzyme, free from A, B, or Le^a-decomposing enzymes, destroyed the H activity of group O red cells (Watkins and Morgan, 1954) and of the water-soluble H substance, with development of type XIV specificity and liberation primarily of L-fucose (Watkins, 1955; Tyler and Watkins, 1960). These results therefore support the inference from serological inhibition (see Section V, A, 1) and enzyme inhibition (see Section V, A, 2) experiments that fucose is an important part of the H determinant structure. Naylor and Baer (1959), working with the H-decomposing enzyme from *B. fulminans*, also reported that fucose was the only sugar released from H substance by the action of the enzyme.

The chemical changes induced by the B-decomposing enzyme from *B. cereus* were not investigated, but Iseki and Ikeda (1956) observed that loss of B serological activity was accompanied by an increase in H activity. A purified enzyme preparation from *T. foetus* which destroyed B specificity was independently shown to give rise to enhanced H activity (Watkins, 1956), and this change was accompanied by the liberation of galactose with only traces of fucose and *N*-acetylhexosamine. The action of the enzyme preparation from *C. maebashi* on B substance also leads to loss of B activity, development of H activity, and release of galactose (Iseki *et al.*, 1959b). Employing the third method of approach, Zarnitz and Kabat (1960) examined the action on B substance of a purified α-galactosidase from coffee beans and found that a release of galactose was accompanied by complete destruction of the capacity of the substance to inhibit hemagglutination. The nondiffusible material remaining after the action of the coffee bean preparation showed considerably enhanced H activity (Watkins *et al.*, 1962a), thus confirming that H active groupings are exposed as the result of the removal of terminal α-linked galactosyl units.

The presence of structures in A substance closely similar to, or identical with, the specific determinant groupings in H substance was confirmed with an A-decomposing enzyme from *T. foetus* (Watkins, 1960, 1962). Le^a substance did not develop any capacity to inhibit anti-H sera when the Le^a activity was destroyed by a *T. foetus* enzyme preparation free from H-decomposing enzyme; on the other hand, certain H substances developed considerable Le^a activity as the result of the action of *T. foetus* H-decomposing enzyme preparations. Since enzymatic destruction of H activity is accompanied by the release mainly of fucose, it can be assumed that removal of this sugar exposes the Le^a reactive structures. Examination of the action of the enzyme on a number of saliva samples, from group O secretors belonging to different Lewis secretor and red cell phenotypes, revealed that saliva from individuals of the red cell phenotypes OLe(a−b−), secretors of H but not Le^a or Le^b

substances, showed no development of Le^a activity, whereas saliva from individuals of the red cell phenotype OLe(a−b+), which normally shows slight Lc^a activity in addition to II and Le^h activity, developed more Le^a activity as the result of the action of the H enzyme. Latent H active structures therefore appear to be present in A and B substances and latent Le^a active structures in certain H substances. By the sequential use of purified B, H, and Le^a enzymes from *T. foetus*, it is possible to bring about the series of changes in the specificity of a human B substance shown in Fig. 1.

The enzyme changes just described have concerned the carbohydrate moiety of the blood-group substances. The proteolytic enzymes trypsin and pepsin have no effect on the serological properties of the blood-group substances, but proteolytic enzymes of plant origin, ficin and papain, have been recently

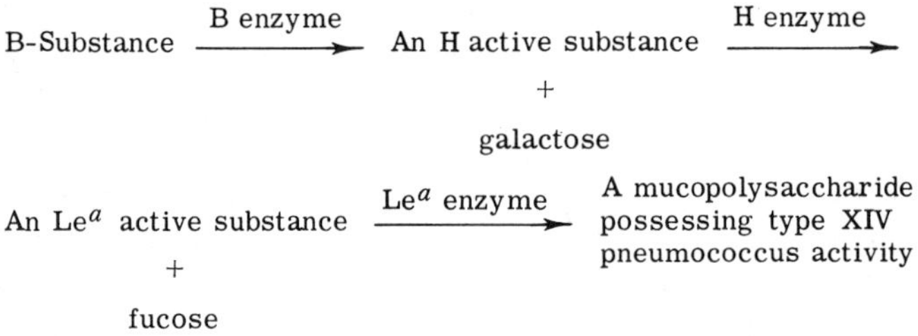

B-Substance —B enzyme→ An H active substance + galactose —H enzyme→

An Le^a active substance + fucose —Le^a enzyme→ A mucopolysaccharide possessing type XIV pneumococcus activity

FIG. 1. Changes in the specificity of human blood-group B substance induced by the sequential action of enzymes from *T. foetus*.

found to bring about a limited, but nevertheless considerable, loss of serological activity (Pusztai and Morgan, 1958, 1961c; Morgan and Pusztai, 1961). None of the carbohydrate components is liberated in a diffusible form and the same changes take place irrespective of the blood-group specificity of the mucopolysaccharide. The fall in serological activity is believed to result from the hydrolysis of a limited number of peptide or ester bonds with the consequent disruption of the secondary molecular structure. These results are of considerable interest because they show that, although the peptide moiety does not play a part in the primary specificity of the molecules, integrity of macromolecular structure is essential for the specific groupings to exert their maximum effect.

4. Partial Acid Hydrolysis of Blood-Group Substances

Mild acid hydrolysis of blood-group A, B, and H substances from animal or human sources results in destruction of blood-group activity as measured by the isoagglutination-inhibition test, marked increase in the capacity of the substances to cross-react with type XIV anti-pneumococcus horse serum (Kabat *et al.*, 1948), and in the case of A substance enhanced capacity to inhibit the hemolysis of sheep cells by rabbit anti-A serum (Aminoff *et al.*, 1948). The materials which are nondialyzable after mild acid hydrolysis of A and B substances also develop a new and independent specificity in addition to the capacity to cross-react with type XIV serum (Allen and Kabat, 1957, 1959). These new specificities have been called AP1 and BP1, but are not related to the P_1 factor of the blood-group P system.

TABLE VIII

OLIGOSACCHARIDE FRAGMENTS ISOLATED FROM HUMAN A SUBSTANCE

Number	Structure	Reference
(1)	*O*-β-D-galactosyl-(1→3)-*N*-acetyl-D-glucosamine	Côté and Morgan (1956); Schiffman *et al.* (1962a)
(2)	*O*-β-D-galactosyl-(1→4)-*N*-acetyl-D-glucosamine	Côté and Morgan (1956); Schiffman *et al.* (1962a)
(3)	*O*-α-*N*-acetyl-D-galactosaminoyl-(1→3)-D-galactose	Côté and Morgan (1956); Schiffman *et al.* (1962a)
(4)	*O*-β-*N*-acetyl-D-glucosaminoyl-(1→3)-D-galactose	Côté and Morgan (1956)
(5)	*O*-α-L-fucosyl-(1→6)-*N*-acetyl-D-glucosamine	Côté and Morgan (1956)
(6)	*O*-β-D-galactosyl-(1→3)-*N*-acetyl-D-galactosamine	Painter *et al.* (1962b)
(7)	*O*-α-*N*-acetyl-D-galactosaminoyl-(1→3)-*O*-β-D-galactosyl-(1→4)-*N*-acetyl-D-glucosamine	Cheese and Morgan (1961)
(8)	*O*-α-*N*-acetyl-D-galactosaminoyl-(1→3)-*O*-β-D-galactosyl-(1→3)-*N*-acetyl-D-glucosamine	Cheese and Morgan (1961); Schiffman *et al.* (1962a)

The oligosaccharides listed in Table VIII have been isolated from the partial acid hydrolysis products of human A substance. Disaccharide No. 2, *O*-β-D-galactosyl-(1→4)-*N*-acetyl-D-glucosamine, was earlier isolated from hog gastric mucin (Yosizawa, 1949, 1950a,b; Tomarelli *et al.*, 1954) and from meconium (Kuhn and Kirschenlohr, 1954). Only one of the six disaccharides, *O*-α-*N*-acetyl-D-galactosaminoyl-(1→3)-D-galactose (No. 3), inhibited in the A system (Côté and Morgan, 1956; Schiffman *et al.*, 1962a) and this disaccharide most probably corresponds to the first two units of the blood-group A antigenic determinant. The two trisaccharides, Nos. 7 and 8, both had the capacity to inhibit a number of anti-A reagents and, on a molar basis, were slightly more active than the active disaccharide (Cheese and Morgan, 1961).

Schiffman *et al.*, (1960) hydrolyzed a specimen of human group B substance by heating with mineral acid at pH 1.6 for 2 hours at 100° and, rather surprisingly, isolated from the hydrolysis products five fucose-containing oligosaccharides. None of the fragments had inhibitory activity in the B system. Hydrolysis of human B substance, with water-soluble polystyrene sulfonic acid as a catalyst in place of mineral acid (cf. Painter, 1960; Painter and

Morgan, 1961a,b), yielded a series of disaccharides of which one was characterized as *O*-α-D-galactosyl-(1→3)-D-galactose (Painter *et al.*, 1962a). This disaccharide was identical to the compound which had previously been demonstrated as the most active inhibitor in the B–anti-B system (see Section V, A, 1), and therefore most probably corresponds to the terminal units of the serologically active structure in group B substance.

Much more structural analysis is required before it will be possible to put forward a definitive structure for the carbohydrate chains of the blood-group mucopolysaccharides. The evidence available at present is compatible with the view that the chains are terminated by the sugar which plays a dominant role in specificity, and that the remainder of the chains are composed of alternating galactose and hexosamine units with fucose and sialic acid attached as branching units to this backbone chain. The presence of other sugars as branching units cannot, however, be excluded. As yet nothing is known of the structure and sequence of amino acids in the peptide part of the molecules, nor is it known how the carbohydrate and peptide units are linked together.[1]

B. A and B Substances from Red Cells

The most highly active blood-group A preparations isolated from red cells by Koscielak (1962) (see Section IV, C) have not been subjected to direct structural analysis. Indirect evidence that the serologically active groupings in the A and B substances isolated from red cells are chemically similar to the active structures in the secreted A and B substances, however, was obtained from serological and enzyme inhibition experiments and by an examination of the behavior of the two types of A substance in double diffusion tests in agar gel (Watkins *et al.*, 1962b). The inhibition data indicated that a nonreducing α-*N*-acetylgalactosaminoyl grouping is present in the A glycolipid blood-group substance, and a nonreducing α-galactosyl grouping in the B glycolipid blood-group substance. Therefore, at least insofar as the terminal nonreducing sugars which make an important contribution to specificity are concerned,

[1] The number of fragments isolated from the partial acid hydrolysis products of the water-soluble blood-group substances has now been increased by the isolation of two serologically active trisaccharides from B substance, *O*-α-D-galactopyranosyl-(1→3)-*O*-β-D-galactopyranosyl-(1→3)-*N*-acetyl-D-glucosamine and *O*-α-D-galactopyranosyl-(1→3)-*O*-β-D-galactopyranosyl-(1→4)-*N*-acetyl-D-glucosamine (Painter *et al.*, 1963a), four disaccharides from B, H, and Le^a substances (Painter *et al.*, 1963b) which are identical with four of the disaccharides previously isolated from A substance (Nos. 1, 2, 4, and 6; Table VIII), and three trisaccharides from A, B, H, and Le^a substances, *O*-β-D-galactopyranosyl-(1→3)-*O*-(*N*-acetyl-β-D-glucosaminoyl)-(1→3)-D-galactose, *O*-β-D-galactopyranosyl-(1→4)-*O*-(*N*-acetyl-β-D-glucosaminoyl)-(1→3)-D-galactose, and *O*-(*N*-acetyl-β-D-glucosaminopyranosyl)-(1→3)-*O*-β-D-galactopyranosyl-(1→3)-*N*-acetyl-D-galactosamine (Rege *et al.*, 1963). On the basis of these, and the earlier results, possible sequences for the sugar units in the carbohydrate chains of the blood-group substances have been proposed (Rege *et al.*, 1963).

the same structures appear to be present in the glycolipid A and B substances as in the secreted mucopolysaccharide substances.

In double diffusion tests in agar gel, the A substance isolated from the red cell gave a pattern of fusion with the mucopolysaccharide A substance when tested with an immune rabbit serum prepared by injection with group A cells. Such a pattern is normally interpreted as indicating that the antigens reacting with the antibody are identical. In this instance the substances are thought to be chemically dissimilar in overall composition, but the fusion of the precipitin bands suggests that the serologically active groupings associated with the two types of macromolecule are chemically identical.

C. M and N Substances from Red Cells

1. Serologically Active Structures

Springer and Ansell (1958) and, independently, Mäkelä and Cantell (1958) found that treatment of red cells with influenza virus or the receptor-destroying enzyme (RDE) from *Vibrio cholera* destroyed the M and N activity of the cells. The enzyme produced by the influenza virus and by *V. cholera* has been identified as a neuraminidase which specifically cleaves the ketosidic linkage joining *N*-acetylneuraminic acid (sialic acid) to another sugar or sugar derivative (cf. Gottschalk, 1960). These enzyme preparations had no action on A, B, H, P, or Rh activity and it was therefore concluded that *N*-acetylneuraminic acid forms an essential part of the M and N receptors.

Treatment of the isolated M and N substances with influenza virus (Romanowska, 1959a, 1960) or RDE (Klenk and Uhlenbruck, 1960) similarly resulted in loss of M and N specificity, and *N*-acetylneuraminic acid was shown to be the only component of the mucopolysaccharides liberated by the action of these enzymes. Therefore, unless the enzyme preparations are bringing about changes in the secondary structure of the M and N substances which result in loss of reactivity, it must be assumed that *N*-acetylneuraminic acid forms part of the serologically active structures responsible for both M and N specificities.

Nagai and Springer (1962), by treatment of isolated M substance with swine influenza virus, succeeded in destroying M activity with a concomitant increase in N activity. A similar increase in the N activity of M substance was observed after mild acid hydrolysis. These results suggest that N specific structures are latent in M substance.

2. Degradation with Proteolytic Enzymes

Treatment of M and N substances isolated by the phenol-saline method (see Section III, B, 2) with trypsin, α-chymotrypsin, pepsin, and papain, causes a fall in the M and N inhibition titers with the release of amino acids and peptides (Klenk and Uhlenbruck, 1960; Lisowska, 1960). The content of *N*-acetylneuraminic acid and other sugar components is not demonstrably changed, and it was suggested (Lisowska, 1960) that the action of the proteolytic enzymes involves the splitting of the macromolecule into smaller nondialyzable fragments. Therefore, although M and N active fragments can be obtained from red cells by the use of proteolytic enzymes (see Section III, B, 2), this procedure is not to be recommended as a method of preparation.

3. Isolation of Fragments by Partial Acid and Alkaline Hydrolysis

Very little direct structural work has been carried out on M and N substances and the value of such studies is, in any case, limited because none of the preparations so far described was shown to be homogeneous. Romanowska (1961) examined the products of mild acid and alkaline hydrolysis of M and N substances, and from the diffusible products after alkaline hydrolysis, isolated two disaccharides. One was identified as *N*-acetylneuraminoylgalactose, and the second as *N*-acetylneuraminoyl-*N*-acetylhexosamine. The M and N preparations therefore contain *N*-acetylneuraminic acid joined to both galactose and *N*-acetylhexosamine residues.

M substance, isolated by the phenol-saline method and further purified by fractional centrifugation, was subjected (Nagai and Springer, 1962) to partial acid hydrolysis with a nondiffusible acidic resin (cf. Painter, 1960) as the hydrolytic agent. Sialic acid, hexose, and at least two oligosaccharides were detected in the hydrolysis products, but free amino sugars and amino acids were absent. The hydrolysis products strongly inhibited a plant seed anti-N reagent.

D. Serologically Active Structures in P_1 Substance

The destruction of blood-group P_1 receptors on the red cell surface by treatment with dilute sodium periodate (Morgan and Watkins, 1951) indicated that the specific structures were carbohydrate in nature and, to investigate this possibility, 70 different simple sugars and polysaccharide materials were tested for capacity to inhibit the agglutination of P_1 cells by human anti-P_1 serum (Watkins and Morgan, 1962b). Only two compounds, 3-*O*-α- and 4-*O*-α-digalactoside, had the capacity to neutralize the agglutinating action of the anti-P_1 serum. An α-D-galactosyl unit may therefore be involved in P_1 specificity. A role for D-galactose in P_1 specificity was also supported by the observation that the enzymatic destruction of P_1 activity by an extract of *T. foetus* is specifically inhibited by D-galactose.

VI. Possible Genetical Pathways for the Biosynthesis of Blood-Group Substances

A. A, B, H, and Le^a Substances

The uncomplicated manner of inheritance of the blood-group antigens and the apparent absence of interaction of genes at different loci led earlier workers to suggest that the blood-group substances were the immediate products of the controlling genes (cf. Haldane, 1937). According to current theories, however, the gene is constituted of deoxyribonucleic acid (DNA), which carries information for the precise determination of the amino acid sequence of proteins (cf. Crick, 1958); proteins are therefore considered to be the only direct products of gene action. The formation of the carbohydrate structures which determine blood-group specificity is therefore at least one stage removed from the blood-group genes, and one must assume the function of these genes to be the formation of specific protein enzymes which subsequently effect, or control, the carbohydrate synthesis.

Possible pathways for the later stages of the biosynthesis of the A, B, H, and Le^{a} blood-group substances, which attempt to bring together the known biochemical, serological, and genetical data, have been proposed (Watkins, 1958, 1959; Watkins and Morgan, 1959; Ceppellini, 1959). A summary of the pathways which could account for the appearance of A, B, H, and Le^{a} activities in secretions and on the red cells is given in Fig. 2. Four independent gene systems, *L* and *l*; *H* and *h*; *A*, *B*, and *O*; and *Se* and *se*, are believed to control certain stages in the conversion of a precursor substance to the specific products which appear in the secretions. The substance found in the secretions of individuals who are nonsecretors of A, B, H, Le^{a}, or Le^{b} substances ("inactive substance, Fl" in Table IV) is believed to constitute the precursor substance which is converted into the blood-group active mucopolysaccharides. The genes, *L*, *H*, *A*, and *B* are active transforming genes; their respective alleles, *l*, *h*, and *O*, play no part in the conversion of the precursor materials, i.e., as far as the scheme is concerned they may be considered as inactive genes.

The gene *L* controls the conversion of the precursor mucopolysaccharide into Le^{a} substance, and the gene *H* the conversion of either Le^{a} or the precursor mucopolysaccharide into H substance. The transformation steps controlled by the *L* and *H* genes involve the addition of α-L-fucosyl units to different sugars in the precursor substance. The genes *Se* and *se* are the secretor genes of Schiff (see Section I, A), which operate at the level of the conversion of the precursor, or Le^{a} substance, into H substance. The gene *Se* may be considered to activate the *H* gene or, alternatively, the genes *se se* to suppress the action of the *H* gene. The net result is that in individuals homozygous for the gene *se*, H substance is not formed. Since H is the substrate on which the changes influenced by the *A* and *B* genes take place, failure to produce H substance results in the absence of A and B substances even if the corresponding genes are present. When H substance is formed, the A gene controls the addition of α-*N*-acetylgalactosaminoyl units to give A specific structures, and the *B* gene the addition of α-galactosyl units to give B active structures. In heterozygous AB individuals, the *A* and *B* genes both act on the H substrate to convert it to an AB substance. The inactive *O* gene brings about no further change in the H substance. It will be seen from Fig. 2 that the presence of various combinations of genes belonging to the four systems can account for the known secretor types (Table II).

Ceppellini (1955) suggested that Le^b specificity is the product of the interaction of the genes *Se* and *L*. If one considers that Le^b results from the inter-

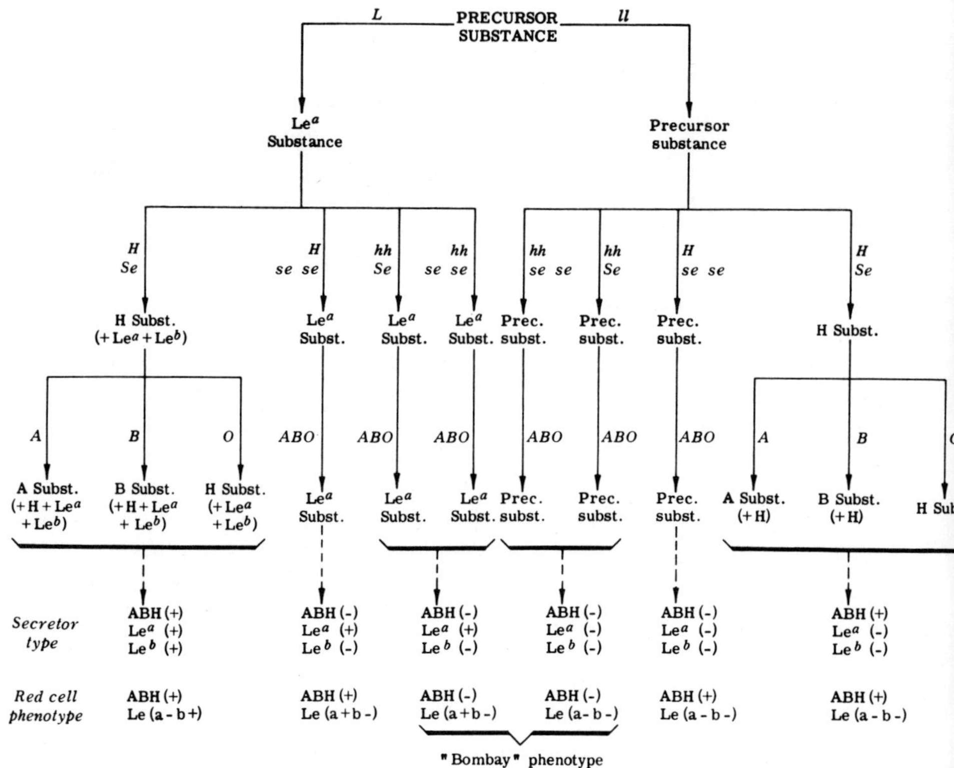

FIG. 2. Possible genetical pathways for the biosynthesis of blood-group A, B, H, Le^a, and Le^b substances.

action of the genes *H* and *L*, in place of Se and L, then it can be visualized that the addition of L-fucosyl units mediated by the *H* gene to Le^a substance, in which fucosyl groupings are already present, could result in the formation of a new specificity which does not result from the action of either gene alone.

The suggested scheme could account for the presence of the A, B, and H antigens on the red cell surface if it is assumed that the secretor genes *Se se* do not function at the red cell level, so that H substance is always formed from a precursor glycolipid when the corresponding *H* gene is present; the subsequent transformations to A and B can then proceed when the individual possesses the appropriate gene. Those very rare individuals who lack A, B, and H reactivity both in their secretions and on their red cells, i.e. the "Bombay" phenotype (cf. Race and Sanger, 1962), would be homozygous for the rare allele of *H*, namely *h*, which fails to provide a substrate for the *A* and *B* genes.

B. *M and N Substances*

Speculation on the pathway of biosynthesis of M and N substances may be premature when relatively so little is known of the chemical nature and structure of these substances. However, the presence of N activity in isolated M preparations derived from *MM* cells (Uhlenbruck, 1961b), the finding that both the M and N activity were associated with the same molecule (Uhlenbruck, 1961b), and the observation that the N activity of M preparations is enhanced after treatment with certain viruses or by hydrolysis with weak acid (Nagai and Springer, 1962) would be compatible with the suggestion that N formed the basic substrate on which the changes carried out under the influence of the *M* gene occur. The *N* gene would then have to be considered as an inactive gene, analogous to the *O* gene in the ABO system; in *NN* individuals the precursor substrate would appear unchanged, in *MN* individuals partial conversion to M would occur, and in *MM* individuals the conversion would be almost complete. The mechanism could be envisaged as the addition of *N*-acetylneuraminic acid units to certain chains in the basic N substance.

VII. Summary and Conclusions

The picture which can be given at present of the chemical nature of the blood-group substances is far from complete. Certain general concepts, however, have emerged from the facts established so far. One is that blood-group substances cannot be regarded as discrete molecular entities which, if obtained from individuals of the same group and freed from inactive materials, have a constant defined qualitative and quantitative composition. The weight of evidence suggests that the blood-group genes act late in the synthesis of the specific substances and do not control the formation of the complete blood-group active molecule. The A and B substances isolated from red cells, for example, appear to be glycolipid in nature, whereas in secretions the same specificities are associated with mucopolysaccharide substances. Moreover, as far as the secreted A, B, H, and Le^a substances are concerned, variations in fine structure and chemical composition occur according to the genetic constitution of the individuals from whom they are derived, because more than one specificity can be associated with the same mucopolysaccharide molecule.

Blood-group substances have in consequence to be regarded, to some extent, as molecules which carry chemical structures that are serologically specific rather than as substances which can in themselves be accurately defined. The evidence at present available, however, indicates that the chemical structures which confer blood-group activity on the macromolecules are identical for substances showing the same specificity, irrespective of the origin and overall chemical composition of the materials. The information gained from a study of the serologically active structures in blood-group specific materials derived from sources other than red cells can therefore be used to suggest the nature of the active structures in the red cell antigens. A summary of the units which have been implicated in the blood-group specificities investigated up to the present is given in Table IX. The A and B specific groupings are most firmly established because the active structures have been isolated and characterized from the partial acid hydrolysis products of mucopolysaccharide A and B substances. The units suggested for the other blood-group specificities are based on indirect evidence. In no one instance is it believed that the complete serologically determinant structure is yet elucidated.

TABLE IX

STRUCTURES PRESENT AS TERMINAL UNITS OF THE SEROLOGICALLY ACTIVE GROUPINGS IN BLOOD-GROUP SUBSTANCES

Blood group	Terminal units of specific grouping
A	*O*-α-*N*-acetyl-D-galactosaminoyl-(1→3)-D-galactosyl-
B	*O*-α-D-galactosyl-(1→3)-D-galactosyl-
H	*O*-α-L-fucosyl-?(1→2)- } *O*-β-*N*-acetyl-D-glucosaminoyl- }
Le[a]	*O*-α-L-fucosyl-(1→4)— > *O*-β-D-galactosyl-(1→3)— > *N*-acetyl-D-glucosaminoyl-
Le[b]	| *O*-α-L-fucosyl-R[a] | *O*-α-L-fucosyl-R |
M	*N*-acetylneuraminoyl-
N	*N*-acetylneuraminoyl-
P_1	*O*-α-D-galactosyl-
Type XIV pneumococcus reactivity of blood-group substances	*O*-β-D-galactosyl-(1→4)-*N*-acetylglucosaminoyl-

[a] Nature of sugar R not established.

Despite the demonstration that the specificity of the blood-group substances resides in the carbohydrate parts of the mucopolysaccharide or glycolipid substance, evidence has been obtained which shows that integrity of the complete macromolecule is essential if the maximum blood-group activity is to be obtained. Both the A, B, H, and Le^a mucopolysaccharides and the M and N mucopolysaccharides, for example, lose activity when treated with certain proteolytic enzymes which depolymerize the molecule by breaking a limited number of peptide bonds without changing the specific carbohydrate structures. Similarly, loss of activity of the glycolipid A and B substances can occur through the removal of inactive glycolipid material which presumably influences the state of aggregation of the active material and does not chemically alter the serologically reactive sites (see Section III, B, 1). The secondary structure of the molecules, or of the complexes formed by interaction of lipid molecules, must therefore play an important part in maintaining either (1) sufficient numbers of active groupings, and/or (2) the correct spatial orientation of the active groupings, and/or (3) secondary binding groupings, for firm combination with the homologous antibody to occur. The difficulties encountered in obtaining blood-group substances from the red cell which are highly active in hemagglutination-inhibition tests, may be due to the fact that the methods used for liberating the substances from the cell membrane destroy this secondary structure at the outset.

The function of the blood groups remains obscure. It is doubtful whether the groupings synthesized under the influence of the blood-group genes have a fundamental physiological function, because the absence of a product of a particular gene, for example, the *A* gene in the *ABO* system, does not give rise to a pathological condition. The macromolecules which carry blood-group specificity, however, undoubtedly have a function either as structural units of the red cell membrane or as constituents of the mucin which protects or lubricates normal epithelial surfaces; it is therefore possible that the changes produced under the influence of the blood-group genes enhance or suppress the normal physiological function of the macromolecules to which the specific structures are attached.

Advances in the elucidation of the chemical basis of blood-group specificity have lagged far behind the discoveries of the blood-group systems and the unravelling of their serological and genetical relationships. One factor which may have contributed to the slow advance is that the biochemist who undertakes the task of isolating a blood-group antigen has until recently found himself working with very small quantities of material and, in addition, may be confronted with problems in fields of organic chemistry in which he has previously had little experience; indeed he may find himself pioneering research on a new type of macromolecule for which there are no parallels in the chemical literature. However, with the rapidly developing interest in the chemistry of biologically active macromolecules and the recognition of the important contribution that a study of blood-group specificity can make to human biochemical genetics, there is little doubt that many of the present gaps in our knowledge will be filled within the next decade.

References

Allen, P. Z., and Kabat, E. A. (1957). *Federation Proc.* **16**, 404.

Allen, P. Z., and Kabat, E. A. (1958). *J. Immunol.* **82**, 358.

Allen, P. Z., and Kabat, E. A. (1959). *J. Am. Chem. Soc.* **81**, 340.

Aminoff, D., and Morgan, W. T. J. (1951). *Biochem. J.* **48**, 74.

Aminoff, D., Morgan, W. T. J., and Watkins, W. M. (1948). *Biochem. J.* **43**, xxxvi.

Aminoff, D., Morgan, W. T. J., and Watkins, W. M. (1950). *Biochem. J.* **46**, 426.

Andresen, P. H. (1948). *Acta Pathol. Microbiol. Scand.* **25**, 728.

Annison, E. F., and Morgan, W. T. J. (1952a). *Biochem. J.* **50**, 460.

Annison, E. F., and Morgan, W. T. J. (1952b). *Biochem. J.* **52**, 247.

Baer, H., Kabat, E. A., and Knaub, V. (1950). *J. Exptl. Med.* **91**, 105.

Baranowski, T., Lisowska, E., and Romanowska, E. (1956). *Arch. Immunol. Terapii Doswiadczalnej* **4**, 45.

Baranowski, T., Lisowska, E., Morawiecki, A., Romanowska, E., and Strozecka, K. (1959). *Arch. Immunol. Terapii Doswiadczalnej* **7**, 15.

Bendich, A., Kabat, E. A., and Bezer, A. E. (1946). *J. Exptl. Med.* **83**, 485.

Bernstein, F. (1924). *Klin. Wochschr.* **3**, 1495.

Bhende, Y. M., Deshpande, C. K., Bhatia, H. M., Sanger, R., Race, R. R., Morgan, W. T. J., and Watkins, W. M. (1952). *Lancet* **i**, 903.

Bird, G. W. G. (1959). *Brit. Med. Bull.* **15**, 165.

Boorman, K. E., and Dodd, B. E. (1943). *J. Pathol. Bacteriol.* **55**, 329.

Boyd, W. C. (1962). "Introduction to Immunochemical Specificity." Wiley (Interscience), New York.

Boyd, W. C., and Boyd, L. G. (1934). *J. Immunol.* **26**, 489.

Bray, H. G., Henry, H., and Stacey, M. (1946). *Biochem. J.* **40**, 124.

Brown, P. C., Glynn, L. E., and Holborow, E. J. (1959). *Vox Sanguinis* **4**, 1.

Buchanan, D. J., and Rapoport, S. (1951). *J. Biol. Chem.* **192**, 251.

Cameron, G. L., and Staveley, J. M. (1957). *Nature* **179**, 147.

Caspary, E. A. (1954). *Biochem. J.* **57**, 295.

Ceppellini, R. (1955). *Proc. 5th Intern. Congr. Blood Transfusion, Paris, 1954*, p. 207.

Ceppellini, R. (1959). *In* "Ciba Foundation Symposium on Biochemistry of Human Genetics" (G. E. W. Wolstenholme and C. M. O'Connor, eds.), p. 242, Little, Brown, Boston, Massachusetts.

Cheese, I. A. F. L., and Morgan, W. T. J. (1961). *Nature* **191**, 149.

Côté, R. H., and Morgan, W. T. J. (1956). *Nature* **178**, 1171.

Crick, F. H. C. (1958). *Symp. Soc. Exptl. Biol.* **12**, 138.

Decastello, A. von, and Sturli, A. (1902). *Muench. Med. Wochschr.* **49**, 1090.

Dungern, E. von, and Hirszfeld, L. (1910). *Z. Immunitaetsforsch.* **6**, 284.

Epstein, A. A., and Ottenberg, R. (1908). *Proc. N. Y. Pathol. Soc.* **8**, 117.

Gibbons, R. A., and Morgan, W. T. J. (1954). *Biochem. J.* **57**, 283.

Gibbons, R. A., Morgan, W. T. J., and Gibbons, M. (1955). *Biochem. J.* **60**, 428.

Glynn, L. E., and Holborow, E. J. (1959). *Brit. Med. Bull.* **15**, 150.

Gottschalk, A. (1960). "The Chemistry and Biology of Sialic Acids and Related Substances." Cambridge Univ. Press, London and New York.

Grubb, R. (1948). *Nature* **162**, 933.

Grubb, R. (1951). *Acta Pathol. Microbiol. Scand.* **28**, 61.

Grubb, R., and Morgan, W. T. J. (1949). *Brit. J. Exptl. Pathol.* **30**, 198.
Hakomori, S., and Jeanloz, R. W. (1961). *J. Biol. Chem.* **236**, 2827.
Haldane, J. B. S. (1937). *In* "Perspectives in Biochemistry" (J. Needham and D. E. Green, eds.), p. 1. Cambridge University Press.
Hallauer, C. (1934). *Z. Immunitaetsforsch.* **83**, 114.
Hirsch, W., Moores, P., Sanger, R., and Race, R. R. (1957). *Brit. J. Haematol.* **3**, 134.
Hiyama, N. (1962). *In* "Biochemistry and Medicine of Mucopolysaccharides" (F. Egami and Y. Oshima, eds.), p. 161. Maruzen, Tokyo.
Hohorst, H. J. (1954). *Z. Hyg. Infektionskrank.* **139**, 561.
Iseki, S., and Ikeda, T. (1956). *Proc. Japan Acad.* **32**, 201.
Iseki, S., and Masaki, S. (1953). *Proc. Japan Acad.* **29**, 460.
Iseki, S., and Okada, S. (1951). *Proc. Japan Acad.* **27**, 455.
Iseki, S., and Tsunoda, S. (1952). *Proc. Japan Acad.* **28**, 370.
Iseki, S., Furukawa, K., and Yamamoto, S. (1959a). *Proc. Japan Acad.* **35**, 507.
Iseki, S., Furukawa, K., and Yamamoto, S. (1959b). *Proc. Japan Acad.* **35**, 513.
Joysey, V. C. (1959). *Brit. Med. Bull.* **15**, 158.
Kabat, E. A. (1956). "Blood Group Substances; Their Chemistry and Immunochemistry." Academic Press, New York.
Kabat, E. A., and Leskowitz, S. (1955). *J. Am. Chem. Soc.* **77**, 5159.
Kabat, E. A., and Schiffman, G. (1962). *J. Immunol.* **88**, 782.
Kabat, E. A., Baer, H., Bezer, A. E., and Knaub, V. (1948). *J. Exptl. Med.* **87**, 295.
Kekwick, R. A. (1950). *Biochem. J.* **46**, 438.
Kekwick, R. A. (1952a). *Biochem. J.* **50**, 471.
Kekwick, R. A. (1952b). *Biochem. J.* **52**, 259.
Kent, P. W., and Whitehouse, M. W. (1955). "Biochemistry of Amino Sugars." Butterworths, London.
Klenk, E. (1941). *Z. Physiol. Chem.* **268**, 50.
Klenk, E., and Uhlenbruck, G. (1960). *Z. Physiol. Chem.* **319**, 151.
Knox, K., and Morgan, W. T. J. (1954). *Biochem. J.* **58**, V.
Koscielak, J. (1962). *Nature* **194**, 751.
Koscielak, J., and Zakrzewski, K. (1959). *In* "International Symposium on Biologically Active Mucoids", p. 21. Polish Acad. Science, Warsaw.
Koscielak, J., and Zakrzewski, K. (1960). *Nature* **187**, 516.
Kosjakov, P. N., and Tribulev, G. P. (1939). *J. Immunol.* **37**, 283.
Kuhn, R. (1957). *Angew. Chem.* **60**, 23.
Kuhn, R., and Baer, H. H. (1956). *Chem. Ber.* **89**, 504.
Kuhn, R., and Gauhe, A. (1958). *Ann. Chem.* **611**, 249.
Kuhn, R., and Gauhe, A. (1960). *Chem. Ber.* **93**, 647.
Kuhn, R., and Kirschenlohr, W. (1954). *Chem. Ber.* **87**, 560.
Kuhn, R., Baer, H. H., and Gauhe, A. (1956). *Chem. Ber.* **89**, 2514.
Kuhn, R., Baer, H. H., and Gauhe, A. (1958). *Chem. Ber.* **91**, 364.
Landsteiner, K. (1900). *Zentr. Bakteriol. Parasitenk. Abt. I*, **27**, 357.
Landsteiner, K. (1901). *Wien. Klin. Wochschr.* **14**, 1132.
Landsteiner, K. (1920). *Biochem. Z.* **104**, 280.
Landsteiner, K., and Levine, P. (1927a). *Proc. Soc. Exptl. Biol. Med.* **24**, 600.
Landsteiner, K., and Levine, P. (1927b). *Proc. Soc. Exptl. Biol. Med.* **24**, 941.
Landsteiner, K., and Levine, P. (1928a). *J. Exptl. Med.* **47**, 457.
Landsteiner, K., and Levine, P. (1928b). *J. Exptl. Med.* **48**, 731.
Landsteiner, K., and Scheer, J. van der (1925). *J. Exptl. Med.* **42**, 123.
Lehrs, H. (1930). *Z. Immunitaetsforsch.* **66**, 175.

Leskowitz, S., and Kabat, E. A. (1954). *J. Am. Chem. Soc.* **76**, 4887.
Levine, P., Bobbit, O. B., Waller, R. K., and Kuhmichel, A. (1951). *Proc. Soc. Exptl. Biol. Med.* **77**, 403.
Levine, P., Ottensooser, F., Celano, M. J., and Pollitzer, W. (1955). *Am. J. Phys. Anthropol.* **13**, 29.
Levine, P., Celano, M. J., and Staveley, J. M. (1958). *Vox Sanguinis* **3**, 434.
Lisowska, E. (1960). *Arch. Immunol. Terapii Doswiadczalnej* **8**, 235.
Mäkelä, O., and Cantell, K. (1958). *Ann. Med. Exptl. Biol. Fenniae (Helsinki)* **36**, 366.
Moore, S., and Stein, W. H. (1954). *J. Biol. Chem.* **211**, 893.
Morgan, W. T. J. (1959). *In* "International Symposium on Biologically Active Mucoids" p. 1. Polish Acad. Sci. Warsaw.
Morgan, W. T. J. (1960). *Proc. Roy. Soc. (London) Ser. B* **151**, 308.
Morgan, W. T. J. (1963). *Ann. N. Y. Acad. Sci.* **106,** 177.
Morgan, W. T. J., and Heyningen, R. van (1944). *Brit. J. Exptl. Pathol.* **25**, 5.
Morgan, W. T. J., and King, H. K. (1943). *Biochem. J.* **37**, 640.
Morgan, W. T. J., and Pusztai, A. (1961). *Biochem. J.* **81**, 648.
Morgan, W. T. J., and Watkins, W. M. (1948). *Brit. J. Exptl. Pathol.* **29**, 159.
Morgan, W. T. J., and Watkins, W. M. (1951). *Brit. J. Exptl. Pathol.* **32**, 34.
Morgan, W. T. J., and Watkins, W. M. (1953). *Brit. J. Exptl. Pathol.* **34**, 94.
Morgan, W. T. J., and Watkins, W. M. (1956). *Nature* **177**, 521.
Morgan, W. T. J., and Watkins, W. M. (1962). *Proc. 9th Intern. Congr. Blood Transfusion, Mexico City, 1962*, p. 225. Karger, Basel/New York.
Morton, J. A., and Pickles, M. M. (1951). *J. Clin. Pathol.* **4**, 189.
Mourant, A. E. (1946). *Nature* **158**, 237.
Mourant, A. E. (1954). "The Distribution of the Human Blood Groups." Blackwell, Oxford.
Nagai, Y., and Springer, G. F. (1962). *Federation Proc.* **21**, 67.
Naylor, I., and Baer, H. (1959). *J. Bact.* **77**, 771.
Painter, T. J. (1960). *Chem. & Ind. (London)* 1214.
Painter, T. J., and Morgan, W. T. J. (1961a). *Nature* **191**, 39.
Painter, T. J., and Morgan, W. T. J. (1961b). *Chem. & Ind. (London)* 437.
Painter, T. J., Watkins, W. M., and Morgan, W. T. J. (1962a). *Nature* **193**, 1042.
Painter, T. J., Cheese, I. A. F. L., and Morgan, W. T. J. (1962b). *Chem. & Ind. (London)* 1535
Painter, T. J., Watkins, W. M., and Morgan, W. T. J. (1963a). *Nature* **199**, 282.
Painter, T. J., Rege, V. P., and Morgan, W. T. J. (1963b). *Nature* **199**, 569.
Pettenkofer, H. J. (1955). *Proc. 5th Intern. Congr. Blood Transfusion, Paris, 1954*, p. 91.
Prokop, O., and Oesterle, P. (1958). *Blut* **4**, 157.
Pusztai, A., and Morgan, W. T. J. (1958). *Nature* **182**, 648.
Pusztai, A., and Morgan, W. T. J. (1961a). *Biochem. J.* **78**, 135.
Pusztai, A., and Morgan, W. T. J. (1961b). *Biochem. J.* **80**, 107.
Pusztai, A., and Morgan, W. T. J. (1961c). *Biochem. J.* **81**, 639.
Pusztai, A., and Morgan, W. T. J. (1963). *Biochem. J.* **88,** 546.
Putkonen, T. (1930). *Acta Soc. Med. Fenn.* **A14**, No. 2, 107.
Race, R. R., and Sanger, R. (1962). "Blood Groups in Man," 4th ed. Blackwell, Oxford.
Radin, N. S. (1957). *Federation Proc.* **16**, 825.
Rapoport, S., and Buchanan, D. J. (1950). *Science* **112**, 150.
Rege, V. P., Painter, T. J., Watkins, W. M., and Morgan, W. T. J. (1963). *Nature* **200,** 532.
Roberts, F. (1959). *Brit. Med. Bull.* **15**, 119.
Romanowska, E. (1959a). *Arch. Immunol. Terapii Doswiadczalnej* **7**, 749.
Romanowska, E. (1959b). *Arch. Immunol. Terapii Doswiadczalnej* **7**, 759.

Romanowska, E. (1960). *Naturwissenschaften* **47**, 66.
Romanowska, E. (1961). *Nature* **191**, 1408.
Rondle, C. J. M. (1954). "The Action of Hypoiodous Acid on Blood Group Substances," Thesis for Ph.D. degree. Univ. London.
Rosenfield, R., and Vogel, P. (1951). *Trans. N. Y. Acad. Sci.* **13**, 213.
Ruszkiewicz, M. (1958). "A Contribution to the Technique of Analyzing Mucopolysaccharides," Thesis for Ph.D. degree. Univ. London.
Sanger, R. (1955). *Nature* **176**, 1163.
Schiff, F., and Adelsberger, L. (1924). *Z. Immunitaetsforsch.* **40**, 335.
Schiff, F., and Sasaki, H. (1932). *Klin. Wochschr.* **34**, 1426.
Schiffman, G., Kabat, E. A., and Leskowitz, S. (1960). *J. Am. Chem. Soc.* **82**, 1122.
Schiffman, G., Kabat, E. A., and Leskowitz, S. (1962a). *J. Am. Chem. Soc.* **84**, 73.
Schiffman, G., Kabat, E. A., and Thompson, W. (1962b). *J. Am. Chem. Soc.* **84**, 463.
Sneath, J. S., and Sneath, P. H. A. (1959). *Brit. Med. Bull.* **15**, 154.
Springer, G. F. (1958). *In* "Ciba Foundation Symposium on Chemistry and Biology of Mucopolysaccharides," p. 200. Churchill, London.
Springer, G. F., and Ansell, N. J. (1958). *Proc. Natl. Acad. Sci. U.S.* **44**, 182.
Stalder, K., and Springer, G. F. (1960). *Federation Proc.* **19**, 70.
Stalder, K., and Springer, G. F. (1961). *Proc. Congr. European Soc. Haematol, 8th Vienna, 1961* p. 489.
Szulman, A. E. (1960). *J. Exptl. Med.* **111**, 785.
Szulman, A. E. (1962). *J. Exptl. Med.* **115**, 977.
Thomsen, O., Friedenreich, V., and Worsaae, E. (1930). *Acta Path. Microbiol. Scand.* **7**, 157.
Tomarelli, R. M., Hassinen, J. B., Eckhardt, E. R., Clark, R. H., and Bernhardt, F. W. (1954). *Arch. Biochem. Biophys.* **48**, 225.
Tyler, H. M., and Watkins, W. M. (1960). *Biochem. J.* **74**, 2P.
Uhlenbruck, G. (1961a). *Nature* **190**, 181.
Uhlenbruck, G. (1961b). *Z. Immunitaetsforsch.* **121**, 420.
Watkins, W. M. (1953). *Biochem. J.* **54**, xxxiii.
Watkins, W. M. (1955). *Proc. 5th Intern. Congr. Blood Transfusion, Paris, 1954*, p. 306.
Watkins, W. M. (1956). *Biochem. J.* **64**, 21P.
Watkins, W. M. (1958). *Proc. 7th Intern. Congr. Blood Transfusion, Rome, 1958*, p. 692.
Watkins, W. M. (1959). *In* "Ciba Foundation Symposium on Biochemistry of Human Genetics" (G. E. W. Wolstenholme and C. M. O'Connor, eds.), p. 217. Little, Brown, Boston, Massachusetts.
Watkins, W. M. (1960). *Bull. Soc. Chim. Biol.* **42**, 1599.
Watkins, W. M. (1962). *Immunology* **5**, 245.
Watkins, W. M., and Morgan, W. T. J. (1952). *Nature* **169**, 852.
Watkins, W. M., and Morgan, W. T. J. (1954). *Brit. J. Exptl. Pathol.* **35**, 181.
Watkins, W. M., and Morgan, W. T. J. (1955a). *Vox Sanguinis* **5** (old series), 1.
Watkins, W. M., and Morgan, W. T. J. (1955b). *Nature* **175**, 676.
Watkins, W. M., and Morgan, W. T. J. (1956). *Nature* **178**, 1289.
Watkins, W. M., and Morgan, W. T. J. (1957a). *Acta Genet. Statist. Med.* **6**, 521.
Watkins, W. M., and Morgan, W. T. J. (1957b). *Nature* **180**, 1038.
Watkins, W. M., and Morgan, W. T. J. (1959). *Vox Sanguinis* **4**, 97.
Watkins, W. M., and Morgan, W. T. J. (1962a). *Vox Sanguinis* **7**, 129.
Watkins, W. M., and Morgan, W. T. J. (1962b). *Proc. 9th Intern. Congr. Blood Transfusion, Mexico City, 1962*, p. 230. Karger, Basel/New York.
Watkins, W. M., Zarnitz, M. L., and Kabat, E. A. (1962a). *Nature* **195**, 1204.

Watkins, W. M., Koscielak, J., and Morgan, W. T. J. (1962b). *Proc. 9th Intern. Congr. Blood Transfusion, Mexico City, 1962*, p. 213. Karger, Basel/New York.

Westphal, O., Luderitz, O., and Bister, F. (1952). *Z. Naturforsch.* **7b**, 148.

Wiener, A. S. (1943). "Blood Groups and Transfusion," 3rd ed. Thomas, Springfield, Illinois.

Yamakami, K. (1926). *J. Immunol.* **12**, 185.

Yamakawa, T., and Iida, T. (1953). *Jap. J. Exptl. Med.* **23**, 327.

Yamakawa, T., and Suzuki, S. (1951). *J. Biochem* (*Tokyo*) **38**, 199.

Yamakawa, T., and Suzuki, S. (1952). *J. Biochem.* (*Tokyo*) **39**, 393.

Yamakawa, T., Matsumoto, M., Suzuki, S., and Iida, T. (1956). *J. Biochem.* (*Tokyo*) **43**, 41.

Yamakawa, T., Ohta, R., Ichikawa, Y., and Osaki, J. (1958). *Compt. Rend. Soc. Biol.* **152**, 1288.

Yamakawa, T., Irie, R., and Iwanaga, M. (1960). *J. Biochem.* (*Tokyo*) **48**, 490.

Yosida, K. (1928). *Z. Ges. Exptl. Med.* **63**, 331.

Yosizawa, Z. (1949). *Tohoku J. Exptl. Med.* **51**, 51.

Yosizawa, Z. (1950a). *Tohoku J. Exptl. Med.* **52**, 111.

Yosizawa, Z. (1950b). *Tohoku J. Exptl. Med.* **52**, 145.

Zacho, A. (1932). *Z. Immunitaetsforsch.* **77**, 520.

Zarnitz, M. L., and Kabat, E. A. (1960). *J. Am. Chem. Soc.* **82**, 3953.

CHAPTER 11

Metabolic Processes Involved in the Formation and Reduction of Methemoglobin in Human Erythrocytes

Ernst R. Jaffé

I. Introduction[1]

Intraerythrocytic methemoglobin is incapable of serving in the transportation of oxygen to the tissues because the iron of the heme moiety has been

[1] In this discussion, the following abbreviations have been used:
NAD and NADH: the oxidized and reduced forms, respectively, of nicotinamide adenine dinucleotide (diphosphopyridine nucleotide). NADP and NADPH: the oxidized and reduced forms, respectively, of nicotinamide adenine dinucleotide phosphate (triphosphopyridine nucleotide). GSSG and GSH: the oxidized and reduced forms, respectively, of glutathione. G-6-P: glucose-6-phosphate. FAD: flavin adenine dinucleotide. FMN: flavin mononucleotide.

oxidized to the ferric state. Methemoglobin (ferric protoporphyrin IX-globin) imparts a brownish color to the blood and has an absorption spectrum with a characteristic maximum at about 632 mμ. The problem of methemoglobin formation has been reviewed extensively by Lemberg and Legge (1949) and Bodansky (1951), while the clinical and therapeutic implications of methemoglobinemia have been summarized by Finch (1948), Gibson (1954), and Gerald (1960). Parenthetically, it must be emphasized that "methemoglobinemia" is a misnomer, for the pigment under discussion here is intraerythrocytic, not circulating in the plasma. The present discussion will be restricted to a consideration of "normal" methemoglobin that apparently involves only the valence change of the iron without alteration in the globin moiety. An entirely different problem is presented by the genetically determined abnormal methemoglobins (hemoglobin M's) in which abnormal absorption spectra (Hörlein and Weber, 1948), altered electrophoretic mobility (Gerald, 1958), and amino acid substitutions in the protein (Gerald and Efron, 1961) have been described.

The concentration of methemoglobin in erythrocytes at any given moment must result from the equilibrium between the rate of formation of methemoglobin and the rate of reduction to hemoglobin. Although it is difficult to dissociate these two processes, much recent investigative effort has been directed toward understanding the mechanisms by which methemoglobin is reduced to hemoglobin. Considerable species variation in susceptibility to methemoglobin-producing agents and in ability of erythrocytes to reduce methemoglobin to hemoglobin has been described (Lester, 1943; Kiese and Weis, 1943; Matthies, 1957a; Malz, 1961–1962). The sensitivity of intracorpuscular hemoglobin to oxidation and the rate of reduction of methemoglobin to hemoglobin appear to differ in the erythrocytes of human subjects with various clinical disorders (Jalavisto and Salmela, 1961; Metcalf, 1962). Because of these complicating factors, this discussion will consider,.primarily, the mechanisms involved in the protection of hemoglobin against oxidation and in the reduction of methemoglobin to hemoglobin in human erythrocytes of normal subjects. Studies of human erythrocytes with metabolic abnormalities have contributed to the understanding of normal mechanisms and, where pertinent, such studies will be included.

II. Biological Effects of Methemoglobin

A. *Physiological Effects in Man*

Methemoglobin comprises 1% or less of the total hemoglobin content of normal human erythrocytes (Bodansky, 1951; Gibson, 1954). Man can tolerate a moderate degree of methemoglobinemia with only mild symptoms attributable to the lowered oxygen-carrying capacity of the blood. Cyanosis becomes apparent when methemoglobin is present in a concentration of about 1.5 gm./100 ml. blood (Finch, 1948). In the rare disorder, hereditary methemoglobinemia associated with an enzymatic deficiency, concentrations of 20–45% methemoglobin are tolerated with only mild exertional dyspnea, occasional headache, and minimal compensatory polycythemia (Gibson and Harrison, 1947; Finch, 1948; Eder *et al.*, 1949; Jaffé, 1959). Similar concentrations of methemoglobin, resulting from the administration of appropriate drugs, can be tolerated (Bodansky, 1951; Beutler and Mikus, 1961a, b). A concentration of 85–90% methemoglobin has been found to be lethal in dogs (Vandenbelt *et al.*, 1944), but the concentration of methemoglobin at which coma and death occur in man is unknown.

In addition to the obvious effect of lowering the oxygen-carrying capacity of the erythrocytes, methemoglobin has been implicated in altering the oxygen dissociation curve of the remaining hemoglobin (Gibson, 1954). Drug-induced methemoglobinemia apparently results in a shift in the oxygen dissociation curve to the left with decreased release of oxygen to the tissues (Darling and Roughton, 1942; Beutler and Mikus, 1961a). In contrast, normal oxygen dissociation curves have been obtained with erythrocytes from several cases of hereditary methemoglobinemia (Eder *et al.*, 1949; Waisman *et al.*, 1952), while abnormal curves have been found with cells from other cases (Gibson, 1954). Whether these differences between hereditary and acquired methemoglobinemia result from oxidation of different numbers of the four hemes of each hemoglobin molecule, or whether there may exist aberrations in the globin which interfere with normal heme-heme interactions, remains to be determined. Further investigations are warranted to resolve the apparently contradictory observations about the influence of methemoglobin on the oxygen dissociation curve (see also Chapter 9).

Therapy for toxic methemoglobinemia may be required, if severe symptoms are present. Methylene blue (Steele and Spink, 1933; Williams and Challis, 1933) is effective when administered in a dose of 1–2 mg./kg. body weight. In hereditary methemoglobinemia associated with an enzymatic deficiency, treatment with ascorbic acid, 500 mg. per day (Lian *et al.*, 1939; King *et al.*, 1947; Gibson and Harrison, 1947), or with methylene blue may be indicated for cosmetic reasons. The probable mechanisms of action of these compounds are discussed below.

B. Effect on the Life Span of Erythrocytes

As an isolated change, the presence of methemoglobin did not shorten the life span of human erythrocytes. Erythrocytes of subjects with hereditary methemoglobinemia due to an enzymatic defect survived normally in the circulation of a normal recipient (Hurley *et al.*, 1954) and in the subject's own circulation (Harris, 1963). Beutler and Mikus (1961a) observed a slight increase in the apparent life span of erythrocytes in subjects with sickle cell disease in whom concentrations of greater than 20% methemoglobin were maintained by the administration of sodium nitrite. Rats given sodium nitrite did not manifest evidence of accelerated erythrocyte destruction (Beutler and Mikus, 1961b) and dogs did not become anemic during chronic sodium nitrite administration (Clark and Morrissey, 1951). In contrast, mice fed sodium nitrite did develop a hemolytic anemia and Heinz bodies were noted in most of the erythrocytes (Richardson, 1941). Thus, species variation appears to play a role in the influence of methemoglobin on the *in vivo* destruction of erythrocytes. The presence of methemoglobin did not increase the spontaneous hemolysis of human erythrocytes *in vitro* (Jaffé, 1959; Vella, 1959).

C. Role of Methemoglobin in the Catabolism of Hemoglobin

Although the formation of methemoglobin, choleglobin, and Heinz bodies is discussed in Chapter 8, it is pertinent to consider here the role of methemoglobin in the breakdown of hemoglobin. Lemberg and Legge (1949) suggested that methemoglobin was an intermediate in the pathway leading from hemoglobin to "sulfhemoglobin" or choleglobin, and Webster (1949) implicated methemoglobin formation in the drug-induced hemolytic anemias. Methemoglobin formation preceded Heinz body formation and hemoglobin denaturation in rats intoxicated with nitrobenzol (Magos and Sziza, 1959). Harley and Mauer (1961) never observed destruction of intact hemoglobin without production of methemoglobin upon incubating human erythrocytes with various oxidant compounds. These findings led to the suggestion that methemoglobin was an essential stage in the destruction of hemoglobin. Jandl and his associates (Jandl *et al.*, 1960; Allen and Jandl, 1961) have described a sequence of changes in human erythrocytes and solutions of hemoglobin incubated with acetylphenylhydrazine in which methemoglobin formation preceded oxidation of the sulfhydryl groups of hemoglobin. However, this latter group of investigators emphasized that damage to enzymes and the erythrocyte membrane may actually account for hemolysis *in vivo* and spherocytosis *in vitro* (Allen and Jandl, 1961; Jacob and Jandl, 1962), a possibility which was also suggested by Beutler (1959). Recent studies have indicated that methemoglobin formation may not be an essential step in the degradation of hemoglobin or the destruction of erythrocytes (Beutler and Baluda, 1962; Beutler, 1962).

Further investigations will be required to establish whether methemoglobin formation is a necessary or just a possible step in the degradation of hemoglobin. The exact relationship of methemoglobin formation to the destruction of human erythrocytes *in vivo*, upon exposure to certain drugs or at the end of the normal life span of these cells, also remains to be determined. Perhaps the formation of methemoglobin takes place coincidentally with irreversible alterations in the essential structures of the erythrocyte membrane.

III. Formation of Methemoglobin

The oxidation of hemoglobin to methemoglobin, involving the loss of an electron and a proton, is still incompletely understood. The various processes that may lead to oxidation of the ferrous iron of the heme moiety have been discussed in detail by Lemberg and Legge (1949) and Bodansky (1951). Direct oxidation of the ferrous iron can be effected by such compounds as ferricyanide, chlorate, nitrate, quinones, and certain dyes with high oxidation-reduction potential. Just how nitrite, one of the most widely used methemoglobin-forming compounds, oxidizes the heme has not been defined completely. An electron hiatus between molecular oxygen and intracellular electron donors exists in the mature mammalian erythrocyte, for this cell lacks cytochrome oxidase and an intact cytochrome system (Rubinstein *et al.*, 1956). This hiatus, however, may be filled by substances in the plasma that already are or that can be converted to forms that can serve as hydrogen acceptors. Thus, extensive methemoglobin formation can result from the formation of active intermediates from aromatic amino or nitro compounds, ascorbic acid, or metabolic products of bacteria and tissues. Although the formation of hydrogen peroxide or equivalent free radicals has been implicated in the coupled oxidation of hemoglobin and a reducing agent in the presence of oxygen (Rostorfer and Cormier, 1957), actual formation of hydrogen peroxide during the autoxidation of hemoglobin has not been demonstrated (Keilin, 1961). Autoxidation of hemoglobin to methemoglobin may occur, perhaps through the formation of intermediates of oxyhemoglobin or reduced hemoglobin. Itano and Robinson (1958) have been able to separate, electrophoretically, intermediate compounds during partial oxidation of carbonmonoxyhemoglobin. Methemoglobin may be formed, therefore, through the direct action of oxidants, through the coaction of hydrogen donors and atmospheric oxygen, or through the autoxidation of hemoglobin.

Oxidation of hemoglobin to methemoglobin *in vitro* occurs at a slow rate. Intact human erythrocytes, incubated at 37°C. without added substrate, contain about 70% methemoglobin after 7 days, while a solution of crystalline human hemoglobin is completely oxidized in the same period of time (Jandl *et al.*, 1960). In hemolyzed erythrocytes, oxidation proceeds to completion in about 5 days (Eder *et al.*, 1949). These studies on the oxidation of hemoglobin *in vitro* do not indicate the true extent to which methemoglobin is formed *in vivo*. There is little direct evidence that extensive methemoglobin formation actually takes place in the normal human erythrocyte while in the circulation. The presence of a small but definite amount of methemoglobin in normal human

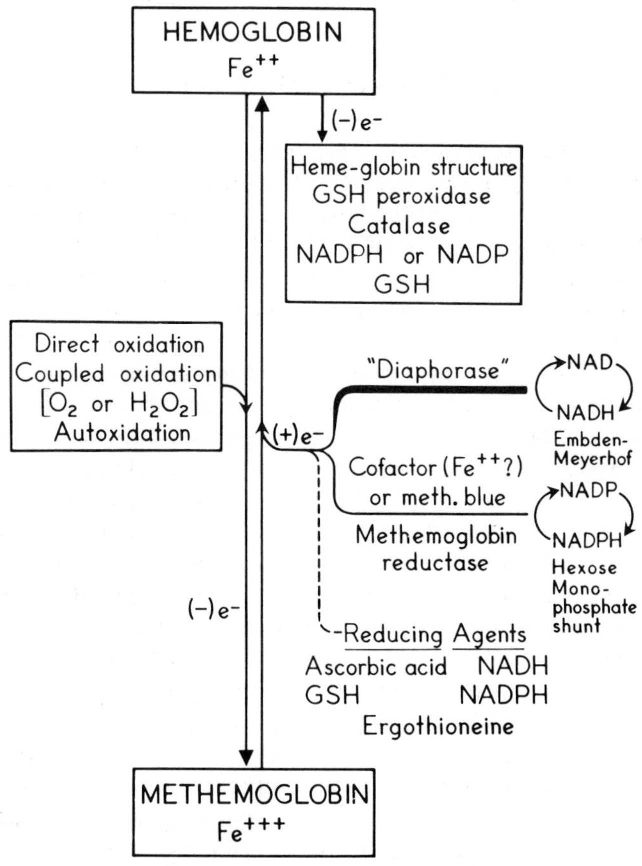

FIG. 1. Schematic representation of the metabolic processes involved in the oxidation of hemoglobin to methemoglobin, the protection against oxidation, and the reduction of methemoglobin to hemoglobin in human erythrocytes.

blood suggests that some tendency for oxidation does exist. Perhaps the best evidence for methemoglobin formation in the circulating erythrocyte comes from studies on patients with hereditary methemoglobinemia due to an enzymatic defect. It has been observed that approximately 0.5–3% of the hemoglobin is oxidized per day, after all the methemoglobin has been reduced to hemoglobin by the administration of methylene blue (Eder *et al.*, 1949;

Waisman *et al.*, 1952). An equilibrium between hemoglobin and methemoglobin formation appears to be attained in the erythrocytes of these subjects at a methemoglobin concentration of 30–40% (Finch, 1948).

The possible mechanisms for the oxidation of hemoglobin to methemoglobin are presented schematically in Fig. 1.

IV. Protection against Formation of Methemoglobin

Several mechanisms appear to exist within human erythrocytes to prevent the oxidation of hemoglobin. Oxyhemoglobin is more resistant to oxidation than is reduced hemoglobin. The availability of the heme groups may, therefore, influence the susceptibility to oxidation. The heme groups lie within hydrophobic groups of globin in an environment of relatively low dielectric constant where they may be protected. The electron hiatus between molecular oxygen and the intracellular electron donors, such as heme, globin, ferrous iron, and sulfhydryl compounds, may prevent extensive oxidation under normal conditions. These factors could account for the rather slow oxidation of hemoglobin that is observed under *in vitro* conditions. However, a number of active protective mechanisms have been the subject of extensive investigation in recent years.

A. Glutathione Peroxidase

Mills has demonstrated the presence of an enzyme, glutathione peroxidase, in rat and bovine erythrocytes that catalyzes the reaction:

$$H_2O_2 + 2GSH \longrightarrow 2H_2O + GSSG$$

Glutathione peroxidase does not appear to be a heme enzyme; its activity is not inhibited by azide (a catalase inhibitor) and it can be separated from both hemoglobin and catalase by cellulose anion exchange column chromatography (Mills, 1959). Evidence has been presented (Mills, 1957, 1959, 1962; Mills and Randall, 1958) that this enzyme system protects hemoglobin against coupled oxidation to methemoglobin and choleglobin by ascorbic acid, cysteine, epinephrine, or acetylphenylhydrazine. Glutathione peroxidase activity is dependent upon regeneration of adequate amounts of GSH through the glutathione reductase reaction:

$$GSSG + NADPH + H^+ \longrightarrow 2GSH + NADP$$

NADPH is generated through the reactions of the hexose monophosphate shunt pathway that are indicated in Fig. 1 and that are described in detail in Chapters 4, 5, and 6.

Cohen and Hochstein (1961, 1963) have presented evidence that glutathione peroxidase played the major role in the destruction of hydrogen peroxide in human and duck erythrocytes. They observed (1961) that the steady state perfusion of hydrogen peroxide through suspensions of normal human erythrocytes failed to lower the concentration of GSH when glucose was provided in the incubation medium. Human erythrocytes deficient in G-6-P dehydrogenase activity and, therefore, unable to regenerate adequate amounts of NADPH, were studied under similar experimental conditions. A marked drop in GSH concentration and an increase in methemoglobin concentration occurred in these enzyme-deficient erythrocytes, even in the presence of an adequate supply of glucose. Although Szeinberg and Marks (1961) were unable to demonstrate glutathione peroxidase activity in human erythrocytes, Hill *et al.* (1962) obtained suggestive evidence for the existence of this enzyme in the nonhemoglobin protein fraction of human erythrocytes.

Because of the failure to demonstrate hydrogen peroxide formation during autoxidation of hemoglobin, it is unclear how important the glutathione peroxidase system is in protecting hemoglobin against oxidation under physiological conditions. The significance of this enzyme system in protecting hemoglobin against oxidative damage by various drugs appears to have been more definitely established.

B. Catalase

Human erythrocytes are rich in the enzyme catalase that can decompose hydrogen peroxide (Lemberg and Legge, 1949). The activity of catalase, favored at high concentration of hydrogen peroxide, is represented as:

$$2H_2O_2 \longrightarrow 2H_2O + O_2$$

Peroxidatic activity of catalase, favored at low concentration of hydrogen peroxide, might function physiologically to remove any hydrogen peroxide formed within erythrocytes:

$$H_2O_2 + R\begin{matrix}/OH\\ \backslash OH\end{matrix} \longrightarrow 2H_2O + R\begin{matrix}/\!\!/O\\ \backslash\!\!\backslash O\end{matrix}$$

Bingold (1933) attempted to prove that the function of catalase in the erythrocyte was to protect the hemoglobin against oxidation, but he employed unphysiologically high concentrations of hydrogen peroxide. Keilin and Hartree (1945) observed no protection against methemoglobin formation from catalase activity when hydrogen peroxide was generated slowly by glucose oxidase. Cohen and Hochstein (1963) found that acatalasic duck and azide-blocked human erythrocytes were protected against methemoglobin formation as long as an adequate supply of glucose was present. These latter observations suggested that catalase may be unimportant in preventing oxidation of hemoglobin. However, erythrocytes obtained from human subjects with hereditary acatalasemia were much more susceptible to the formation of methemoglobin upon the addition of hydrogen peroxide (Takahara *et al.*, 1960) or upon x-ray irradiation (Aebi *et al.*, 1962) than were normal human erythrocytes. Thus, the role of catalase in the protection of hemoglobin against oxidation to methemoglobin under physiological conditions remains unknown.

C. Other Possible Protective Mechanisms

If the formation of hydrogen peroxide was essential for the oxidation of hemoglobin to methemoglobin, the two enzymes whose activities were summarized above, glutathione peroxidase and catalase, could serve to remove this oxidant upon its formation within the cell. Other protective mechanisms have been suggested. A direct protective effect of GSH has been implied (Allen and Jandl, 1961; Harley and Mauer, 1961), but not established. Recent studies with acetylphenylhydrazine (Desforges, 1962) and with sodium nitrite (Harley and Robin, 1962b) have demonstrated the formation of methemoglobin without a decrease in the concentration of GSH. Harley and Robin (1962b) suggested that methemoglobin formation buffered the intact erythrocyte against nitrite-induced depletion of the GSH. Beutler and Kelly (1963) have reported that the apparent destruction of erythrocyte GSH by sodium nitrite may be an artifact produced during the protein precipitation step in the determination of GSH. Although GSH and cysteine could reduce methemoglobin to hemoglobin (Morrison and Williams, 1938; Holmquist and Vinograd, 1963), these compounds may be of greater importance in protecting the sulfhydryl groups of enzymes and other proteins and in preventing "sulfhemoglobin" or choleglobin formation than in protecting against oxidation of hemoglobin to methemoglobin.

Ergothioneine, another sulfhydryl compound, was reported to be present in normal human erythrocytes in a concentration of about 10 mg./100 ml. erythrocytes (Touster and Yarbro, 1952), about 12–17% of the concentration of GSH. Spicer and his associates (1951) found that erythrocytes from rabbits depleted of ergothioneine by dietary restriction were more susceptible to methemoglobin formation upon exposure to nitrite than were erythrocytes from nondepleted rabbits. No alteration in concentration of GSH in the blood of the depleted rabbits was noted. Just what significance ergothioneine may have in human erythrocytes has not been investigated, although Klebanoff (1962) described an ergothioneine-dependent oxidation of NADH by a hemolysate of human erythrocytes.

NADP and NADPH, but not GSH, have been found to be important to the stability of such proteins as G-6-P dehydrogenase (Marks *et al.*, 1961; Kirkman, 1959). Szeinberg and Marks (1961) found that NADP and NADPH could protect hemoglobin against denaturation to choleglobin by ascorbic acid. The nicotinamide nucleotides may, therefore, afford protection against oxidation of hemoglobin without mediation through GSH formation.

Future investigations should provide more information about the relative importance of the various mechanisms by which hemoglobin may be shielded against oxidation. These protective mechanisms are indicated in Fig. 1.

Despite the relative stability of oxyhemoglobin and the incompletely unraveled protective mechanisms, a small amount of methemoglobin is present in human erythrocytes under normal conditions. Methemoglobin is most certainly formed after exposure of erythrocytes, either *in vivo* or *in vitro*, to certain drugs and chemicals. Toxic methemoglobinemia does not persist for more than 12–24 hours after the offending agent is withdrawn or metabolized (Finch, 1948; Bodansky, 1951). It is apparent, therefore, that there must exist within normal human erythrocytes processes that can reduce methemoglobin to functional, oxygen-carrying hemoglobin.

V. Reduction of Methemoglobin to Hemoglobin

A. General Considerations

That methemoglobin could be reduced to hemoglobin *in vivo* has been known since at least the end of the nineteenth century (Dittrich, 1892; Haldane *et al.*, 1897). That this reduction occurred within erythrocytes and would take place *in vitro* was demonstrated later (Sakurai, 1925; Warburg *et al.*, 1930; Wendel, 1931). Further studies developed from the observations of Barron and Harrop (Barron and Harrop, 1928; Harrop and Barron, 1928) that methylene blue increased the oxygen utilization of erythrocytes. The early investigations of Warburg and his associates on the effects of methylene blue later led to the isolation of the nicotinamide nucleotides and to studies on G-6-P dehydrogenase and the hexose monophosphate shunt pathway. It soon became apparent that the normal process of methemoglobin reduction was dependent upon the structural integrity of the erythrocyte (Warburg *et al.*, 1930; Warburg and Christian, 1931), was associated with carbohydrate metabolism (Kiese, 1944; Drabkin, 1946), and required the regeneration of reduced nicotinamide nucleotides (Kiese, 1944; Gutmann *et al.*, 1947). Mammalian erythrocytes reduced methemoglobin to hemoglobin when the cells were incubated with glucose (Warburg *et al.*, 1930), lactate (Wendel, 1931), glyceraldehyde or fructose (Kiese, 1944), fumaric or malic acid (Kiese and Schwartzkopff-Jung, 1947), mannose or galactose (Spicer *et al.*, 1949), formaldehyde (Matthies, 1956), other aliphatic or aromatic aldehydes (Matthies, 1957b), and purine nucleosides and ribose (Jaffé, 1959). The results are shown in Fig. 2 of a typical experiment with normal human erythrocytes in which 65% of the hemoglobin had been converted to methemoglobin by treatment with sodium nitrite before the washed cells were incubated with various compounds. Except for the effect of ascorbic acid, the reduction of

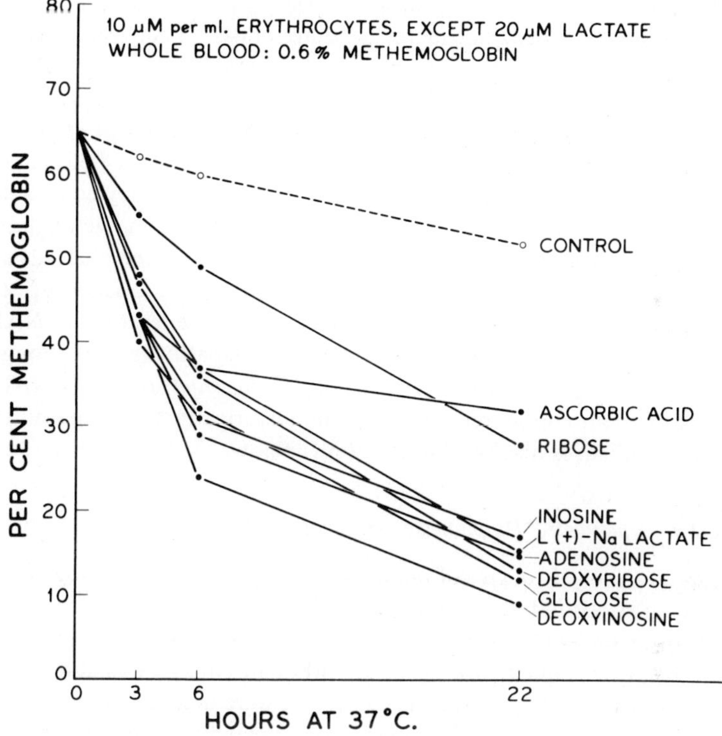

FIG. 2. The reduction of methemoglobin to hemoglobin in normal human erythrocytes during incubation with various compounds. (From Jaffé, 1959.)

methemoglobin to hemoglobin was associated with the metabolism of the purine nucleosides and sugars to lactic acid or the disappearance of added lactic acid. The investigations of Kiese (1944) and Gibson (1948) led to the suggestion that there were two pathways in normal human erythrocytes by which methemoglobin could be reduced to hemoglobin in association with carbohydrate metabolism. The reduction of methemoglobin upon incubation of human erythrocytes with glucose or lactate was accompanied by the formation of an amount of pyruvate equivalent to the amount of methemoglobin reduced. The addition of iodoacetate inhibited methemoglobin reduction by glucose, but not by lactate, while the addition of fluoride did not inhibit reduction by either substrate. High concentrations of pyruvate inhibited reduction of methemoglobin when lactate was the substrate, but did not affect reduction with glucose. Gibson (1948, 1954) suggested, therefore, that the reaction catalyzed by glyceraldehyde-3-phosphate dehydrogenase and requiring triose phosphate derived from glucose was of principal importance for the reduction of methemoglobin in human erythrocytes. He postulated the existence of an intermediate carrier (coenzyme factor I, "diaphorase"[2]) between NADH and methemoglobin, for the rate of the direct reaction between NADH and methemoglobin had been shown by Gutmann and co-workers (1947) to be too slow to account for significant reduction of methemoglobin in erythrocytes. The nature of this NADH-dependent "diaphorase" system is discussed in Section B below. Gibson's observation (1948) that erythrocytes of subjects with hereditary methemoglobinemia were able to reduce methemoglobin to hemoglobin as rapidly as could normal cells, when methylene blue was added to the glucose substrate, led him to suggest that the dye opened up a new reaction pathway. This latter pathway, involving the generation of NADPH via reactions of the hexose monophosphate shunt pathway, was thought to require coenzyme factor II or Kiese's *Hämiglobinreduktase*. This NADPH-dependent methemoglobin reductase system, historically the earliest and most extensively studied, is discussed in Section C below.

B. NADH-Dependent "Diaphorase" System

Studies on the erythrocytes of patients with hereditary methemoglobinemia not due to an abnormal methemoglobin have led to a partial understanding of the NADH-dependent "diaphorase" system, first postulated by Gibson (1948) and later by Rossi-Fanelli *et al.* (1957). Although Gibson was able to obtain circumstantial evidence that such erythrocytes were deficient in a "coenzyme factor" and observed that the deficiency was corrected by addition of a solution containing the Straub flavoprotein, Eder *et al.* (1949) found a normal level of FAD in the erythrocytes of their patient. Numerous investigations have demonstrated that the metabolism of glucose by these erythrocytes was normal. Specific assays of activities of various enzymes of the Embden-Meyerhof and

[2] Diaphorase may be defined as a flavoprotein enzyme that catalyzes the reduction of a dye, but not of cytochrome c, in the presence of NADH. The imprecise application of the name, diaphorase, has become customary in discussions of the NADH-dependent system for the reduction of methemoglobin to hemoglobin in erythrocytes. There is disagreement about the existence of flavins in human erythrocytes, and the nature of the enzyme systems for the reduction of methemoglobin have not been characterized completely. The designation, methemoglobin reductase, has been pre-empted for the NADPH-dependent system for the reduction of methemoglobin. In order to minimize confusion, the term "diaphorase" in quotation marks is used in this presentation.

hexose monophosphate shunt pathways, of catalase, and of concentrations of organic phosphate esters and nicotinamide nucleotides have yielded normal values (Gibson, 1948; Eder *et al.*, 1949; Scott and Hoskins, 1958; Waller and Löhr, 1961–1962; Jaffé, unpublished). However, as can be seen in Fig. 3, such erythrocytes were unable to reduce methemoglobin to hemoglobin when incubated with the nucleosides and sugars that promoted the reduction of

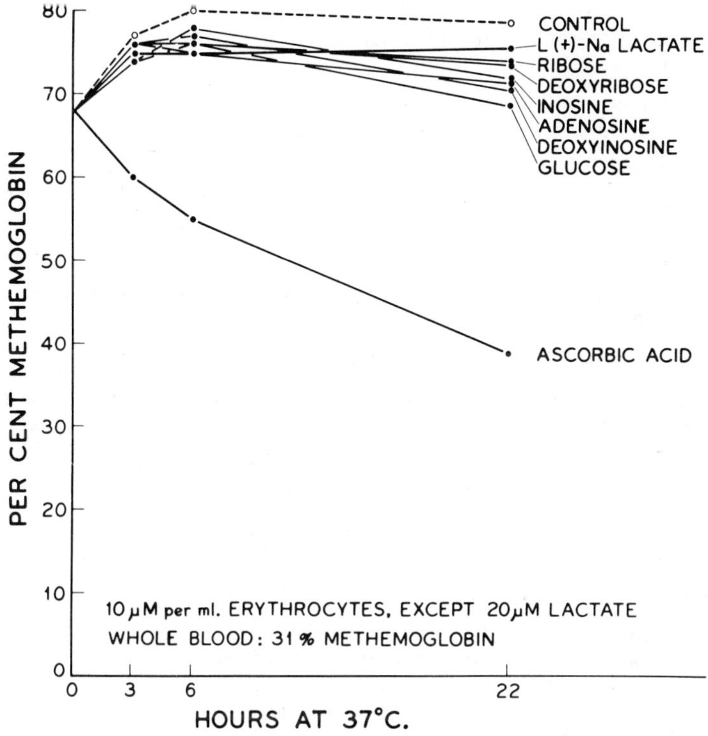

FIG. 3. The reduction of methemoglobin to hemoglobin in erythrocytes of a patient with hereditary methemoglobinemia due to an enzymatic defect, during incubation with various compounds. (From Jaffé, 1959.)

methemoglobin in normal erythrocytes (Fig. 2). Nitrite-treated erythrocytes of hereditary methemoglobinemia formed less pyruvate (Gibson, 1948) and slightly more lactate (Jaffé, 1959) from glucose than did normal erythrocytes treated similarly. These latter findings may be explained by the greater availability of NADH for the lactic dehydrogenase reaction in the abnormal cells where it was not utilized for the reduction of methemoglobin.

Scott and Hoskins (1958) discovered a high incidence of hereditary methemoglobinemia among Alaskan Eskimos and Indians. A severe deficiency in an enzyme system that reduced the dye 2,6-dichlorobenzenone indophenol with NADH was demonstrated in the erythrocytes of affected subjects (Scott and Griffith, 1959). Intermediate enzyme activities were observed in hemolysates of the erythrocytes of the parents of children with the disorder. The evidence was compatible with a recessive mode of inheritance of hereditary methemoglobinemia (Scott, 1960). Similar evidence of intermediate enzyme activity or intermediate ability to reduce methemoglobin to hemoglobin *in vitro* has been obtained with erythrocytes from presumed heterozygous individuals of European and Puerto Rican origin (Betke *et al.*, 1962; Cawein *et al.*, 1962; Jaffé and Neumann, 1964).

The enzyme, called a "diaphorase," was isolated from normal human erythrocytes by ammonium sulfate and calcium phosphate gel fractionation (Scott and McGraw, 1962). Only a small amount of enzyme activity could be isolated from the erythrocytes of subjects with hereditary methemoglobinemia (Scott, 1962). The reaction of this "diaphorase" system was thought to involve rapid transfer of electrons to the enzyme and slower reduction of the final acceptor. The reaction can be represented as below and as in Fig. 1:

$$\text{NADH} \xrightarrow{e-} \text{“Diaphorase”} \xrightarrow{e-} \text{Methemoglobin}$$

The relative rates at which several electron acceptors could be reduced by the purified enzyme system were: methemoglobin, 1.0; oxygen, 4.6; cytochrome c, 23; 2,6-dichlorobenzenone indophenol, 9200. For this reason, the reduction of the dye has been employed to measure the activity of this system in whole hemolysates. Heme-containing protein, a constant impurity during the isolation procedure, decreased in proportion as the purification proceeded. The enzyme appeared to contain flavin that resembled FAD and it was calculated that the "diaphorase" could account for only about 5% of the total flavin in erythrocytes. This low value may explain the failure to find a decreased FAD content in the erythrocytes of patients with hereditary methemoglobinemia. The enzyme was relatively specific for NADH. The purified preparation had with NADPH, only about 1.5% of the activity with NADH. In hemolysates the activity with NADPH was 10–15% that with NADH. The purified enzyme was inhibited by *p*-hydroxymercuribenzoate, but not by cyanide. The preparation had no appreciable dihydrolipoic dehydrogenase or glutathione reductase activity. This "diaphorase" system, capable of reducing methemoglobin to hemoglobin in the absence of methylene blue or other artificial electron carriers, appears to represent the major pathway for methemoglobin reduction in normal human erythrocytes.

C. *NADPH-Dependent Methemoglobin Reductase System*

Partial purification, identification, and characterization of an enzyme system from human erythrocytes, whose existence was implied by the investigations of Warburg and Christian (1931) and which was named methemoglobin reductase (*Hämiglobinreduktase*) by Kiese (1944), have been reported (Kiese *et al.*, 1957; Huennekens *et al.*, 1957, 1958). Huennekens postulated that the enzyme had two prosthetic groups: (1) an unknown carrier, perhaps ionic iron, which was detached upon hemolysis and purification and could be substituted for by methylene blue or other autoxidizable dyes, and (2) a tightly bound iron porphyrin moiety. This system was believed to require the transfer of electrons from NADPH to methylene blue or unknown natural cofactor and then to a heme enzyme. The reduced enzyme could then reduce either cytochrome c, which was the preferred acceptor, or oxygen or methemoglobin. A recent investigation by Shrago and Falcone (1963) indicated that the component of the isolated enzyme that was responsible for a 406-mμ peak on spectral analysis played no role in the functioning of the enzyme. Therefore, the postulated mechanism involving a heme moiety may be questioned. The reaction sequence, as outlined by Huennekens, is summarized in Fig. 1 and below:

$$\text{NADPH} \xrightarrow{e-} \begin{array}{c}\text{methylene blue}\\ \text{or}\\ \text{natural cofactor}\end{array} \xrightarrow{e-} \text{heme enzyme} \xrightarrow{e-} \text{methemoglobin}$$

The enzyme, isolated by ethanol-chloroform and ammonium sulfate fractionation, had an absolute requirement for methylene blue, appeared to be distinct from NADH-dependent "diaphorase" and hemoglobin, and had a minimum molecular weight of 185,000. The activity of the methemoglobin reductase with NADH was about 20% of the activity with NADPH. Kiese and his co-workers (1957) reported that the enzyme contained an amount of FAD representing 20–30% of the total FAD content of human erythrocytes. Huennekens and his associates (1958) were unable to detect bound flavin at any stage of purification. The activity of the enzyme system could be inhibited by several divalent ions, and the pattern of inhibition was similar to that observed with NADH oxidase isolated from pig heart. A search for the physiological cofactor or electron carrier was unrevealing. Riboflavin, FMN, FAD, GSH, ascorbic acid, and ergothioneine were without effect. Methemoglobin reductase isolated from beef erythrocytes in crude form appeared to contain a natural cofactor that was lost on further purification. Ultraviolet light-absorbing material was noted in the crude preparation, but disappeared upon ammonium sulfate fractionation or passage through resin columns. Ferric iron was found to be able to function as a cofactor in the reduction of methemoglobin in some crude enzyme preparations without methylene blue being required (Huennekens *et al.*, 1958). However, the physiological significance of this latter finding remains unknown. Although the turnover number of the enzyme isolated from human erythrocytes is small, it was calculated that the amount of enzyme present would adequately dispose of the methemoglobin presumed to be formed each day *in vivo*.

Methylene blue can accelerate greatly the rate of reduction of methemoglobin to hemoglobin both *in vitro* and *in vivo*. The activity of the hexose monophosphate shunt pathway in human erythrocytes is also greatly accelerated by methylene blue (Brin and Yonemoto, 1958), probably through oxidation of the NADPH regenerated through the reactions of this pathway (Szeinberg and Marks, 1961). The oxidation of NADPH may be mediated through the methemoglobin reductase that can function as a NADPH oxidase. Menadione sodium bisulfite (vitamin K_3) promotes limited acceleration of methemoglobin reduction (Harley and Robin, 1962a) and somewhat accelerates oxidation of NADPH with isolated methemoglobin reductase (Sass-Kortsak *et al.*, 1962). These observations support Gibson's (1948) suggestion that methylene blue can open up a new pathway for the reduction of methemoglobin. By serving as an electron carrier between NADPH and methemoglobin reductase, methylene blue and other artificial electron carriers accelerate the activity of the hexose monophosphate shunt pathway and facilitate the reduction of methemoglobin to hemoglobin. In the absence of methemoglobin, the reduced methemoglobin reductase may reduce oxygen to water or, perhaps, to hydrogen peroxide (Huennekens *et al.*, 1957). The NADPH-dependent methemoglobin reductase, however, appears to be a reserve system for the reduction of methemoglobin.

D. Other Possible Mechanisms for Methemoglobin Reduction

Ascorbic acid may act directly upon methemoglobin *in vivo* and *in vitro* (Barcroft *et al.*, 1945; King *et al.*, 1947; Jaffé, 1959). Ascorbic acid promotes the reduction of methemoglobin to hemoglobin in the erythrocytes of a patient with hereditary methemoglobinemia (Fig. 3), in normal erythrocytes (Fig. 2), and in hemolysates (Jaffé, 1959). The mechanism of this reaction is not completely understood (Kiese, 1944; Gibson, 1954). It is conceivable that methemoglobin is reduced to hemoglobin, while the ascorbic acid is oxidized to dehydroascorbic acid. The latter compound may, in turn, be reduced to ascorbic acid by GSH. The rate of methemoglobin reduction by ascorbic acid is so slow that it is unlikely that this agent plays a major role in normal erythrocytes (Finch, 1948; Thal and Lachhein, 1961). Some patients with hereditary methemoglobinemia have low serum ascorbic acid levels (Eder *et al.*, 1949; King *et al.*, 1947; Scott and Hoskins, 1958). The concentration of methemoglobin in the erythrocytes of such subjects can be maintained at 9–13% with oral ascorbic acid therapy. The Puerto Rican patient studied by the author has had normal serum ascorbic acid levels on several occasions when her erythrocytes contained about 20% methemoglobin, but ascorbic acid therapy is still effective in reducing the methemoglobinemia. A seasonal variation in the extent of the methemoglobinemia in the Alaskan Eskimos with this disorder has been attributed to a seasonal variation in the intake of ascorbic acid (Scott and Hoskins, 1958).

Although GSH reduced methemoglobin to hemoglobin *in vitro* (Morrison and Williams, 1938), the rate and efficiency of this reaction was limited (Finch, 1948; Allen and Jandl, 1961). Strömme and Eldjarn (1962), however, interpreted their studies with human erythrocytes as indicating that whatever methemoglobin reduction resulted from activity of the hexose monophosphate shunt pathway could be explained by a direct nonenzymatic reduction of methemoglobin by GSH. The oxidized glutathione formed would be reduced to GSH by glutathione reductase with NADPH generated by reactions of the hexose monophosphate shunt pathway. Low concentration of GSH, decreased production of lactate from glucose, and inability of glucose to promote reduction of methemoglobin *in vitro* were observed with erythrocytes from a case of hereditary methemoglobinemia in which erythrocyte NADH-dependent "diaphorase" activity was normal (Townes and Morrison, 1962). It was postulated, but not proven, that inadequate synthesis of GSH resulted in impaired glyceraldehyde-3-phosphate dehydrogenase activity which led to insufficient generation of NADH. A study of the family of this patient suggested a dominant mode of inheritance. Müller and associates (1963) reported a somewhat similar case whose erythrocytes were able to reduce methemoglobin normally upon incubation with lactate, but failed to do so upon incubation with glucose. These investigators noted a normal erythrocyte GSH concentration and suggested that the mode of inheritance was recessive. Although a hereditary deficiency of NADPH-dependent methemoglobin reductase activity was implied, the patient's methemoglobinemia disappeared after administration of methylene blue. As in the case reported by Townes and Morrison (1962), the erythrocytes appeared to have an impaired ability to utilize glucose for the reduction of methemoglobin. Further investigations of these variants of hereditary methemoglobinemia may disclose other metabolic abnormalities that will explain the diverse findings. Patients with hereditary absence of GSH in erythrocytes apparently did not have methemoglobinemia (Oort *et al.*, 1961). A decreased concentration of GSH in erythrocytes of hereditary methemoglobinemia was found by Eder and associates (1949), but normal levels were noted in cells of the Alaskan Eskimos (Scott and Hoskins, 1958) and of the Puerto Rican patient.

Other sulfhydryl compounds, such as cysteine (Holmquist and Vinograd, 1963) and ergothioneine (Klebanoff, 1962), can reduce methemoglobin to hemoglobin. What physiological roles these compounds play in human erythrocytes is unknown.

Both NADH and NADPH can effect the reduction of methemoglobin *in vitro* without addition of an artificial electron carrier (Gutmann *et al.*, 1947;

Scott and Hoskins, 1958). The rate of the reaction, however, appears to be too slow to contribute significantly to physiological methemoglobin reduction.

E. Relative Importance of Various Mechanisms for Methemoglobin Reduction

The relative importance of the various mechanisms for the reduction of methemoglobin to hemoglobin has been evaluated, for the most part, from indirect evidence. The observations that persistent methemoglobinemia occurs in patients whose erythrocytes are deficient in NADH-dependent "diaphorase" activity, and that normal methemoglobin levels are attained after administration of methylene blue which activates the NADPH-dependent methemoglobin reductase system, have provided strong evidence that the former pathway is of major physiological importance. Erythrocytes deficient in the capacity to generate NADPH (G-6-P-dehydrogenase-deficient) contain normal concentrations of methemoglobin, are able to reduce methemoglobin to hemoglobin normally *in vitro* in the absence of methylene blue (Beutler *et al.*, 1954; Dawson *et al.*, 1958; Jaffé, 1963), and have a normal NADH-dependent "diaphorase" system (Jaffé, 1963). The marked acceleration of methemoglobin reduction that results from addition of methylene blue to normal erythrocytes *in vitro* does not occur in G-6-P-dehydrogenase-deficient erythrocytes (Dawson *et al.*, 1958; Ross and Desforges, 1959; Löhr and Waller, 1958; Brewer *et al.*, 1960; Jaffé, 1963). Since it is the NADPH-dependent methemoglobin reductase system that is accelerated most strikingly by methylene blue (Gibson, 1948; Huennekens *et al.*, 1957, 1958), the limited acceleration observed in erythrocytes incapable of reducing NADP to NADPH as readily as normal cells would be expected. A deficiency in methemoglobin reductase activity in G-6-P-dehydrogenase-deficient erythrocytes has also been reported (Bonsignore *et al.*, 1960; Jaffé, 1963). The decreased ability of G-6-P-dehydrogenase-deficient erythrocytes to reduce methemoglobin upon incubation with glucose and methylene blue may not be due only to a deficient source of NADPH, but may also result from a defect in the methemoglobin reductase system itself. Brewer *et al.* (1962) have noted that male Negro subjects whose erythrocytes are deficient in G-6-P dehydrogenase activity develop higher levels of methemoglobin upon administration of sodium nitrite than do normal individuals. They have also observed a less rapid fall in the concentration of methemoglobin in enzyme-deficient erythrocytes than in normal cells when whole blood, mixed with acid-citrate-dextrose solution and sodium nitrite, is incubated for 16 hours. These latter experiments involve both the formation and the reduction of methemoglobin. They do not, therefore, permit an evaluation of the mechanisms that may protect against oxidation of hemoglobin, as contrasted with mechanisms responsible for the reduction of methemoglobin. Harley and Robin (1962b) have found no striking difference in the rate of methemoglobin formation resulting from a given concentration of sodium nitrite under experimental conditions with various activity levels of the hexose monophosphate shunt pathway. Future investigations will be required to resolve these apparently contradictory observations.

The susceptibility of young infants to develop methemoglobinemia upon exposure to certain chemicals led to studies that demonstrated a deficiency in NADH-dependent "diaphorase" activity in cord blood erythrocytes (McDonald and Huisman, 1962; Ross, 1963). Lonn and Motulsky (1957) isolated a diminished amount of a nonhemoglobin erythrocyte constituent that possessed NADPH-dependent methemoglobin reductase activity upon paper electrophoresis of cord blood hemolysates. McDonald and Huisman (1962), however, demonstrated normal NADPH-dependent methemoglobin reductase activity in cord blood erythrocytes. These latter investigators also reported increased glutathione reductase activity and normal concentrations of GSH in cord blood erythrocytes. They concluded that the accumulation of methemoglobin in these erythrocytes was prevented by increased reduction of methemoglobin by GSH. It might also be true that the enhanced availability of GSH simply prevented oxidation of hemoglobin, perhaps through the activity of glutathione peroxidase.

The studies of DeLoecker and Prankerd (1961), in which the enhanced oxygen utilization observed in nitrite-treated human erythrocytes was prevented by the formation of cyanmethemoglobin, were interpreted as indicating that the hexose monophosphate shunt pathway provided an additional mechanism for the normal reduction of methemoglobin. Erythrocytes of patients with thyrotoxicosis reduced methemoglobin at a higher rate upon incubation with glucose than did erythrocytes of euthyroid subjects (Jalavisto and Salmela, 1961). Necheles and Beutler (1959) demonstrated that triiodothyronine enhanced glucose consumption and oxygen utilization of normal human erythrocytes *in vitro*. Enhanced hexose monophosphate shunt activity may, therefore, be involved in the accelerated reduction of methemoglobin in the erythrocytes of thyrotoxic subjects. Although triiodothyronine was not capable of replacing NADP in the electron transfer system of the erythrocyte (Necheles and Beutler, 1959), the effect of this compound on the methemoglobin reductase system itself has not been investigated.

These various divergent observations emphasize the difficulty in determining the relative roles of the presumed protective and reductive mechanisms in maintaining hemoglobin in a functional state. Perhaps the most direct evidence for the relative contributions of the reductive mechanisms was provided recently by Scott and his associates (1963). They compared the rates of reduction of purified methemoglobin by the different reducing systems with the substrate or enzyme concentrations found in normal human erythrocytes. The relative rates were: NADH-dependent "diaphorase" 73, ascorbic acid 12,

GSH 9, and NADPH-dependent "diaphorase" (methemoglobin reductase) 6.

The tentative conclusion to be drawn from these various investigations is that in intact normal human erythrocytes the major pathway for reduction of methemoglobin to hemoglobin proceeds by way of the NADH-dependent "diaphorase" system. Reduction of methemoglobin by ascorbic acid and by GSH may occur under conditions where the capacity of the normal reductive mechanism is exceeded. The NADPH-dependent methemoglobin reductase appears to be a reserve system that requires an artificial electron carrier, such as methylene blue, to become fully effective in reducing methemoglobin to hemoglobin.

VI. Relation of Methemoglobin Content and Methemoglobin Reduction to Age of Erythrocyte

A. General Consideration of Erythrocyte Aging

Several excellent reviews have detailed the physical, chemical, and biological differences between nucleated erythrocytes (normoblasts), reticulocytes, young mature erythrocytes, and senescent cells of man and other species (London, 1961; Prankerd, 1961; Marks, 1962; Harris, 1963). The capacity to synthesize deoxyribonucleic acid and, therefore, the ability to divide appear to be lost at the polychromatophilic normoblast stage. Loss of the ability to synthesize heme, proteins, lipids, and purine and pyrimidine nucleotides from small molecule precursors accompanies the disappearance of mitochondria, ribosomes, and ribonucleic acid from reticulocytes. The ability to incorporate nicotinic acid and nicotinamide into the nicotinamide nucleotides appears to decrease with maturation of the reticulocyte. An intact Krebs tricarboxylic acid cycle and a complete cytochrome system are not present in mature mammalian erythrocytes. These changes of maturation are distinct from the alterations that occur with aging of the mature erythrocyte. Young erythrocytes may contain more potassium and sodium, have a greater cell volume, and have a lower density than do older cells. Immature erythrocytes appear to be more resistant to hemolysis in hypotonic media than are the older erythrocytes. A progressive decrease in activities of several enzymes of the glycolytic pathway and of the hexose monophosphate shunt pathway and in concentrations of organic phosphate esters is associated with aging of mature mammalian erythrocytes *in vivo*. Decreases in activities of G-6-P dehydrogenase and of glyceraldehyde-3-phosphate dehydrogenase appear to be the most prominent alterations in enzyme activity that have been described. Although the variations in methods used to evaluate the effect of aging of erythrocytes make it difficult to compare the various investigations, it is apparent that a general decrease in metabolic capabilities of these cells does take place. What finally determines that the senescent erythrocyte will be removed from the circulation remains unknown. It is not unreasonable to speculate that the survival of the erythrocyte *in vivo* may be determined by the stability of the enzyme proteins required for one or more critical metabolic reactions.

B. Relation of Methemoglobin Content to Erythrocyte Age

Jung (1949) found a higher concentration of methemoglobin in osmotically more fragile and, presumably, older human erythrocytes than in the younger, more resistant cells. Waller *et al.* (1959), employing differential agglutination to recover transfused human erythrocytes, reported that a progressive increase in methemoglobin concentration occurred after 40 days of aging *in vivo* and that it attained a level of about 8% after 80 days. The rise in methemoglobin concentration appeared to take place after the decrease in activity of glyceraldehyde-3-phosphate dehydrogenase became apparent and before the concentration of adenosine triphosphate declined. These authors concluded that an even higher level of methemoglobin was not present in older cells because the diffusion of lactate from younger, actively metabolizing cells into the older cells permitted generation of NADH by lactic dehydrogenase, whose activity did not decline with aging. NADH was thereby made available for reduction of methemoglobin by the "diaphorase" reaction. Beutler and Mikus (1961a) found that the osmotically more fragile erythrocytes of two patients with sickle cell anemia who were made methemoglobinemic contained more methemoglobin than did the younger, more resistant cells. Brewer *et al.* (1962), using differential centrifugation to separate erythrocytes of different average age, noted higher methemoglobin concentrations in the denser, older cells of subjects with normal and with G-6-P-dehydrogenase-deficient erythrocytes after the subjects were given sodium nitrite or primaquine. Contradictory results, however, have been reported. Beutler and Mikus (1961b) failed to demonstrate a difference in methemoglobin concentration in erythrocytes of normal subjects given a methemoglobin-producing drug, *p*-aminopropriophenone, when the cells were fractionated by differential osmotic lysis. Betke and his associates (1960) separated normal untreated human erythrocytes by differential centrifugation and by differential hypotonic lysis and were unable to detect differences in methemoglobin concentrations. Thus, the question of the extent to which methemoglobin accumulates within human erythrocytes as they age normally *in vivo* remains unsettled.

C. Influence of Age of Erythrocyte on Capacity to Reduce Methemoglobin

Matthies (1956) found that the ability of rabbit reticulocytes to reduce methemoglobin to hemoglobin was 6–20 times greater than that of mature erythrocytes. The most striking differences were noted with glucose and, especially, with glucose plus methylene blue, but no differences were apparent when lactate or formaldehyde was used as substrate. He concluded that the activity of the NADPH-dependent methemoglobin reductase declined with maturation of the immature erythrocyte. Jalavisto and associates (Jalavisto and Solantera, 1959; Jalavisto, 1960) demonstrated that the methemoglobin reduction rate of rabbit, dog, and guinea pig erythrocytes was a function of cell age and that a logarithmically decreasing age decay curve could be employed for calculating the methemoglobin reduction rates. These studies utilized reticulocytes produced in response to a bleeding anemia. Similar results were obtained by Berger *et al.* (1960) with erythrocytes and reticulocytes from rabbits made anemic by administration of phenylhydrazine. Löhr and his co-workers (1958), utilizing differential agglutination to recover transfused human erythrocytes, described a decrease in capacity to reduce methemoglobin as the erythrocytes aged. This decline in activity, determined with intact erythrocytes incubated with glucose and toluidine blue, was much less striking than the decrease in activities of G-6-P dehydrogenase and glyceraldehyde-3-phosphate dehydrogenase. Although Betke *et al.* (1960) failed to find a significant difference in rate of reduction of methemoglobin in human erythrocytes separated by differential centrifugation, they did note a higher oxygen utilization in the younger cells at the top of the centrifuged column.

The apparent decrease in capacity to reduce methemoglobin to hemoglobin that occurs with aging of mammalian erythrocytes can be explained by the decrease in metabolic activity associated with erythrocyte aging. Decreased metabolic activity might limit the available supplies of reduced nicotinamide nucleotides required for the reduction of methemoglobin. Since lactic dehydrogenase activity does not decrease markedly with aging of erythrocytes (Marks, 1962), oxidation of lactate to pyruvate in the presence of excess lactate might provide NADH for the NADH-dependent "diaphorase" system. Such a mechanism might explain Matthies' (1956) finding that the ability of lactate to promote methemoglobin reduction does not decrease with maturation of rabbit reticulocytes.

Rigas and Koler (1961) observed a moderate age-dependent decrease in activities of the NADH-dependent "diaphorase" and NADPH-dependent methemoglobin reductase systems. These systems were assayed as NADH or NADPH oxidases in lysates of human erythrocytes, prepared after separation by differential centrifugation. Similar changes were noted in erythrocytes of two subjects with hemoglobin H disease, although the relatively younger average age of these cells apparently contributed to the higher overall activity of the two systems. These age-dependent alterations in "diaphorase" and methemoglobin reductase activities, however, appeared to be less prominent and, perhaps, less important than the general decrease in glycolytic activity that accompanied aging of erythrocytes *in vivo*.

If the content of methemoglobin does increase with aging of normal mammalian erythrocytes, it is still not possible to decide whether the increase is the result of decrease in mechanisms that may protect against oxidation or in systems that reduce methemoglobin to hemoglobin.

VII. Conclusions

Although extensive investigations have provided information on the occurrence of methemoglobin, the oxidation of hemoglobin, and the reduction of methemoglobin to hemoglobin, many unanswered questions remain. To what extent does the hemoglobin contained in the circulating normal human erythrocyte actually undergo oxidation? What factors are present in the erythrocyte or in the plasma that promote the oxidation of hemoglobin? The contribution of copper in the coupled oxidation of hemoglobin has not been studied. How does the presence of methemoglobin in the erythrocyte influence the oxygen affinity of the remaining hemoglobin? What is the relative importance of the various mechanisms that appear to protect hemoglobin against oxidation in relation to those that reduce methemoglobin back to hemoglobin? What are the precise mechanisms involved in the transfer of electrons from reduced nicotinamide nucleotides to methemoglobin by way of methemoglobin reductase or "diaphorase"? What other physiological functions, beside reduction of methemoglobin, may the two methemoglobin reductase systems described perform in erythrocytes? Is the formation of methemoglobin an essential step in the degradation of hemoglobin under normal conditions, or is the oxidation of hemoglobin just a coincidental event in the denaturation of essential enzymes or erythrocyte membrane components? Alterations in erythrocyte proteins not as readily apparent as changes in the hemoglobin could be of vital importance to the viability of the cell. Hopefully, future studies will provide solutions to these problems and to other questions not yet proposed.

Acknowledgments

The investigations of the author have been supported by grants from the U.S. Public Health Service, H-2803; the Atomic Energy Commission, Contract AT (30-1) 1855; the Office of Naval Research, Contract Nonr-1765 (00); and the Health Research Council of the City of New York, U-1315 and I-169. The expert assistance of Miss Gertrude Neumann is also gratefully acknowledged. The author is a Career Scientist of the Health Research Council of the City of New York.

References

Aebi, H., Heiniger, J. P., and Suter, H. (1962). *Experientia* **18**, 129.

Allen, D. W., and Jandl, J. H. (1961). *J. Clin. Invest.* **40**, 454.

Barcroft, H., Gibson, Q. H., Harrison, D. C., and McMurray, J. (1945). *Clin. Sci.* **5**, 145.

Barron, E. S. G., and Harrop, G. A., Jr. (1928). *J. Biol. Chem.* **79**, 65.
Berger, H., Zuber, C., and Miescher, P. (1960). *Gerontologia* **4**, 220.
Betke, K., Baltz, A., Kleihauer, E., and Scholz, P. (1960). *Blut* **6**, 203.
Betke, K., Steim, H., and Tönz, O. (1962). *Deut. Med. Wochschr.* **87**, 65.
Beutler, E. (1959). *Blood* **14**, 103.
Beutler, E. (1962). *Nature* **196**, 1095.
Beutler, E., and Baluda, M. C. (1962). *Acta Haematol.* **27**, 321.
Beutler, E., and Kelly, B. M. (1963). *Experientia* **19**, 96.
Beutler, E., and Mikus, B. J. (1961a). *J. Clin. Invest.* **40**, 1856.
Beutler, E., and Mikus, B. J. (1961b). *Blood* **18**, 455.
Beutler, E., Dern, R. J., and Alving, A. S. (1954). *J. Lab. Clin. Med.* **44**, 177.
Bingold, K. (1933). *Klin. Wochschr.* **12**, 1201.
Bodansky, O. (1951). *Pharmacol. Revs.* **3**, 144.
Bonsignore, A., Fornaini, G., Segni, G., and Fantoni, A. (1960). *Giorn. Biochim.* **9**, 345.
Brewer, G. J., Tarlov, A. R., and Alving, A. S. (1960). *Bull. World Health Organ.* **22**, 633.
Brewer, G. J., Tarlov, A. R., Kellermeyer, R. W., and Alving, A. S. (1962). *J. Lab. Clin. Med.* **59**, 905.
Brin, M., and Yonemoto, R. H. (1958). *J. Biol. Chem.* **230**, 307.
Cawein, M., Behlen, C. H., and Lappat, E. J. (1962). *Blood* **20**, 786.
Clark, B. B., and Morrissey, R. E. (1951). *Blood* **6**, 532.
Cohen, G., and Hochstein, P. (1961). *Science* **134**, 1756.
Cohen, G., and Hochstein, P. (1963). *Biochemistry* **2**, 1420.
Darling, R. C., and Roughton, F. J. W. (1942). *Am. J. Physiol.* **137**, 56.
Dawson, J. P., Thayer, W. W., and Desforges, J. F. (1958). *Blood* **13**, 1113.
DeLoecker, W. C. J., and Prankerd, T. A. J. (1961). *Clin. Chim. Acta* **6**, 641.
Desforges, J. F. (1962). *Blood* **20**, 186.
Dittrich, P. (1892). *Arch. Exptl. Pathol. Pharmakol.* **29**, 247.
Drabkin, D. L. (1946). *Federation Proc.* **5**, 132.
Eder, H. A., Finch, C., and McKee, R. W. (1949). *J. Clin. Invest.* **28**, 265.
Finch, C. A. (1948). *New Engl. J. Med.* **239**, 470.
Gerald, P. S. (1958). *Blood* **13**, 936.
Gerald, P. S. (1960). *In* "The Metabolic Basis of Inherited Disease" (J. B. Stanbury *et al.*, eds.), pp. 1068–1085. McGraw-Hill, New York.
Gerald, P. S., and Efron, M. L. (1961). *Proc. Natl. Acad. Sci. U. S.* **47**, 1758.
Gibson, Q. H. (1948). *Biochem. J.* **42**, 13.
Gibson, Q. H. (1954). *In* "The Chemical Pathology of Animal Pigments" (R. T. Williams, ed.), Biochemical Society Symposia No. 12, pp. 55–70. Cambridge Univ. Press, London and New York.
Gibson, Q. H., and Harrison, D. C. (1947). *Lancet* **2**, 941.
Gutmann, H. R., Jandorf, B. J., and Bodansky, O. (1947). *J. Biol. Chem.* **169**, 145.
Haldane, J., Makgill, R. H., and Mavrogordato, A. E. (1897). *J. Physiol.* (*London*) **21**, 160.
Harley, J. D., and Mauer, A. M. (1961). *Blood* **17**, 418.
Harley, J. D., and Robin, H. (1962a). *Nature* **193**, 478.
Harley, J. D., and Robin, H. (1962b). *Blood* **20**, 710.
Harris, J. W. (1963). "The Red Cell. Production, Metabolism, Destruction: Normal and Abnormal," pp. 206–215, 229. Harvard Univ. Press, Cambridge, Massachusetts.
Harrop, G. A., Jr., and Barron, E. S. G. (1928). *J. Exptl. Med.* **48**, 207.
Hill, A. S., Jr., Haut, A., Cartwright, G. E., and Wintrobe, M. M. (1962). *Blood* **20**, 785.
Hörlein, H., and Weber, G. (1948). *Deut. Med. Wochschr.* **73**, 476.
Holmquist, W. R., and Vinograd, J. R. (1963). *Biochim. Biophys. Acta* **69**, 337.

Huennekens, F. M., Caffrey, R. W., Basford, R. E., and Gabrio, B. W. (1957). *J. Biol. Chem.* **227**, 261.
Huennekens, F. M., Caffrey, R. W., and Gabrio, B. W. (1958). *Ann. N. Y. Acad. Sci.* **75**, 167.
Hurley, T. H., Weisman, R., Jr., and Pasquariello, A. E. (1954). *J. Clin. Invest.* **33**, 835.
Itano, H. A., and Robinson, E. (1958). *Biochim. Biophys. Acta* **29**, 545.
Jacob, H. S., and Jandl, J. H. (1962). *J. Clin. Invest.* **41**, 1514.
Jaffé, E. R. (1959). *J. Clin. Invest.* **38**, 1555.
Jaffé, E. R. (1963). *Blood* **21**, 561.
Jaffé, E. R., and Neumann, G. (1964). *Federation Proc.* **23**, 470.
Jalavisto, E. (1960). *Ann. Acad. Sci. Fennicae Ser. A V.* **74**, 1.
Jalavisto, E., and Salmela, H. (1961). *Ann. Acad. Sci. Fennicae Ser. A V.* **75**, 1.
Jalavisto, E., and Solantera, L. (1959). *Acta Physiol. Scand.* **46**, 273.
Jandl, J. H., Engle, L. K., and Allen, D. W. (1960). *J. Clin. Invest.* **39**, 1818.
Jung, F. (1949). *Deut. Arch. Klin. Med.* **195**, 454.
Keilin, D. (1961). *Nature* **191**, 769.
Keilin, D., and Hartree, E. F. (1945). *Biochem. J.* **39**, 293.
Kiese, M. (1944). *Biochem. Z.* **316**, 264.
Kiese, M., and Schwartzkopff-Jung, W. (1947). *Arch. Exptl. Pathol. Pharmakol.* **204**, 267.
Kiese, M., and Weis, B. (1943). *Arch. Exptl. Pathol. Pharmakol.* **202**, 493.
Kiese, M., Schneider, C., Waller, H.-D. (1957). *Arch. Exptl. Pathol. Pharmakol.* **231**, 158.
King, E. J., White, J. C., and Gilchrist, M. (1947). *J. Pathol. Bacteriol.* **59**, 181.
Kirkman, H. N. (1959). *Nature* **184**, 1291.
Klebanoff, S. J. (1962). *Biochim. Biophys. Acta* **64**, 554.
Lemberg, R., and Legge, J. W. (1949). "Hematin Compounds and Bile Pigments," pp. 218–222, 389–396, 515–532. Wiley (Interscience), New York.
Lester, D. (1943). *J. Pharmacol. Exptl. Therap.* **77**, 154.
Lian, C., Frumusan, P., and Sassier. (1939). *Bull. mém. soc. méd. hôp. Paris* **55**, 1194.
Löhr, G. W., and Waller, H. D. (1958). *Klin. Wochschr.* **36**, 865.
Löhr, G. W., Waller, H. D., Karges, O., Schlegel, B., and Müller, A. A. (1958). *Klin. Wochschr.* **36**, 1008.
London, I. M. (1961). *Harvey Lectures, Ser.* **56** (*1960–1961*), pp. 151–189.
Lonn, L., and Motulsky, A. G. (1957). *Clin. Res. Proc.* **5**, 157.
McDonald, C. D., Jr., and Huisman, T. H. J. (1962). *Clin. Chim. Acta* **7**, 555.
Magos, L., and Sziza, M. (1959). *Acta Haematol.* **22**, 51.
Malz, E. (1961–1962). *Folia Haematol.* **78**, 510.
Marks, P. A. (1962). *In* "Biological Interactions in Normal and Neoplastic Growth" (M. J. Brennan and W. L. Simpson, eds.), pp. 481–498. Little, Brown, Boston, Massachusetts.
Marks, P. A., Szeinberg, A., and Banks, J. (1961). *J. Biol. Chem.* **236**, 10.
Matthies, H. (1956). *Arch. Exptl. Pathol. Pharmakol.* **229**, 331.
Matthies, H. (1957a). *Wiss. Z. Humboldt-Univ. Berlin, Math. Naturw. Reihe* **6**, 489.
Matthies, H. (1957b). *Biochem. Z.* **329**, 341.
Metcalf, W. K. (1962). *Phys. Med. Biol.* **6**, 437.
Mills, G. C. (1957). *J. Biol. Chem.* **229**, 189.
Mills, G. C. (1959). *J. Biol. Chem.* **234**, 502.
Mills, G. C. (1962). *J. Biochem. (Tokyo)* **51**, 41.
Mills, G. C., and Randall, H. P. (1958). *J. Biol. Chem.* **232**, 589.
Morrison, D. B., and Williams, E. F., Jr. (1938). *Science* **87**, 15.
Müller, J., Murawski, K., Szymanowska, Z., Koziorowski, A., and Radwan, L. (1963). *Acta Med. Scand.* **173**, 243.

Necheles, T., and Beutler, E. (1959). *J. Clin. Invest.* **38**, 788.
Oort, M., Loos, J. A., and Prins, H. K. (1961). *Vox Sanguinis* **6**, 370.
Prankerd, T. A. J. (1961). "The Red Cell. An Account of its Chemical Physiology and Pathology," pp. 1–12. Blackwell, Oxford.
Richardson, A. P. (1941). *J. Pharmacol. Exptl. Therap.* **71**, 203.
Rigas, D. A., and Koler, R. D. (1961). *J. Lab. Clin. Med.* **58**, 417.
Ross, J. D. (1963). *Blood* **21**, 51.
Ross, J. D., and Desforges, J. F. (1959). *J. Lab. Clin. Med.* **54**, 450.
Rossi-Fanelli, A., Antonini, E., Mondovì, B. (1957). *Clin. Chim. Acta* **2**, 476.
Rostorfer, H. H., and Cormier, M. J. (1957). *Arch. Biochem. Biophys.* **71**, 235.
Rubinstein, D., Ottolenghi, P., and Denstedt, O. F. (1956). *Can. J. Biochem. Physiol.* **34**, 222.
Sakurai, K. (1925). *Arch. Exptl. Pathol. Pharmakol.* **107**, 278.
Sass-Kortsak, A., Thalme, B., and Ernster, L. (1962). *Nature* **193**, 480.
Scott, E. M. (1960). *J. Clin. Invest.* **39**, 1176.
Scott, E. M. (1962). *Biochem. Biophys. Research Commun.* **9**, 59.
Scott, E. M., and Griffith, I. V. (1959). *Biochim. Biophys. Acta* **34**, 584.
Scott, E. M., and Hoskins, D. D. (1958). *Blood* **13**, 795.
Scott, E. M., and McGraw, J. C. (1962). *J. Biol. Chem.* **237**, 249.
Scott, E. M., Duncan, I. W., and Ekstrand, V. (1963). *Federation Proc.* **22**, 467.
Shrago, E., and Falcone, A. B. (1963). *Biochim. Biophys. Acta* **67**, 147.
Spicer, S. S., Hanna, C. H., and Clark, A. M. (1949). *J. Biol. Chem.* **177**, 217.
Spicer, S. S., Wooley, J. G., and Kessler, V. (1951). *Proc. Soc. Exptl. Biol. Med.* **77**, 418.
Steele, C. W., and Spink, W. W. (1933). *New Engl. J. Med.* **208**, 1152.
Strömme, J. H., and Eldjarn, L. (1962). *Biochem. J.* **84**, 406.
Szeinberg, A., and Marks, P. A. (1961). *J. Clin. Invest.* **40**, 914.
Takahara, S., Hamilton, H. B., Neel, J. V., Kobara, T. Y., Ogura, Y., Nishimura, E. T., Ozaki, K., and Ito, K. (1960). *J. Clin. Invest.* **39**, 610.
Thal, W., and Lachhein, L. (1961). *Klin. Wochschr.* **39**, 1022.
Touster, O., and Yarbro, M. C. (1952). *J. Lab. Clin. Med.* **39**, 720.
Townes, P. L., and Morrison, M. (1962). *Blood* **19**, 60.
Vandenbelt, J. M., Pfeiffer, C., Kaiser, M., and Sibert, M. (1944). *J. Pharmacol. Exptl. Therap.* **80**, 31.
Vella, F. (1959). *Experientia* **15**, 433.
Waisman, H. A., Bain, J. A., Richmond, J. B., and Munsey, F. A. (1952). *Pediatrics* **10**, 293.
Waller, H. D., and Löhr, G. W. (1961–1962). *Folia Haematol.* **78**, 588.
Waller, H. D., Schlegel, B., Müller, A. A., and Löhr, G. W. (1959). *Klin. Wochschr.* **37**, 898.
Warburg, O., and Christian, W. (1931). *Biochem. Z.* **242**, 206.
Warburg, O., Kubowitz, F., and Christian, W. (1930). *Biochem. Z.* **227**, 245.
Webster, S. H. (1949). *Blood* **4**, 479.
Wendel, W. B. (1931). *Proc. Soc. Exptl. Biol. Med.* **28**, 401.
Williams, J. R., and Challis, F. E. (1933). *J. Lab. Clin. Med.* **19**, 166.

CHAPTER 12

Life Span of the Red Cell

Nathaniel I. Berlin

I. Introduction

Satisfactory methods for measuring the red cell life span are widely available. The use of thymidine has made feasible satisfactory measurements of the life span of other cells. However, it is only for the red cell that a large number of measurements in man and experimental animals have been reported in both the normal and disease state. Although practical attempts to measure the red cell life span were begun by Todd and White (1911), it has only been with the introduction of isotopic techniques that these determinations were carried out in many laboratories. A number of methods have been proposed for the determination of red cell life span. Many of these are of historical interest only; some were not physiologically sound and others were technically difficult. The Ashby differential agglutination technique provided satisfactory measurements of the life span of donor cells in the recipient environment (1919). This method has been applied almost exclusively to man, although a few studies have been carried out with this technique in the dog (Stohlman and Schneiderman, 1956; Swisher *et al.*, 1953) and in the rat (Smith *et al.*, 1959). Red cells from normal donors have been transfused into normal recipients and into patients with various diseases and in turn patients' red cells have been transfused into normal recipients. In this way, intra-corpuscular defects could be differentiated from extra-corpuscular defects. Technical requirements restricted the usefulness of the Ashby method. A relatively small number of investigators contributed a large amount of information. In 1946 Shemin and Rittenberg reported the measurement of red cell life span with N^{15}-labeled glycine. This method was not widely applied because of the requirement of a mass spectrometer. C^{14}-labeled glycine was also utilized, but the techniques for measuring C^{14} were also not widely available (Grinstein *et al.*, 1949; Berlin *et al.*, 1951). Then in 1950 Gray and Sterling demonstrated that Cr^{51} could be used to label red cells. Since then Cr^{51} has come into widespread use for measurement of red cell survival but elution of the isotope from intact surviving cells makes interpretation of the results difficult. Diisopropylfluorophosphate (DFP) labeled with P^{32} (Cohen and Warringa, 1954; Bove and Ebaugh, 1958; Garby, 1962; Eernisse and Van Rood, 1961; and Van Putten, 1958) or tritium (Cline and Berlin, 1962b) has been shown to provide a satisfactory measurement of the red cell life span. It is predicted that isotopically labeled DFP will become the method of choice where the measurement of red cell life span is required.

There are several reviews of the red cell life span that are of particular value. Schiodt (1938) reviewed the results of many of the older studies, principally those involving the rate of return of the red count to normal following either phlebotomy or some other applied variable. Eadie and Brown (1953) and Dornhorst (1951) have discussed in detail the mathematical aspects of the red cell survival curves. General reviews are those of Ashby (1948), Strumia (1956), Mollison (1961a), and Berlin *et al.* (1959). The present chapter should be considered as both a brief recapitulation of the latter review and a survey of the work published since 1958.

II. Methods

The methods of historical interest will not be considered here; they have been reviewed previously in detail (Berlin *et al.*, 1959).

Red cell labeling methods for measurement of the red cell life span can be divided into two classes: (1) those in which the cells are labeled randomly, that is, all the cells are equally labeled, and (2) those in which a cohort of cells of similar age are labeled. The Ashby differential agglutination method, Cr^{51}, and isotopically labeled DFP label cells randomly. Cohort labeling can be achieved with the use of glycine labeled with either N^{15} or C^{14}, radioactive iron, and a combination of unlabeled and isotopically labeled DFP (see Section II, B, 3). In some situations it is desirable to have cells doubly labeled. This may be accomplished by a combination of an immunological and isotopic marker, or by two isotopic labels.

The red cell life span is most satisfactorily measured when the total red cell volume is constant as a result of a constant rate of production and removal of red cells (RBC). Most investigators measure the amount of label per unit red cell as either isotope per milliliter RBC or isotope per milliliter blood. As generally applied, all methods depend upon the replacement of labeled cells by non labeled cells.

The random labeling methods are, in general, more sensitive to changes in the rate of production of red cells than are the cohort labeling techniques. Three cases need to be considered: (1) a decreasing rate of synthesis of red cells, (2) absence of erythropoiesis, and (3) an increasing rate of production (see Fig. 1).

For the random labeling methods, if it is assumed that the rate of red cell production is constant when in fact it is actually decreasing and hence the total red cell volume is also decreasing, then the rate of change of label per milliliter RBC is factitiously low. The red cell life span will therefore be estimated as longer than it really is. In the absence of erythropoiesis there is no change in label content per milliliter RBC and the red cell life span appears to be infinite; when the rate of production increases and the total red cell volume increases, the calculated red cell life span is falsely short. For the cohort labeling methods, when the red cell life span is finite and the total red cell volume is decreasing, the plateau portion of the curve will not be flat but will show a tendency to rise; in the absence of erythropoiesis, the red cells will not be labeled since the cohort labeling with labeled glycine or Fe^{59} requires biosynthetic incorporation of the label into hemoglobin. Cohort labeling with DFP requires the synthesis of unlabeled red cells. When the total red cell volume is increasing, the plateau portion will have a negative slope of a magnitude dependent upon the rate of increase in total red cell volume. Repeated measurements of the total red cell volume with another red cell label, e.g. $NaH_2P^{32}O_4$, and calculation of total circulating label are the only reliable solution to the problem of the measurement of red cell life span in the nonsteady state. It is becoming increasingly apparent that investigators are taking into consideration the necessity for measuring the rate of deviation from the steady state when this occurs. Examples of correction for blood volume changes in which the blood volume was either measured or assumed are those of Dancis *et al.* 1959; Birkeland, 1958; Kaplan and Hsu, 1961; and Turnbull *et al.*, 1957.

A new direct method that has been proposed for measurement of red cell life span is from the rate of clearance of bilirubin (Lewis and Gershow, 1961). This has been tested in the rabbit and data from the literature applied to man. Bilirubin was given intravenously and the rate of decrease in the blood determined. If total circulating bilirubin and rate of turnover of bilirubin are

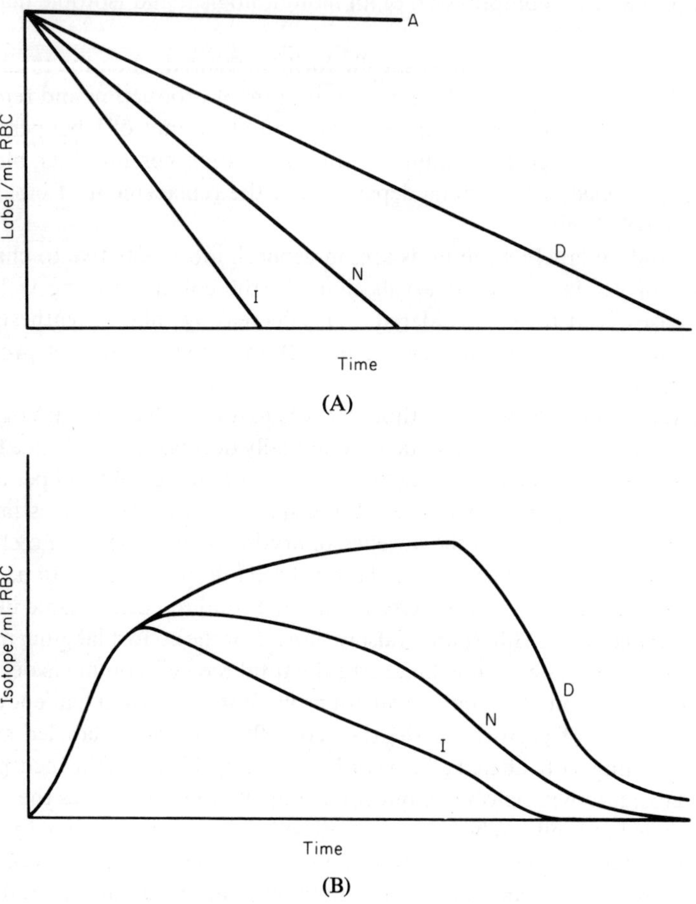

FIG. 1. Schematic presentation of the effect of a changing total red cell volume on the measurement of red cell life span. (A) Effect when a random labeling method is used. A = absence of erythropoiesis, D = decreasing total red cell volume, I = increasing total red cell volume, N = normal (total red cell volume is constant as a result of a constant rate of induction and destruction of red cells). (B) Effect when a cohort labeling method is used.

known, the turnover rate of red cells and hence the mean red cell life span can be calculated. This method assumes that the clearance of the added bilirubin from the blood follows first order kinetics within both the normal range of plasma concentrations and that achieved with the intravenously injected bilirubin. In the rabbit, the calculated red cell life span is in good agreement with those obtained by other methods. In man, analysis by Lewis and Gershow (1961) of the data of Kornberg (1942) yielded values in good agreement with other values of the red cell life span of man. However, in both situations values for the blood volume and body weight had to be assumed. This particular method will probably give results that are only approximately correct. It will probably not find widespread use but it would be desirable to have a method which measures bilirubin turnover. The most likely possibility is that with the use of radioactive bilirubin this goal may be achieved.

A. Random Labeling Methods

1. Ashby Differential Agglutination Technique

The Ashby differential agglutination technique is the oldest of the satisfactory methods for the measurement of red cell life span. Considerable effort has been devoted to the development of this procedure (Mollison, 1961a). Careful technique is required. While the Ashby differential technique has contributed much to our knowledge, it has been displaced by the isotopic methods. The Ashby differential agglutination technique consists in the transfusion from donor to recipient of compatible but immunologically identifiable cells. This precludes measurement of the red cell survival in its normal environment and is a basic criticism of the Ashby method. The number of surviving donor cells in the recipient is determined after either agglutination or hemolysis of the recipient cells.

2. Chromium-51

The development by Gray and Sterling (1950) of the technique for labeling red cells with Cr^{51} opened a new era in measurement of red cell survival. The technique is simple. Red cells are labeled *in vitro* with Cr^{51}-labeled sodium chromate. The excess unincorporated isotope is then removed by washing the cell, or uptake of the isotope is stopped by reduction of the chromate with ascorbic acid. The labeled cells are then reinfused and the survival determined. The total circulating red cell volume can also be calculated (Read, 1954).

This technique labels red cells randomly and, if the red cell life span is finite, there should be a linear decrease with time in the isotope content of the red cells. However, in the normal human and experimental animal, the isotope content of the red cell decreases more rapidly than would be predicted from the known red cell life span. This is due to elution of Cr^{51} from intact surviving cells. Mollison (1961b) has reviewed the differences in rate of elution in normal subjects calculated from an equation which assumes a normal red cell life span of 115 days. He has brought together data indicating that the mean Cr^{51} half-time is 32 days if the cells are washed in citrate buffered to pH 6.4–6.9, whereas if washed in heparin or acid-citrate-dextrose the half-time is of the order of 25 days. He suggests that cells be washed in this buffer before being labeled.

There are relatively few direct measurements of the rate of elution of chromium from intact red cells. In the normal individual it is possible to approximate the elution rate from an assumed mean life span (Eadie and Brown, 1955; Mollison, 1961b; Rigas and Koler, 1961). However, in order to calculate the elution rate from the following equations, an independent measurement of red cell life span is required. There are three possible cases to consider (Cline and Berlin, 1963a): (1) red cell life span is finite; (2) red cells are randomly destroyed and none reaches the potential life span; and (3) a combination of a finite life span and random destruction of some of the cells.

If the red cell life span is finite, then

$$N = N_0\left(1-\frac{t}{T}\right)\exp(-k_e t) \tag{1}$$

where $N = Cr^{51}$ c.p.m./ml. RBC at time t, $N_0 = Cr^{51}$ c.p.m./ml. RBC at $t = 0$, $T =$ mean life span, and $k_e = Cr^{51}$ elution rate constant.
If T is known, then k_e can be determined from the slope of the line

$$\ln N/[1-(t/T)] \text{ against } t.$$

If T is determined from a random labeling method and N' is the quantity of random label per ml. red cells at time t, k_e can be determined from the slope of the line of $\ln (N/N')$ as a function of time. If red cell destruction is random and none survives to time T, then

$$N = N_0 \exp[-(k_e+k_d)t] \tag{2}$$

where $k_d =$ rate of random destruction.

The difference between the slopes of line $\ln N$ and line $\ln N'$ versus time is k_e.

If red cell destruction is partially random, k_e can be calculated by the method of Eadie *et al.* (1960) where the slope of the line $\ln (N/N')$ against time is k_e, if N' is derived from a random labeling technique.

In 12 normal subjects the rate of elution was 0.57–1.28 %/day and averaged 0.93 %/day (Eadie and Brown, 1955; Ebaugh *et al.*, 1953; Read *et al.*, 1954). In 34 patients with various hematological diseases, the red cell elution rate was 0.62–2.27 %, and averaged 1.29 %/day (Cline and Berlin, 1963a). In four of these 34 patients there were two chromium elution rate constants. The first had a half-time of approximately 4 days and represented 8–19 % of the chromium eluted. The rate of elution has been calculated to be 1.3 %/day by assuming a red cell life span of 115 days (Birkeland, 1958; Rigas and Koler, 1961). In two sheep there was a rapid component of elution at the rate of 40 %/day for half the Cr^{51}, followed by a slower rate of elution of 2.2–3.5 %/day (Eadie *et al.*,

1960). Elution rates have also been calculated for the rat (1–2%/day) (Smith *et al.*, 1959), (1.88%/day) (Jones and Cheney, 1961); hamster (3.08%/day) (Brock, 1960); rabbit (1.5%/day) (Jones, 1961), (2%/day) (Marvin and Lucy, 1957), (3%/day) (Sutherland *et al.*, 1959); dog (1.35%/day) (Stohlman and Schneiderman, 1956), (1.77%/day) (Weissman *et al.*, 1960), pigeon (4%/day) (Marvin and Lucy, 1957) and duck (3%/day) (Marvin and Lucy, 1957).

There are several methods of analysis of the Cr^{51} survival data. The most common method is to plot the logarithm of isotopic content per milliliter red cells as a function of time, and force the data for the first 30 or 40 days to fit to a straight line, thus deriving a half-time. A more precise method is to plot the change in isotopic content with time on Cartesian coordinates and to extrapolate the final portion to the abscissa. In this case, the mean life span can be determined. Physical decay of the isotope, limitations as to quantity of chromium which can be added to the red cell, and difficulty in curve fitting make this particular method more difficult. It is also time-consuming, requiring 110–120 days in man as compared to the 25–40 days required for a determination of the Cr^{51} survival half-time. Eadie and Brown (1955) fitted the data to Eq. (1) by a series of successive approximations obtaining a best fit for T and k_e. This method has also been used by others, e.g. Rigas and Koler (1961), Hall (1960). Horwitt *et al.*, (1963) suggest that the time required for the red cell Cr^{51} content to decrease by 90–95% may be more reliable than extrapolation to the abscissa.

The recurring problem of the measurement of survival of red cells in the first 24 hours posttransfusion has been the subject of considerable study. Most workers agree that there appears to be an increased removal of labeled cells in the first 24 hours. This has been attributed in the case of Cr^{51}-labeled cells to elution and to loss of viability of some cells in the process of labeling. From data obtained with a double-labeling technique (Cr^{51} and Ashby techniques), Strumia *et al.* (1962) concluded that there is removal of cells in addition to elution of Cr^{51}.

Schenk and Bow (1961) labeled dog cells with Cr^{51}, then induced hemolysis with acetylphenylhydrazine, and showed there was no reutilization of Cr^{51}, which had been assumed.

Van Kampen and Heerspink (1961) have suggested that the lifespan of the red cell can be calculated from *in vitro* uptake of Cr^{51} by the red cell. They interpret the data as evidence that reticulocytes take up little Cr^{51}, and that elution from intact surviving cells does not occur. Elution from intact surviving cells is accepted. This method will probably not be widely used.

3. Diisopropylfluorophosphate (P^{32}- and H^3-labeled)

Diisopropylfluorophosphate (DFP) belongs to the class of compounds known as phosphofluoridates. DFP interacts with biological materials to form esters, probably with the hydroxyl groups of serine. It combines with cholinesterase which it irreversibly inhibits. During the labeling process the phosphorus-fluorine bonds are broken and the resultant diisopropylphosphate is no longer capable of reacting with proteins to label them. In 1954 Cohen and Warringa were the first to report the use of DFP^{32} to measure the red cell life span. Since then a number of studies have shown this to be a satisfactory, and possibly the best, label for the measurement of red cell life span in the experimental animal and in man (Van Putten, 1958; Eernisse and Van Rood, 1961; Garby, 1962; Brewer *et al.*, 1961; Cline and Berlin, 1963d; Bove and Ebaugh, 1958, and Eadie *et al.*, 1960). The red cells may be labeled *in vivo* by administration intramuscularly or intravenously of DFP, or cells may be labeled *in vitro*. Isotopic labeling of the DFP with P^{32} and tritium is available. C^{14}-labeled material is theoretically possible but has not been prepared. In the first 7–10 days following administration of labeled DFP, or after *in vitro* labeling, there is elution of isotope from intact surviving cells (Bove and Ebaugh, 1958; Hjort *et al.*, 1960). The amount eluted varies with the method of labeling, the preparation used, and the quantity of DFP used (Eernisse and Van Rood, 1961; Garby, 1962; Bove and Ebaugh, 1958; Cline and Berlin, 1963d, and Hjort *et al.*, 1960). There appears to be an upper maximum of the amount of DFP which can bind irreversibly to the cell; this varies from species to species (Van Putten, 1958; Hjort *et al.*, 1960).

The initial difficulties with the DFP^{32} method probably stemmed from the lack of a consistently satisfactory preparation. Its synthesis is difficult. In addition, Cohen and Warringa (1954) measured the isotope content in terms of P^{32} content per milligram red cell nitrogen. This required a separate determination of the red cell nitrogen. Subsequently, the isotope content has been measured in terms of either hemoglobin content or volume of red cells. This has considerably simplified the procedure. In the normal, following the initial elution period, the red cell specific activity declines in a linear manner, yielding a red cell life span in good agreement with data obtained by other methods (Bove and Ebaugh, 1958; Eernisse and Van Rood, 1961; Garby, 1962; Cline and Berlin, 1962a; Van Putten, 1958).

B. *Cohort Labeling*

1. Labeled Glycine (N^{15}, C^{14})

Cohort labeling consists in the preparation of a cohort of cells of similar age that are identifiable. This can be achieved with either labeled glycine (Shemin and Rittenberg, 1946), radio-iron (Burwell *et al.*, 1953), or DFP (Cline and Berlin, 1962a). The labeled glycine and radio-iron techniques label the cells as a result of the biosynthesis of isotopically labeled hemoglobin. A cohort of cells is labeled because the specific activity of the precursor decreases rapidly and thus only the cells produced during a relatively short period of time are labeled. With respect to radio-iron, the precursor specific activity decreases rapidly with a half-time of approximately 90 minutes and 80–90 % of the isotope is taken up by cells of the normoblastic series in the marrow (Huff *et al.*, 1950). This is, for this purpose, "flash" labeling. In the experimental animal the body iron stores can be flooded by parenteral administration of large doses of iron. This markedly reduces the specific activity of the nonhemoglobin iron (Burwell *et al.*, 1953). When the red cells reach the end of their life span, the specific activity of the hemoglobin iron is greatly reduced by admixture with the increased body iron stores; thus good cohort labeling is achieved (Burwell *et al.*, 1953; I. W. Brown and Eadie, 1953). This is not possible in man. Determination of the percentage of radio-iron-labeled red cells by autoradiographic means has also been used to measure the red cell life span in the rat (Belcher and Harriss, 1959).

Precursor labeled glycine of high specific activity is available for a longer period of time, and thus the period in which the specific activity of circulating hemoglobin increases is longer than with radio-iron. Labeled precursor is available, albeit at a low level, during the entire time required for the measurement. A small correction is necessary when the red cell life span is finite (Berlin *et al.*, 1954). A larger correction may be necessary when random destruction occurs (Berlin *et al.*, 1959). These corrections can be calculated if the precursor-glycine specific activity variations with time are known.

3. Diisopropylfluorophosphate

Cohort labeling with DFP is achieved in the following way. A dose of unlabeled DFP sufficient to combine with the available red cell binding sites is administered. Several days later a dose of isotopically labeled DFP is given (Cline and Berlin, 1962a). The isotopically labeled dose combines with protein of the cells produced subsequent to the first dose. Thus a cohort of cells of maximum age range equivalent to the interval between the two doses is produced. This method has been applied in the normal dog and following acute hemorrhage in the dog (Cline and Berlin, 1962a).

C. *Doubly Labeled Cells*

1. Immunological and Isotopic

Several workers have studied the fate of red cells doubly labeled by immunological and isotopic means, e.g., Eadie and Brown (1955), Read *et al.* (1954), and Smith *et al.* (1959). Chromium^{51}-labeled cells and the Ashby differential agglutination technique were used. The Ashby differential agglutination technique was used to provide a standard for comparison with Cr^{51} and to permit the calculation of the rate of elution of Cr^{51} from intact surviving red cells. The difficulties of the Ashby differential agglutination technique and the availability of other isotopic methods for labeling cells make this combination of immunological and isotopic labels unnecessarily difficult from the standpoint of technique. Berlin *et al.* (1957) compared Fe^{59} and C^{14} labeled cells with the Ashby technique.

2. Double Isotope

Red cells labeled with two isotopes have been used for simultaneous measurement of the survival of two populations of red cells (Munker *et al.*, 1961; Eadie *et al.*, 1960; Cline and Berlin, 1963c). The double labeling technique permits a comparison of the two methods or a simultaneous measurement of the survival of two populations of cells. Doubly labeled cells provide a method for differentiating between intracorpuscular and extracorpuscular defects which lead to the shortening of the red cell life span. Both Munker *et al.* (1961) and Eadie *et al.* (1960) and their collaborators labeled cells with DFP and Cr^{51}. DFP^{32} and H^3-DFP can be used to label two populations of red cells with the same chemical but different isotopic markers (Cline and Berlin, 1963c). This eliminates the need for some independent measurement or some assumption of the rate of elution of chromium in studies such as those of Munker *et al.* (1961) and Eadie *et al.* (1960) and their collaborators.

Red cells can be labeled with two isotopes of iron but biosynthetic incorporation of the isotope into red cells is necessary. Cells doubly labeled with Fe^{55} and Fe^{59} have been used to measure the immediate posttransfusion survival of red cells but not the red cell life span (Gibson *et al.*, 1947; Gabrio and Finch, 1954).

D. Comparison and Evaluation of Methods

A comparison and evaluation of methods for determining the life span of the red cell must rest upon several factors. These are the availability of the equipment necessary, the precision with which it is desired to determine the red cell life span, and the time available. In the normal mammal and healthy man, the time required for determination of red cell life span by the cohort-labeling method varies from approximately 50 to 200 days. It is longer in poikilotherms (Cline and Waldmann, 1962a, 1962b; Altland and Brace, 1962). With random labeling methods, shorter periods of time may be utilized since it is only necessary to determine the rate at which the label is replaced. The time required for a satisfactory measurement depends upon the number of measurements possible, the precision of each estimate, and the slope. This can be determined by statistical means. Garby (1962) has suggested that a period of time as short as 2 weeks may be utilized, although a precise measurement of the red cell life span is not obtained.

At present, it is suggested that isotopically labeled DFP is the method of choice for determining red cell life span (Brewer *et al.*, 1961; Garby, 1962; Eernisse and Van Rood, 1961). DFP labeled with P^{32} is readily available. The high-energy β-rays make the measurement of P^{32} technically easy. The specific activity of the available DFP^{32} is adequate. The only problem with the use of DFP^{32} is elution from cells labeled *in vitro* and the occasional elution observed after *in vivo* labeling. Elution is observed in all cases of *in vitro* labeling. With *in vivo* labeling the quantity eluted appears to be dependent upon the preparation and the quantity used. Elution is an infrequent occurrence after *in vivo* labeling (Garby, 1962; Eernisse and Van Rood, 1961; Brewer *et al.*, 1961, and Cline and Berlin, 1963d). DFP can be used to label the cells either randomly or by cohort labeling. The latter has been demonstrated in the dog but has not yet been applied to man (Cline and Berlin, 1962a). The relatively small (compared to the toxic) dose of DFP required to block further uptake by red cells of DFP for cohort labeling, and the dose of isotopically labeled DFP required, appear to make this method feasible in man. The Cr^{51} method as generally applied does not yield a red cell life span but only an apparent survival half-time. The increasing availability of liquid scintillation spectrometers and the development of a satisfactory method of counting barium carbonate make the labeled glycine method more widely available (Nathan *et al.*, 1958). However, the time required to process a single sample is considerably longer than with DFP^{32}, but comparable to H^3-DFP. This requirement of a mass spectrometer for N^{15} measurements limits the usefulness of N^{15}-labeled glycine. The radio-iron method is limited in man since the large doses of iron required to achieve good cohort labeling are usually not justified on clinical grounds.

III. Red Cell Life Span Data

A. Patterns of Red Cell Survival

In the normal state the red cell survives for a fixed period of time, i.e., its lifespan is finite. In addition, there is a variable degree and rate of random destruction of the red cells. This is minimal in man and dog and probably most pronounced in the pig (Bush *et al.*, 1955) and llama (Cornelius and Kaneko, 1962).

With the exception of hibernating mammals (Brace, 1953; Brock, 1960), and poikilotherms (Cline and Waldmann, 1962a, 1962b) taken from a warm to a cold environment, all variations in red cell survival involve a decreased survival. Two patterns of decreased survival are observed, a finite but shortened life-span and random destruction. The intensity of the random destructive process can vary within rather wide limits—from that where only a small fraction of the cells are randomly destroyed to the extent that, for practical purposes, all red cells are randomly destroyed.

B. *Equations*

The equations describing red cell survival for the random labeling and cohort labeling methods have been reviewed by Eadie and Brown (1953), Dornhorst (1951), Sheets *et al.* (1951), and Berlin *et al.* (1959).

The principal equations are as follows:

A. For randomly labeled cells where the red cell life span is finite

$$N_t = N_0\left(1-\frac{t}{T}\right) \tag{3}$$

where N_0 = numbers of cells at time 0, and T = red cell life span.
When the red cells are destroyed randomly and none of the cells survives to T for that species

$$N_t = N_0 e^{-kt} \tag{4}$$

where k = rate of random destruction. When some of the cells are randomly destroyed and some survive to T

$$N_t = N_0\left(1-\frac{t}{T}\right) e^{-kt}. \tag{5}$$

B. The general equation for hemoglobin isotope content following biosynthetic incorporation of label is

$$N_{(t)} = C \int_0^t rf(B)\, \alpha(t-B)\, dB \tag{6}$$

where C = proportionality constant, r = rate of red cell formation, $f(B)$ = isotope content of red cells formed at time B, and $\alpha(t)$ = probability that a red cell formed at $t_{(0)}$ will live beyond time t.

When red cell destruction is random and few cells survive to the potential life span, the decreasing portion of the curve may be approximated as

$$N_t = N_0 e^{-kt} \tag{7}$$

When some of the cells are randomly destroyed and some survive to T, the declining portion of the curve may be approximated as

$$N_t = \frac{N_0 e^{-kt}}{1+e^{\alpha(t-T)}} \tag{8}$$

where α = coefficient of uniformity around T of cells destroyed by senescent processes.

Equation 8 is modified from that developed by Brown and Eadie (1953), for the case where there is no reutilization of the label.

These are the basic equations necessary to describe red cell survival. They do not provide for reutilization of label, except for Eq. (6), for elution of label from intact surviving cells, and for variation in distribution of cell age seen under certain conditions.

C. Values in Normal Man and in Animals

The values published since 1958 of red cell life span for man and a number of experimental animals are detailed in Table I.

There is apparently no change in red cell life span in elderly subjects (Hurdle and Rosin, 1962), in children (Remenchik *et al.*, 1958), or in the last half of pregnancy (Pritchard and Adams, 1960).

From studies of the survival of red cells from placental blood and from premature and full-term infants by the Ashby method (Mollison, 1961a), Cr^{51}-labeled autologous and homologous transfusions (Foconi and Sjolin, 1959; Hollingsworth, 1955; Kaplan and Hsu, 1961), and N^{15}-labeled glycine (Dancis *et al.*, 1959), the following conclusions can be drawn.

(1) Full-term infants at birth produce cells that have a normal survival.

(2) Red cells derived from premature infants have a shortened survival.

(3) Red cells from infants 3–9 weeks of age have a shortened survival when transfused into adults; this is due to a decrease in the rate of erythropoiesis following birth; thus at the age of 3–9 weeks of age the circulating cells contain a disproportionate number of older cells and hence when transfused into normal adults would have a shortened survival.

D. Values in Disease States and Applied Variables

With the possible exception of the hibernating marmot (Brace, 1953), hamster (Brock, 1960), and squirrel (Marvin, 1963), there is no evidence that the red cell life span can be significantly increased beyond the normal for that species in mammals.

Red cells may have a shorter life span than the normal because of a defect within the cell (intracorpuscular defect), or because there is some factor operative in the milieu that removes red cells before they reach the end of their potential life span (extracorpuscular defect). A few selected examples of alterations in red cell life span are given in the following paragraphs.

Two sheep given molybdenum for long periods of time showed a pattern consistent with two populations of red cells, one having a life span consistent

TABLE I

RED CELL LIFE SPAN DATA[a]

Animal	Method	Analytical method	Mean	Range	Remarks	Reference
Mouse	—	$T\frac{1}{2}$	20	±2.5	—	Smith and Toha (1958)
	—	$T\frac{1}{2}$	—	15–20	—	Goodman and Smith (1961)
	Cr^{51}	Extinction point	—	50–55	—	Goodman and Smith (1961)
	Glycine-C^{14}	—	41	40–43	—	Ehrenstein (1958)
	DFP^{32}	—	42	40–51	—	Edmondson and Wyburn (1963)
			40.7	±1.9		Van Putten (1958)
Rat	Cr^{51}	$T\frac{1}{2}$	19	—	—	Goodman and Smith (1961)
	—	—	18	±2.5	—	Smith and Toha (1958)
	—	—	17.1	±2.33	—	Brown *et al.* (1961)
	—	—	20.7	±2.5	—	Belcher and Harriss (1959)
	—	—	17	—	—	Smith *et al.* (1959)
	—	—	18	—	—	Thompson *et al.* (1961)
	—	Extinction point	approx. 60	—	—	Goodman and Smith (1961)
	—	Extinction point	65	—	—	Smith *et al.* (1959)
	Ashby differential agglutination	—	65	—	—	Smith *et al.* (1959)
	Fe^{59}	—	60	50–75	Fe^{59} cohort labeling	Jones (1961)
	Fe^{59}	—	59	—	Fe^{59} cohort labeling	Belcher and Harriss (1959)
	Glycine-C^{14}	—	55	—	—	Forssberg and Tribukait (1962)
	DFP^{32}	—	65	56–90	—	Edmondson and Wyburn (1963)
			60	±3.2		Van Putten (1958)

Hamster	Cr^{51}	$T\frac{1}{2}$	14.5	—	—	Rigby *et al.* (1961a)
	Cr^{51}	$T\frac{1}{2}$	12–20	—	—	Rigby *et al.* (1961b)
	Cr^{51}	Extinction point	60–70	—	—	Rigby *et al.* (1961b)
	Cr^{51}	Extinction point	78.5	—	—	Brock (1960)
Squirrel	Cr^{51}	Extinction point	60	—	—	Marvin (1963)
Guinea pig	Cr^{51}	$T\frac{1}{2}$	20	—	—	Grönroos (1960)
	Cr^{51}	$T\frac{1}{2}$	16	—	Autologous, isologous	Smith and McKinley (1962)
	Cr^{51}	$T\frac{1}{2}$	12	—	Homologous	Smith and McKinley (1962)
	Cr^{51}	Extinction point	65	—	—	Grönroos (1960)
	Cr^{51}	—	80–90	—	—	Smith and McKinley (1962)
	Cr^{51}	—	80	—	—	Edmondson and Wyburn (1963)
	DFP^{32}	Extinction point	79	—	—	Edmondson and Wyburn (1963)
Sloth (*Choloepus didactylus*)	Cr^{51}	Extinction point	130, 135	—	2 Animals	Marvin and Shook (1963)
Rabbit	Cr^{51}	$T\frac{1}{2}$	12	8–17	—	Gardner *et al.* (1961)
	—	$T\frac{1}{2}$	13.5	—	—	Sutherland *et al.* (1959)
	—	—	19.0	± 5.9	—	Marvin and Lucy (1957)
	—	Extinction point	68	± 5	—	Marvin and Lucy (1957)
	—	Extinction point	—	55–60	—	Gardner *et al.* (1961)
	—	Extinction point	65	60–68	—	Sutherland *et al.* (1959)
	Fe^{59}	—	65	50–80	Fe^{59} cohort labeling	Jones and Cheney (1961)
	Glycine-C^{14}	—	57	± 0.2	Fe^{59} cohort labeling	Gower and Davidson (1963)
	—	—	50	± 0.2	—	Gower and Davidson (1963)

TABLE I—*continued*

Animal	Method	Analytical method	Mean	Range	Remarks	Reference
Dog	Glycine-C^{14}	—	108	97–133	—	Weissman *et al.* (1960)
	Cr^{51}	$T\frac{1}{2}$	24.3	±2.8	—	Weissman *et al.* (1960)
	Cr^{51}	$T\frac{1}{2}$	18.7	±1.0	—	Wellington and Gardner (1962)
	Cr^{51}	$T\frac{1}{2}$	—	22–35	Intravenous administration	Rochlin *et al.* (1961)
	Cr^{51}	$T\frac{1}{2}$	—	24–32	Intraperitoneal administration	Rochlin *et al.* (1961)
	Cr^{51}	Extinction point	—	96–110	Intravenous administration	Rochlin *et al.* (1961)
	—	Extinction point	—	102–110	Intraperitoneal administration	Rochlin *et al.* (1961)
	Cr^{51}	Extinction point	104	±10.4	Autologous cell, intraperitoneal	Clark and Woodley (1959)
	—	Extinction point	98	8.9	Autologous cell, intraperitoneal	Clark and Woodley (1959)
	—	Extinction point	96.5	11.6	Isologous cell	Clark and Woodley (1959)
	—	Extinction point	98.8	10.5	Puppy	Clark and Woodley (1959)
	—	Extinction point	108.6	—	Intramedullary administration	Clark and Woodley (1959)
Mule deer	Glycine-C^{14}	—	95	—	1 Animal	Cornelius *et al.* (1960)
Llama	Glycine-C^{14}	—	225	—	30% cells destroyed randomly	Kaneko and Cornelius (1962)
Sheep						
Auodad	Glycine-C^{14}	—	65, 170	—	2 Populations of cells (20 and 80% resp.)	Cornelius *et al.* (1960)

Domestic	Glycine-C^{14}	—	64, 94	—	2 Animals	Kaneko *et al.* (1961b)
Domestic	Glycine-C^{14}	—	131, 150, 157	—	3 Animals	Judd and Matrone (1962)
Karakul	Glycine-C^{14}	—	118, 130	—	2 Animals	Kaneko *et al.* (1961b)
Bighorn	Glycine-C^{14}	—	147	—	1 Animal	Kaneko *et al.* (1961b)
	DFP^{32}	—	100	—	—	Eadie *et al.* (1960)
Antelope	Glycine	—	80	—	1 Animal	Cornelius *et al.* (1959)
Goat						
Himalayan	Glycine-C^{14}	—	160, 165	—	2 Animals	Kaneko and Cornelius (1962)
Domestic	Glycine-C^{14}	—	125	—	1 Animal	Kaneko and Cornelius (1962)
Monkey	Cr^{51}	Extinction point	91, 98, 101	—	5 Animals	Marvin *et al.* (1960)
Pig	Glycine-C^{14}	—	86	—	Lifespan	Bush *et al.* (1955)
	Cr^{51}	$T\frac{1}{2}$	17	—	Homologous cells	Bush *et al.* (1956)
	Cr^{51}	$T\frac{1}{2}$	13.8	± 5.7	Homologous cells	Talbot and Swenson (1963)
	—	—	28.0	± 4.0	Autologous cells	Talbot and Swenson (1963)
Man	DFP^{32}	—	127	114–136	8 Subjects	Eernisse and Van Rood (1961)
	DFP^{32}	—	122	112–133	6 Subjects	Garby (1962)
	DFP^{32}	—	132	118–154	5 Subjects	Brewer *et al.* (1961)
	DFP^{32}	—	124	118–127	8 Subjects	Bove and Ebaugh (1958)
Cattle	DFP^{32}	—	107	—	—	Mizuno *et al.* (1959)
	Cr^{51}	$T\frac{1}{2}$	11.7	10.5–13.0	—	Baker *et al.* (1961)

TABLE I—*continued*

Animal	Method	Analytical method	Mean	Range	Remarks	Reference
Horse	Glycine-C^{14}	—	140, 150	—	2 Animals	Cornelius *et al.* (1960)
Birds						
Duck	Glycine-C^{14}	—	39	—	—	Brace and Altland (1956)
	Cr^{51}	Extinction point	42	—	—	Rodnan *et al.* (1957)
	—	—	42	± 2	—	Marvin and Lucy (1957)
Chicken	Glycine-C^{14}	—	20	—	Random destruction	Brace and Altland (1956)
	Glycine-N^{15}	—	28	—	1 Animal	Shemin (1948)
	P^{32b}	—	28	—	2 Animals	Hevesy and Ottesen (1945)
	P^{32b}	—	32	—	1 Animal	Ottesen (1948)
Pigeon	Cr^{51}	$T\frac{1}{2}$	10.8	± 2.9	—	Marvin and Lucy (1957)
	—	Extinction point	44.0	± 3	—	Marvin and Lucy (1957)
Turkey	Cr^{51}	$T\frac{1}{2}$	12.5	9–16	—	Silber *et al.* (1961)
Alligator	DFP-H^3	—	184, 260, 437	—	3 Animals	Cline and Waldmann (1962b)
Frog	DFP^{32}	—	200	—	—	Cline and Waldmann (1962a)
Toad	Glycine	—	1000–1400	—	—	Altland and Brace (1962)
Turtle	Glycine	—	600–800	—	—	Altland and Brace (1962)

[a] With some exceptions this table is intended to supplement the data presented by Berlin *et al.* (1959)

[b] Measured by incorporation of $NaH_2P^{32}O_4$ into cell nucleic acid.

with red cells in normal sheep, the other short, 20–28 days, and involving 30–40% of the red cells (Kaneko *et al.*, 1961a).

Monkeys on a vitamin E-deficient diet are anemic and the red cell life span is markedly shortened (Marvin *et al.*, 1960).

In splenectomized rats with *Bartonella* infection, the red cell life span is reduced. When these cells are given to normal recipients, the survival is also reduced even if the *Bartonella* infection is treated with Terramycin. This study indicates that *Bartonella* induces a hemolytic anemia with irreversible damage to the red cell (Rudnick and Hollingsworth, 1959). Red cells from *Bartonella*-infected Long-Evan rats given to *Bartonella*-free Sprague-Dawley rats had a decreased survival presumably due to the development of a *Bartonella* infection (Thompson *et al.*, 1961). In experimental *Anaplasma marginale* infection in cattle the red cell life span is markedly reduced (Baker *et al.*, 1961).

Chronic administration of phenacetin can result in a nephritis accompanied by an anemia. This anemia is due in part to a reduction in red cell life span. Red cells from normal subjects, given to patients taking phenacetin and with phenacetin renal insufficiency and anemia, have a shortened survival, while red cells from phenacetin habitues have a normal survival in normal subjects. This indicates that there is some extracorpuscular factor operating to reduce the red cell life span. The nature of the factor is not known (Friis *et al.*, 1960a,b).

Patients with macroglobulinemia have an increased serum viscosity which can be reduced by plasmapheresis (Schwab and Fahey, 1960). In two patients, the red cell life span was shown to be reduced when the plasma viscosity was increased, and was increased—but not to normal—when the viscosity was reduced (Cline *et al.*, 1963). This is the first demonstration that viscosity of the plasma can influence the red cell life span.

In iron-deficient anemic patients, the data on red cell life span vary. Temperley and Sharp (1962) found a normal Cr^{51} half-time in 13 subjects; in 7 subjects Verloop *et al.* (1960) found a decreased survival. Two of Verloop's subjects presented in detail had complex courses, the other five were described as having an insufficient response to iron therapy. This may explain the difference. Rasch *et al.* (1958) reported that the Cr^{51} half-time of autologous cells was decreased in 14 iron-deficient infants, but all subjects had gastro-intestinal bleeding which could account in part for the decreased Cr^{51} half-time.

In a study of the anemia of neoplastic disease, Ehrenstein (1958) measured the red cell life span in normal mice, mice bearing a transplanted tumor, and mice with a spontaneous mammary carcinoma. Following transplantation of the Ehrlich ascites tumor in a solid form, on the fifth day after administration of labeled glycine the life span of the circulating cells was reduced from approximately 40 to 26 days. If transplantation was done 10 days before the tracer was given, red cells were produced at an increased rate and were randomly destroyed with a half-time of 10 days. The red cells of C_3H mice with spontaneous mammary carcinoma were randomly destroyed with a half-time of 11 days. The data have been interpreted as indicating that both extra-corpuscular and intracorpuscular defects occur in these tumor-bearing animals, leading to considerable reduction in the red cell life span.

IV. Determinants of Red Cell Life Span

One of the interesting recent approaches to an understanding of the factors determining red cell life span has been the calculations of Lemez and Kopecky (1962) and Allison (1960) on the number of recirculations of the red cell. Data are available from the rat, rabbit, cat, dog, and man. In these five mammals, the number of recirculations was calculated from the product of the cardiac output and the mean red cell life span divided by the blood volume. The number of recirculations varied from 1.60×10^5 in man to approximately 2×10^5 in the rabbit. In these five species the cardiac output was approximately 80–170 ml./kg./min., the red cell life span 50–120 days, and the total red cell volume 2.2–3.8 ml./100 g. body weight. These variations make it surprising that the calculated number of recirculations falls in this narrow range. There is one significant assumption, namely, that the circulation of cells is random. A large fraction of the cardiac output is delivered to brain, liver, and kidneys. The rest of the visceral organs and the extremities receive in the resting state a relatively small proportion of the cardiac output. Studies of the rate of mixing of red cells indicate that there are at least two mixing components if not more (Strajman *et al.*, 1957). Then the distribution may not be random, but the patterns are probably similar in the species studied. However, it is possible that the assumption is met in large measure. The fact that the numbers do prove to be similar supports this view.

A. Role of Spleen

The role of the spleen in the removal of effete red blood cells has been demonstrated by a number of investigators in different ways. The principal methods have been the localization of isotope following administration of labeled cells in the spleen and, in particular, in cells that have been altered *in vitro* (Harris *et al.*, 1958; Jacob and Jandl, 1962). In the normal animal the red cell life span is unchanged following splenectomy, with the possible exception of the slight increase noted by Belcher and Harriss (1956) and Thompson *et al.* (1961) in the rat. In the rabbit there is some suggestion of very slight prolongation in the red cell life span after splenectomy (Gardner *et al.*, 1961). In the dog the red cell life span following splenectomy is normal (Waldmann *et al.*, 1960) and in man in at least one instance it is normal post-splenectomy

(Gevirtz *et al.*, 1962). The normal red cell life span after splenectomy suggests that the other segments of the reticuloendothelial system have the capacity to assume the function of removal of effete cells.

In patients with hemoglobin H there is an increase in red cell survival, but not to normal, following splenectomy (Rigas and Koler, 1961).

The longer, but shorter than normal, survival of influenza-treated rabbit red cells in splenectomized rabbits again points to the role of the spleen in removal of red cells (Gardner *et al.*, 1961).

B. Role of Metabolic Rate

Rodnan *et al.* (1957) showed a good interspecies correlation between basal metabolic rate and red cell life span. Subsequently Allison (1960), using similar data, showed a good correlation between red cell survival and body weight. Allison (1960) calculated that red cell survival in the mammal could be fitted to the following equation

$$T = 23.95 \log m - 1.89 \tag{9}$$

where T is the red cell life span in days, and m is the body weight in grams. This holds for data obtained in the mouse, rat, rabbit, cat, dog, sheep, and man.

Red cells from hypothyroid and hyperthyroid patients have a normal survival in normal recipients by the Ashby method, but autologous Cr^{51}-labeled cells in hyperthyroid patients have a diminished survival (McClellan *et al.*, 1958). The dog with experimentally induced hyperthyroidism becomes polycythemic as a result of an increased rate of production of red cells, but there is no change in the red cell life span (Waldmann *et al.*, 1962). There is also no change or at most a very small decrease (Marvin, 1963) in the red cell life span in the hypermetabolic rat (Hall *et al.*, 1957). In the hypothyroid dog there is an approximate 38% decrease in total red cell volume due to decrease in red cell production, but again no change in red cell life span (Cline and Berlin, 1963b). If the environmental temperature of the alligator is changed from 31°C. to 16°C., there is an apparent prolongation of the red cell life span. However, there is considerable reduction, if not almost complete suppression, of red cell synthesis at 16°C. (Cline and Waldmann, 1962b). In the hibernating golden hamster, there is also considerable reduction in erythropoiesis (Brock, 1960). Without determination of changes in total red cell volume, it is not possible to make a definite statement as to the red cell life span in the hibernating hamster. The observed data have been interpreted as indicating prolongation of red cell life span, but the numerical values may need to be revised (Brace, 1953; Brock, 1960; Marvin, 1963).

These data indicate that there is good correlation from species to species between metabolic rate and red cell life span, but that in a given species the predominant effect of variation in metabolic rate is on the rate of erythropoiesis—not the red cell life span.

C. *Abnormal Hemoglobins*

The abnormal hemoglobins are associated with a reduction in red cell life span. The mechanisms involved have not been worked out (Frick *et al.*, 1962; Hillcoat and Waters, 1962; Pearson and McFarland, 1962; Rigas and Koler, 1961; Scott *et al.*, 1960; Malamos *et al.*, 1962).

D. *Enzymatic Defects in Red Cell*

The principal enzymatic system which has been studied in relationship to red cell life span is glucose-6-phosphate dehydrogenase. A deficiency of this enzyme is associated with an increased sensitivity to primaquine (Kellermeyer *et al.*, 1962). In the primaquine-sensitive individual the red cell life span is shortened in the normal state and after the administ.ation of primaquine (Brewer *et al.*, 1961). The degree of shortening is dependent upon the dose of primaquine (Kellermeyer *et al.*, 1962). Conrad *et al.*, (1960) suggested that in hereditary nonspherocytic hemolytic disease, a disease characterized by decrease in red cell life span, there may be an enzymatic or metabolic defect, which in the type II variant has been shown to be a pyruvate kinase deficiency (Tanaka *et al.*, 1962).

E. *Ineffective Erythropoiesis*

Ineffective erythropoiesis is defined as the production of red cells which are either destroyed in the marrow or have a very short survival in the peripheral circulation (Finch, 1959). These are cells defective in the sense that they either do not complete maturation or do not survive. In the normal individual given glycine labeled with either C^{14} or N^{15}, there is an early peak of incorporation of the isotope into bile pigment and stercobilin, reaching a maximum specific activity at 3–5 days (London *et al.*, 1950; Gray *et al.*, 1950; Gray and Scott, 1959). There is then a second peak in approximately 100–120 days. The second peak is derived from the excretion of bilirubin derived from the catabolism of senescent cells that have been labeled 100–120 days previously. The early peak of incorporation of isotope indicates that stercobilin is not derived exclusively from the catabolism of hemoglobin of senescent cells and that there is at least one other source of bile pigment (Gray *et al.*, 1950; London *et al.*, 1950). In a patient with aplastic anemia and with no evidence of incorporation of radioiron or glycine into hemoglobin, the early peak of incorporation of isotope into stercobilin was markedly reduced, if not absent (Barrett, *et al.*, 1964).

In two patients who temporarily failed to produce red cells and then resumed production of red cells when subjected to adrenal cortical steroid therapy, the early peak was absent during the period of erythropoietic failure and considerably increased during the period of erythropoiesis. These studies indicate that the early peak of stercobilin incorporation is almost entirely associated with erythropoiesis. Therefore, quantitation of the amount of isotope excreted during the early peak when compared to the second peak yields an estimate of the amount of ineffective erythropoiesis. Thus some 10–15% of red cells produced in a healthy man are defective. An alternative interpretation would be that hemoglobin is formed in excess and is removed from the cell but that anatomically the cell persists. A second type of ineffective erythropoiesis is seen in the response to acute blood loss. In the rabbit (Neuberger and Niven, 1951), the rat (Stohlman, 1961; Berlin and Lotz, 1951), and the dog (Cline and Berlin, 1962a) following extensive blood loss the red cells produced have a shorter than normal life span. In the rat this has been shown to be associated with a macrocytosis (Brecher and Stohlman, 1961), and appears to be time dependent. It was not observed in cells produced on the third day after hemorrhage in the rat (Forssberg and Tribukait, 1962), but was observed in cells produced within 8 hours after hemorrhage (Berlin and Lotz, 1951). It was not observed in cells produced in a dog on the ninth day after acute loss, but was observed in cells produced on the third and sixth days after hemorrhage (Cline and Berlin, 1962a).

There are patients with a refractory anemia associated with a markedly increased amount of ineffective erythropoiesis. The central pattern appears to be anemia with a hyperplastic normoblastic marrow, normal or low reticulocyte count, increased bile pigment excretion (fecal urobilinogen), and some reduction in the red cell life span (Greendyke, 1962; Verloop *et al.*, 1962). The red cells and normoblasts may contain iron granules (Dacie *et al.*, 1959). The bile pigment excretion appears to be much greater than can be accounted for by accelerated destruction of circulating red cells (Haurani and Tocantins, 1961; Dacie *et al.*, 1959).

F. Extracorpuscular Factors

It has become apparent that in approximately 30% of transfusions in man of a small volume of labeled homologous cells (Kaplan and Hsu, 1961; Adner and Sjolin, 1957; Mollison, 1959; Jandl and Greenberg, 1957; Adner *et al.*, 1963) the cells are rapidly removed beginning in approximately 2 weeks. This phenomenon has also been observed in the dog (Stohlman and Schneiderman, 1956) and rat (Belcher and Harriss, 1959; Thompson *et al.*, 1961) and pigeon (Marvin, 1959). This is best explained by the development of antibodies, even though the cells were cross-matched before transfusions and antibodies could not be demonstrated by the usual immunological techniques in all instances studied.

In the mouse and dog, transfusion of homologous cells results in a red cell survival in the normal range but shorter than that of autologous cells (Thompson *et al.*, 1961; Goodman and Smith, 1961). In the pig homologous Cr^{51} labeled cells had a shorter than normal survival (Talbot and Swenson, 1963). This has also been observed in man (Cline and Berlin, 1963c; Richmond *et al.*, 1961), but additional confirmatory data are required. A satisfactory explanation is not available, although several possibilities exist.

Rabbit red cells exposed to influenza or Newcastle disease virus have a markedly shortened survival which was increased if the spleen was removed (Gardner *et al.*, 1961). If the cells were washed in saline or media without virus the survival was normal. The rat given trypan blue develops an acute anemia (D. V. Brown *et al.*, 1961). Normal recipients given red cells derived from an acutely anemic animal had a shortened survival, whereas cells derived from a long-term trypan blue-treated animal had a normal survival. If the recipient was acutely anemic the cells derived from a normal animal had a markedly decreased survival. The occurrence of splenomegaly and lymphadenopathy suggests that the red cells coated with proteins by these means may be susceptible to early removal from the reticuloendothelial system.

Red cells coated with Rh agglutinins are removed by the spleen, whereas red cells exposed to ABO agglutinins are removed mainly by the liver (Jandl *et. al*, 1957, 1960).

G. Blood Loss

Clinical hookworm infestation in the dog resulted in markedly decreased red cell survival (Clark and Woodley, 1959). Subclinical hookworm infestation did not result in a mean shortened red cell survival; however, from the data given it is evident that some of the dogs did have a shortened red cell life span. This is attributed to blood loss through parasites. The study points out that one of the mechanisms of decrease in red cell survival is loss of cells from the vascular tree before removal by the normal processes of senescence. This complication in a red cell survival study is often overlooked. Chemical and/or isotopic measurements of urinary and fecal blood losses are possible, but measurement of the quantity of blood lost into tissues is not possible.

V. Summary and Conclusions

The red cell life span is probably most easily measured with isotopically labeled DFP by either random or cohort labeling.

The red cell life span is finite but the degree and rate of random destruction of red cells in all species are variable.

With the exception of the hibernating mammal and poikilotherms taken from a warm to a cold environment, the only variation in red cell life span is shortening. The red cell life span may be shortened but finite, or the cells may be randomly removed. When the red cell life span is shortened, the defect may be intracorpuscular or extracorpuscular. Intracorpuscular defects and extracorpuscular defects can be differentiated by simultaneous measurement of the survival of two populations of red cells in the same subject.

References

Adner, P. L., and Sjölin, S. (1957). *Scand. J. Clin. Lab. Invest.* **9**, 265.

Adner, P. L., Foconi, S., and Sjölin, S. (1963). *Brit. J. Haematol.* **9**, 288.

Allison, A. C. (1960). *Nature* **188**, 37.

Altland, P. D., and Brace, K. C. (1962). *Am. J. Physiol.* **203,** 1188.

Ashby, W. (1919). *J. Exptl. Med.* **29**, 267.

Ashby, W. (1948). *Blood* **3**, 486.

Baker, N. F., Osebold, J. W., and Christensen, J. F. (1961). *Am. J. Vet. Res.* **22**, 590.

Barrett, P. V. D., Cline, M. J., and Berlin, N. I., (1964). *Clin. Res.* **12,** 108.

Belcher, E. H., and Harriss, E. B. (1959). *J. Physiol. (London)* **146**, 217.

Berlin, N. I., and Lotz, C. (1951). *Proc. Soc. Exptl. Biol. Med.* **78**, 788.

Berlin, N. I., Meyer, L. M., and Lazarus, M. (1951). *Am. J. Physiol.* **165,** 565.

Berlin, N. I., Hewitt, C., and Lotz, C. (1954). *Biochem. J.* **58**, 498.

Berlin, N. I., Beeckmans, M., Elmlinger, P. J., and Lawrence, J. H. (1957). *J. Lab. Clin. Med.* **50**, 558.

Berlin, N. I., Waldmann, T. A., and Weissman, S. M. (1959). *Physiol. Rev.* **39**, 577.

Birkeland, S. (1958). *Scand. J. Clin. Lab. Invest.* **10,** 122.

Bove, J. R., and Ebaugh, F. G., Jr. (1958). *J. Lab. Clin. Med.* **51**, 916.

Brace, K. C. (1953). *Blood* **8**, 648.

Brace, K. C., and Altland, P. D. (1956). *Proc. Soc. Exptl. Biol. Med.* **92**, 615.

Brecher, G., and Stohlman, F., Jr. (1961). *Proc. Soc. Exptl. Biol. Med.* **107**, 887.

Brewer, G. J., Tarlov, A. R., and Kellermeyer, R. W. (1961). *J. Lab. Clin. Med.* **58**, 217.

Brock, M. A. (1960). *Am. J. Physiol.* **198**, 1181.

Brown, D. V., Boehni, E. M., and Norlind, L. M. (1961). *Blood* **18**, 543.

Brown, I. W., Jr., and Eadie, G. S. (1953). *J. Gen. Physiol.* **36**, 327.

Burwell, E. L., Brickley, B. A., and Finch, C. A. (1953). *Am. J. Physiol.* **172**, 718.

Bush, J. A., Berlin, N. I., Jensen, W. N., Brill, A. B., Cartwright, G. E., and Wintrobe, M. M. (1955). *J. Exptl. Med.* **101**, 451.

Bush, J. A., Jensen, W. N., Athen, J. W., Ashenbrucher, H., Cartwright, G. E., Wintrobe, M. M. (1956). *J. Exptl. Med.* **103**, 701.

Clark, C. H., and Woodley, C. H. (1959). *Am. J. Vet. Res.* **20**, 1069.

Cline, M. J., and Berlin, N. I. (1962a). *Blood* **19**, 715.

Cline, M. J., and Berlin, N. I. (1962b). *J. Lab. Clin. Med.* **60**, 826.

Cline, M. J., and Berlin, N. I. (1963a). *Blood* **21**, 63.

Cline, M. J., and Berlin, N. I. (1963b). *Am. J. Physiol.* **204,** 415.

Cline, M. J., and Berlin, N. I. (1963c). *J. Lab. Clin. Med.* **61,** 249.

Cline, M. J., and Berlin, N. I. (1963d). *Blood* **22,** 459.

Cline, M. J., and Waldmann, T. A. (1962a). *Am. J. Physiol.* **203**, 401.
Cline, M. J., and Waldmann, T. A. (1962b). *Proc. Soc. Exptl. Biol. Med.* **111**, 716.
Cline, M. J., Solomon, A., Berlin, N. I., and Fahey, J. L. (1963). *Am. J. Med.* **34**, 213.
Cohen, J. A., and Warringa, M. G. P. J. (1954). *J. Clin. Invest.* **33**, 459.
Conrad, M. E., Jr., Crosby, W. H., and Howie, D. L. (1960). *Am. J. Med.* **29**, 811.
Cornelius, C. E., and Kaneko, J. J. (1962). *Science* **137**, 673.
Cornelius, C. E., Kaneko, J. J., and Benson, D. C. (1959). *Am. J. Vet. Res.* **20**, 917.
Cornelius, C. E., Kaneko, J. J., Benson, D. C., and Wheat, J. D. (1960). *Am. J. Vet. Res.* **21**, 1123.
Dacie, J. V., Smith, M. D., White, J. C., and Mollin, D. L. (1959). *Brit. J. Haematol.* **5**, 56.
Dancis, J., Danoff, S., Zabriskie, J., and Balis, M. E. (1959). *J. Pediat.* **54**, 748.
Dornhorst, A. C. (1951). *Blood* **6**, 1284.
Eadie, G. S., and Brown, I. W., Jr. (1953). *Blood* **8**, 1110.
Eadie, G. S., and Brown, I. W., Jr. (1955). *J. Clin. Invest.* **34**, 629.
Eadie, G. S., Smith, W. W., and Brown, I. W., Jr. (1960). *J. Gen. Physiol.* **43**, 825.
Ebaugh, F. G., Jr., Emerson, C. P., and Ross, J. F. (1953). *J. Clin. Invest.* **32**, 1260.
Edmondson, P. W., and Wyburn, J. R. (1963). *Brit. J. Exptl. Path.* **44**, 72.
Eernisse, J. G., and Van Rood, J. J. (1961). *Brit. J. Haematol.* **7**, 382.
Ehrenstein, G. V. (1958). *Acta Physiol. Scand.* **44**, 80.
Finch, C. A. (1959). *Ann. N.Y. Acad. Sci.* **77**, 410.
Foconi, S., and Sjölin, S. (1959). *Acta Paediat.* **48**, 18.
Forssberg, A., and Tribukait, B. (1962). *Acta Physiol. Scand.* **54**, 152.
Frick, P. G., Hitzig, W. H., and Betke, K. (1962). *Blood* **20**, 261.
Friis, T., Fogh, J., and Nissen, N. I. (1960a). *Acta Med. Scand.* **167**, 253.
Friis, T., Fogh, J., and Nissen, N. I. (1960b). *Acta Med. Scand.* **168**, 127.
Gabrio, B. W., and Finch, C. A. (1954). *J. Clin. Invest.* **33**, 242.
Garby, L. (1962). *Brit. J. Haematol.* **8**, 15.
Gardner, E., Jr., Wright, C. S., and Williams, B. Z. (1961). *J. Lab. Clin. Med.* **58**, 743.
Gevirtz, N. R., Nathan, D. G., and Berlin, N. I. (1962). *Am. J. Med.* **32**, 148.
Gibson, J. G., Seligman, A. M., Peacock, W. C., Fine, J., Aub, J. C., and Evans, R. D. (1947). *J. Clin. Invest.* **26**, 126.
Goodman, J. W. and Smith, L. H. (1961). *Am. J. Physiol.* **200**, 764.
Gower, D. B., and Davidson, W. M., (1963). *Brit. J. Haematol.* **9**, 132.
Gray, C. H., and Scott, J. J. (1959). *Biochem. J.* **71**, 38.
Gray, C. H., Neuberger, A., and Sneath, P. H. A. (1950). *Biochem. J.* **47**, 87.
Gray, S. J., and Sterling, K. (1950). *J. Clin. Invest.* **29**, 1604.
Greendyke, R. M. (1962). *Am. J. Med.* **32**, 611.
Grinstein, M., Kamen, M. D., and Moore, C. V. (1949). *J. Biol. Chem.* **179**, 359.
Grönroos, P. (1960). *Australian J. Sci.* **23**, 195.
Hall, C. A. (1960). *Am. J. Med.* **28**, 541.
Hall, C. E., Nash, J. B., and Hall, O. (1957). *Texas Rept. Biol. Med.* **15**, 890.
Harris, I. M., McAlister, J., and Prankerd, T. A. (1958). *Brit. J. Haematol.* **4**, 97.
Haurani, F. I., and Tocantins, L. M. (1961). *Am. J. Med.* **31**, 519.
Hevesy, G., and Ottesen, J. (1945). *Nature* **156**, 534.
Hillcoat, B. L., and Waters, A. H. (1962). *Australasian Ann. Med.* **11**, 55.
Hjort, P. F., Paputchis, H., and Cheney, B. (1960). *J. Lab. Clin. Med.* **55**, 416.
Hollingsworth, J. W. (1955). *J. Lab. Clin. Med.* **45**, 469.
Horwitt, M. K., Century, B., and Zeman, A. A. (1963). *Am. J. Clin. Nutr.* **12**, 99.
Huff, R. L., Hennessy, T. G., Austin, R. E., Garcia, J. F., Roberts, B. M., and Lawrence, J. W. (1950). *J. Clin. Invest.* **29**, 1041.

Hurdle, A. D., and Rosin, A. J. (1962). *J. Clin. Pathol.* **15**, 343.

Jacob, H. S., and Jandl, J. H. (1962). *J. Clin. Invest.* **41**, 1514.

Jandl, J. H., and Greenberg, M. S. (1957). *J. Lab. Clin. Med.* **49**, 233.

Jandl, J. H., and Kaplan, M. E. (1960). *J. Clin. Invest.* **39**, 1145.

Jandl, J. H., Jones, A. R., and Castle, W. B. (1957). *J. Clin. Invest.* **36**, 1428.

Jones, N. C. Hughes, (1961). *Clin. Sci.* **20**, 315.

Jones, N. C. Hughes, and Cheney, B. (1961). *Clin. Sci.* **20**, 323.

Judd, J. T., and Matrone, T. (1962). *J. Nutr.* **77**, 264.

Kaneko, J. J., and Cornelius, C. E. (1962). *Am. J. Vet. Res.* **23**, 913.

Kaneko, J. J., Cornelius, C. E., and Baker, N. F. (1961a). *Proc. Soc. Exptl. Biol. Med.* **107**, 924.

Kaneko, J. J., Cornelius, C. E., and Heuschele, W. P. (1961b). *Am. J. Vet. Res.* **22**, 683.

Kaplan, E., and Hsu, K. S. (1961). *Pediatrics* **27**, 354.

Kellermeyer, R. W., Tarlov, A. R., Brewer, G. J., Carson, P. E., and Alving, A. S. (1962). *J. Am. Med. Assoc.* **180**, 388.

Kornberg, A. (1942). *J. Clin. Invest.* **21**, 299.

Lemez, L., and Kopecky, M. (1962). *Physiol. Bohemoslov.* **1**, 93.

Lewis, A. E., and Gershow, J. (1961). *J. Appl. Physiol.* **16**, 1140.

London, I. M., West, R., Shemin, D., and Rittenberg, D. (1950). *J. Biol. Chem.* **184**, 351.

McClellan, J. E., Donegan, C., Thorup, O. A., and Leavell, B. S. (1958). *J. Lab. Clin. Med.* **51**, 91.

Malamos, B., Gyftaki, E., Binopoulos, D., and Kesse, M. (1962). *Acta Haematol.* **28**, 124.

Marvin, H. N. (1959). *J. Cell. Comp. Physiol.* **53**, 13.

Marvin, H. N. (1963). *Am. J. Clin. Nutr.* **12**, 88.

Marvin, H. N., and Lucy, D. D. (1957). *Acta Haematol.* **18**, 239.

Marvin, H. N., and Shook, B. R. (1963). *Comp. Biochem. Physiol.* **8**, 187.

Marvin, H. N., Dinning, J. S., and Day, P. L. (1960). *Proc. Soc. Exptl. Biol. Med.* **105**, 473.

Mizuno, N. S., Perman, V., Bates, F. W., Sautter, J. H., and Schultze, M. O. (1959). *Blood* **14**, 708.

Mollison, P. L. (1959). *Brit. Med. J.* **2**, 1035.

Mollison, P. L. (1961a). "Blood Transfusion in Clinical Medicine." 3rd ed., p. 135. Blackwell, Oxford.

Mollison, P. L. (1961b). *Clin. Sci.* **21**, 21.

Munker, T., Matzke, J., and Videbaek, A. (1961). *Acta Med. Scand.* **170**, 607.

Nathan, D. G., Davidson, J. D., Waggoner, J. G. and Berlin, N. I. (1958). *J. Lab. Clin. Med.* **52**, 915.

Neuberger, A., and Niven, J. S. F. (1951). *J. Physiol. (London)* **112**, 292.

Ottesen, J. (1948). *Nature* **162**, 730.

Pearson, H. A., and McFarland, W. (1962). *J. Lab. Clin. Med.* **59**, 147.

Pritchard, J. A., and Adams, R. H. (1960). *Am. J. Obstet. Gynecol.* **79**, 750.

Rasch, C. A., Cotton, E. K., Griggs, R. C., and Harris, J. W. (1958). *J. Lab. Clin. Med.* **52**, 938.

Read, R. C. (1954). *New Engl. J. Med.* **250**, 1021.

Read, R. C., Wilson, G. M., and Gardner, F. H. (1954). *Am. J. Med. Sci.* **228**, 40.

Remenchik, A. P., Schuckmell, N., Dyniewicz, J. M., and Best, W. R. (1958). *J. Lab. Clin. Med.* **51**, 753.

Richmond, J., Alexander, W. R., Potter, J. L., and Duthie, J. J. (1961). *Ann. Rheumatic Diseases* **20**, 133.

Rigas, D. A. and Koler, R. D. (1961). *Blood* **18**, 1.

Rigby, P. G., Emerson, C. P., Betts, A., and Friedell, G. H. (1961a). *J. Lab. Clin. Med.* **58**, 854.

Rigby, P. G., Emerson, C. P., and Friedell, G. H. (1961b). *Proc. Soc. Exptl. Biol. Med.* **106,** 313.

Rochlin, D. B., Rawnsley, H., Duhring, J. H., and Blakemore, W. S. (1961). *Surg. Gynecol. Obstet.* **112**, 675.

Rodnan, G. P., Ebaugh, F. G., Jr., and Fox, M. R. S. (1957). *Blood* **12**, 355.

Rudnick, P., and Hollingsworth, J. W. (1959). *J. Infect. Diseases* **104**, 24.

Schenk, W. G., Jr., and Bow, T. M. (1961). *Arch. Surg.* **82**, 391.

Schiodt, E. (1938). *Acta Med. Scand.* **95**, 49.

Schwab, P. J., and Fahey, J. L. (1960). *New Engl. J. Med.* **263**, 574.

Scott, J. L., Haut, A., Cartwright, G. E., and Wintrobe, M. M. (1960). *Blood* **16**, 1239.

Sheets, R. F., Janney, C. D., Hamilton, H. E., and DeGowin, E. L. (1951). *J. Clin. Invest.* **30**, 1272.

Shemin, D. (1948). *Cold Spring Harbor Symp. Quant. Biol.* **13**, 185.

Shemin, D., and Rittenberg, D. (1946). *J. Biol. Chem.* **166**, 627.

Silber, R., Hedberg, S. E., Akeroyd, J. H., and Feldman, D. (1961). *Blood* **18**, 207.

Smith, L. H., and McKinley, T. W., Jr. (1962). *Proc. Soc. Exptl. Biol. Med.* **111**, 768.

Smith, L. H., and Toha, J. (1958). *Proc. Soc. Exptl. Biol. Med.* **98**, 125.

Smith, L. H., Odell, T. T., Jr. and Caldwell, B. (1959). *Proc. Soc. Exptl. Biol. Med.* **100**, 29.

Stohlman, F., Jr. (1961). *Proc. Soc. Exptl. Biol. Med.* **107**, 884.

Stohlman, F., Jr., and Schneiderman, M. A. (1956). *J. Lab. Clin. Med.* **47**, 72.

Strajman, E., Berlin, N. I., Elmlinger, P. J., and Robinson, J. (1957). *Acta Med. Scand.* **157**, 263.

Strumia, M. M. (1956). *Progr. Hematol.* **1**, 74.

Strumia, M. M., Dugan, A., and Colwell, L. S. (1962). *Blood* **19**, 115.

Sutherland, D. A., Minton, P., and Lanz, H. (1959). *Acta Haematol.* **21**, 36.

Swisher, S. N., Izzo, M. J., and Young, L. E. (1953). *J. Lab. Clin. Med.* **41**, 946.

Talbot, R. B., and Swenson, M. J. (1963). *Proc. Soc. Exptl. Biol. Med.* **112**, 573.

Tanaka, K. R., Valentine, W. N., and Miwa, S. (1962). *Blood* **19**, 267.

Temperley, I. J., and Sharp, A. A. (1962). *J. Clin. Pathol.* **15**, 346.

Thompson, J. S., Gurney, C. W., Hanel, A., Ford, E., and Hofstra, D. (1961). *Am. J. Physiol.* **200**, 327.

Todd, C., and White, R. G. (1911). *Proc. Roy. Soc.* (*London*) Ser. B, **84**, 255.

Turnbull, A., Hope, A., and Verel, D. (1957). *Clin. Sci.* **16**, 389.

Van Kampen, E. J., and Heerspink, W. (1961). *Clin. Chim. Acta* **6**, 630.

Van Putten, L. M. (1958). *Blood* **13**, 789.

Verloop, M. C., Wolk, M. Van der, and Heier, A. J. (1960). *Blood* **15**, 791.

Verloop, M. C., Bierenga, M., and Diezeraad-Njoo, A. (1962). *Acta Haematol.* **27**, 129.

Waldmann, T. A., Weissman, S. M., and Berlin, N. I. (1960). *Blood* **15**, 873.

Waldmann, T. A., Weissman, S. M., and Levin, E. H. (1962). *J. Lab. Clin. Med.* **59**, 926.

Weissman, S. M., Waldmann, T. A., and Berlin, N. I. (1960). *Am. J. Physiol.* **198**, 183.

Wellington, J. S., and Gardner, R. E. (1962). *Arch. Surg.* **84**, 491.

CHAPTER 13

Use of the Erythrocyte in Functional Evaluation of Vitamin Adequacy[1]

Myron Brin

I. General Introduction

For the most part, vitamin adequacy in experimental animals and man has been assessed by evaluating clinical appearance and behavior, by measuring growth rates, or by determining blood levels and urinary excretion levels of particular nutrients. A knotty problem has been the evaluation of a marginal state of deficiency in which clinical status is not clearly abnormal, and in which biochemical data are marginal according to current criteria (ICNND, 1957). Deficiency criteria have been established on the basis of biochemical data obtained from normal and from clinically ill individuals, and the values suggested for the marginal state have been interpolated. These criteria have served admirably well for population surveys (ICNND, 1956–1962).

It is well recognized that many vitamins function as cofactors which are essential for the activity of specific enzyme systems at the cellular level. It is to be expected, therefore, that as deficiency of a vitamin progresses the coenzyme becomes more limiting, and ultimately inadequate coenzyme is available to satisfy the enzymatic requirements of the cell. A biochemical enzyme defect is therefore established, and this defect must precede the development of clinical deficiency disease. We like to refer to this state as the

[1] Acknowledgment is made to the Williams-Waterman fund, and the Nutrition Study Section of the National Institutes of Health for the financial support of these studies.

biochemical stage of vitamin deficiency and feel that it is the core of any studies on the marginal vitamin-deficiency state. At this point we must recognize that the threshold concentration of vitamin necessary to maintain normal enzymatic activity in cells may vary with different individuals. Therefore it is to be expected that a blood level or urinary excretion level of a nutrient in the low range of the criteria may be a deficiency level for one person, but not for another.

Consider the equation:

$$\underset{\text{(protein)}}{\text{Apoenzyme}} + \underset{\substack{\text{(vitamin}\\\text{derivative)}}}{\text{Coenzyme}} \rightleftharpoons \underset{\substack{\text{(active}\\\text{catalyst)}}}{\text{Holoenzyme}}$$

Assuming a normal physiological and nutritional state, the concentration of holoenzyme in a tissue cell would be maintained at a level necessary to preserve the biochemical integrity of the tissue. In a vitamin-deficiency state, there is inadequate coenzyme to saturate the apoenzyme and, therefore, the holoenzyme activity is reduced. As the severity of the deficiency develops, the reduced enzyme activity becomes detrimental to cellular integrity.

This enzyme-coenzyme relationship would permit two types of functional analysis for vitamin adequacy: (a) determination of reduced enzyme activity in the vitamin-deficient tissue and (b) determination of the effects on the activity of the enzyme in the deficient tissue of adding the limiting coenzyme to the deficient system. The first test would lend sensitivity to the assay and the second would lend specificity for the nutrient being studied.

The effect of vitamin deficiency on tissue enzymes has been studied extensively in tissues obtained from experimental animals for thiamine (Peters and Thompson, 1934; Olson *et al.*, 1948; Brin *et al.*, 1958, 1960a), riboflavin (Warburg and Christian, 1932; Burch *et al.*, 1956), pyridoxine (Schlenk and Fisher, 1947; Caldwell and McHenry, 1953; Brin *et al.*, 1954, 1960b; Marsh *et al.*, 1955), etc. However, blood is the tissue most readily available from man. Presented in this chapter are some beginnings in the development of functional enzyme tests for vitamin adequacy by the use of erythrocytes. Only by the development of such tests can we strive to reveal marginal biochemical deficiencies of vitamins before the appearance of clinical signs. Furthermore, the use of these functional specific techniques would permit diagnosis of a specific biochemical deficiency in an individual with complicated clinical malnutrition.

II. Thiamine

A. Intact Erythrocytes

At the turn of the century Warburg (1909) demonstrated that mammalian erythrocytes showed negligible oxidation of glucose to CO_2. Twenty years later it was shown by Barron and Harrop (1928) that glucose was oxidized by erythrocytes in the presence of methylene blue, and by Warburg and Christian (1931) that hexose monophosphate under proper experimental conditions was oxidized by rat erythrocyte preparations in the presence of triphosphopyridine nucleotide. Almost a decade later it was reported by Dische (1951) that when pentoses were incubated with hemolysates, about 70% of the material added as pentose was recovered from the system as hexose. Although these observations had been extended and confirmed, a precise explanation of the methylene blue effect on the respiration of intact erythrocytes was not forthcoming. Suggestions were: (a) increased oxidation of a degradation product of glucose (Barron and Harrop, 1928), (b) oxidation of lactate (De Meio *et al.*, 1934), (c) increased reversible conversion of hemoglobin to methemoglobin (Warburg *et al.*, 1930), (d) conversion of lactic acid to pyruvate (Wendel, 1929). None of these explanations, however, accounted for the magnitude of the increased respiration which resulted from the addition of methylene blue to intact erythrocytes.

1. Effects of Methylene Blue on Metabolism of Glucose Specifically Labeled with C^{14}

Following the rigorous elucidation of the glucose oxidative pathway in yeast (reviewed by Racker, 1954), it was feasible to re-evaluate the previous observations in erythrocyte metabolism. This was done with the aid of isotopic glucose (Brin *et al.*, 1956). It was shown that virtually no $C^{14}O_2$ was released from glucose labeled with C^{14} by intact erythrocytes. However, in the presence of methylene blue significantly large quantities of $C^{14}O_2$ were recovered as shown in Table I (Brin and Yonemoto, 1958). Furthermore, under these conditions the recovery of $C^{14}O_2$ from the second carbon of glucose appeared to be approximately one half of that obtained from the first (aldehyde) carbon. From additional studies employing glucose labeled in the number 6 position and glucose labeled uniformly with C^{14}, it was concluded that in the presence of methylene blue the oxidation of glucose in intact erythrocytes was confined to the upper half of the glucose molecule. This was based on the observation that virtually no C^{14} was obtained as CO_2 from the sixth carbon of the glucose molecule, and that the total activity obtained from the first two carbons of the molecule was almost equivalent to that obtained from the use of uniformly labeled glucose. With the recognition that 6-phosphogluconic acid dehydrogenase could selectively remove only the first carbon of glucose as CO_2, and yet $C^{14}O_2$ from the second carbon of glucose was also recovered, it appeared that the addition of the dye to intact erythrocytes expedited a continuous availibility of pentose phosphate which was recycled to hexose and ultimately oxidized as such. This assumed that the second carbon of the original glucose became the first carbon of the pentose; therefore, the second carbon of the original glucose could be released as $C^{14}O_2$ only by traversing the glucose oxidative cycle a second time. Additional evidence for the latter proposition was obtained from studies which showed that the lactic acid formed from glucose-1-C^{14} by intact erythrocytes in the presence of methylene blue contained significantly less radioactivity than that produced by erythrocytes in the absence of the dye (Brin and Yonemoto, 1958).

a. Effects of Thiamine Deficiency in Rat Erythrocytes. The definitive reactions of glycolysis and the glucose oxidative pathway referred to are

TABLE I[a]

RECOVERY OF $C^{14}O_2$ FROM C^{14} DIFFERENTIALLY LABELED GLUCOSE INCUBATED WITH HUMAN ERYTHROCYTES

Experiment	Molecule[b]	Counts added	Counts recovered (total)	Counts recovered (%)	C-1 counts/ C-2 counts
1. With methylene blue, 0.0033%	Glucose-1-C^{14}	20,777	4954	23.9	2.15
	Glucose-2-C^{14}	9,450	1045	11.1	—
	Glucose-6-C^{14}	28,861	10	0.0	—
	Glucose-U-C^{14}	32,646	2056	6.3	—
2. With methylene blue, 0.0033%	Glucose-1-C^{14}	20,777	5544	26.8	2.01
	Glucose-2-C^{14}	9,450	1253	13.3	2.01
	Glucose-6-C^{14}	28,861	8	0.0	—
	Glucose-U-C^{14}	32,646	2192	6.7	—
3. No methylene blue	Glucose-1-C^{14}	20,777	144	0.69	9.4
	Glucose-2-C^{14}	9,450	7	0.07	—
	Glucose-6-C^{14}	28,861	6	0.02	—
	Glucose-U-C^{14}	32,646	36	0.11	—

[a] Reproduced by permission from the *Journal of Biological Chemistry* (Brin and Yonemoto, 1958).

[b] Glucose-1-C^{14}, glucose-2-C^{14}, and glucose-6-C^{14} refer to three solutions in which the glucose was labeled independently with C^{14} in carbons 1, 2, and 6, respectively. Glucose-U-C^{14} designates a solution in which the glucose was labeled with C^{14} equally in all positions.

described more fully in other chapters of this book (4, 5, and 6). A diagrammatic presentation of these metabolic reactions is shown in Fig. 1. It had been previously observed that the enzyme responsible for the metabolism of pentose phosphate, namely transketolase, required thiamine pyrophosphate (TPP) as a cofactor (Horecker and Smyrniotis, 1953; Racker *et al.*, 1953). It appeared to us that, were the rate of these reactions in the presence of methylene blue to be retarded by thiamine deficiency, it would serve as additional proof that the dye did activate a recycling glucose oxidative pathway in intact erythrocytes. Under these conditions one would expect that (a) pentose phosphate would accumulate in the cells, and (b) the recovery of $C^{14}O_2$ from glucose-2-C^{14} would be depressed. This was tested by placing rats on a low thiamine diet for increasing periods of time and assaying intact erythrocytes for transketolase activity in the Warburg apparatus with methylene blue and isotopic glucose. It was observed (Table II) that as the deficiency became more severe, more pentose accumulated in the cells and less $C^{14}O_2$ from glucose-2-C^{14} was recovered (Brin *et al.*, 1956, 1958). It was therefore

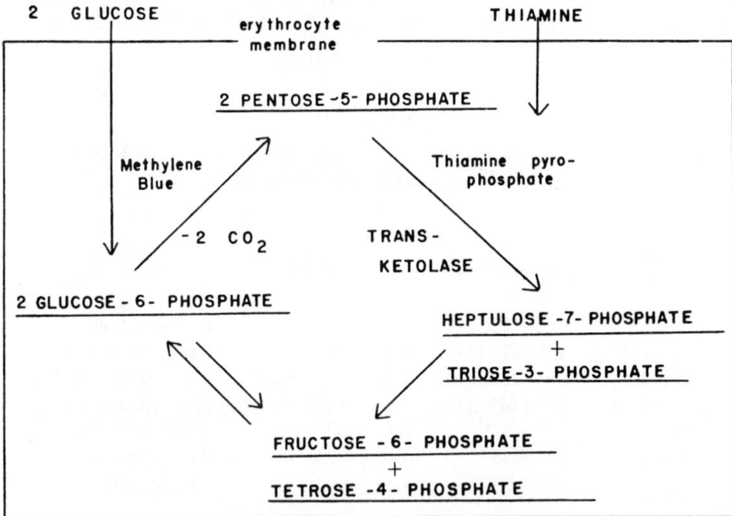

FIG. 1. A diagrammatic presentation of the principal reactions involved in the glucose oxidative pathway used in the assay of transketolase as related to thiamine deficiency. Glucose and thiamine are phosphorylated when utilized as metabolic mediators within the cell. The oxidation of glucose with concomitant production of carbon dioxide is not measured in the hemolysate procedure (reproduced by permission of the *Journal of Nutrition*, Brin *et al.*, 1960a).

apparent that the recycling of glucose through the pathway was markedly depressed in thiamine deficiency. This served to support the argument that methylene blue activated the pentose phosphate pathway in intact erythrocytes, and also showed that the TPP cofactor for transketolase was functional for the enzyme. The functional role that TPP played in the transketolase reaction was supported by additional studies in which the decreased transketolase activity observed in deficient red cells was largely restored when thiamine was added (a) *in vitro* to the cells before they were incubated in the Warburg flask and (b) *in vivo* to the animals (Brin *et al.*, 1958). The specificity of the thiamine effect was supported by these data, therefore.

In addition to elucidation of the methylene blue effect on erythrocyte respiration, it was apparent from these studies that an enzyme had been encountered in the rat which was both sensitive and specific for a nutritional deficiency of thiamine. Furthermore this enzyme was present in the erythrocyte, a cell very readily available without detriment to the host, whether experimental animal or man. Coincidentally, the erythrocyte was uniquely suited as an assay tissue for transketolase activity because it is virtually devoid of an active endogenous oxidative metabolism. Therefore there were few extraneous reactions to interfere with the assay of transketolase. It occurred to us, then, that the erythrocyte might be useful as a biopsy material in the assessment of thiamine adequacy in man.

TABLE II[a]

EFFECT OF THIAMINE DEFICIENCY ON GLUCOSE OXIDATIVE PATHWAY IN RAT ERYTHROCYTES IN PRESENCE OF METHYLENE BLUE

Days on diet	Oxygen consumption (μl.)	Pentose accumulation (μg. per flask)	C-1 recovery (fraction)	C-2 recovery (fraction)	No. of observations
0	116±5.3[b]	126±7.2	0.52±0.03	0.139±0.008	26
1–7	116 (81–141)	128 (97–149)	0.38 (0.267–0.434)	0.095 (0.086–0.111)	4
8–10	98 (92–114)	136 (130–144)	0.453 (0.394–0.565)	0.073 (0.036–0.115)	6
11–15	106 (89–117)	177 (141–230)	0.462 (0.179–0.759)	0.057 (0.003–0.110)	7
16–29	98±4	173±5.2	0.49±0.02	0.047±0.003	17
30–44	89±4.5	263±35	0.46±0.02	0.030±0.003	29
45–58	84±7	353±38	0.45±0.04	0.020±0.004	10

[a] Reproduced by permission from the *Journal of Biological Chemistry* (Brin *et al.*, 1958).
[b] Standard error of the mean; where there are fewer than eight values, the range is given in parentheses.

b. Effects of Thiamine Deficiency in Human Erythrocytes. A study was made of 17 individuals suspected of thiamine insufficiency due to excessive alcoholism and malnutrition (Wolfe *et al.*, 1958). Nine of the 17 had Wernicke's encephalopathy and 7 or more showed each of the following: nystagmus, peripheral neuritis, confusion and delirium, and ataxia. The other 8 subjects were suspected of thiamine deficiency but lacked ophthalmoplegia. Twenty controls were included in the study, of which 11 were hospital convalescents and 9 were laboratory personnel. Intact erythrocytes from all of these individuals were assayed for transketolase activity as previously described (Brin *et al.*, 1958); the data are summarized in Table III. It was clearly apparent that the recovery of $C^{14}O_2$ from glucose-2-C^{14} in intact erythrocytes obtained from the individuals with Wernicke's encephalopathy was markedly depressed below that of the controls. The accumulation of pentose was elevated in this group. These data, therefore, indicated the failure of the second carbon of glucose to recycle through the glucose oxidative pathway and suggested a biochemical block at the transketolase step. Presumably this block was due to a deficiency of thiamine at the enzyme level. Following treatment of the Wernicke group with thiamine for varying periods of time, increased $C^{14}O_2$ recovery and decreased pentose accumulation resulted in erythrocytes obtained from the treated individuals. These data

TABLE III[a]

C^{14} RECOVERIES AND PENTOSE ACCUMULATION OF VARIOUS GROUPS STUDIED[b]

Group	C-2 recovery % counts added (%)	Pentose accumulation (μg. per flask)	No. of experiments
Controls	16.6±2.3	133±13	20
Wernicke group			
Before treatment	10.2±2.1[c]	172±18[c]	8
After treatment (maximum recovery)	13.8±2.1	148±21	8
Suspected thiamine deficiency	15.3±1.0	146±21	8

[a] Reproduced by permission from the *Journal of Clinical Investigation* (Wolfe *et al.*, 1958).
[b] Figures represent mean±S.D.
[c] $P = 0.01$.

supported the proposition that the biochemical defect in thiamine deficiency included reduction of transketolase activity. It appeared, then, that a biochemical differentiation between thiamine deficiency at the cellular level and nonspecific clinical disease could be made.

B. *Hemolyzed Erythrocytes*

1. Transketolase Assay Procedure

Although the intact erythrocyte assay for study of thiamine deficiency proved useful in man, it was not appropriate for routine clinical use. This was because the oxidative metabolism of the cells as stimulated by the presence of methylene blue deteriorated rapidly after the cells were shed, and also because the use of the Warburg apparatus and the use of isotopes required special equipment and technical skill. Additional studies, however, showed that the transketolase enzyme in erythrocytes was relatively stable to freezing. The enzyme assay was therefore modified to use these hemolyzed cells (Brin *et al.*, (1959, 1960a). In short, heparinized blood was centrifuged to a constant cell volume, the plasma removed, and a volume of water equal to the volume of packed cells added. The cells were resuspended and frozen. This served to assure complete hemolysis of the cells and permitted storage in the frozen state until it was convenient to assay the samples. For the transketolase assay the hemolysate was thawed and an aliquot was incubated with ribose-5-phosphate for 1 hour, at which time the reaction was terminated with trichloroacetic acid (TCA). After TPP (thiamine pyrophosphate) was added, the hemolysate was incubated for 20 minutes before the substrate was added to the system. In both cases, with and without TPP, the TCA filtrate was analyzed for both amount of pentose utilized in the reaction and amount of hexose formed during the incubation period.

2. Effects of Thiamine Deficiency

a. Young and Older Rats. Typical data obtained from a study in which groups of rats were fed thiamine-deficient diets for increasing periods of time

TABLE IV[a]

EFFECT OF THIAMINE DEFICIENCY ON APPEARANCE OF HEXOSE (FROM PENTOSE) IN RAT RED CELL HEMOLYSATES[b]

Days on test	Control rats (μg. hexose/ml./hr.)		Deficient rats (μg. hexose/ml./hr.)		Depression from control (%)
	No addition	+TPP[c]	No addition	+TPP[c]	
7	897±14	898±44 (0)	680±53	749±36 (9)	24
9	859±26	936±34 (9)	667±78	776±52 (17)	22
11	922±24	955±22 (3)	460±50	590±32 (28)	50
13	922±46	1017±40 (10)	491±75	650±47 (33)	46
20	978±17	941±18 (0)	371±36	487±28 (31)	61

[a] Reproduced by permission from the *Journal of Nutrition* (Brin *et al.*, 1960a).

[b] Rats were FDRL strain. Each value represents mean ± S.E. of 6 rat blood hemolysates.

[c] To each hemolysate 100 μg. TPP was added. Values in parentheses represent percentage change due to the TPP effect.

are presented in Table IV. It was apparent that after but 3 weeks on a deficient diet, the formation of hexose by hemolysates obtained from the deficient animals had dropped to 39% of that of the appropriate control group. Whereas the addition of TPP to hemolysates of thiamine-adequate rats resulted in little change in transketolase activity (10% or less), marked increases were observed for the deficient samples (up to 33%). This is referred to as the "TPP effect." Additional groups of thiamine-depleted rats were repleted with thiamine by injection or by feeding. The data obtained from transketolase assays on erythrocytes of these rats are shown in Table V.

Note that the amount of hexose formed by hemolysates from rats fed the deficient diet for but 9 days was depressed and that a greater depression was observed at 16 days. However, treatment of the deficient rats with thiamine either by injection or by feeding resulted in essentially normal transketolase values. Furthermore, although a significant enhancement of transketolase activity was elicited by adding TPP to the deficient hemolysates, virtually no TPP effect was observed in erythrocytes of either control or thiamine-treated groups. It was apparent, therefore, that the hemolysate assay for transketolase was also both sensitive and specific for thiamine deficiency.

TABLE V[a]

REPLETION *in Vivo* OF THIAMINE-DEFICIENT RATS

Group	Days on test	Number and sex	Hexose appearance[b] (μg./ml. blood/hr.) No addition	+TPP[c]	TPP effect (%)
Control	6	5F	1119±28	1099±23	0
	16	3F	1456 (1339–1611)	1430 (1263–1533)	0
Deficient	9	5F	732±37	974±18	33
	16	3F	501 (443–559)	805 (675–947)	60
Injected[d]	9	3F	1087 (1035–1132)	1061 (997–1073)	0
	12	3F	1237 (1108–1301)	1224 (1070–1340)	0
Fed[e]	13	5F	1054 (963–1238)	1011 (839–1330)	0

[a] Reproduced by permission of the *Journal of Nutrition* (Brin *et al.*, 1960a).

[b] Data are presented as mean ± S.E. or mean with range of values. CFN rats.

[c] Thiamine pyrophosphate (100 μg.) added *in vitro* to the hemolysates.

[d] Four intraperitoneal injections of 2 mg. thiamine·HCl daily over a 5-day period to rats fed the deficient diets for 9 and 12 days.

[e] After 13 days on the deficient diet the control diet was fed for 14 days.

It has been noted in a series of studies that normal growth was obtained in rats fed a thiamine-deficient diet over a 2-week period (Brin *et al.*, 1958, 1960a; Salcedo *et al.*, 1948). Yet transketolase was depressed 30 and 24% at 1 week and 50 and 51% at 2 weeks for the intact cell and the hemolysate systems, respectively (Brin *et al.*, 1958, 1960a). These data demonstrated therefore that the biochemical defect in transketolase was demonstrable before any other adverse clinical signs were noted in the rat, including the very sensitive measure of nutritional adequacy, namely, growth.

Up to this point all studies were done on young, rapidly growing rats. It was therefore of interest to evaluate the sensitivity of the erythrocyte transketolase assay for thiamine deficiency in heavier, slower growing animals. Female rats weighing approximately 250 gm. were divided into 2 groups and fed thiamine-deficient and supplemented diets, respectively, for periods of up to 4 weeks. The data are presented in Table VI (Brin, 1962a). It was observed that the body weights of these animals increased for 12 days in a manner similar to that previously observed in younger animals. However, the transketolase activity in the thiamine-deficient group was depressed about 50% at 2 weeks and a positive TPP effect was observed. It appeared therefore that the erythrocyte was useful in evaluating thiamine lack in older, as well as in rapidly growing, experimental animals.

TABLE VI[a]

EFFECTS OF THIAMINE DEFICIENCY ON ERYTHROCYTE HEMOLYSATE TRANSKETOLASE ACTIVITY IN HEAVY RATS

Days on test	Body weight (gm.)	Formation of hexose[b] (μg./ml. hemolysate/hr.)	
		No addition	+TPP
0	259	1068	1072
12	271	549	709
19	264	160	292
26	223	187	243

[a] Reproduced by permission of New York Academy of Sciences (Brin, 1962a).

[b] Assayed as described previously. Each transketolase value represents mean for 3 rats at zero days and 4 rats subsequently.

(i) Effects of varying level of dietary thiamine. The demonstration of an enzyme defect in thiamine-deficient rats before growth was retarded was of interest because nutritionists have, with much profit, used the growth of young rats as a measure of dietary adequacy. It is reasonable, however, that in a nutritional insufficiency the biochemical defect would precede other pathology, whether clinical or cellular. It was desirable then to determine the effects of graded levels of dietary thiamine on rat erythrocyte transketolase activity during a 2-week period of marginal deficiency. The results of these studies are presented in Table VII (Brin and Owens, 1960; Brin, 1962a). There were no significant differences in body weight of groups of rats fed diets containing 0.0, 0.1, 0.5, and 1.0 μg. thiamine/gm. purified diet. However, the transketolase activity of the hemolysates obtained from these groups increased as the dietary level of thiamine increased. It is to be noted that these are suboptimal levels of thiamine for the rat. These data demonstrated that the effect of thiamine deficiency on erythrocyte transketolase was not an all-or-none effect, but that within the given range of dietary thiamine the activity of the enzyme varied with the thiamine content of the diet.

(ii) Biological availability of thiamine in food. It was then of interest to determine whether the graded response of erythrocyte transketolase to graded levels of dietary thiamine could be utilized to evaluate the thiamine content of food supplements. Accordingly, 3 groups of 5 rats each were fed purified diets containing 3 levels of thiamine, namely, 0.3, 0.5, and 0.8 μg./gm. diet, respectively. Three additional groups of 5 rats each were fed the basal purified diets supplemented with unenriched flour, enriched flour, and cracked corn. The supplements were added to the diets to approximate a thiamine concentration of 0.5 μg. thiamine/gm. diet as determined by the thiochrome

TABLE VII[a]

EFFECTS OF GRADED LEVELS OF DIETARY THIAMINE ON ERYTHROCYTE TRANSKETOLASE IN RATS[b]

Level of thiamine in diet (μg./gm.)	Body weight (gm.)	Transketolase activity (μg. hexose/ml. hemolysate/hr.)
0.0	129.9	541.3
0.1	134.0	679.3
0.5	129.1	802.0
1.0	133.7	905.8

[a] Reproduced by permission of New York Academy of Sciences (Brin, 1962a).

[b] Each value for body weight represents 10 rats, for transketolase activity 5 rats. Animals were on test diet for 12 days.

assay (Hennesey and Cerecedo, 1939) as modified (ICNND, 1957). In each case the supplements were substituted for an equivalent weight of dextrose in the basal mixture. All rats were fed for a period of 14 days in wire-bottomed cages with food and water available *ad libitum*. At the end of the 2-week feeding period, erythrocyte transketolase was determined in each group. Values for erythrocyte transketolase activity, obtained from the groups fed the supplements, were interpolated on the dose-response curve (Fig. 2) to determine the thiamine content of each supplement. The results are shown in Table VIII. For the 3 materials tested, the values obtained by both measures of transketolase activity were within the range of values obtained by chemical assay with the thiochrome technique.

In addition, erythrocyte transketolase has been used to measure, by the biological means described above, the extent of destruction of thiamine in foods preserved by x-irradiation. By use of the transketolase assay it was shown that the availability of thiamine in pork was reduced at exposure levels of 3–6 megarads (Brin *et al.*, 1961b). However, it was also shown that the adverse effects on erythrocyte transketolase were eliminated by adding thiamine to diets containing the x-irradiated food (Brin *et al.*, 1961a).

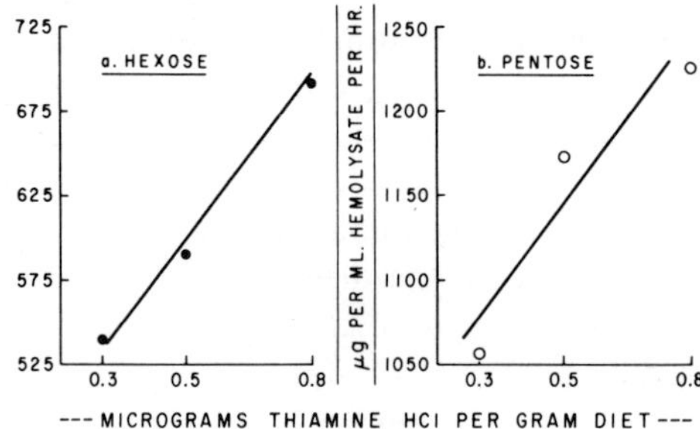

FIG. 2. A diagrammatic plot from which the thiamine content of unenriched flour, enriched flour, and cracked corn was determined in the assay for biological availability of thiamine by the use of erythrocyte transketolase in rats (data previously presented in abstract, Brin and Owens, 1960).

(iii) Effects of pyridoxine, riboflavin, and protein deficiencies. It had now been demonstrated that the activity of erythrocyte transketolase was very sensitive to the development of thiamine deficiency in the rat and man and that the addition of TPP to the hemolysate system restored a large portion

TABLE VIII[a]

ERYTHROCYTE TRANSKETOLASE AS A BIOASSAY FOR THIAMINE IN FOODS[b]

	Transketolase activity (μg./ml. hemolysate/hr.)		Thiamine content (μg./gm. product)		
Group	Hexose	Pentose	Hexose	Pentose	Thiochrome
0.1 μg. B_1/gm. diet	542	1057	—	—	—
0.5 μg. B_1/gm. diet	590	1172	—	—	—
0.8 μg. B_1/gm. diet	692	1225	—	—	—
Unenriched flour	652	1158	2.9	2.4	2.2
Enriched flour	599	1148	5.3	5.4	5.2
Cracked corn	610	1156	5.0	5.0	4.6

[a] Data previously reported in abstract (Brin and Owens, 1960).
[b] Three control groups of 10 rats each and 3 test groups of 5 rats; samples were air dried.

of the depressed activity. Nevertheless, additional data on the nutritional specificity of the effect were desired, because it was recognized that malnourishment is rarely confined to one nutrient. Accordingly, pyridoxine, riboflavin, and protein deficiencies were studied in rats as follows: an appropriately supplemented group and a deficient group were studied for each vitamin, and the effects of protein deficiency were studied at 5 graded levels. All animals were maintained on the appropriate diets for 2 weeks, at which time erythrocyte hemolysates were prepared for transketolase assay. The assay data are presented in Table IX (Brin, 1961, 1962a). It was noted that body weight was maintained in the group fed the thiamine-deficient diet, as was shown previously. Erythrocyte transketolase in this group was markedly depressed, however. In both pyridoxine- and riboflavin-deficient rats, body weight was markedly depressed during the experimental period. However, normal erythrocyte transketolase activity prevailed in these deficiencies. In

TABLE IX[a]

EFFECTS OF GRADED LEVELS OF DIETARY PROTEIN AND OF PYRIDOXINE AND RIBOFLAVIN DEFICIENCIES ON RAT ERYTHROCYTE HEMOLYSATE TRANSKETOLASE[b]

Nutrient	Level	Transketolase activity (μg. hexose/ml./hr.)	Body weight (gm.)
(1) Thiamine	Complete diet	837	110.9
	B_1-deficient diet	296	109.1
(2) Pyridoxine	Complete diet	930	103.7
	B_6-deficient diet	989	88.2
(3) Riboflavin	Complete diet	994	114.4
	B_2-deficient diet	992	94.1
(4) Protein (casein)	5% of diet	1168	99.3
	10% of diet	1200	116.8
	15% of diet	1085	134.2
	20% of diet	1165	126.8
	25% of diet	1220	139.2

[a] Reproduced by permission of New York Academy of Sciences (Brin, 1962a).

[b] Each value represents 10 animals per group. Duration of test was 14 days.

the protein-deficient groups it appeared that body weight increased as the level of dietary protein was increased from 5 to 15% of the diet. Transketolase activity, however, appeared to be constant and normal despite the varied protein level in the several diets. It was evident from these studies that the activity of erythrocyte transketolase was a sensitive reflection of a lack of thiamine but was not sensitive to deficiencies of pyridoxine, riboflavin, or protein during the experimental period.

(iv) Effects on other tissues of thiamine deficiency and of oxythiamine. Although the erythrocyte was a most convenient tissue for study of the effects of thiamine deficiency on transketolase activity, it was desirable to determine the effects on the transketolase activity of other tissues. Only then could one conclude that the erythrocyte may be used as a reflection of thiamine adequacy in other cells of the body. Furthermore, it was of interest to determine whether thiamine antagonists affected transketolase activity adversely. Groups of rats were maintained on thiamine-adequate and thiamine-deficient diets both with and without the addition of oxythiamine (Brin, 1962b). The rats were sacrificed after 13 days of treatment and red cells, brain, heart, kidney, muscle, lung, intestine, and spleen were assayed for transketolase activity. The data are shown in Fig. 3. With the exception of brain, the tissues of all rats fed the thiamine-deficient diet showed reduced transketolase activity at the end of

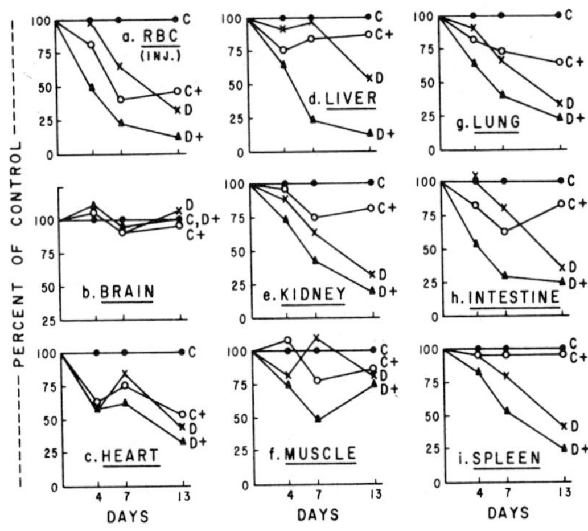

FIG. 3. Effects of injected oxythiamine (+) on transketolase activity (formation of hexose) of 9 tissues in control (C) and thiamine-deficient (D) rats. Data are expressed as percentage of the control group (reproduced by permission of the *Journal of Nutrition*, Brin, 1962b).

the experimental period. In most cases, too, the injection of oxythiamine resulted in reduced transketolase activity in both thiamine-adequate and thiamine-deficient rats. Normal transketolase activity was maintained in brain for the experimental period whether or not oxythiamine was administered to rats fed thiamine-adequate or thiamine-deficient diets. It appeared, therefore, that the brain reserved its thiamine against an adverse gradient. This was in confirmation of earlier studies by Salcedo *et al.* (1948), in which it was shown that normal thiamine content of brain was retained for at least 2 weeks in rats placed on thiamine-deficient diets. These studies demonstrated that the effect of thiamine deficiency on decreasing erythrocyte transketolase was a reflection of similar effects in other body tissues.

b. Man. (i) Controlled studies in young men. More recently, in order to better evaluate the effects of marginal thiamine deficiency on erythrocyte transketolase in man, a controlled study was done with men maintained on an intake of 200 μg. thiamine per day in an otherwise relatively palatable diet. Subjective and objective clinical determinations were made weekly on these

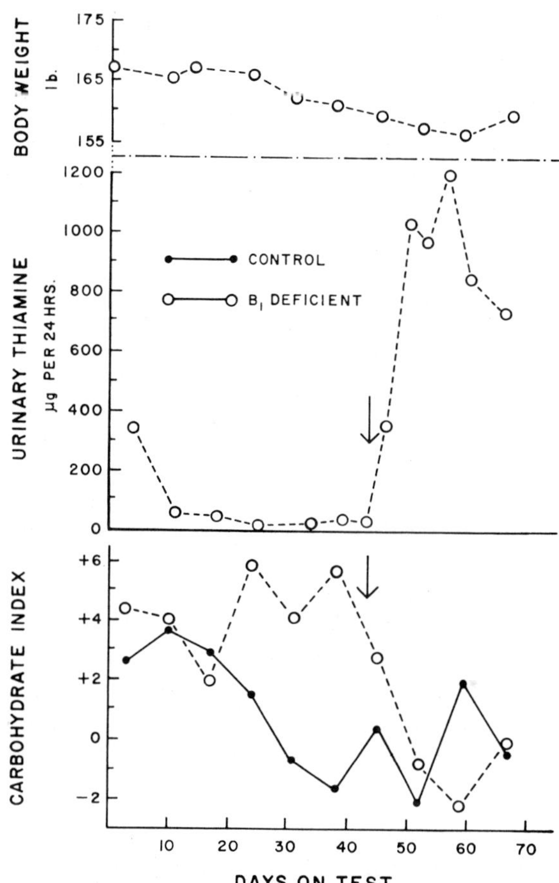

FIG. 4. Effects of thiamine deficiency in man on body weight, urinary excretion of thiamine, and carbohydrate index. The deficient group of four men consumed approximately 190 μg. thiamine daily, and were repleted (shown by arrow) after 6 weeks on the diet (reproduced by permission of New York Academy of Sciences, Brin, 1962a).

volunteers under conditions in which neither the men, nor the attending physician, nor the analysts knew which individuals were supplemented with thiamine. No objective clinical signs were found for the entire deficient period with the exception of weight loss. This began after the twenty-first day of the study as shown in Fig. 4 (Brin, 1962a, c). It was at this time, too, that subjective effects were found. These included diminished concentration ability, fatiguability, some insomnia, and loss of appetite. Biochemically, it was apparent that the urinary thiamine had dropped to about 20 μg. per day by the second week and that it remained at this level for the remainder of the study (Fig. 4). Values for carbohydrate index[2] (Horwitt *et al.*, 1948) were within normal limits, although the values for the deficient men were higher than those for the supplemented men after 3 weeks (Fig. 4). The data for erythrocyte transketolase assayed at intervals during the study are presented in Fig. 5 (Brin, 1962a, c). In the upper curve are transketolase assay data for formation of hexose/ml. hemolysate for each group, expressed as percentage of pentose

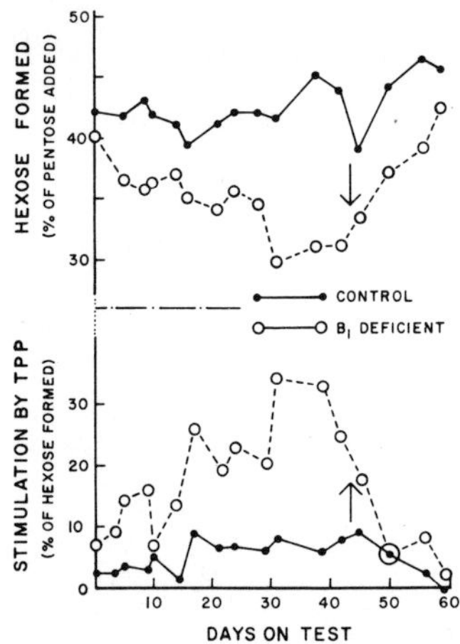

FIG. 5. Effects of thiamine deficiency in man on erythrocyte hemolysate transketolase activity as shown by depressed formation of hexose and the enhanced activity observed after adding TPP to the hemolysate. The deficient group was repleted at 6 weeks (shown by arrow) (reproduced by permission of New York Academy of Sciences, Brin, 1962a).

added as substrate. The curves diverged after but 8 days of the experimental regimen. The divergence between control and deficient groups became more marked as the deficiency became more severe. Presented in the lower set of curves in Fig. 5 are data on the effect of adding TPP to the hemolysates *in vitro*. These are expressed as percentage stimulation of the hexose formation observed upon addition of TPP to the incubating hemolysates. It was apparent that the TPP effect was less than 10% in the control group for the duration

[2] The carbohydrate index was devised to reflect the biochemical defect in the metabolism of pyruvic acid due to thiamine deficiency, and served to minimize the effects of varying levels of glucose and lactic acid in blood. It is expressed as $\text{C.I.} = [(\text{L}-0.1\text{G})+(15\text{P}-0.1\text{G})]/2$, where L, P, and G correspond to the blood levels of lactic acid, pyruvic acid, and glucose, respectively, expressed in mg./100 ml. blood. It was suggested that an index in excess of 15 was indicative of thiamine deficiency (Horwitt *et al.*, 1948).

of the study. In the deficient group, however, the TPP effect was 15% on day 8 and 35% on day 30. All values were rapidly restored to normal following treatment of the deficient individuals with thiamine.

It was apparent from these data that the effects of thiamine deficiency on erythrocyte transketolase in man occurred earlier than any other clinical or subjective findings, and before an effect was observed on pyruvate metabolism.

TABLE X[a]

CLINICAL STATUS OF PATIENTS WITH SUSPECTED THIAMINE DEFICIENCY: HEMOLYSATE STUDY

Status	Patient			
	TY	MG	TS	RE
(a) Findings[b]				
Alcoholism	+	+	+	+
Incoherent	+	—	+	—
Polyneuropathy	+	+	+	+
Ophthalmoplegia	—	—	+	—
Nystagmus	+	—	—	—
Hyperkeratosis	+	—	—	+
Ataxia	+	—	—	—
Edema	—	—	+	+
(b) Vitamin therapy[c]	*	*	**	*
(c) Time for clinical improvement[d]	3 days	2 days	3 days	2 months

[a] Reproduced by permission of New York Academy of Sciences (Brin, 1962a).

[b] Physical and neurological findings upon admission to the hospital.

[c] Routine diets were fed after drawing of initial blood sample; * denotes supplement of thiamine alone and ** denotes multivitamin supplement as follows: TY—50 mg. thiamine daily intramuscularly, MG—25 mg. thiamine daily orally, TS—300 mg. thiamine plus multivitamins intravenously on first day followed by 25 mg. thiamine daily orally, RE—therapeutic multivitamin capsule daily orally.

[d] TY, MG, and TS showed marked clinical improvement and ability for self care in time shown. RE regained partial muscular strength in time shown.

Furthermore, the TPP effect was evident after but 8 days, This again demonstrated the sensitivity of the transketolase assay and the specificity of the TPP effect in the evaluation of thiamine insufficiency in man.

(ii) Patients suspected of beriberi. The hemolysate assay has been applied to the evaluation of patients suspected of thiamine deficiency. In Table X are presented clinical findings on four of the patients studied (Brin, 1962a). The transketolase assay findings are shown in Table XI. Data presented for controls were obtained from 29 clinically healthy male outpatients. Before thiamine therapy, reduced transketolase activity was observed in all patients.

The TPP effect ranged from 27 to 66% in these individuals, and the effect disappeared after thiamine therapy. In the individuals with ophthalmoplegia and/or nystagmus (TY and TS) the enzyme activity increased within 24–48 hours after treatment. In the case of RE clinical improvement was slow, as

TABLE XI[a]

EFFECTS OF ADMINISTRATION OF THIAMINE TO SUBJECTS WITH SUSPECTED THIAMINE DEFICIENCY ON ERYTHROCYTE HEMOLYSATE TRANSKETOLASE

Subject, sex, age, and treatment	Transketolase activity (μg. hexose/ml. hemolysate/hr.)	
	No addition	+TPP
(1) TY (male, 65)		
Before treatment	606	1004
After treatment		
2 days	1002	1087
4 days	937	1032
(2) MG (female, 67)		
Before treatment	812	1034
After treatment		
6 days	1015	1101
(3) TS (male, 41)		
Before treatment	466	708
After treatment		
2 days	998	1024
8 days	945	974
(4) RE		
Before treatment	598	841
After treatment		
1 day	684	895
3 days	662	716
6 days	1054	1012
(5) Controls	1051±24[b]	1106

[a] Reprinted by permission of New York Academy of Sciences (Brin, 1962d).

[b] Mean±S.E. in 29 healthy subjects.

was the case with the transketolase enzyme. It was evident that the erythrocyte apotransketolase was not saturated in these individuals, and that measuring both (a) absolute transketolase activity and (b) TPP effect is useful diagnostically. The use of erythrocyte transketolase to evaluate thiamine deficiency in rats and man has recently been confirmed (Dreyfus, 1962) and discussed (anon., 1962; Brin, 1962d.)

C. Recommendation

The evaluation of marginal thiamine deficiency in man has been recognized to be a very difficult problem. These difficulties have been recently reviewed in some detail (Plough and Bridgforth, 1960). The use of blood levels of thiamine or TPP in man is difficult technically for field work (Burch *et al.*, 1952). Furthermore the percentage depression of blood thiamine or TPP in man even in frank beriberi is very small (Burch *et al.*, 1950) and for this reason their use has been described as being impractical (Bessey, 1954). The measurement of the pyruvate defect in carbohydrate metabolism in the intact individual by the carbohydrate index (Horwitt *et al.*, 1948) has contributed much, but it may not be feasible for evaluation of physically handicapped persons or for field use.

A biochemical defect in the transketolase activity of erythrocytes from thiamine-deficient rats or man has been demonstrated before onset of other clinical signs, including cessation of growth. The TPP effect (an *in vitro* therapeutic trial), the treatment of deficient subjects with the limiting vitamin (an *in vivo* therapeutic trial), and studies with protein, pyridoxine, and riboflavin deficiencies support the concept of a specific relationship between thiamine nutrition and transketolase activity at the enzyme or cellular level. It is suggested that the technique be used (a) to evaluate marginal thiamine deficiency in the absence of clinical signs, and (b) to aid in the differential diagnosis of thiamine inadequacy in the face of complicated malnutrition.

III. Pyridoxine

Clinical pyridoxine deficiency has been encountered in man only under special circumstances. Because of its relative infrequency, a minimum daily requirement for vitamin B_6 has not yet been established. However, the absolute requirement for pyridoxine was established when the deficiency appeared in babies fed a purified B_6-deficient diet. Normal clinical status was re-established in this case when pyridoxine was administered to the children (Snyderman *et al.*, 1950). A variety of clinical pyridoxine deficiency may be attained in man following high dosage therapy with isonicotinic hydrazide (INH) in the treatment of tuberculosis (Sass and Murphy, 1958). Although INH is a chemical analog of niacin, it appears to act biochemically as an antagonist for pyridoxine. Moreover, clinical signs of pyridoxine deficiency have also been obtained in man following administration of large doses of deoxypyridoxine (Vilter *et al.*, 1953). Pyridoxine is involved in certain cases of hyperemesis or toxemia of pregnancy which are relieved by administration of large amounts of the vitamin (McGanity *et al.*, 1949). The curious finding is that, although these individuals may have a normal dietary intake of pyridoxine and show no other clinical signs of B_6 deficiency, an abnormal tryptophan load test is observed; that is, abnormally large amounts of xanthurenic acid are excreted in the urine by these individuals after oral administration of 10 gm. DL-tryptophan (Wachstein and Gudaitis, 1952). The abnormal tryptophan metabolism can be corrected by increasing the daily dose of pyridoxine beyond what is considered normal. The higher daily need for pyridoxine in these cases of abnormal tryptophan metabolism in pregnancy has not yet been explained.

The involvement of vitamin B_6 in the transaminase enzymes was demonstrated in 1947 (Schlenk and Fisher) following a period of much controversy over this problem. The relationship was subsequently confirmed (Caldwell and McHenry, 1953; Brin *et al.*, 1954; Marsh *et al.*, 1955). It was shown that the activity of the alanine transaminase enzyme in pyridoxine-deficient rat and duck tissues was reduced about twice as much as that of the aspartic enzyme.

A. Effects of Pyridoxine Deficiency on Plasma Transaminases in Rats

A marked reduction in activity of both plasma alanine and plasma aspartic transaminase enzymes occurred in pyridoxine-deficient rats (Brin *et al.*, 1960b). The data in Table XII show that the alanine and the aspartic transaminase enzymes in pyridoxine-deficient rat plasma were depressed 85% and 63%, respectively, after 2 weeks on the deficient diet.

TABLE XII[a]

EFFECT OF PYRIDOXINE DEFICIENCY ON PLASMA TRANSAMINASES IN YOUNG RATS[b]

		Alanine enzyme		Aspartic enzyme	
		No addition	Depression[c]	No addition	Depression[c]
Group	Number of rats	(units)	(%)	(units)	(%)
Control	13	378 ± 74[d]	—	831 ± 211[d]	—
Deficient	6	55 ± 24[d]	85	333 ± 87[d]	63

[a] Reprinted by permission of *Journal of Nutrition* (Brin *et al.*, 1960b).
[b] Rats were on test 2–4 weeks at time of assay. Data are presented as mean ± S.E.
[c] Percentage of depression calculated as (control − deficient)/control × 100.
[d] $P < 0.01$.

1. Biological Availability of Pyridoxine in Food

This technique was utilized to study the biological availability of pyridoxine in foods exposed to x-irradiation. These data, presented in Table XIII, show that the alanine transaminase enzyme was depressed in rats fed diets in which x-irradiated pork was the only source of pyridoxine. Yet the animals maintained a normal growth rate (Brin *et al.*, 1961c). An additional study demonstrated that when adequate pyridoxine was added to these diets, both growth rate and plasma transaminase activity were normal (Brin *et al.*, 1961a). The use of the plasma transaminase system under these very controlled conditions demonstrated that a marginal deficiency of pyridoxine caused by feeding

TABLE XIII[a]

EFFECT ON PLASMA TRANSAMINASES IN RATS[b] OF FEEDING CONTROL AND IRRADIATED PORK

Diet	Glutamic-aspartic transaminase[c]	Glutamic-alanine transaminase[d]	Body weight of males (gm.)
(a) DPO[e]	583 ± 40[f]	246 ± 24	365.4
(b) DPO-P	610 ± 43	172 ± 17	360.8
(c) DP3-P	593 ± 50	142 ± 16	363.7
(d) DP6-P	574 ± 76	109 ± 11	347.5

[a] Reprinted by permission of the *Journal of Nutrition* (Brin *et al.*, 1961c).

[b] 18–20 rats (males plus females) per group. Na pyruvate produced in μg./ml. plasma/hr.

[c] No statistically significant differences between any groupings.

[d] Statistical significance of differences: (1) not significant, (c) – (d), (b) – (c); (2) P = 0.05, (a) – (b); (3) P = 0.01, (b) – (d); (4) P = 0.001, (a) – (c), (a) – (d).

[e] DPO denotes diets with unirradiated pork but adequate in pyridoxine. DP3 and DP6 denote diets containing pork irradiated with 3 and 6 megarads, respectively. P indicates that no pyridoxine was added beyond that present in the pork.

[f] Mean ± S.E.

foods exposed to 3 and 6 megarads of ionizing radiation could be revealed by a reduced transaminase activity, despite normal growth.

B. *Effects of Pyridoxine Deficiency on Erythrocyte Transaminases in Rats*

It is recognized that the activity of serum transaminases in normal individuals is highly variable. The serum enzymes are also known to vary widely in the presence of pathology of the heart or liver or in alcoholism, whether intermittent or chronic, and these effects serve to complicate the problem (White, 1958; Greenberg and Harper, 1960). This daily variability, coupled with analytical difficulties in the assay of samples of low activity, renders impractical the use of plasma or serum transaminases to assess pyridoxine adequacy in man.

Presented here are data to show additional relationships between plasma transaminases, erythrocyte transaminases, and pyridoxine deficiency. In Table XIV are data on the effects of pyridoxine deficiency on plasma alanine transaminase and erythrocyte alanine transaminase in rats, and of injecting the rats with pyridoxine. The animals were maintained on pyridoxine-deficient diets for a period of 14 days, following which 1 mg. pyridoxine hydrochloride was injected into one-half the control group and one half the deficient group daily for a period of 4 days. The alternate half of each group was injected with physiological saline (0.9% NaCl in water). After 18 days of pyridoxine deficiency the activity of plasma alanine transaminase dropped to approximately 35% of normal in the pyridoxine-deficient rats. Hemolysate alanine

TABLE XIV[a]

EFFECTS OF PYRIDOXINE REPLETION ON PLASMA AND HEMOLYSATE TRANSAMINASES IN B_6-DEFICIENT RATS[b]

Group injected	Alanine transaminase activity (units)	
	Plasma	Hemolysate
Control		
Saline	234.9 ± 21.5	723.8 ± 23.0
Pyridoxine	241.2 ± 15.1	741.2 ± 36.9
Deficient		
Saline	68.6 ± 17.2	332.8 ± 17.8
Pyridoxine	250.8 ± 15.8	397.4 ± 28.7

[a] Data previously presented in abstract (Albert and Brin, 1960).

[b] Groups of 7–8 rats. Na pyruvate produced in μg./ml. sample/hr. Data are means ± S.E.

transaminase was also significantly decreased in this period in the B_6-deficient animals. However, although plasma transaminase of the B_6-deficient rats was increased to normal after but 3 days of pyridoxine therapy, the hemolysate transaminase was not.

A second study was performed to compare the rates of recovery to normal values of plasma and hemolysate transaminases in pyridoxine-deficient rats, following placement on the control diet. The data are presented diagrammatically in Fig. 6. The values for the control groups are presented as 100% and the values for plasma and hemolysate alanine transaminase activity are presented as percentages of the control activity at the time of analysis. In the group of rats maintained on the pyridoxine-deficient diet for a period of 2 weeks, plasma alanine transaminase activity was reduced to 27% of normal and the hemolysate enzyme to 47% of normal. The plasma enzyme in the deficient animals had returned to normal activity within 1 week of pyridoxine therapy. However, hemolysate alanine enzyme activity was not completely restored to normal until the third week of therapy. The difference in response may be resolved as follows: It is recognized that transaminases in a number of tissues are restored to normal activity in the pyridoxine-deficient animal shortly after treatment with pyridoxine (Caldwell and McHenry, 1953; Brin *et al.*, 1954, 1960b; Marsh and Greenberg, 1955). Furthermore, it is conceived that plasma enzymes are derived by exudation from other tissues of the body, particularly the liver (White, 1958). Rapid return of the plasma enzyme to normal activity might therefore be expected. The erythrocyte, then, is somewhat independent of the plasma enzyme. Either it cannot convert the vitamin to pyridoxal phosphate, or the apoenzyme content of the

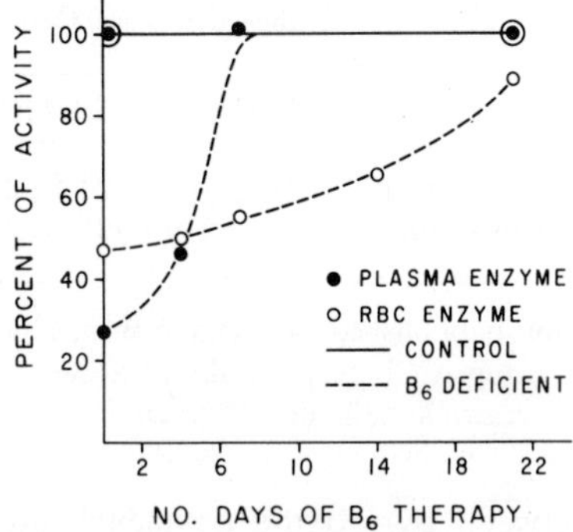

FIG. 6. A diagrammatic presentation of the difference in rate of recovery to normal activity of plasma and erythrocyte (RBC) alanine transaminase activities in pyridoxine-deficient rats, following placement on the pyridoxine-adequate diet (data previously presented in abstract, Albert and Brin, 1960).

cell is reduced and cannot be synthesized by the mature cell, or both. It is conceivable, though, that erythrocytes formed after pyridoxine adequacy is re-established would have a normal enzyme titer. The rate at which the hemolysate transaminase recovered following treatment of the deficient rats with pyridoxine suggested that recovery to normal activity was related to red cell turnover.

1. Effects of Administering Carbon Tetrachloride on Plasma and Erythrocyte Transaminase Activity

Because of the disparity between rates of recovery of hemolysate and plasma alanine transaminase enzymes in treated pyridoxine-deficient rats, it was considered desirable to investigate further the differentiation between these two sources of enzyme. A group of rats was divided into two subgroups, one of which was treated with carbon tetrachloride by oral administration at a dose of 1 gm./kg. body weight, and the other with physiological saline. The rats were then maintained on a chow diet for a period of 48 hours, when plasma and hemolysate alanine transaminase activities were determined. The data are shown in Table XV. The injection of carbon tetrachloride resulted in very marked increase in plasma transaminase activity. No change in hemolysate alanine transaminase activity was observed, however, nor was there an effect on body weight of these groups. The nonidentity of the alanine transaminase enzyme of the red cell with that in the plasma was therefore confirmed.

TABLE XV[a]

EFFECTS OF CARBON TETRACHLORIDE (*per os*) ON PLASMA AND HEMOLYSATE ALANINE TRANSAMINASE ACTIVITY IN RATS[b]

Group	Alanine transaminaes activity (units)		Body weight (gm.)
	Plasma	Hemolysate	
Control	220.0 ± 16	724.4 ± 28.4	233.7 ± 5.1
Carbon tetrachloride-treated	1862.6 ± 379	701.8 ± 41.3	237.8 ± 5.4

[a] Data not previously published (Albert and Brin, 1960).

[b] Nine rats per group. CCl_4 given orally at a dose of 1 gm./kg. body weight and samples drawn at 48 hours. Data are means ± S.E.

The relationship between pyridoxine deficiency and whole blood transaminase was established by Marsh *et al.* (1955), despite variable results. A number of studies with human subjects have also demonstrated a positive though variable relationship between pyridoxine deficiency and the serum aspartic enzyme (Vilter *et al.*, 1953; Sass and Murphy, 1958). Other effects of pyridoxine deficiency on the enzymes required for heme synthesis in nucleated erythrocytes have been demonstrated (Richert and Shulman, 1959; Richert *et al.*, 1960), although the use of these to evaluate pyridoxine adequacy has not been studied.

C. Recommendation

It is apparent that hemolysate alanine transaminase activity is very sensitive to pyridoxine deficiency. While the activities of the plasma transaminase enzymes return to normal following treatment of pyridoxine-deficient rats with pyridoxine, recovery of the erythrocyte enzyme appears to be more directly related to red cell turnover. In view of the sensitivity of the transaminase enzymes to pyridoxine deficiency, it would appear that the additional work necessary to develop useful assays in man may prove very worthwhile.

IV. Summary

In view of the wealth of information now being collected concerning the enzyme distribution in plasma and in formed elements of blood (White, 1958), it is anticipated that additional enzyme systems will be studied with a view toward their use for functional evaluation of vitamin adequacy. The advantages of the use of a functional enzyme test for vitamin adequacy over the use of a static determination of the level of a vitamin in blood or urine are described. Data are presented to support the use of erythrocyte transketolase activity as a functional test for thiamine adequacy in man, and of erythrocyte alanine transaminase for evaluation of pyridoxine. It is anticipated that further work in this rather new field will result in the development of additional functional tests for vitamin adequacy.

References

Albert, D., and Brin, M. (1960). *Federation Proc.* **19**, 321.
Anonymous. (1962). *New Engl. J. Med.* **267**, 623.
Barron, E. S. G., and Harrop, G. A. (1928). *J. Biol. Chem.* **79**, 65.
Bessey, O. A. (1954). *In* "Methods for Evaluation of Nutritional Adequacy and Status" (H. Spector and M. S. Peterson, eds.), Symposium, Quartermaster Food and Container Inst., p. 59, Nat. Acad. Sci.—Natl. Res. Council, Washington, D.C.
Brin, M. (1961). *Federation Proc.* **20**, 228.
Brin, M. (1962a). *Ann. N. Y. Acad. Sci.* **98**, 528.
Brin, M. (1962b). *J. Nutr.* **78**, 179.
Brin, M. (1962c). *Federation Proc.* **21**, 468.
Brin, M. (1962d). *New Eng. J. Med.* **267,** 1265.
Brin, M., and Owens, B. A. (1960). *Federation Proc.* **19**, 321.
Brin, M., and Yonemoto, R. H. (1958). *J. Biol. Chem.* **230**, 307.
Brin, M., Olson, R. E., and Stare, F. J. (1954). *J. Biol. Chem.* **210**, 435.
Brin, M., Shohet, S. S., and Davidson, C. S. (1956). *Federation Proc.* **15**, 224.
Brin, M., Shohet, S. S., and Davidson, C. S. (1958). *J. Biol. Chem.* **230**, 319.
Brin, M., Tai, M., and Ostashever, A. S. (1959). *Federation Proc.* **18**, 518.
Brin, M., Ostashever, A. S., Tai, M., and Kalinsky, H. (1960a). *J. Nutr.* **71**, 273.
Brin, M., Tai, M., Ostashever, A. S., and Kalinsky, H. (1960b). *J. Nutr.* **71**, 416.
Brin, M., Ostashever, A. S., and Kalinsky, H. (1961a). *Toxicol. Appl. Pharmacol.* **3**, 600.
Brin, M., Ostashever, A. S., Tai, M., and Kalinsky, H. (1961b). *J. Nutr.* **75**, 29.
Brin, M., Ostashever, A. S., Tai, M., and Kalinsky, H. (1961c). *J. Nutr.* **75**, 35.
Burch, H. B., Salcedo, J., Jr., Carrasco, E. O., Intengen, C. D., and Caldwell, A. B. (1950). *J. Nutr.* **42**, 9.
Burch, H. B., Bessey, O. A., Love, R. H., and Lowry, O. H. (1952). *J. Biol. Chem.* **198**, 477.
Burch, H. B., Lowry, O. H., Padilla, A. M., and Combs, A. M. (1956). *J. Biol. Chem.* **223**, 29.
Caldwell, E. F., and McHenry, E. W. (1953). *Arch. Biochem. Biophys.* **45**, 97.
DeMeio, R. H., Kissin, M., and Barron, E. S. G. (1934). *J. Biol. Chem.* **107**, 579.
Dische, Z., in McElroy, W. D. (1951). *Symp. Phosphorous Metabol. Baltimore* **1**, 171.
Dreyfus, P. M. (1962). *New Engl. J. Med.* **267**, 596.

Greenberg, D. M., and Harper, H. A. (1960). "Enzymes in Health and Disease." Thomas, Springfield, Illinois.

Hennesey, D. J., and Cerecedo, L. R. (1939). *J. Am. Chem. Soc.* **61**, 179.

Horecker, B. L., and Smyrniotis, P. Z. (1953). *J. Amer. Chem. Soc.* **75**, 1009.

Horwitt, M. K., Liebert, E., Kreisler, O., and Wittman, P. (1948). "Investigations of Human Requirements for B Complex Vitamins," Bull. Natl. Res. Council, No. 116. Washington, D.C.

ICNND (1956–1962). Summary reports on nutrition surveys. Interdepartmental Committee on Nutrition for National Defense, Washington 25, D.C.

ICNND (1957). "Manual for Nutrition Surveys," Interdepartmental Committee on Nutrition for National Defense, Washington 25, D.C.

ICNND (1962). Revised biochemical methods. Interdepartmental Committee on Nutrition for National Defense, Washington 25, D.C.

Marsh, E. M., Greenberg, L. D., and Rinehart, J. F. (1955). *J. Nutr.* **56**, 115.

McGanity, W. J., McHenry, E. W., VanWyck, H. B., Watt, G. L. (1949). *J. Biol. Chem.* **178**, 511.

Olson, R. E., Pearson, O. H., Miller, O. N., and Stare, F. J. (1948). *J. Biol. Chem.* **175**, 489.

Peters, R. A., and Thompson, R. H. S. (1934). *Biochem. J.* **28**, 916.

Plough, I. C., and Bridgforth, E. B. (1960). *Public Health Rept.* **75**, 699.

Racker, E. (1954). *Advances Enzymol.* **15**, 141.

Racker, E., de La Haba, G., and Leder, I. G. (1953). *J. Am. Chem. Soc.* **75**, 1010.

Richert, D. A., and Schulman, M. P. (1959). *Am. J. Clin. Nutr.* **7**, 416.

Richert, D. A., Pixley, B. Q., and Schulman, M. P. (1960). *J. Nutr.* **71**, 289.

Salcedo, J., Jr., Najjar, V. A., Holt, L. E., Jr., and Hutzler, E. W. (1948). *J. Nutr.* **36**, 307.

Sass, M., and Murphy, G. T. (1958). *Am. J. Clin. Nutr.* **6**, 12.

Schlenk, F., and Fisher, A. (1947). *Arch. Biochem.* **12**, 69.

Snyderman, S. E., Carretero, R., and Holt, L. E., Jr. (1950). *Federation Proc.* **9**, 371.

Vilter, R. W., Mueller, J. F., Glazer, H. S., Jarrold, T., Abraham, J., Thompson, C., and Hawkins, V. R. (1953). *J. Lab. Clin. Med.* **42**, 335.

Wachstein, M., and Gudaitis, A. (1952). *J. Lab. Clin. Med.* **40**, 550.

Warburg, O. (1909). *Z. Physiol. Chem.* **59**, 112.

Warburg, O., and Christian, W. (1931). *Biochem. Z.* **242**, 207.

Warburg, O., and Christian, W. (1932). *Naturwissenschaften* **20**, 688.

Warburg, O., Kubowitz, F., and Christian, W. (1930). *Biochem. Z.* **227**, 245.

Wendel, W. B. (1929). *Proc. Soc. Exptl. Biol. Med.* **26**, 865.

White, L. P., ed. (1958). *Ann. N. Y. Acad. Sci.* **75**, 1.

Wolfe, S. J., Brin, M., and Davidson, C. S. (1958). *J. Clin. Invest.* **37**, 1476.

CHAPTER 14

Approaches to Red Cell Preservation in the Liquid State

John G. Gibson II

I. Introduction

Having read, marked, and inwardly digested the preceding chapters, the reader will have gained some comprehension of the complexity of the organization of the normal red cell as a functioning entity. Its morphology, composition, interactions with its environment, selective permeability, metabolism, role in respiration (but not in blood coagulation), its clannishness (blood groups), genetics, and life span, all adequately described, serve as a basis for understanding the performance of its several duties in support of the total organism.

In the consideration of factors influencing the preservation of the red cell for purposes of replacement therapy, the maintenance of its chief function, gas transport, is of primary importance. From an engineering point of view the red cell may be regarded as a "single purpose machine," having a multiplicity of parts enmeshed and entrained to perform a comparatively simple operation under completely automated control. The preservation of the red cell would therefore appear to be a maintenance problem: keeping all the parts in good repair and the machine in running order.

Yet in terms of practical clinical medicine (and blood preservation is an intensely practical matter), this has turned out to be very difficult indeed. The introduction of citrate made possible the "indirect" transfusion, and initiated the requirement of preservation in the liquid state for the operation of a blood bank. Modification of the citrate solution by acidification and addition of glucose (acid-citrate-dextrose, ACD) provided a blood which, under adequate refrigeration (4°C.) was "safe" for transfusion for a period of 21 days. But little real progress in improving the maintenance of viability of red cells during storage has been made since. Probably no field of research, in which so many workers have been engaged and upon so which much money has been spent, has been so unrewarding.

The chief reason for this failure has been the lack of appreciation of the changes that occur during blood collection in an anticoagulant solution and during subsequent refrigerated storage, since they affect the fate of the captive red cell on return to the circulation—rarely does the practicing physician consider the effect of these changes on quality of the blood he prescribes.

Another reason lies in the differences in viewpoint of the personnel investigating and dispensing blood. The director of a blood bank has not the basic training, time, or facilities for studying the behavior of red cells under the conditions in which he uses them. His interest lies in the selection of compatible bloods and the proper clinical use thereof. The investigator with adequate basic training has by and large taken an "ivory tower" viewpoint, with little or no interest in the practical application of his findings. Rarely has a working association been established between the basic scientist and the dispenser of the object of his investigation. Better liaison between these groups is a *sine qua non*. In all probability much of the specific information contained in this volume, if incorporated into the design of experiments directed towards the clinical use of blood, would result in significant improvement in the preservation of the red cell.

II. Red Cell Viability

Preservation of red cells implies maintenance of normal functional capacity to such an extent that, after return to the body, they will stay in circulation and do their job. *In vitro* tests, while useful as screening procedures, are not sufficiently reliable for evaluation. Judgment of the efficiency of any preservation system must therefore be based on transfusion experiments in human subjects, designed to quantitate the percentage of red cells remaining in the circulation. The term "survival" is generally accepted as referring to the percentage of cells retained in circulation 24 hours after infusion.

A. Methods of Determining Posttransfusion Survival

The oldest and still the most reliable and informative method is the differential agglutination technique developed by Ashby (1919) in studies of the normal life span of the erythrocyte. Group O cells are infused into an A recipient. The A cells of subsequent blood samples are precipitated with anti-A serum and the unagglutinated O cells counted in a hemocytometer. The cell count that would result from dilution of the infused O cells in the total red cell volume (determined prior to infusion) is calculated, and the cell count of samples, divided by the above value, gives the percentage of cells remaining in the circulation. Normal cells disappear from the circulation as a linear function of time. Preserved bloods show varying degrees of loss in the first 24 hours, after which a linear curve is found. The method not only quantitates immediate (within 24 hours) survival, but also the life span of the remaining cells, information not obtainable by any other method. The technique is difficult and time-consuming. It requires transfusion of a large quantity of homologous blood with the ever attendant risk of a reaction.

Several methods using radioisotopes have been developed for tagging red cells. Radioiron (Fe^{59}, Fe^{55}) was extensively used during the war in the study of red cell preservation (Gibson *et al.*, 1947a). Since radioiron does not tag cells *in vitro* it is necessary to "build up" a donor by infusing the isotope, which then becomes incorporated in the hemoglobin of the developing erythrocyte. To obtain adequate specific activity of recipients' red cells after infusion, fairly large quantities of isotope are necessary for donor build-up. Again there is the danger inherent in all homologous transfusions. Efficient radiation detection apparatus has been developed to permit counting of both Fe^{59} and Fe^{55}, making possible the highly useful "double tracer" experiment in which the fate of cells of different ages or other characteristics can be followed. The chief limitation of the method is the rapid reutilization of the radioiron from destroyed cells for the synthesis of hemoglobin, detectable within 24 hours. Thus the plotted data yielded two parameters: the loss of cells from the circulation and the advent of new cells from the bone marrow.

Two isotopes can be used to tag red cells *in vitro*, thus eliminating the build-up donor. The first of these to be used was radiophosphate (P^{32}), which tagged the cell by entering the normal phosphate metabolism (Hahn and Hevesy, 1942). It is not, as in the case of iron, a permanent tag, and therefore is of limited use for evaluating anything but immediate posttransfusion survival. Its prime use is in the determination of the recipient's red cell volume prior to transfusion. (Donahue *et al.*, 1955; Ebaugh *et al.*, 1953; Finch and Gabrio, 1954; Gibson and Scheitlin, 1955).

The isotope commonly used today is radiochromium (Cr^{51}) which is bound to globin *in vitro*. The permanence of this tag is not definitely known. While tagged cells do not lose Cr^{51} during refrigerated storage, the shape of the disappearance curve after infusion suggests a loss of the isotope from cells still in circulation. While the method is acceptable for assaying immediate post-transfusion survival, it is unreliable for determining the life span of residual viable cells.

One essential is common to all techniques, namely, the calculation of the "100% retention value": the cell count or radioactivity level that would result from complete retention in the blood stream of all the infused test cells. This requires measurement of the recipient's red cell volume prior to infusion, and should always be done with a method different than that used for tagging the test cells. Plasma volume can be measured with Evans blue (Gibson and Evans, 1934), radioiodine (I^{131}) (Crispell *et al.*, 1949), and red cell volume calculated from the plasma volume and plasmatocrit. Red cell volume may be determined directly with P^{32} (Hahn and Hevesy, 1942).

III. The Lesion of Collection

Throughout its life span the red cell enjoys a degree of protection from the cradle to the grave never equalled by citizens of the most socialistic state. Its exterior environment, plasma, assures optimal temperature and chemical conditions for maintenance of water balance, nutrient supply, and electrolyte transport. Regulation of acid-base balance of plasma and extracellular fluid, by the respiratory and renal functions and lymphatic circulation, assures high efficiency of gas exchange. Its energy-transfer mechanism is adequately supported (in ways not completely understood), levels of high-energy phosphates, substrate, enzymes and cofactors, and metal catalysts being kept at well-balanced adequate levels. In other words, the battery is kept in a good state of charge.

Concentration differences of the several measurable physiochemical characteristics have been found in relation to age distribution. But the precise degree of change from neonatal values leading to senescence and death is not known.

When the red cell is removed from the body and plunged into an anticoagulant solution, it goes into a state of shock—of thermal, osmotic, and chemical origin. Sudden lowering of the temperature deranges the steady state of electrolyte flux. Dilution of plasma by the anticoagulant solution lowers the tonicity of the exterior milieu to a degree never encountered in the normal state, with a profound effect on water balance. If the solution is acid and hypotonic (as in ACD) these changes are pronounced and result in immediate alteration of membrane permeability and osmotic resistance. Since the concentration of dextrose (in ACD) is much higher than that of normal plasma, the intracellular level is raised three- to fourfold. All of these changes are interrelated and disturb the steady state which anaerobic glycolysis requires. These are some of the measurable changes; doubtless there are others too subtle to detect, but probably important. And, finally, the battery has been disconnected from the "charger."

It is the usual practice to draw blood into a volume of fluid intended to act as an anticoagulant for the total donation. It follows that the ratio of red cells to diluent is lowest at the onset of collection and rises as collection proceeds. Thus the degree of "shock" to which the cells are exposed varies directly with the sequence of collection. The extent of immediate damage during collection is a random phenomenon bearing no relationship to the age distribution of the cells, a fact having an important bearing on the design of preservative solutions.

Let us examine in more detail what occurs during collection of blood from the initial to the final phase (Gibson *et al.*, 1956). Suppose that five separate aliquots of blood are collected in ACD in amounts corresponding to 100, 200, 300, 400, and 500 ml. of blood in 75 ml. of ACD. The five aliquots represent the situation as it obtains from beginning to end of collection. Each sample is assayed for pH, MCHC (mean corpuscular hemoglobin concentration), percent hemolysis in 0.6% NaCl, and intracellular dextrose, K^+, and P_i (inorganic phosphate). Results obtained in a series of experiments are shown in Table I.

TABLE I

OSMOTIC AND CHEMICAL CHANGES TO WHICH THE RED CELL IS SUBJECTED DURING COLLECTION OF BLOOD IN ACD AND CPD

Blood collected (ml.)	Plasma pH	MCHC (gm./100 ml.)	Hemolysis in 0.6% NaCl (%)	Intracellular: Dextrose (mg./100 ml.)	Intracellular: Potassium (meq./liter)	Inorganic phosphorus (whole blood) (mmoles/liter)
In 75 ml. of ACD (pH 5.0, hypotonic)						
Control	7.48	33.0	0	94	95.0	0.813
100	5.78	22.2	48.6	861	112.3	1.026
200	6.26	24.0	13.3	675	109.3	0.929
300	6.64	25.8	1.8	572	105.3	0.949
400	6.85	27.6	0.2	448	107.6	1.001
500	7.00	29.7	0	340	104.4	0.950
In 70 ml. of CPD (pH 5.65, isotonic)						
Control	7.46	32.5		78	98.0	
100	6.50	30.5	0	802	102.2	—[a]
200	6.82	30.7	0	660	101.8	—
300	7.05	30.8	0	500	100.9	—
400	7.10	31.0	0	420	100.1	—
500	7.20	31.5	0	300	99.8	—

[a] Due to added phosphate of solution (CPD), a valid comparison cannot be made.

It is apparent that a series of progressive changes related to the sequence of collection has occurred. As the blood enters the solution the plasma pH, initially 7.4, has precipitately dropped to 5.8; it rises progressively during collection, due to buffering of proteins and hemoglobin, and finally equilibrates at 7.0. Concomitantly there is an initial swelling of the red cell of about 30%, decreasing during collection but not to the control value. Thus the cells have undergone a drastic and continuous change in pH and water content, with a pronounced and changing effect on osmotic resistance. Whereas none of the cells of a sample at the end of collection hemolyzed in 0.6% NaCl, about one half of these in the early phase had reached the critical stage of membrane tensile strength.

Both intracellular potassium and inorganic phosphate increase immediately, possibly in relation to the influx of water. In the case of K^+, this is certainly evidence of a disturbance of the steady state. As collection continues the K^+ values fall but not to normal, while P_i values remain unchanged, indicating no measurable degree of breakdown of inorganic phosphate.

There is little doubt as to the superiority of ACD as a preservative solution over sodium citrate or citrate dextrose. The 70% survival value of cells of citrated blood is reached in 3–5 days, of citrate-dextrose blood in 10–12 days, but not until 21 days in ACD blood.

However, the data presented emphasize an important fact. The collection of blood in the preservative solution exposed the red cells to extracellular conditions which markedly altered the integrity of the membrane. Subsequent experiments in which a series of aliquots stored 28 days at 4°C., similar to those described, were assayed by the Cr^{51} method in normal human volunteers, showed the posttransfusion survival of a sample of a complete collection to be about 60% (an expected value), whereas the survival of the highest dilution aliquot was only 30%, the bloods of the intermediate dilution ratios falling closely on the overall slope. It is evident that there is a great differential in the ability of the cells to maintain viability during storage, and that this is related to the sequence of collection.

In contrast a similar series of experiments, in which blood was collected in citrate-phosphate-dextrose (CPD) (pH 5.65 and isotonic), showed far less damage throughout collection (Gibson *et al.*, 1957). As shown in Table I, the changes in pH were less violent; water imbibition and membrane stress were less, as was the disturbance of K^+ flux.

Yet the differences between the two solutions are slight. CPD contains 20% less citrate than ACD, is adjusted to slightly higher pH (5.65 as against 5.0), has a small amount of added phosphate, but is *isotonic*. Several survival experiments similar to those described showed no significant differences with respect to the dilution ratios.

But these minor differences had a significant effect on maintenance of viability during storage. In a large series of experiments, the mean survival of cells in ACD blood stored at 4°C. for 21 and 28 days was 83 and 70%, respectively, whereas the survival of cells in CPD blood stored 30 days was 75%. It is apparent that the changes determining the deterioration of red cells during refrigerated storage are *all initiated during collection.*

IV. The Lesion of Storage

Figure 1 shows the progressive alterations from normal that occur in ACD blood over a 30-day period. Refrigeration retards the rate of all chemical

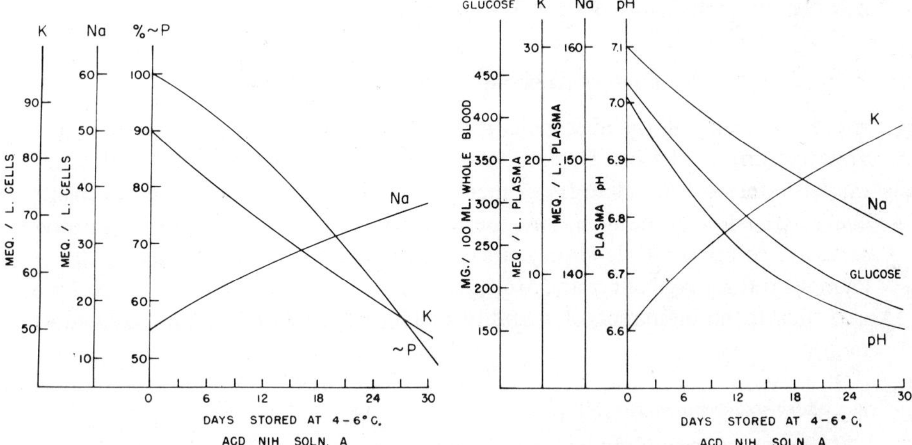

FIG. 1. The lesion of storage. Changes in composition of plasma (right-hand chart) and intracellularly (left-hand chart) in ACD blood during refrigerated storage. Lactate from continuing glycolysis progressively lowers plasma pH and high-energy phosphate level falls; as a result of these changes glycolysis is inhibited. Loss of selective permeability of the membrane disrupts the steady state of ion transport, with reversal of the normal cell-plasma sodium-potassium gradient differential. These changes, all parameters of deterioration of the red cell, take place simultaneously with progressive loss of red cell viability.

reactions. But glycolysis continues throughout storage with continuous consumption of high-energy phosphates.

Glucose concentration falls and lactate (not shown) rises, bringing about a progressive fall in pH to a level which in itself is rate-limiting, possibly through inhibition of enzymes at some intermediary stage. ATP is consumed and since the normal feedback mechanism is retarded or inhibited, the supply of high-energy phosphates drops to a critical level and glycolysis grinds to a halt.

The selective permeability of the membrane is progressively lost, transport characteristics approaching the Donnan state of equilibrium. Other changes occur but these are the measurable ones. Again, in shop language, the battery has run down.

All of these changes are deterimental to maintenance of the functional capacity of the red cell. This is clearly shown by the fact that as the period of refrigerated storage is prolonged, fewer of the red cells remain in circulation after reinfusion, as shown by postinfusion survival studies (Gibson *et al.*, 1947b).

These changes also impair the functional efficiency of the viable red cell. During storage there is a significant shift to the left in the oxygen dissociation curve (Valtis and Kennedy, 1954), interfering with normal respiratory exchange.

After 3 weeks of refrigerated storage, the material issued for transfusion can be only euphemistically described as blood.

V. Factors Affecting Maintenance of Viability

It is clear that all the above changes proceed concurrently, nor is there any apparent primary lesion. Three factors appear to exert demonstrable influences on cell integrity: the changes in membrane permeability, the changes in the energy-transfer mechanism, and the hydrogen ion concentration of the preservative solution. Table II presents the normal red cell characteristics, shows changes during collection and storage, and then lists applicable *in vitro* tests and aids to maintenance of viability of red cells, related to the controlling factors.

A. Membrane Permeability

The simplest test of the integrity of the membrane is its behavior in solutions of varying concentrations of NaCl. In the normal so-called "fragility" curve, hemolysis is first observed at a concentration of 0.67%, rises rapidly as the concentration is reduced further, and is complete at 0.3% NaCl. When this sigmoid curve is plotted as a frequency distribution curve, it is apparent that there are varying degrees of resistance to lysis throughout the cell population. Cell dimensions exhibit a similar type of distribution about a mean (Strumia, 1956). In the normal red cell a steady state of transport of water, electrolytes, etc., is maintained, rates of efflux equalling rates of influx.

As stated above, the collection of blood in ACD produces marked swelling, as evidenced by the values for MCHC and cell diameter (Rapaport, 1947), but not (at the end of collection) to the critical point of rupture. As storage is prolonged, there is a progressive loss of osmotic resistance, and a rough correlation between the increased fragility and posttransfusion survival of the red cells.

B. Metabolism

In the early phases of work on the preservation of red cells, investigators were only vaguely aware of the importance of the glycolytic mechanism.

TABLE II

FACTORS INVOLVED IN MAINTENANCE OF VIABILITY OF RED CELL DURING REFRIGERATED STORAGE

Parameter	Normal characteristics	Changes during collection and storage	*In vitro* tests	Aids to maintenance of viability
Cell membrane	Presence of phospholipid and protein; MCD[a] 7.4–9.4 μ; MCV[b] 74–98 μ^3; MCHC 30–34 gm./100 ml.	Changes in MCD, MCV, MCHC (water content)	Microscopy; hemoglobin; hematocrit	Isotonicity of medium
Membrane permeability	Hemolysis in 0.6–0.3% NaCl; steady-state ion transport	Decrease in osmotic resistance; loss of K^+; gain in Na^+	Osmotic and mechanical fragility tests; measurement of rates of influx and efflux	Isotonicity; lipid-rich plasma fractions
Respiratory function	Normal O^2 dissociation curve	Shift to left in O^2 dissociation curve	O^2 dissociation curve	Maintenance of normal pH
Metabolism	10% Aerobic and 90% anaerobic glycolysis (Emden-Meyerhof-Paras)	Progressive loss of high-energy phosphates	Assay of ATP, ADP, AMP; chromatography	Glucose phosphate; lower pH; purine ribosides
Acid-base balance	Plasma pH 7.24–7.45; red cell pH 7.14–7.725	Initial lowering and progressive fall to pH 6.8–6.6	Determination of whole blood or plasma pH (glass electrode)	Adjustment of pH (organic buffers, ion-exchange resins)
Viability (posttransfusion survival)	Life span 120 (110–130) days	Progressive loss of viability, rate accelerating with time of storage	Post-transfusion survival tests: Ashby, I^{131}, P^{32}, Cr^{51}	Better preservative solution based on theory and experiment

[a] Mean cell diameter. [b] Mean cell volume.

Although the complex chemistry of the breakdown of glucose to lactate was not as well worked out, a relationship was apparent between the failure of the system, as evidenced by phosphate partition studies (Rapaport, 1947), and the ability of the red cell to maintain viability during storage (Gibson *et al.*, 1947b).

Studies of the nucleotide pattern of red cells during storage in ACD have now clearly shown a consistent degradation: ATP→ADP→AMP→IMP (inosine monophosphate)→hypoxanthine (Bishop, 1961). A similarity in trend has been demonstrated between the lowering of ATP concentration and the percentage of viable red cells after transfusion. The percentage decrease in ATP, however, exceeds the percentage loss of viability of the red cells. Thus after 3-week storage of ACD blood the ATP level falls about 50% (Bishop, 1961), whereas the posttransfusion survival of red cells in ACD blood stored in plastic bags declines only 15% (Walter *et al.*, 1957).

C. Acid-Base Balance

The effect of the initial pH of collected blood on the rate of glycolysis during refrigerated storage has been known for some time (Parpart *et al.*, 1947), and the controlled lowering of pH by citrate buffer was the first major improvement in blood preservation (Loutit *et al.*, 1947), namely, ACD.

There can be little doubt that the observed behavior of the three measurable parameters, i.e., membrane permeability, nucleotide metabolism, and pH, are reflections of a single degenerative process.

It should be emphasized that under routine conditions blood is stored in the sedimented state, and that as the formed elements settle the lighter leucocytes and platelets form a film at the red cell-plasma interface. To what extent this "buffy coat" acts as a diffusion barrier between the packed red cells and supernatant plasma is not known. It is of interest, however, that the posttransfusion survival of red cells, concentrated by sedimentation or centrifugation, from which the supernatant plasma has been removed within 24 hours after collection, is equally good, throughout a 21-day storage period, as that of red cells stored as whole blood (Gibson, 1960).

VI. Aids to Maintenance of Viability

A. Membrane Protection

Efforts to protect the membrane have not received a great deal of attention.

1. Proteolytic Inhibitors

Substances known to exhibit antiproteolytic activity have been found to increase the osmotic resistance of the red cell. Phenergan hydrochloride added to ACD blood decreased the percent hemolysis of bloods stored 14 and 37 days by about 50 and 25%, respectively (Schales, 1953). *In vivo* experiments, however, did not demonstrate an improvement in posttransfusion survival over controls (Chaplin *et al.*, 1952).

2. Lipid-Rich Plasma Fractions

More hopeful has been the addition of lipid-rich plasma fractions. Fraction IV-3-4 (method 6 of Cohn), added to citrate-dextrose solution buffered to pH 6.0 and used as a resuspension medium for separated red cells of blood collected in 4% sodium citrate, afforded 70–80% survival up to 28 days of refrigerated storage, a value significantly higher than that for cells stored in the solution without added protein (Gibson *et al.*, 1947b).

B. Metabolic Adjuvants

1. Glucose

Glucose is the normal substrate for red cell metabolism, and was, quite naturally, the first adjuvant to be added to the preservative solution. The rate of utilization, even when retarded by refrigeration, is sufficient to consume practically all of the cell native glucose in 24–48 hours. The amounts usually employed raise the intracellular level to 300–400 mg./100 ml. The rate of utilization appears to be independent of the initial concentration. Long before the glucose is completely utilized, glycolysis has been retarded to a level at which the red cell is nonviable. In all probability, less added glucose would suffice. Other sugars, such as fructose, have not improved preservation.

2. Purine Ribosides

Adenosine or inosine, added to an ACD solution, appears to improve preservation, as evidenced by satisfactory transfusion survival for periods up to 30–40 days (Finch and Gabrio, 1954). Discussion of the metabolism of the purine ribosides is beyond the scope of this chapter (see Chapters 4–6). But for the first time a means has been found for supporting the glycolytic process by supplying another nutrient, a riboside, to boost the energy potential. Important is the fact that the breakdown of riboside does not involve the initial hexokinase reaction, thus conserving ATP.

It is known that most of the deteriorative changes in stored blood are reversible if not too far advanced. All the red cells of a 21-day stored ACD blood have suffered some degree of damage. On transfusion, those cells damaged irreversibly are rapidly culled from the circulation. But the residual cells are restored to complete normality, as evidenced by the finding (by the Ashby technique) that these cells remain in the blood stream for 120 days from the day of transfusion, not collection. The addition of purine ribosides to ACD blood stored 21 days (with an expected cell survival of not over 70%) rejuvenated the blood to the extent that additional 1–2-week storage was feasible, thus demonstrating for the first time that such repair could, to some extent, be accomplished *in vitro*. This concept holds promise of better preservation of red cells in the liquid state.

C. *Acid-Base Balance*

1. Initial Control of pH

The rate-limiting effect of lowered pH on glycolysis has been commented on. Deferment of the period at which this level is reached definitely prolongs maintenance of viability of the red cells. As an example, the initial pH of ACD blood is 7.0, falling to 6.8 at 14 and to 6.75 at 21 days of storage. The initial pH of CPD blood is 7.2, 6.85 at 21 and 6.75 at 28 days of storage. The average survival of ACD and CPD bloods at 28 days of storage is 70 (Walter *et al.*, 1957), and 75% (Gibson *et al.*, 1957), respectively. This slight difference affords an additional week of safe refrigerated storage.

2. Continuous Control of pH

Preliminary investigations (Bishop, 1962) have shown that when lactic acid is neutralized during storage, glycolysis continues for longer periods with better maintenance of ATP levels than in untreated controls.

The preservation of red cells has always been handicapped by the finality of collecting blood in a given solution. Once blood is collected, events proceed—relentlessly—and the matter is in the lap of the refrigerator! Continuous adjustment of pH may offer great possibilities.

VII. Practical Considerations

This chapter may be criticized as merely a recapitulation of the mistakes and progress of the past, and not an approach to the problem of preservation of red cells stored under refrigeration in the liquid state. The work proceeded empirically, of necessity. There was an occasional "lucky strike," but steady improvement came only when the influence of variations in the anticoagulant solution on basic physiochemical characteristics of the cell was assayed by *in vivo* determination for the effect on maintenance of viability.

But it must be borne in mind that what proves to be an important advance in the laboratory may not be readily accepted in practice. Blood is a life-saving tissue, but hospitals are extremely cost conscious. To be acceptable, innovations must not involve complicated and time-consuming procedures.

The objectives for prolonging the safe storage period of red cells (blood) are threefold: (1) to afford the largest quantity of red cells in the best possible functional state; (2) to conserve the inventory of the rare bloods, with reference to either the OAB system or the complex of antigen-antibody characteristics of red cells; and (3) to eliminate the cost of wastage through outdating. The clinician is vitally interested in the first, the director of the blood bank in the second, and the hospital accountant in the third objective. Any system for improving the preservation of the red cell must run the gauntlet of this "conflict of interest."

Acknowledgment

This chapter is based to a large extent on work supported by a grant-in-aid from the National Heart Institute of the National Institutes of Health, and by a contract with the Office of the Surgeon General, U.S. Army.

The author expresses his gratitude to the Editor of the *American Journal of Clinical Pathology* for permission to include Fig. 1.

References

Ashby, W. (1919). *J. Exptl. Med.* **29**, 267.

Bishop, C. (1961). *Transfusion* **1**, 349.

Bishop, C. (1962). *Transfusion* **2**, 408.

Chaplin, H., Jr., Cutbush, C. H., and Mollison, P. L. (1952). *J. Clin. Pathol.* **5**, 91.

Crispell, K. R., Porter, B., and Nieset, R. T. (1949). *J. Clin. Invest.* **24**, 513.

Donohue, D. M., Motulsky, A. G., Giblett, E. R., Pirzio-Biroli, G., Viranoratto, V., and Finch, C. A. (1955). *Brit. J. Hematol.* **1**, 249.

Ebaugh, F. G., Jr., Emerson, C. P., and Ross, J. H. (1953). *J. Clin. Invest.* **32**, 1260.

Finch, C. A., and Gabrio, B. W. (1954). *J. Clin. Invest.* **33**, 932.

Gibson, J. G., IInd (1960). *New Engl. J. Med.* **263**, 634.

Gibson, J. G., IInd, and Evans, W. A., Jr. (1934). *J. Clin. Invest.* **16**, 301.

Gibson, J. G., IInd, and Scheitlin, W. A. (1955). *J. Lab. Clin. Med.* **46**, 679.

Gibson, J. G., IInd, Aub, J. C., Evans, R. D., Peacock, W. C., Irvine, J. W., Jr., and Sack, T. (1947a). *J. Clin. Invest.* **16**, 704.

Gibson, J. G., IInd, Evans, R. D., Aub, J. C., Sack, T., and Peacock, W.C. (1947b). *J. Clin. Invest.* **26**, 704.

Gibson, J. G., IInd, Murphy, W. P., Jr., Scheitlin, W. A., and Rees, S. B. (1956). *Am. J. Clin. Pathol.* **26**, 855.

Gibson, J. G., IInd, Rees, S. B., McManus, T. J., and Scheitlin, W. A. (1957). *Am. J. Clin. Pathol.* **28**, 589.

Hahn, L., and Hevesy, G. (1942). *Acta. Physiol. Scand.* **1**, 3.

Loutit, J., Jr., Mollison, P. L., and Young, I. M. (1940). *Quart. J. Exptl. Physiol.* **32**, 183.

Parpart, A. K., Lorenz, P. B., Parpart, E. R., and Chase, A. M. (1947). *J. Clin. Invest.* **16**, 636.

Rapaport, S. (1947). *J. Clin. Invest.* **26**, 591.

Schales, O. (1953). *Proc. Soc. Exptl. Biol. Med.* **83**, 593.

Strumia, M. M. (1956). *Bibliotheca Haematol.* **7**, 303.

Valtis, D. J., and Kennedy, A. C. (1954). *Lancet* **i**, 119.

Walter, C. W., Button, L. N., and Ritts, R. E., Jr. (1957). *Surg. Gynecol. Obstet.* **105**, 365.

CHAPTER 15

Red Cell Storage in the Frozen State[1]

James L. Tullis

I. Historical Background

Attempts to alter the natural course of human life, notably the inevitable decay of aging, have interested man since the dawn of history. In different cultures this has assumed widely divergent forms: from the golden apples of Greek mythology—to the necromancy of Egyptian mummies. Yet, until comparatively modern times, little attempt was made to prolong life by the obvious expediency of freezing. This seeming paucity of experiments on preservation of viability in the frozen state probably was the simple accident of history which placed essentially all scientific thought, education, and study in a narrow geographic band around the world (between the 20th and 30th parallels), where it remained for some 3000 years. Since natural ice did not exist in this area, no recorded reference can be found to its effect on living tissue until the time when science shifted northward and Sir Robert Boyle (1665) successfully revived a fish frozen in ice for two days. Little further reference to the effect of freezing temperatures appears until the empirical observation of Polge *et al.* (1949) that spermatozoa, treated with glycerol, did not lyse following freezing and thawing.

[1] Some of the material in this chapter appeared earlier in an editorial entitled "Transfusion" by James L. Tullis, *Transfusion* **3**, 155 (1963). The Editors.

II. Effects of Freezing Unprotected Blood

Unprotected blood cooled to temperatures below freezing shows massive destruction of nearly all, but curiously not quite all, viable cells. This damage is largely a result of the phase change from a liquid to solid state. Careful supercooling to several degrees below zero without ice crystal formation is essentially free of damaging effect. This seeming paradox, wherein the random distribution of particles, solutes, and solvents is more "natural" than the orderly state of crystal formation, has prompted much work on the harmful effects of ice on viability. At least the three following explanations have been proposed. None is wholly in agreement with the accepted facts.

(1) *Effect of extracellular ice crystals.* Extracellular ice crystals may exert a physical grinding action on cells, especially at the time of thawing. This concept is based on observations in industry, especially meat packing, which demonstrate the disruptive effect of large extracellular ice crystals randomly distributed through muscle fibers. Much of the protective action of various substances, such as polyhydric alcohols, was thought for a time to be due to the small, more uniform crystals which form in their presence. However, in the blood specimens studied *in vitro* there is roughly an equal proportion of cells to solute, and there is no rigidly confined space within which sheer forces can work. Moreover, the red cells, despite their biconcave shape, probably can and do withstand much greater physical stress and change of shape *in vivo* than occurs from melting ice crystals *in vitro.*

(2) *Effect of high salt concentration.* Water crystallizes in a pure state, leaving behind local concentrations of salt in the extracellular compartment. Evidence increasingly supports the view that this is the principal damage from freezing. Lovelock (1953) was the first to suggest that much of the harmful effect of ice formation on blood cells was due to the combined protein-denaturing effect and intracellular hypertonicity. Here again, however, theory does not fit all of the data. Meryman (1960) has shown that whereas freezing and thawing of unprotected sperm cause lysis, similar specimens can be frozen and then dehydrated from the frozen state with subsequent rehydration and return of viability.

(3) *Effect of intracellular ice crystals.* The formation of intracellular ice crystals may disrupt important spatial relationships in cells. Although the nonnucleated red cell is relatively free of the structural complexity and morphological differentiation of a cell like the leucocyte, it is possible that high-energy loci and other important elements of the erythrocyte must retain their spatial integrity in order properly to continue their function. Even small intracellular ice crystals could profoundly affect these relationships during the physical torque which accompanies crystallization. Still other effects, of a type more chemical than physical, result from low temperature. For example,

certain oxidative enzymes have differing preferential temperatures of optimal activity. At low temperatures this may lead to unequal cessation of certain chemical reactions and resultant piling up of degradation products. The effect of low temperature upon dissolved gases in blood has not even been approached experimentally, but may be still another factor of importance in the damage from low temperature to unprotected cells.

III. Methods of Blood Protection at Temperatures below Freezing

Largely on an empirical basis, four methods have been studied which make it possible to lower temperatures below freezing without ice crystal formation: dehydration; replacement of the free intracellular water by an additive such as glycerol or dimethyl sulfoxide (DMSO) which penetrates the cells; ultra-rapid freezing at a rate too fast for ice crystals to form; and high pressure gradients to permit cooling to below freezing without crystal formation. To these basic techniques may be added at least three modifications: (*a*) A rapid freeze method under study by Rinfret and associates at Linde Laboratories, wherein nonpenetrating macromolecular substances are added as hydrogen-bonding agents to "lock" water outside of the cells (Doebbler and Rinfret, 1962); (*b*) a combined approach under study by Pert *et al.* (1963) of the American Red Cross, wherein both a penetrating additive, such as glycerol, and a non-penetrating osmotic additive, such as sucrose, permit the use of lesser concentrations of each agent than would otherwise be necessary; (*c*) a rapid freeze method under study by Meryman of Naval Medical Research Institute, wherein high concentrations of glucose are used, which can be quickly removed after thawing.

The dehydration method, suggested earlier by Meryman, has the greatest esthetic and scientific appeal. If one could preserve a pint of blood like powdered coffee on a shelf, no complex storage equipment would be required. An individual's lifetime needs could be met by a half-dozen containers of autologous blood. Unfortunately, this technique as yet can be applied only to thin films of dried blood.

The method of rapid freezing also proved unsuitable when volumes as large as one pint were used. The blood yields obtained were low, unless some type of protective substance was added to the blood before cooling.

The use of high pressures to avoid crystal formation will probably never become practical. The level of 35,000 p.s.i. pressure, needed to maintain a liquid state at $-22°$C., is so great as to be impractical in large volume and is cytotoxic from the pressure itself.

Thus, for practical purposes, only three approaches to the freezing problem currently can be considered sufficiently advanced to permit developmental study: the use of slow or random freezing in the presence of "penetrating" additives, such as glycerol and DMSO; the use of rapid freezing in the presence of "nonpenetrating" or "slowly penetrating" additives, such as PVP (polyvinylpyrrolidone), dextran, gelatin, sucrose, lactose, or glucose; and the aforementioned combination of the two methods. Each of these methods requires that something be added to blood before freezing. Moreover, each of these methods appears to require that the additive be removed again after thawing. The most important considerations in evaluating the relative merits of the different techniques, therefore, are:

(*a*) What additive can be instilled and removed most effectively?

(*b*) What additive is most protective to the cells during freezing and thawing and thus gives rise to a final post-thaw transfusion unit of optimal stability?

The principal lesion of low-temperature blood preservation appears to be that which occurs during freezing and thawing, and it is chiefly here that the different additives exert their protective action. Once the eutectic point (warmest temperature at which total crystallization of a frozen solution still exists) of the mixture has been passed, the exact temperature of storage below freezing becomes of lesser importance. The length of time the blood is preserved also appears to be of limited significance. For example, in the case of glycerol-preserved cells the circulatory viability after 5 years in storage is roughly comparable to 5 days in storage, although the total cell yield appears to be somewhat decreased.

IV. Physical Changes during Freezing of Simple Solutions

The manner in which these divergent techniques exert their protective effects is only beginning to be understood. However, studies on the freezing of simple aqueous solutions help significantly to improve our understanding of the complex behavior of cellular functions at low temperatures. (They include the following observations.)

(1) *Temperature Range for Ice Crystal Formation.* In an aqueous solution, crystallized ice can form only within a relatively narrow temperature zone, 0°C. to about −20°C. At lower temperatures the molecules do not have sufficient mobility to assume the crystalline state.

(2) *Crystallization Requires a Finite Time.* If rates of cooling through the narrow crystallization zone and subsequent rates of thawing are ultrarapid, crystals do not have time to form. The liquid passes directly into the vitreous state and back again. For stark drama there is little in all of nature that exceeds the speed and force necessary suddenly to convert a drop of water into ice. Luyet (1960) has calculated that the distance between water molecules in ice is 3 Å., and that the material needed to construct a crystal only 1 micron in size is 27 billion molecules. Each of these molecules must be moved from

its random location in the liquid phase to a precise geometric pattern in a fraction of a second. In terms of human work-equivalents, this is analogous to the construction in 1 second of a brick wall long enough to circle the earth about 10 times.

(3) *Speed of Crystal Formation Is Proportional to Water Content.* The velocity of cooling or warming, which must be achieved in order to exceed the rate of crystal formation during passage through the eutectic point, is related to the water content of the tissue and the nature of the solute. Each reduction of 20–30% in water content lessens approximately tenfold the necessary rate of heat exchange which must be achieved to avoid crystallization. For example, a rate of 1000°C./second is necessary for 80% pure water; 100°C./second is necessary for 60% pure water; and 20°C./second is necessary for 30% pure water. Once a level below 20–30% intracellular water is reached, the remaining liquid is so tightly bound to protein that freezing will not only occur at any rate of temperature.

(4) *Achievable Velocities Are Related to Heat Capacity of the Tissue.* Luyet (1949) has shown experimentally that the heat capacity of blood is closely related to the thickness of the film being cooled. He was able to vitrify, without crystal formation, a solution containing 80% water in layers 0.01 mm. thick. If the water content was reduced to 60%, the thickness could be increased to 0.1 mm. without crystal formation. Meryman and Kafig (1955), utilizing this principle, were able to freeze blood successfully without additives by spraying it in small particle size directly into liquid nitrogen.

(5) *Crystal Size Is Related to Thermal History of the Sample.* In aqueous systems to which no protective agent is added, the size and shape of crystals are markedly influenced by the rate at which the crystals are formed. After quick freezing, the crystals show a small uniform size and are probably chiefly extracellular. The commercially successful Birdseye system for quick freezing of food products takes advantage of this fact. With slower rates, the number of crystals is smaller, but the size of the crystals increases. Their characteristic hexagonal shape is unchanged. If the crystals grow slowly, they release latent heat of crystallization which in turn modifies the distribution of temperature gradients throughout the freezing mixture.

(6) *Phase Change from Liquid to Ice Is Related to Both Temperature and Pressure.* By the use of very high pressures, it is possible for aqueous solutions to retain a liquid state when cooled to increments considerably below zero. Thus Taylor (1960) was able to maintain the liquid state at −22°C. with 35,000 p.s.i. pressure. Viable cells can tolerate such pressures for only a few seconds, which, as noted earlier, seems to preclude any practical benefit from this observation. By employing such a model, Taylor was able to study, through pressure release, the effect of phase changes independent of temperature variation.

When these experimental observations (1–6) on the freezing of simple aqueous solutions are translated into complex biological multiphase systems, there is a tendency to forget that all freezing is not potentially deleterious. Although most biological systems, such as blood, appear to be damaged by crystal formation, certain bacteria, viruses, and yeasts that often contaminate blood are unaffected by repeated freezing and thawing. The nature of their resistance to low temperature damage remains elusive; but the suggestion has been advanced that their large surface area, in relation to total mass, may permit sufficiently rapid water diffusion to allow intracellular dehydration to the level of "bound" water and thus preclude intracellular crystal formation. As noted earlier, a few enzyme systems are activated, rather than destroyed, by freezing. Woodruff and Shelor (1949) report that a number of oxidative enzymes are markedly stimulated by freezing, and of course the change of blackberries to a red color in the deep freeze and the riotous colors of a New England autumn owe their existence to ice crystal formation. Regrettably, no one as yet has put such observations to purposeful work in a blood bank.

V. Results Achieved by Red Cell Storage at Temperatures below Freezing

The manifold benefits which can accrue from long-term preservation of human red cells at subzero temperatures are patent. To mention but a few, there are the elimination of all wastage from outdating; elimination of public appeals for rare blood types; and, with the development of autotransfusion, an elimination of isosensitization, tissue "reject" phenomenon, homologous serum hepatitis and all other diseases potentially transmissible through transfusion. Which of the methods discussed above gives promise of earliest and safest large-scale use? What are the problems and pitfalls inherent in each?

VI. Penetrating Additives

A. Glycerol

The first protective agent in the low temperature field (glycerol) has thus far proven highly acceptable. Considerably more data have been reported with this method than with others, reflecting only the much longer period it has been under study. Glycerol is cheap, stable, easy to procure, and, as a normal metabolite, essentially free of toxicity. It must be fully removed from red cells before transfusion, but this is due solely to its slow rate of exosmosis ($\frac{1}{4}$ that of water) which creates osmotic imbalance in an aqueous system such as plasma. The protection afforded by glycerol is so great that no control over rate of freezing and thawing is necessary. A corollary of this is the fact that power failure or temporary refrigeration breakdown does not lead to significant loss of the stockpile of stored blood. This remarkable protective action of the penetrating additives is reflected even more in the post-thaw stability of previously glycerolized and frozen cells. After thawing, removal of glycerol, and resuspension in autologous plasma, the cells can be kept an additional fortnight at ordinary refrigeration temperatures for cross-matching, sterility checking, shipment to areas of use, or reshipment to other areas in the event of nonutilization. The logistics of effective blood banking would seem to necessitate a reasonable period of post-thaw stability such as this for any method of freezing to have significant importance in blood transfusion therapy.

The principal disadvantage of the glycerol method is the length of time required for its installation and removal (> 30 and > 45 minutes, respectively).[2] Major efforts have been directed, therefore, to the development of automated sterile centrifuge equipment for carrying out the glycerol processing. The Cohn-ADL centrifuge, originally built as a research tool for a totally different use, was adapted by Tullis and associates (1956) to this type of sterile processing. Human red cells and plasma processed through such equipment and stored at temperatures between −80° and −120°C. have been extensively studied in diverse clinical situations. Details of *in vivo* and *in vitro* experience with such blood have been published (Tullis *et al.*, 1958; Ketchel *et al.*, 1958; Tullis, 1959; Tullis and Pyle, 1960; Haynes *et al.*, 1960). The clinical aspects of frozen blood are outside the scope of this review and have been summarized fully elsewhere (Tullis, 1963). However, it should be noted that in addition to the obvious practical benefits following long-term storage, there are certain favorable features deriving from the sterile washing process which accompanies deglycerolization. Such features probably would be present in any freezing method accompanied by a washing step.

Modification by Sproul and Zemp (1962) of the solutions used for glycerolization has led to a more stable post-thaw population of red cells. Recent studies by Henderson and associates point out that variable numbers of ghosts still remain at the end of deglycerolization. A more recent type of automated equipment utilizing disposable plastic centrifuge bowls is under development by Arthur D. Little, Inc., Cambridge, Massachusetts.

1. Immunological Competence

Isoantigenicity appears to be unimpaired by repeated freezing and thawing of red cells, and one of the first practical applications of cryobiology was the banking of panels of rare blood groups. Compared with biochemical integrity, the immunological specificity of a red cell is a relatively stable function and bears no relation to viability.

[2] Recent data indicate this time can be reduced to the range of 15 to 18 minutes.

2. Cationic Flux

Sodium and potassium exchange in previously glycerolized and frozen red cells has been extensively studied by Wallach and associates (1962) and Zemp (1963) and found to compare closely with fresh cells collected in heparin or acid-citrate-dextrose (ACD). Potassium leakage occurs after deglycerolization and to a lesser extent during storage at −80°C. as well. However, this leakage during post-thaw storage at +4°C. in low extracellular potassium media is less than that which occurs in ordinary ACD blood stored at +4°C., and shows an average increase of 23.1 meq./liter after 21 days at +4°C. compared with 25.2 meq./liter for ACD cells. When the thawed red cells are incubated at +37°C. in the presence of dextrose, there is prompt reincorporation of intracellular potassium. Cells with a net deficit of intracellular potassium can be specially prepared by glycerolizing and freezing cells previously stored at +4°C. Such cells when subsequently transfused into hyperkalemic recipients act as a potassium sponge and serve to lower the circulating cationic excess. The intracellular sodium content of previously frozen red cells is within the upper limits of normal. The ratio of Na:K exchange of thawed cells is highly unpredictable. Fresh non-frozen cells show on the average one sodium atom in compared to two potassium atoms out, whereas in thawed deglycerolized cells the ratio can vary from 1:2 to 2:1.

3. Inorganic Phosphate

Zemp and O'Brien (1962) have studied the partition of organic phosphorus in deglycerolized red cells. Analyses for labile phosphate, hydrolyzable phosphate derived from hexose diphosphate and adenosine monophosphate, and stable phosphate which is primarily 2,3-diphosphoglycerate, show no essential differences from similar phosphate studies on fresh red cells collected in ACD and CPD (citrate-phosphate-dextrose). ACD cells actually show a greater decrease in stable phosphate than thawed deglycerolized red cells or CPD cells. This is probably due to the lower pH of ACD cells and somewhat increased inorganic phosphate present in the media used for resuspension of the thawed deglycerolized cells. The addition of phosphate apparently exerts a protective effect on the organic esters of phosphate within the red cell. The high-energy phosphate appears to be one of the few things altered appreciably by low temperature storage. Both intracellular ATP (adenosine triphosphate) and membrane ATP appear to be lowered. Unpublished work by Zemp (1964) suggests that the ATP is only 60–70% of normal, but the lowering appears to be more related to the processing than to the long-term storage.

4. Gas Transport

The primary function of red cells is the transport of gas. Glycerolized frozen blood shows no significant methemoglobin content, and the gas transport and release appear normal. O'Brien and Watkins (1960), using thawed red cells in pump-oxygenator experiments *in vitro*, found an O_2 uptake of 2.22 ml./disk/minute, compared with 2.0 ml./disk/minute for fresh ACD blood. Of perhaps still greater import was the finding of a normal oxyhemoglobin dissociation curve. Studies by Valtis and Kennedy (1954) on ACD blood, stored for short periods above freezing, showed a significant shift to the left in the oxyhemoglobin dissociation curve after 1-week storage at +4°C. An oxygen tension of 20 mm. Hg must be reached before hemoglobin will release 34% of its oxygen from such 1-week-old blood. Although this is of little physiological significance in the patient requiring an occasional transfusion, such an anoxic tissue pO_2 could be of critical importance in a critically ill or multiply transfused patient. O'Brien and Watkins (1960) found no such shift in deglycerolized blood, irrespective of previous low temperature storage time over periods ranging from 1 month to 3 years. If the thawed deglycerolized blood is subsequently stored at +4°C., an exactly similar Valtis-Kennedy effect appears after 1 week. This suggests that blood stored at −80°C., unlike that in the liquid state, remains nearly in a state of suspended viability.

B. Dimethyl Sulfoxide

Another type of penetrating additive, DMSO, possesses characteristics suggesting that it may eventually supplant glycerol as a protective agent if its toxicity does not preclude large-scale use. Lovelock and Bishop (1959) showed that the rapidity with which this substance crosses the red cell membrane is so fast that one cannot remove an aliquot of cells for assay. Subsequent work by Pyle (1963) demonstrated that DMSO was an optimal agent for protecting bone marrow and leucocytes for storage in the frozen state, and possessed no gross human toxicity. However, it proved difficult to remove from the nonnucleated human red cell. Recently Huggins (1963a, b) made the important observation that it can be "washed" from red cells by the simple expedient of causing red cell aggregation and sedimentation in low electrolyte high-sugar media. The obvious advantages of this unique approach are speed of processing and simplicity of the equipment needed for handling the cells before freezing and again after thawing. Several years of study will be needed to ascertain if the cells have the storage characteristics and the post-thaw stability of glycerolized cells. Since this material, like glycerol, is a penetrating additive which displaces and binds free water, it would seem likely that satisfactory results will be forthcoming.

Studies on the use of this agent to protect bone marrow during freezing suggest that the benefit is due to partial protection of ATP. By supplying fresh red cells, Pyle (1963) was able to restore the ability of thawed bone marrow to incorporate H_3-thymidine at a level comparable to the prefreezing rate. Exposure of this same *in vitro* system to ouabain, to destroy ATPase, had an effect similar to that of adding red cells.

VII. Nonpenetrating Additives

A major study has been made of the physical characteristics of ice crystal formation during rapid freezing in liquid nitrogen (Rinfret, 1960; Carslaw and Jaeger, 1959; Strumia *et al.*, 1958). Rinfret and associates (1963) have studied the protective action of many hydrogen-bonding agents during such freezing, and a significant amount of knowledge now exists as to the engineering conditions which minimize the accompanying cellular damage. As yet comparatively little has been reported as to the biochemical and physiological competence of cells frozen in this manner. Preliminary transfusion data, however, utilizing chiefly volumes less than one pint, suggests that acceptable numbers of such cells remain in the circulation of recipients at 24 hours (Rinfret *et al.*, 1963). It appears unlikely that blood processed in this manner will ever have the post-thaw stability *in vitro* and the low concentration of free hemoglobin and dead cells that can be achieved with washed deglycerolized red cells resuspended in native plasma, but it should be borne in mind that the goal of the direct-freeze liquid nitrogen is specifically pointed toward a method which will permit direct freezing, thawing, and transfusion without removal of the protective agent. The military requirements for mass casualty management would best be served if no final centrifugation or reconstitution were necessary before use.

The philosophy underlying such an approach is quite different from that which obtains for a hospital blood bank. Under conditions of stress, one can justify a certain compromise in quality in favor of increase in quantity. Regrettably, the transfusion unit, thus far proved best *in vitro*, contains nearly 35 gm. PVP per pint of blood, as well as high extracellular potassium and free supernatant hemoglobin (300 mg.). This makes it unlikely that such a transfusion unit will have significant utilization, unless it too is washed before use. Although it probably could be tolerated unwashed by a normovolemic recipient, the possibility of sludging of the renal microcirculation by the macromolecular additive and cell ghosts would seem real, especially to the recipient who is hypovolemic or in shock. Further work in this field will doubtless be in the direction of continuing search for a more acceptable additive. High concentrations of glucose alone will exert partial protection. Preliminary studies in progress by Meryman (1963) suggest that this simple sugar is effective, if one is willing to accept a decreased cell yield and the inconvenience of a short wash after thawing. Glucose is of course actively transported across the cell membrane, but in high extracellular concentrations it is unlikely that full penetration occurs. Its primary role would thus be that of a nonpenetrating additive, i.e., binding of water extracellularly and prevention of high concentrations of salt.

VIII. General Problems of Blood Storage at Temperatures below Freezing

The problem of free supernatant hemoglobin is common to all types of blood freezing. The clinical importance of supernatant hemoglobin and its possible toxicity are under active discussion. Some reports suggest that pure hemoglobin is nontoxic to a healthy recipient (not in need of blood), but that hemoglobin in the presence of denatured cellular constituents can affect renal function. Even if it is free of toxicity, however, its presence in thawed blood can only indicate an instability of at least part of the cell population and an inherent probability that some of the remaining cells have decreased stability both *in vitro* and *in vivo*. One of the errors which must be avoided in assessing the future progress of any of the methods of low temperature storage is the assumption that blood is safe merely because it is tolerated intravenously by a series of volunteer recipients.

The question of sterility must always be satisfied whether one is preparing a unit of red cells for *in vitro* experiment or for transfusion. Cryophilic organisms have been known to produce profound complications in blood stored at +4°C. At the temperatures used for subzero storage, there has been an overreliance on the assumption that bacterial growth will not prove a hazard. Moreover, all the proposed methods require a finite time during which the blood is in the liquid state before freezing and after thawing, and many of the additives are optimal for the support of bacterial and viral growth. If one accepts the likelihood that the various methods will also entail centrifugation after blood collection, addition of a protective agent, and finally repeated centrifugation and washing after storage, many potential lapses in sterile technique exist.

Despite these common problems, however, it appears that knowledge and methodology have now progressed far enough for low temperature red cell preservation soon to reach the level of broad applicability. It seems reasonable to predict that the large-scale application of the provocative findings, already uncovered in the study of frozen blood, will have a revolutionary impact on blood banking logistics, unequalled since the evolution of blood grouping knowledge.

ACKNOWLEDGMENTS

This work was supported by Grants H 5979, H 6302, and A 2089 from the National Institutes of Health, U.S. Public Health Service, Department of Health, Education, and Welfare, by Contract Nonr-1852(00), Office of Naval Research, by grants to Protein

Foundation, Inc. from other charitable trusts, and by contributions from industries interested in the alleviation and cure of human disease.

References

Boyle, R. (1665). *J. Crook*, p. 184. London.

Carslaw, H. S., and Jaeger, J. D. (1959). *In* "Conduction of Heat in Solids," pp. 282–296. Oxford Univ. Press (Clarendon), London and New York.

Doebbler, G. F., and Rinfret, A. P. (1962). *Biochim. Biophys. Acta* **58**, 449.

Haynes, L. L., Tullis, J. L., Pyle, H. M., Wallach, S., and Sproul, M. T. (1960). *J. Am. Med. Assoc.* **173**, 1657.

Huggins, C. (1963a). *Surgery* **50**, 191.

Huggins, C. (1963b). *Science* **139**, 504.

Ketchel, M. M., Tullis, J. L., Tinch, R. J., Driscoll, S., and Surgenor, D. M. (1958). *J. Am. Med. Assoc.* **168**, 399.

Lovelock, J. (1953). *Biochim. Biophys. Acta* **11**, 28.

Lovelock, J., and Bishop, M. W. (1959). *Nature* **183**, 1394.

Luyet, B. J. (1949). *In* "Preservation of the Formed Elements and of the Proteins of the Blood," p. 141. American Red Cross, Washington, D.C.

Luyet, B. J. (1960). *Ann. N. Y. Acad. Sci.* **85**, 552.

Meryman, H. T. (1960). *Ann. N. Y. Acad. Sci.* **85**, 504.

Meryman, H. T. (1963). Personal communication.

Meryman, H. T., and Kafig, E. (1955). *Proc. Soc. Exptl. Biol. Med.* **90**, 587.

O'Brien, T. G., and Watkins, E., Jr. (1960). *J. Thoracic Surg., St. Louis* **40**, 611.

Pert, J. H., Schork, P. K., and Moore, R. (1963). *Clin. Res.* **11**, 197.

Polge, C., Smith, A. U., and Parkes, A. S. (1949). *Nature* **164**, 666.

Pyle, H. M. (1963). *Vox Sanguinis.* **8**, 100.

Rinfret, A. P. (1960). *Ann. N. Y. Acad. Sci.* **85**, 576.

Rinfret, A. P., Cowley, C. S., Doebbler, G. F., and Schreiner, H. R. (1963). *Proc. 9th Intern. Congr. Blood Transfusion, Mexico City, 1962* (in press).

Sproul, M. T., and Zemp, J. W. (1962). *Vox Sanguinis* **7**, 96.

Strumia, M. M., Colwell, L. S., Strumia, P. V., and Sharpe, J. S. (1958). *Bull. Intern. Inst. Refrig. Suppl.* **3**, 81.

Taylor, A. C. (1960). *Ann. N. Y. Acad. Sci.* **85**, 595.

Tullis, J. L. (1959). *Proc. 5th Congr. Intern. Soc. Blood Transfusion, Rome 1958*, p. 43.

Tullis, J. L. (1963). *Transfusion* **3**, 155.

Tullis, J. L., and Pyle, H. M. (1960). *Vox Sanguinis* **5**, 70.

Tullis, J. L., Surgenor, D. M., Tinch, R. J., D'Hont, M., Gilchrist, F. L., Driscoll, S. G., and Batchelor, W. H. (1956). *Science* **124**, 792.

Tullis, J. L., Ketchel, M. M., Pyle, H. M., Pennell, R. B., Gibson, J. G. 2nd, and Driscoll, S. G. (1958). *J. Am. Med. Assoc.* **168**, 388.

Valtis, D. J., and Kennedy, A. C. (1954). *Lancet* **i**, 119.

Wallach, S., Zemp, J. W., Cavins, J. A., Jenkins, L. J., Jr., Bethea, M., Freshette, L., Haynes, L. L., and Tullis, J. L. (1962). *Blood* **20**, 344.

Woodruff, J. G., and Shelor, E. (1949). *In* "Preservation of the Formed Elements and of the Proteins of the Blood," p. 152. American Red Cross, Washington, D.C.

Zemp. J. W. (1963). Personal communication.

Zemp, J. W. (1964). Personal communication.

Zemp, J. W., and O'Brien, T. G. (1962). *Proc. 8th Intern. Congr. Hematol., Tokyo, 1960*, p. 1189.

Author Index

Numbers in italics refer to pages on which the complete references are listed

A

B

C

E

H

I

L

M

N

O

P

Q

R

S

T

U

V

Y

Z

Subject Index

A

D

E

F

G

I

J

K

L

M

N

O

P

Q

R

S

Y

Z